SAUNDERS TEXT AND REVIEW SERIES

PATHOLOGY

REVIEW

EDWARD F. GOLJAN, M.D.

Chairman
Department of Pathology
College of Osteopathic Medicine of Oklahoma State University

Clinical Professor
Department of Obstetrics and Gynecology
University of Oklahoma College of Medicine
Tulsa, Oklahoma

W.B. SAUNDERS COMPANY
A Harcourt Health Sciences Company
Philadelphia London New York St. Louis Sydney Toronto

W.B. SAUNDERS COMPANY
A Harcourt Health Sciences Company

The Curtis Center
Independence Square West
Philadelphia, Pennsylvania 19106

Library of Congress Cataloging-in-Publication Data

Pathology review / Edward F. Goljan.

p.   cm.

ISBN 0–7216–7024–5

1. Pathology—Examinations, questions, etc.   I. Title.
   [DNLM: 1. Pathology.   QZ 140 G626pa 1998]

RB111.G645   1998 Suppl.   616.07′076—dc21

DNLM/DLC   97–37847

PATHOLOGY REVIEW   ISBN 0–7216–7024–5

Printed in the United States of America

Last digit is the print number: 9   8   7   6   5

To my grandson, Austin Lee,
who truly exemplifies the scripture in Proverbs 17:6,
which states that
"Children's children are a crown to the aged."

PREFACE

Although medical students have access to a number of excellent abbreviated review texts in pathology, this book is designed for the student who desires a more integrated approach to the study of pathology. In addition, it provides the student with 500 questions, more than 100 of which are accompanied by photographs that in the author's extensive experience with national board examinations are representative of those on the United States Medical Licensing Examination (USMLE) Step 1 examination. This review book complements the larger text entitled *Pathology*, which presents pathology as the bridging science that links the basic with the clinical sciences. Hence, these two books contain discussions utilizing principles learned in biochemisty, physiology, anatomy, microbiology, and pharmacology as well as discussions emphasizing pathophysiology, physical examination, and laboratory medicine. A cursory review of the Table of Contents and the quality of the questions and answer discussions should convince the student of the significant differences from other pathology review texts.

Since the concepts in this book and the larger text derive from notes utilized by the author in teaching pathology and board review courses nationwide, they are "student tried and true" and have enjoyed considerable success in helping students attain high scores in pathology and on the USMLE Step 1 and 2 examinations.

I would like to thank the many outstanding medical students both at home and abroad whom I have had the privilege of teaching. I would also like to thank my darling wife, Joyce, who has prayerfully supported me throughout my medical career, and my grandson, Austin Lee, who is a never-ending source of delight in my life.

EDWARD F. GOLJAN, MD

CONTENTS

S E C T I O N   I I I

SYSTEMIC PATHOLOGY   105

S E C T I O N   I V

COMPREHENSIVE EXAMINATION   301

ANSWER KEY   341

OVERVIEW OF

LABORATORY MEDICINE

CHAPTER ONE

GENERAL PRINCIPLES OF LABORATORY MEDICINE

SYNOPSIS

OBJECTIVES

1. To understand the use of laboratory tests in clinical practice.
2. To define the sensitivity, specificity, reliability, and accuracy of a laboratory test.
3. To define the predictive value of positive and negative test results and how they vary with changes in the prevalence of disease.
4. To understand the meaning of the reference interval of a test and how it is manipulated to increase the test's sensitivity and specificity.
5. To understand the principles of anticoagulation in blood collection tubes and the differences between plasma and serum.
6. To define and give examples of preanalytical, analytical, and postanalytical variables that affect laboratory tests.

Objective 1: To understand the use of laboratory tests in clinical practice.

I. Purposes of laboratory tests
 A. They are used for **mass screening** (e.g., phenylketonuria in newborns), **screening asymptomatic patients** (e.g., mammography), and **screening symptomatic patients** (e.g., stress electrocardiogram in a patient with chest pain).
 B. They are used to **confirm a diagnosis** (e.g., coronary angiogram to confirm coronary artery disease in a patient with a positive stress electrocardiogram).
 C. They are used to **monitor a patient's disease status** (e.g., serum glucose in a person with uncontrolled diabetes).

Objective 2: To define the sensitivity, specificity, reliability, and accuracy of a laboratory test.

II. Operating characteristics of laboratory tests
 A. A person with a disease can have either a true-positive (TP) or a false-negative (FN) test result.
   1. A **TP** is a positive (abnormal) test result in a patient with disease (e.g., positive creatine kinase MB isoenzyme in a patient with a myocardial infarction).
   2. An **FN** is a negative (normal) test result in a

patient with disease (e.g., a normal electrocardiogram in a patient with a myocardial infarction).
 B. People without disease (normal) can have either a true-negative (TN) or a false-positive (FP) test result.
   1. A **TN** is a negative (normal) test result in a normal person (e.g., a negative electrocardiogram in a patient without a myocardial infarction).
   2. An **FP** is a positive test result in a normal person (e.g., a positive syphilis serology test in someone who does not have syphilis).
 C. A positive test result either represents a TP or an FP, while a negative test result is either a TN or an FN.
 D. The "**ideal**" **test** is one that always distinguishes disease from nondisease.
 E. The **sensitivity** of a test refers to how often a test is positive in a patient with disease ("positivity in disease").
   1. The formula is

$$\text{Sensitivity (\%)} = \frac{\text{TP}}{\text{TP} + \text{FN}} \times 100$$

   2. The lower the FN rate, the greater the sensitivity of the test.
     a. When a test with 100% sensitivity returns negative in a patient, it must be a TN, since no FNs are associated with the test.
     b. When a test with 100% sensitivity is positive, it represents either a TP or an FP, and additional tests are necessary to distinguish the two possibilities.
   3. Tests with a sensitivity approaching or equal to 100% are used to screen for disease.
     a. In tests with high sensitivity, a negative test result excludes disease (no FNs).
     b. A positive test result includes all patients with disease at the expense of having a few FPs.
 F. The **specificity** of a test refers to how often the test is normal in a patient without disease ("negativity in health").
   1. The formula is

$$\text{Specificity (\%)} = \frac{\text{TN}}{\text{TN} + \text{FP}} \times 100$$

3

2. The lower the FP rate, the greater the specificity of the test.
   a. When a test with 100% specificity returns positive on a patient, it must be a TP rather than an FP, since there no FPs.
   b. However, if the test returns negative, it could represent a TN or an FN result.
3. Tests with a specificity approaching or equal to 100% are most useful in confirming disease, since a positive test result must be a TP rather than an FP.
4. Using the serum antinuclear antibody (ANA) test in systemic lupus erythematosus (SLE) as an example, if the test returns negative, SLE is excluded, since the sensitivity is 100% (no FNs), but if it returns positive, the patient can have SLE or some other collagen vascular disease, so additional tests are necessary to confirm the diagnosis.
   a. The anti-Smith (anti-Sm) and anti–double-stranded DNA (anti-dsDNA) antibodies have a specificity of 100% and 98%, respectively.
   b. If either or both tests are positive, the patient has SLE (TP), while negative results most likely indicate that some other collagen vascular disease is present (e.g., progressive systemic sclerosis).
G. The **reliability**, or **precision**, of a test is established by repeating the same test over a number of times on the same sample.
   1. Calculation of the **standard deviation** (SD) is the best indicator of the reliability of a test, since a low SD indicates that the test is reliable, while a high SD connotes an unreliable test.
      a. Laboratories most commonly use 2 SD from the mean of a test when establishing the test's **reference interval**, or **normal range**.
      b. The **mean** of a test is the sum of the concentrations of a group of test results divided by the total number of tests performed.
      c. In a normal gaussian distribution (bell-shaped curve), 1, 2, and 3 SDs encompass 68%, 95%, and 99.7% of the normal population, respectively.
   2. An example of establishing a reference interval is as follows: if the mean of the serum glucose is 100 mg/dL and 1 SD is 5 mg/dL (2 SD = 10 mg/dL), the reference interval for the test is 90–110 mg/dL (100 mg/dL + 10 mg/dL = 110 mg/dL and 100 mg/dL − 10 mg/dL = 90 mg/dL).
H. The **accuracy** of a test reflects the degree to which the test result reflects the true value of the test.

Objective 3: To define the predictive value of positive and negative test results and how they vary with changes in the prevalence of disease.

III. Predictive value of positive and negative test results
A. The predictive value of a positive test result (**PV+**) refers to the percent probability that a positive test result is a TP rather than an FP.
   1. The formula for the PV+ is

$$PV+ \ (\%) = \frac{TP}{TP + FP} \times 100$$

   2. When a test has a specificity of 100% (0% FP rate), then the PV+ is always 100%, which illus-

trates the importance of using tests with high specificity for confirming disease.
B. The predictive value of a negative test result (**PV−**) refers to the percent probability that a negative test result is a TN rather than an FN.
   1. The formula for the PV− is

$$PV- \ (\%) = \frac{TN}{TN + FN} \times 100$$

   2. When a test with 100% sensitivity (0% FN rate) returns negative, the PV− is always 100%, which underscores why tests with high sensitivity are excellent screening tests.
C. The **prevalence** of disease, or the number of people with disease in the total population under study ([TP + FN/TP + FN + TN + FP] × 100), affects the predictive value of positive and negative test results.
   1. The PV+ is low when the prevalence of disease is low, since FPs outnumber TPs, and it is high when the prevalence is high, because TPs outnumber FPs.
   2. The PV− is high when prevalence of disease is low, since TNs outnumber FNs, and it is low when the prevalence is high, because FNs outnumber TNs.
D. Figure 1–1 exhibits a format that is useful in calculating the sensitivity and specificity as well as the PV+ and PV− of a test.

Objective 4: To understand the meaning of the reference interval of a test and how it is manipulated to increase the test's sensitivity and specificity.

IV. Reference intervals (normal range)
A. Since reference intervals are based on 2 SDs from the mean and encompass 95% of the normal population, 5% of normal people (1 of 20 normal people), could potentially have an FP test result.
B. The reference interval for a test may be adjusted by either the clinician or the laboratory to render it more sensitive or more specific.
   1. The "ideal" test, as depicted in Figure 1–2A, clearly separates the normal from the disease population, since a reference interval from 0 to point A has 100% sensitivity (no FNs) and 100% specificity (no FPs beyond A).
   2. When there is no clear-cut distinction between the normal and disease population (overlap area), a test with 100% sensitivity is obtained by placing the upper limit of the reference interval at the beginning of the disease curve (point A), as depicted in Figure 1–2B.
   3. A test with 100% specificity is obtained by placing the upper limit of the reference interval at the end of the normal curve (point B), as depicted in Figure 1–2C.
   4. In establishing tests with 100% sensitivity or 100% specificity, there is always a trade-off in that an increase in one parameter always results in a decrease in the other, as depicted in Figures 1–2B and C.

	Row C (PV+) → Positive Test	Row D (PV-) → Negative Test	Row E (Prevalence) → Totals	
Row A → Patients with disease	True positives (TP)	False negatives (FN)	Total number with disease	**Sensitivity** TP/TP + FN × 100
Row B → Control group	False positives (FP) $\frac{TP}{TP + FP} \times 100$	True negatives (TN) $\frac{TN}{TN + FN} \times 100$	Total number without disease $\frac{TP + FN}{\text{Total population}}$ (disease + control)	**Specificity** TN/TN + FP × 100

PV+, predictive value of a positive test result (chance that a positive test result is a TP); PV-, predictive value of a negative test result (chance that a negative test result is a TN).

FIGURE 1–1. Format for calculating sensitivity, specificity, predictive values of positive (PV+) and negative (PV−) test results, and prevalence of disease. In this format, note that the calculation of the sensitivity and specificity of a test, or the operating characteristics of the test, is made by moving from left to right. Sensitivity, or positivity of the test in disease, moves across row A, while specificity, or the negativity of the test in people without the disease, moves across row B. The calculations for the PV+ move from top to bottom in row C, while the PV− calculation moves from top to bottom in Row D. The prevalence of disease is calculated by moving from top to bottom in row E.

Objective 5: To understand the principles of anticoagulation in blood collection tubes and the differences between plasma and serum.

V. Blood collection tubes
  A. An **anticoagulant** is added to a blood collection tube in order to prevent clotting when **plasma** is required for a test.
    1. **Chelating agents**, such as citrate, bind calcium, which prevents clot formation.
    2. **Heparin** enhances antithrombin III activity, which neutralizes clotting factors.
  B. Centrifugation of the tube results in three layers that settle out, with plasma at the top, leukocytes and platelets in the middle (also called the buffy coat), and red blood cells (RBCs) at the bottom.
  C. **Plasma** contains all the coagulation factors but does not contain platelets.
  D. When no anticoagulant is added to a blood collection tube, the blood clots and **serum** is harvested after centrifugation of the sample.
  E. Serum is deficient in fibrinogen (factor I), factor II (prothrombin), factor V, factor VIII, and platelets.

Objective 6: To define and give examples of preanalytical, analytical, and postanalytical variables that affect laboratory tests.

VI. Variables affecting laboratory tests
  A. **Preanalytical variables** relate to the collection of the sample (e.g., blood, urine) and patient factors that alter test results, such as age, sex, habits, and underlying diseases.

1. Compared with that of a child, the hemoglobin (Hb) and RBC count in a **newborn** is higher owing to the increased concentration of HbF (fetal Hb) and its effect on left-shifting the oxygen dissociation curve, which leads to tissue hypoxia and the release of erythropoietin.
2. Compared with that of an adult, alkaline phosphatase (located in osteoblasts) and serum phosphate (which drives calcium into bone) concentrations are higher in children because of active bone growth.
3. Adult men have higher Hb, serum iron, and serum ferritin (the circulating fraction of iron that correlates with iron stores) levels than adult women do, since adult women lose iron during menses and pregnancy if they do not take an iron supplement.
4. Pregnant women have notable test variations.
  a. The plasma volume increases three times more than the RBC mass, so the Hb concentration is reduced (dilutional effect).
  b. The increase in plasma volume increases the glomerular filtration rate (GFR), which increases the creatinine clearance and the clearance of analytes such as creatinine, blood urea nitrogen, and uric acid, hence lowering their serum concentrations.
  c. The increase in estrogen results in an increased synthesis of binding proteins such as thyroid-binding globulin and transcortin, which in turn results in an increase in the total thyroxine and total cortisol concentra-

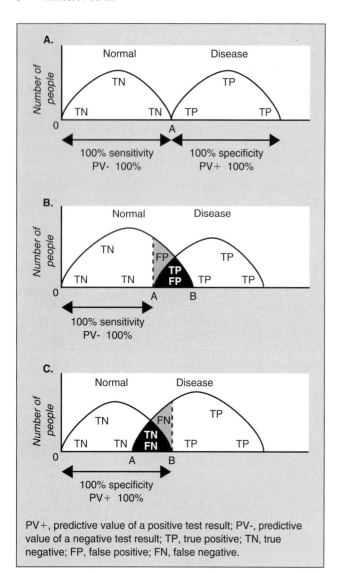

A.

B.

C.

PV+, predictive value of a positive test result; PV-, predictive value of a negative test result; TP, true positive; TN, true negative; FP, false positive; FN, false negative.

FIGURE 1–2. Altering the sensitivity and specificity of a laboratory test by changing the reference intervals. (A) demonstrates a test with 100% sensitivity and 100% specificity when the reference interval is 0 to A. Note how the test clearly distinguishes the normal from the disease population without any overlap between the two populations. A test with 100% sensitivity automatically has a PV− of 100%, since there are no FN test results. This is useful as a screening test. A test with 100% specificity automatically has a PV + of 100%, since there are no FP test results. This is most useful in distinguishing TP from FP test results. Placing the upper limit of the reference interval at the beginning of the disease curve creates a test with 100% sensitivity, as illustrated in **(B)**. Note that all test values between 0 and A are under the normal curve and all are TNs with no FNs. The overlap zone between the A and B test values (shaded area) contains a few normal people who have FP test results and a few individuals who have TP test results. Note how the specificity of the test has decreased owing to the increase in the number of FPs. Placing the upper limit of the reference interval at the end of the normal curve creates a test with 100% specificity, as depicted in **(C)**. Note that no patient value beyond B has an FP test result. In the overlap area between A and B (shaded area), there are a few people with disease, who are FNs, and a few normal people, who are TNs. Note how the sensitivity of the test decreases as a result of the increase in FNs.

tion, respectively, without altering the free hormone levels.

   d. There is a mild glucose intolerance, secondary to the anti-insulin effect of human placental lactogen, and a lower renal threshold for glucose, which often results in glucosuria in the presence of normal serum glucose concentration.

  5. Elderly patients have significant variations in test results that may be misinterpreted as representing disease.

   a. They have a significant drop in the GFR, which renders them susceptible to drug toxicity if they are given drugs that are excreted by the kidneys.

   b. There is a reduction in the number of suppressor CD8 T cells, leading to an increased production of autoantibodies.

   c. An increase in adipose tissue in the elderly down-regulates the synthesis of insulin receptors, thus leading to mild glucose intolerance.

  6. A hemolyzed sample of blood results in a false elevation of serum lactate dehydrogenase, potassium, and iron, since they are present in RBCs.

  7. A fasting blood sample is necessary in order to obtain accurate serum glucose and serum triacylglycerol (TG) levels, since diet affects these two analytes.

  8. Because alcohol enhances the activity of the cytochrome P-450 system in the liver, which is involved in drug metabolism, the serum concentration of a prescribed drug is likely to be lower than expected if alcohol is consumed.

  9. Cimetidine, a histamine blocker used in treating peptic ulcer disease, blocks the cytochrome P-450 system, so there is a potential for drug toxicity by drugs normally metabolized in the liver.

B. **Analytical variables** refer to problems with performance of the test in the laboratory, such as turbidity of the sample (due to excess TG) or hypoalbuminemia, which automatically lowers the total calcium concentration (40% of calcium is normally bound to albumin).

C. **Postanalytical variables** refer to the reporting of the test results to the clinician.

QUESTIONS

DIRECTIONS. (ITEMS 1–6): Each of the numbered items or incomplete statements in this section is followed by answers or by completions of the statement. Select the ONE lettered answer or completion that is BEST in each case. Correct answers and explanations are given at the end of the chapter.

1. The prevalence of disease is equal to the incidence × the duration of the disease. Therefore, if a new drug prolongs the interval between contraction of the human immunodeficiency virus (HIV) and onset of the acquired immunodeficiency syndrome (AIDS) but does not prevent AIDS or lead to its cure, you would expect which of the following?

   (A) Incidence of HIV positivity to increase
   (B) Prevalence of HIV positivity to become lower than the incidence
   (C) Prevalence of HIV positivity to approach the incidence as duration increases
   (D) Prevalence of HIV positivity to increase
   (E) Prevalence and incidence of HIV positivity to both increase

2. A test for coronary artery disease (CAD) is positive in 180 of 200 people with known CAD and negative in 140 of 200 people who do not have CAD. If the test result returns positive on a patient, what is the chance that the patient has CAD?

   (A) 70%
   (B) 75%
   (C) 80%
   (D) 90%
   (E) 95%

3. Assuming the use of 2 standard deviations to establish the reference interval of a test, in a test with a reference interval (normal range) of 10–30 mg/dL, 1 standard deviation equals

   (A) 2.5 mg/dL
   (B) 5.0 mg/dL
   (C) 7.5 mg/dL
   (D) 10 mg/dL
   (E) 20 mg/dL

4. The schematic illustrates a normal control population and a population of people with a 24-hour-old acute myocardial infarction (AMI) who were evaluated with a new serum test to detect myocardial injury. Two different reference intervals for the same test are noted, with the first extending from 0 to 3 and the second from 0 to 4. The areas under the two curves are subdivided into different populations of people, which are represented by letters A through E. Depending upon the reference interval selected, some of these areas will contain people whose test results are true negatives, false negatives, true positives, or false positives.

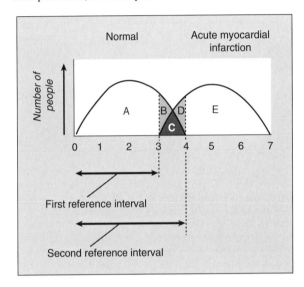

Which of the following correctly describes the lettered patient subpopulations for the two different reference intervals?

	First Reference Interval	Second Reference Interval
(A) Area A	True negatives	False negatives
(B) Area B	False positives	True negatives
(C) Area C	False negatives only	False positives only
(D) Area D	False positives and false negatives	True positives and true negatives
(E) Area E	True positives	False negatives

5. Plasma and serum are similar in that they both contain

   (A) fibrinogen
   (B) coagulation factor XII
   (C) coagulation factor V
   (D) coagulation factor VIII
   (E) platelets

6. You would expect a pregnant woman, who is not taking prenatal vitamins, and a nonpregnant woman of the same age, to both have similar reference intervals for

   (A) serum phosphate
   (B) serum uric acid
   (C) serum blood urea nitrogen
   (D) a 24-hour creatinine clearance
   (E) plasma hemoglobin concentration

DIRECTIONS. (ITEMS 7–8): For each numbered item select the ONE lettered option that is most closely associated with it.

(A) True positive
(B) False positive
(C) True negative
(D) False negative

7. A 65-year-old man with a history of coronary artery disease presents with severe substernal chest pain for the past 12 hours. No acute changes are noted on an electrocardiogram. A blood sample is drawn for electrolytes, serum creatine kinase (CK) isoenzyme MB, and serum lactate dehydrogenase (LDH) isoenzymes. Owing to technical difficulties in collecting the blood, the sample is visibly hemolyzed. The serum potassium, CK isoenzyme MB, and total LDH are elevated, with the isoenzyme results pending. The elevated serum potassium is most likely a _____.

8. A 55-year-old smoker with chronic obstructive lung disease takes theophylline to improve his breathing and cimetidine for peptic ulcer disease. He is taking his medicine as prescribed. A therapeutic drug level of serum theophylline is reported to be in the toxic range. This test result most likely represents a _____.

ANSWERS AND EXPLANATIONS

1. The answer is D: prevalence of HIV positivity to increase. Prevalence equals incidence × duration of the disease (a mnemonic is PID, where P = prevalence, I = incidence, and D = duration). Prevalence is the total number of people with disease in the population under study, while incidence is the number of new cases over a set period of time. Since P = I × D, as duration increases between the onset of HIV positivity and overt AIDS, the prevalence of HIV positivity automatically increases, since more HIV-positive people are living longer. Since prevalence of disease is a function of incidence × duration, it is never lower than the incidence, but as the duration of disease *decreases*, prevalence can approach the incidence. Incidence, which is based on new cases only, remains unchanged.

2. The answer is B: 75%. The question asks for the PV+ test result, or the chance that a test is a TP rather than an FP. The sensitivity of the test (positivity in disease) is 90%, since 180 people of 200 people with coronary artery disease (CAD) had a positive test. The specificity of the test (negativity in health) is 70%, since 140 of 200 people without CAD had a negative test. The PV+ is 75%, and the PV− is ~88% (see calculations below). The prevalence of disease is 50%. This information is charted below along with the calculations for sensitivity, specificity, PV+, PV−, and prevalence of CAD in the population studied.

	Positive Test	Negative Test	Total
Coronary artery disease	True positive 180	False negative 20	200
Control group	False positive 60	True negative 140	200
Total population	240	160	400

Sensitivity (%) = TP/TP + FN × 100
= 180/180 + 20 × 100 = 90%
Specificity (%) = TN/TN + FP × 100
= 140/140 + 60 × 100 = 70%
PV+ (%) = TP/TP + FP × 100 = 180/180 + 60 × 100
= 75% (FP rate is 100 − 75 = 25%)
PV− (%) = TN/TN + FN × 100 = 140/140 + 20 × 100
= ~88% (FN rate is 100 − 88 = 12%)
Prevalence (%) = TP + FN/total population studied × 100
= 180 + 20/400 × 100 = 50%

3. The answer is B: 5.0 mg/dL. The standard deviation (SD) correlates with the reliability (precision) of the test in that a low SD indicates good reliability and a high SD represents poor reliability. The reference interval for this test is 10–30 mg/dL, so the mean of the test is 20 mg/dL, 2 SD is 10 mg/dL, and 1 SD is 5 mg/dL.

4. The answer is B: area B in the first reference interval represents false positives and in the second reference interval represents true negatives. The first reference interval is set for 100% sensitivity, since there are no false negatives in the interval between 0 and 3. The second reference interval is set for 100% specificity, since there are no false positives beyond the reference interval of 0 to 4. Area A, regardless of the reference interval used, contains only normal people with true negative test results. Area B has only normal people; however, with the first reference interval, they all have positive test results (false positives), and with the second reference interval, they are correctly classified as normal (true negatives), since the test results are within the 0 to 4 interval. Other tests will be necessary to document that these patients have false positive test results. Area C contains people who are normal and people who have an acute myocardial infarction (AMI). Using the first reference interval, the normal people are falsely classified as having an AMI (false positives), while the patients with an AMI are correctly classified (true positives). Other tests will be necessary to separate the true from the false positives. Area D has only people with an AMI. Using the first reference interval, they are correctly classified as having true positive test results; however, with the second reference interval, the test results fall within the normal range, so they are now false negatives. Area E, like area D, has only patients with an AMI, and they are correctly classified with both reference intervals.

5. The answer is B: coagulation factor XII. Plasma contains all the coagulation factors. Serum is harvested after blood is allowed to clot in a tube without an anticoagulant. Fibrinogen, factor V, factor VIII, factor II (prothrombin), and platelets are all used up in the formation of a clot. Neither plasma nor serum contains platelets, since in plasma they are part of the buffy coat (which also contains leukocytes), whereas in serum they are consumed in the clot.

6. The answer is A: serum phosphate. Because of a greater increase in plasma volume (PV) than in RBC mass, pregnant women have a lower Hb concentration (diluted)

than nonpregnant women do. The increase in PV increases the GFR and creatinine clearance. This, in turn, increases the clearance of blood urea nitrogen, creatinine, and uric acid, which all have reduced reference intervals. Serum phosphate is not altered in either condition.

7. The answer is B: false positive. A hemolyzed blood sample falsely elevates the serum potassium (a major intracellular cation), lactate dehydrogenase (LDH), and serum iron. The CK-MB is a true positive because it does peak in 24 hours and is not affected by hemolysis. The negative electrocardiogram is a false negative.

8. The answer is A: true positive. Cimetidine, a histamine blocker, inhibits the cytochrome P-450 system in the liver, which is important in the metabolism of drugs. Theophylline is metabolized in the liver, so cimetidine is blocking its metabolism, thus causing a true increase in free levels of the drug.

SECTION II

GENERAL PATHOLOGY

CHAPTER TWO

PATHOPHYSIOLOGY OF

CELL INJURY

AND ADAPTATION

SYNOPSIS

OBJECTIVES

1. To understand the mechanisms of hypoxic cell injury.
2. To understand the formation, neutralization, and clinical significance of free radicals.
3. To understand the differences between cell necrosis and apoptosis and morphologic expressions of these pathologic processes.
4. To describe and give clinical examples of extracellular and intracellular accumulations in cell injury.
5. To define and give examples of cytoskeletal and membrane abnormalities.
6. To understand the pathophysiology of growth alterations.

Objective 1: To understand the mechanisms of hypoxic cell injury.

I. Mechanisms of tissue hypoxia
  A. **Hypoxia** means reduction in the amount of oxygen that is available to tissue.
    1. It is associated with ischemia (most common cause), hypoxemia, hemoglobin (Hb)-related abnormalities, defective or uncoupled oxidative phosphorylation, and arteriovenous shunting.
    2. It leads to decreased synthesis of adenosine triphosphate (ATP) in the mitochondria.
  B. **Ischemia** is a reduction in blood flow to tissue.
    1. Atherosclerotic occlusion of a vessel is the most common cause of hypoxia.
    2. Other causes include a reduction in the cardiac output (e.g., myocardial infarction), torsion of vessels (e.g., twisting of the spermatic cord), and compression of vessels (e.g., herniated temporal lobe pressing against the posterior cerebral artery).
  C. **Hypoxemia** is a reduction in the amount of oxygen (O_2) dissolved in plasma (PaO_2, where the lowercase letter "a" means arterial).
    1. It can be secondary to the following disorders.
      a. Respiratory acidosis, which is secondary to retention of CO_2 in the lungs (e.g., chronic obstructive pulmonary disease).
      b. Ventilation defects, in which air does not reach the respiratory unit for gas exchange (e.g., atelectasis, or the collapse of alveoli).
      c. Perfusion defects characterized by blockage of blood flow through the pulmonary capillaries (e.g., pulmonary embolus).
      d. Diffusion defects, which interfere with gas exchange at the alveolar-capillary interface (e.g., fluid in patients with left heart failure).
    2. As long as the capillary PO_2 is higher than that in the tissue, O_2 will move into the tissue by the process of **diffusion**.
  D. Hb-related abnormalities encompass those associated with a reduction in Hb concentration; decreased O_2 saturation (SaO_2), representing the percentage of heme groups occupied by O_2; and decreased release of O_2 from Hb at the tissue level.
    1. The **O_2 content** is the total amount of O_2 carried in the blood and is equal to 1.34 (Hb g/dL) $\times$ SaO_2 + PaO_2.
    2. In **anemia**, there is a reduction in the Hb concentration, which reduces the total O_2 content (1.34 [$\downarrow$ Hb g/dL] $\times$ SaO_2 + PaO_2) without altering the SaO_2 or the PaO_2, since there is normal O_2 exchange in the lungs.
    3. **Methemoglobin** (metHb) is heme iron in the +3 (ferric) state, which is unable to bind with O_2; iron must be in the ferrous (+2) state to bind with O_2.
      a. MetHb reduces the O_2 content by decreasing the SaO_2 without affecting the PaO_2 (1.34 [Hb g/dL] $\times$ $\downarrow$ SaO_2 + PaO_2).
      b. Oxidizing agents such as nitrites (e.g., nitroglycerin), nitrates converted into nitrites in the gut (e.g., from nitrate-rich well water), and sulfur-containing drugs increase the formation of metHb.
      c. Patients are cyanotic and do not respond to administration of O_2, since the heme iron is in the +3 state.
      d. **Methylene blue** is the treatment of choice, since it enhances the conversion of iron to

the ferrous condition by acting as an artificial electron carrier in the **NADPH** (*not* NADH)-**dependent metHb reductase system**, while **ascorbic acid**, a reducing agent, assumes an ancillary role in treatment.

4. In **carbon monoxide** (CO) **poisoning**, CO competes with O_2 for binding sites on heme iron in place of O_2, thereby decreasing the O_2 content by decreasing the SaO_2 without altering the PaO_2 (1.34 [Hb g/dL] $\times$ ↓ SaO_2 + PaO_2).
   a. The patient will have a cherry red discoloration of the skin owing to the combination of CO with myoglobin.
   b. Administration of O_2 is the treatment of choice in CO poisoning.

5. Factors moving the O_2 dissociation curve to the left (high affinity of Hb for O_2), such as decreased 2,3-bisphosphoglycerate, CO, metHb, hypothermia, and HbF (fetal Hb), decrease the release of O_2 to the tissue.

E. Abnormalities in **oxidative phosphorylation** include those which block the oxidative pathway (e.g., inhibition of cytochrome oxidase by CO and cyanide) and those which produce abnormalities in phosphorylation by damaging mitochondrial membranes (e.g., uncoupling agents such as alcohol and salicylates).
   1. The O_2 content is normal, but ATP synthesis is decreased.
   2. O_2, an electron acceptor, is the last reaction in the electron transport chain, which underscores why tissue hypoxia virtually shuts down ATP synthesis.

F. **Arteriovenous shunting** of blood flow bypasses the delivery of O_2 to the microcirculation without affecting the O_2 content.

II. Ultrastructural and biochemical alterations in hypoxic cell injury
A. There are reversible consequences directly related to a reduction in ATP synthesis.
   1. There is a loss of the ATP-dependent sodium/potassium pump, leading to an influx of water into the cytosol, which is called **cloudy swelling** (the first alteration).
   2. **Anaerobic glycolysis** is increased owing to allosteric activation (alteration of structure and function) of phosphofructokinase by an increased concentration of adenosine monophosphate and a low concentration of citrate.
   3. Reduced protein synthesis occurs secondary to a disruption of ribosomes in the rough endoplasmic reticulum.
   4. Reversible electron microscopic findings are swelling of the smooth endoplasmic reticulum (first alteration) and mitochondria.
   5. Intracellular lactic acidosis is the end result of anaerobic glycolysis.
   6. There is a net gain of 2 ATP without a gain of NADH + H^+, since NADH + H^+ is used to convert pyruvate to lactate to replenish NAD^+ in the glycolytic cycle.
   7. Glycogen stores are depleted in order to supply glucose for anaerobic glycolysis.

B. There are irreversible consequences of hypoxic cell injury.
   1. Most importantly, cell membranes are damaged because of activation of phospholipases in the membrane and alterations produced by lipid peroxidation secondary to free radical damage (see below).
   2. Mitochondria are structurally altered by calcium, which leads to the formation of large amorphous densities that are visible by electron microscopy (EM).
   3. Increased cytosolic concentration of calcium leads to the activation of enzymes, such as endonucleases in the nucleus and phospholipases in the cell membrane, that contribute to cell death.
   4. Nuclear abnormalities noted with the light microscope include **pyknosis** (ink-dot appearance), **karyorrhexis** (nuclear fragmentation), and **karyolysis** (dissolution of nuclear chromatin).
   5. The release of intracellular enzymes from damaged cells is an excellent marker of cell injury (e.g., creatine kinase-MB isoenzyme elevation in a myocardial infarction).

Objective 2: To understand the formation, neutralization, and clinical significance of free radicals.

III. Formation, function, and neutralization of free radicals (FRs)
A. FRs are unstable chemical species that have a single, unpaired electron in their outer orbit.
B. They are produced by ionizing radiation, damaged mitochondria, oxidase reactions, drugs (e.g., acetaminophen), and chemicals (e.g., carbon tetrachloride [CCl_4]).
C. Oxygen-derived FRs include superoxide, hydroxyl ions, and peroxide.
D. FRs injure cell membranes and cell organelles by the process of **lipid peroxidation**, in which lipid FRs combine with molecular O_2.
E. FRs are neutralized by superoxide dismutase; catalase; glutathione peroxidase (which generates glutathione); and antioxidants, such as vitamin E, vitamin C, and selenium.
F. The following are examples of FR injury.
   1. **Retrolental fibroplasia** and blindness in newborns secondary to O_2 FR injury results from 100% O_2 administration.
   2. Damage occurs to tissue in iron overload states (e.g., hemochromatosis), since iron helps generate FRs by the **Fenton reaction**.
   3. Acetaminophen hepatotoxicity is associated with the formation of acetaminophen FRs in the cytochrome P-450 system, leading to liver necrosis and failure.
   4. CCl_4 hepatotoxicity is related to its conversion to CCl_3 FRs in the cytochrome system, leading to liver cell necrosis and fatty change.

Objective 3: To understand the differences between cell necrosis and apoptosis and morphologic expressions of these pathologic processes.

IV. Apoptosis
A. Apoptosis refers to individual cell necrosis (cell death) without an inflammatory reaction.
B. It is operative in the following processes.
   1. It is important in normal embryogenesis, such as the involution of müllerian and wolffian

structures in males and females, respectively, and the development of lumens in hollow organs, such as the heart and bowels.

2. Apoptosis is involved in normal involutional changes (e.g., the retrograde changes of endometrial tissue in menses) and in the reduction of cell mass in atrophy (see below).

3. It is operative in toxin-induced injury and cytotoxic T cell destruction of cells (e.g., hepatocytes infected with hepatitis B virus).

C. Histologic features include cell shrinkage with intense eosinophilia of the cytoplasm, nuclear condensation, loss of cell surface specializations (microvilli), preservation of organelles, and eventual phagocytosis by other cells.

D. Histologic examples of apoptosis include **Councilman bodies** (dead hepatocytes in viral hepatitis) and **red neurons** in the brain (dead neurons that are present in hypoxic injury).

E. Tissue necrosis primarily differs from apoptosis in that there is an inflammatory infiltrate associated with more widespread necrosis.

V. Morphologic types of necrosis

A. **Coagulation necrosis** is secondary to denaturation of both structural and enzymatic proteins by the combined effects of increased lactate anions (intracellular acidosis) and calcium in tissue.

1. It is most commonly due to ischemia secondary to atherosclerosis but can also be associated with heavy metal poisoning (lead) and radiation.

2. Unlike in the process of apoptosis, there is more widespread tissue necrosis, which is called an **infarction**.

3. Infarctions are pale or hemorrhagic depending on the consistency of the tissue.

   a. **Pale (ischemic) infarcts** usually occur in solid organs, such as the heart, spleen, liver, and kidneys.

   b. **Hemorrhagic (red) infarcts** are more likely to occur in loose-textured tissue such as that found in the lungs, bowel, ovaries, and testicles.

   c. Venous occlusion also results in hemorrhagic infarctions (e.g., splenic vein thrombosis).

4. Obstruction of arterial vessels with dichotomous branching (e.g., pulmonary artery with repeated bifurcations) produces wedge-shaped areas of infarction, with the apex pointing to the source of obstruction (usually a blood clot) and the base of the lesion at the periphery of the organ.

5. Histologic findings include the presence of dead tissue with vague outlines of cellular structure, loss of nuclei, and cytoplasmic eosinophilia with standard hematoxylin and eosin (H and E) staining.

6. Brain tissue undergoes liquefactive necrosis (see below) rather than coagulation necrosis as a response to ischemia.

7. **Dry gangrene** is a variant of coagulation necrosis in which the tissue appears mummified (e.g., diabetic foot), whereas wet gangrene refers to a superimposed infection, with liquefactive necrosis (see below) assuming the primary role.

B. **Liquefactive necrosis** is due to the destructive effects of enzymes generated from neutrophils and monocytes in infected tissue (e.g., a lung abscess) or to enzymatic destruction of the brain in infarction.

C. **Enzymatic fat necrosis** refers to the release of pancreatic enzymes (lipases) in association with acute pancreatitis.

1. Fatty acids released by lipolysis of fatty tissue combine with calcium to form chalky white areas (i.e., saponification).

2. The calcified areas are frequently visible on radiographs.

D. **Traumatic fat necrosis**, unlike enzymatic fat necrosis, is not enzyme mediated but is secondary to trauma to fatty tissue (e.g., breast tissue injury or a surgical site).

E. **Caseous necrosis** is a combination of coagulative and liquefactive necrosis with the formation of well-circumscribed granulomas containing macrophages, CD4 T helper cells, and multinucleated giant cells (fusion of macrophages).

1. The caseous material in the center of the granulomas derives from the lipid-rich cell walls of the pathogens (e.g., *Mycobacterium tuberculosis*, systemic fungi) destroyed by activated macrophages.

2. It is a **delayed-type hypersensitivity reaction** (type IV cellular immunity; Chapter 4).

3. Activated macrophages have the appearance of epithelial cells, thus the term **epithelioid cells**.

4. Most granulomas are noncaseating and are present in noninfectious diseases, such as sarcoidosis and Crohn's disease.

F. **Fibrinoid necrosis** is the necrosis of immunologic damage and is characterized by deposits of eosinophilic staining material in tissue (e.g., within vessel walls, synovium, vegetations of rheumatic fever) representing plasma proteins and complement, the latter particularly prominent in immunocomplex diseases (e.g., Henoch-Schönlein purpura).

G. **Gummatous necrosis** is a granulomatous variant of caseous necrosis that is associated with gummas (destructive, rubbery lesions) in tertiary syphilis.

H. **Postmortem necrosis** is due to **autolysis**, or the self-destruction of tissue, secondary to the release of endogenously derived intracellular enzymes moments after death (there is no inflammatory infiltrate, since an inflammatory response occurs only in living tissue).

Objective 4: To describe and give clinical examples of extracellular and intracellular accumulations in cell injury.

VI. Lipid accumulation

A. **Fatty change** is a reversible accumulation of triacylglycerol (TG) in a cell.

1. Alcohol intake is the most common cause of fatty change in the liver.

2. Mechanisms for fatty change in the liver and other tissues involve the excess production of substrates used in TG synthesis (e.g., fatty acids, glycerol 3-phosphate) or abnormalities in excretion of the lipid (e.g., deficiency of apolipoproteins).

3. In the metabolism of alcohol (see below), three substrates contribute to the synthesis of TG in the hepatocyte, namely, NADH + H$^+$, acetate (simple fatty acid), and acetyl-CoA.

$$\text{Alcohol} \xrightarrow{\begin{array}{c}\textit{Alcohol}\\\textit{dehydrogenase}\end{array}} \text{Acetaldehyde} + \text{NADH} +$$

$$H^+ \xrightarrow{\begin{array}{c}\textit{Aldehyde}\\\textit{dehydrogenase}\end{array}} \text{Acetate} + \text{NADH} + H^+ \rightarrow \text{Acetyl–CoA}$$

a. An increase in NADH reverses the NAD $\rightarrow$ NADH reaction in glycolysis in the direction of dihydroxyacetone phosphate (DHAP) rather than in the direction of pyruvate.

b. DHAP is converted to glycerol 3-phosphate (glycerol-3P), the carbohydrate backbone of TG, by glycerol phosphate dehydrogenase.

c. Acetate is added to glycerol-3P to form TG along with other fatty acids mobilized from the adipose tissue by alcohol and synthesized from the excess of acetyl-CoA.

d. TG is packaged into the very low density lipoprotein (VLDL) fraction, which coalesces in the cytoplasm and pushes the hepatocyte nucleus to the periphery.

e. **Microvesicular fatty change** associated with Reye's syndrome does not push the nucleus to the periphery.

4. Alcohol also interferes with apolipoprotein synthesis; therefore, VLDL cannot be excreted, since it needs a water-soluble apolipoprotein coating in order to dissolve in plasma.

5. Increased NADH inhibits the β-oxidation of fatty acids, since the biochemical reactions require a greater concentration of NAD$^+$ rather than NADH + H$^+$.

VII. Protein accumulations
 A. **Amyloid** is a linear, nonbranching protein derived from different proteins (e.g., excess light chains in multiple myeloma).
 B. Excess immunoglobulin production in plasma cells can coalesce to form eosinophilic globules called **Russell bodies**.
 C. Viral envelope proteins can form inclusions in cells (e.g., the Negri body of rabies).

VIII. Pigment accumulations
 A. **Melanin** is synthesized in **melanocytes** within the epidermis when the enzyme tyrosinase converts tyrosine to 3,4-dihydroxyphenylalanine (dopa), which in turn is polymerized in the Golgi apparatus into membrane-bound organelles called **melanosomes**.
  1. Sunlight and adrenocorticotropic hormone (ACTH) stimulate melanin synthesis in the skin.
  2. Clinical conditions associated with excess melanin synthesis resulting from an increase in ACTH secondary to the loss of negative feedback from cortisol include **Addison's disease** (destruction of the adrenal glands) and the **adrenogenital syndrome** (enzyme deficiencies in cortisol synthesis).
  3. **Nevocellular nevi**, or "moles," and **malignant melanomas** are examples of benign and malignant melanocyte disorders, respectively.
 B. Melanin look-alikes, such as **anthracotic pigment** (coal dust, an environmental pollutant) in lung tissue, are often confused with malignant melanoma.
 C. **Bilirubin, hemosiderin,** and **hematin** are derived from the breakdown of Hb by macrophages in the spleen and bone marrow that have phagocytosed red blood cells (RBCs).

1. **Hb** is a combination of heme (iron + protoporphyrin) and globin, which is composed of α, β, δ, and γ chains.
2. **Bilirubin** derives from protoporphyrin and is released from macrophages as **unconjugated** (lipid-soluble) **bilirubin (UCB)**, which is conjugated into water-soluble, **conjugated bilirubin (CB)** in the liver.
 a. An increase in CB or UCB produces **jaundice**.
 b. UCB is primarily increased in hemolytic anemias characterized by macrophage removal of RBCs (e.g., **congenital spherocytosis**) and with abnormalities involving the uptake and conjugation of UCB in the liver (e.g., **physiologic jaundice of the newborn**).
 c. In newborns with Rh hemolytic disease, an increase in unbound UCB may result in **kernicterus** when it enters the central nervous system and dissolves in brain tissue.
 d. CB is primarily increased in viral hepatitis and obstructive jaundice (e.g., gallstone in the common bile duct).
3. **Hemosiderin** consists of packets of **ferritin**, the storage form of iron.
 a. It is primarily located in the fixed macrophages of the bone marrow.
 b. The Prussian blue stain identifies hemosiderin in tissue.
 c. It is increased in the iron overload disorders **hemochromatosis** (autosomal recessive disease with excessive iron reabsorption) and **hemosiderosis** (acquired iron overload).
 d. Hemosiderin is increased in bone marrow macrophages in the **anemia of inflammation** (also called anemia of chronic disease) and in alveolar macrophages in heart failure ("heart failure" cells).
 e. Hemosiderin is absent in bone marrow macrophages in **iron deficiency**.
4. **Hematin** is a Prussian blue-negative, black, crystalline product originating from the oxidation of heme from the ferrous to the ferric state in conditions associated with macrophage removal of RBCs in the spleen (e.g., malaria).

IX. Glycogen and glycosaminoglycans
 A. **Glycogen** is a soluble, branched-chain polysaccharide composed of D-glucose residues held together by α-1,4 linkages.
  1. It is manufactured and primarily stored in the liver and muscle and is easily identified with the PAS stain.
  2. Clinical conditions associated with glycogen accumulation include the hereditary glycogenoses (e.g., von Gierke's disease, with a deficiency of glucose-6-phosphatase) and diabetes mellitus.
 B. **Glycosaminoglycans** (GAGs) are large complexes of negatively charged carbohydrate chains with a small amount of protein (e.g., heparan sulfate) and are increased in lysosomes in hereditary lysosomal enzyme deficiency diseases, such as Hurler's syndrome.

X. Calcium
 A. **Dystrophic calcification** refers to the calcification of previously damaged tissue in the presence of normal serum calcium and phosphorous concen-

trations (e.g., calcified atherosclerotic plaques in the aorta).
B. **Metastatic calcification** is defined as the deposition of calcium into normal tissue (e.g., renal tubular basement membrane) in the presence of hypercalcemia or an increase in the serum phosphate concentration.

Objective 5: To define and give examples of cytoskeletal and membrane abnormalities.

XI. Cytoskeletal abnormalities
  A. The **cytoskeleton** represents the complex network of protein filaments in the cytosol that maintain cell structure (shape) and, in some cases, assist in the motility of the cell.
    1. It is composed of microtubules, actin filaments, and intermediate filaments.
      a. **Microtubules** are polymers composed of the protein **tubulin** that are capable of undergoing rapid assembly and disassembly in the cytosol.
      b. **Actin thick and thin filaments** are present in muscle and nonmuscle cells and are involved in the contractile process.
      c. **Intermediate filaments**, such as keratin, neurofilaments, glial filaments, desmin, and vimentin, are important in the integration of cell organelles.
    2. The **Chédiak-Higashi syndrome** (CHS) is an autosomal recessive cytoskeletal abnormality in which the main defect is in the assembly (polymerization) of microtubules in the cytoplasm.
    3. Alterations occur in certain of the intermediate filaments when damaging stimuli cause cells to release **stress proteins** (also called **heat shock proteins**) that are vital to survival of the cell.
      a. One of these proteins is **ubiquitin**, whose function is to aid in the removal of old or damaged proteins, such as intermediate filaments, by first binding to the protein and then delivering it to proteases for degradation.
      b. **Mallory's bodies** are masses of keratin intermediate filaments in hepatocytes of patients with alcoholic liver disease that have been "ubiquinated," or marked for destruction by proteases.
    4. Immunochemical stains utilizing monoclonal antibodies against individual intermediate filaments (e.g., desmin to identify muscle) are useful in identifying the origin of neoplasms.
  B. The **membrane skeleton** provides structural integrity to the cell membrane.
    1. It is composed of **spectrin**, **actin**, and **protein 4.1**.
    2. **Congenital spherocytosis**, an autosomal dominant disease, is an example of a defect in spectrin resulting in a hemolytic anemia.

Objective 6: To understand the pathophysiology of growth alterations.

XII. Atrophy and other conditions associated with small cell size
  A. **Atrophy** refers to a shrinkage in cell size (organ size and weight as well) with the loss of cell substance and reduction in metabolic activity.
  B. It may be a physiologic (e.g., involution of the thymus with advancing age) or a pathologic process (e.g., cerebral atrophy in atherosclerosis of the carotid artery).
  C. Histologically, cell atrophy is characterized by the destruction of cell organelles and structural proteins without death of the cell in a process called **autophagy**.
    1. In autophagy, cell organelles are encompassed by membranes to form vacuoles wherein they are progressively degraded until only undigestible, lipid-rich material, called **lipofuscin**, remains behind in residual bodies.
    2. In H- and E-stained tissue, lipofuscin, often called the "wear and tear pigment," has a yellow-brown granular appearance, which, if extensive enough, grossly discolors the tissue, producing a condition called **brown atrophy**.
  D. Clinical examples of atrophy include skeletal muscle atrophy in a cast and atrophy of target organs in hypopituitarism as a result of the loss of trophic hormone stimulation.
  E. There are pathologic processes other than atrophy that reduce organ size.
    1. **Agenesis** refers to the absence of an organ resulting from failure to develop any discernible primordial tissue (anlage) during embryonic development (e.g., renal agenesis).
    2. In **aplasia**, the primordium of the organ is present, but there is no further development of the tissue (e.g., aplasia of the adrenal cortex).
    3. **Hypoplasia** refers to incomplete or partial development of an organ or tissue (e.g., hypoplastic left heart) and differs from atrophy in that the latter begins with a normal-sized organ that subsequently becomes smaller as cell mass is lost.

XIII. Hypertrophy and hyperplasia
  A. **Hypertrophy** is defined as an increase in cell size due to an increase in the synthesis of structural components and organelles (e.g., mitochondria, Golgi apparatus), whereas **hyperplasia** refers to an increase in the number of cells.
    1. Both processes are characterized by an increased expression of the **protooncogenes**, which are growth-controlling genes.
    2. It is possible to have the same stimulus promote only hypertrophy (e.g., in nondividing cells, such as cardiac muscle) as well as varying proportions of both hypertrophy and hyperplasia (e.g., in smooth muscle cells or renal epithelial cells).
    3. Clinical examples of physiologic hypertrophy and hyperplasia are hypertrophy of the heart in a well-trained athlete and hyperplasia of endometrial glands during the proliferative phase of the menstrual cycle.
    4. Factors that promote the cell growth involved in hypertrophy and hyperplasia are listed below.
      a. Hormones, such as estrogen, are first released into the blood stream and then stimulate target cells (e.g., ductal epithelium in the breast) to enter the cell cycle for mitosis.
      b. Protooncogenes code for growth factors

(e.g., epidermis-derived growth factor), growth factor receptors, signal transducers (e.g., mitogen-induced protein kinases), and DNA transcription factors to initiate cell mitosis.

   c. Cell growth by **paracrine** stimulation refers to the production of a growth peptide in one cell that attaches to peptide receptors on nearby cells without having to enter the blood stream.

   d. Cell growth by **autocrine** stimulation occurs when the same cell produces growth factors and receptors.

   e. A structural loss of tissue is frequently a stimulus for tissue to begin dividing (e.g., regeneration of liver tissue following partial removal of the liver).

5. In the **cell division cycle**, the main cell cycle regulators are **kinases** (e.g., p34 kinase), which regulate the progression from one phase to the next, and small proteins called **cyclins**, whose main function is to activate these kinases.

   a. Cells in the G_0 **phase** (G = gap), or resting phase of the cell cycle, enter the cycle when one or more of the above-mentioned growth promoter mechanisms are invoked.

   b. In the G_1 **phase** (most variable phase of the cycle), structural proteins are synthesized.

   c. Chromosomal replication occurs in the **S (synthetic) phase**.

   d. In the G_2 **phase**, the mitotic spindle (composed of microtubules) is assembled.

   e. **Mitosis (M phase)** results in division of the cell into two daughter cells; the latter then enter the G_1 phase, which determines whether the cells enter the G_0 phase, remain in the cycle to divide again, or become terminally differentiated and unable to divide again.

6. With reference to the regenerative capacity of cells in tissue, there are three types of cells: labile, stable, and permanent.

   a. Tissues that characteristically have more than 1.5% of their adult cells in active mitosis contain **labile cells** (e.g., skin, hematopoietic cells), which also include in their number stem cells that either self-replicate or differentiate into mature cells.

   b. Tissues with less than 1.5% of their adult cells in active mitosis contain **stable cells** (e.g., liver cells, renal tubular cells, and smooth muscle cells), which must be stimulated to come out of the G_0 phase in order to reenter the cycle.

   c. **Permanent cells** are terminally differentiated and cannot reenter the cell cycle to divide (e.g., neurons, striated and cardiac muscle, and cells in the lens of the eye).

   d. Only labile and stable cells are able to undergo both hypertrophy and hyperplasia, while permanent cells, such as striated and cardiac muscle, are limited to hypertrophy.

7. Clinical examples of hypertrophy are left ventricular hypertrophy due to increased resistance against muscle contraction (e.g., increased peripheral vascular resistance) and hypertrophy of skeletal muscle from weight training.

8. Clinical examples of hyperplasia include lactation, various endocrinologic syndromes (e.g., acromegaly due to excess growth hormone), and prostate hyperplasia.

9. An example of approximately equal amounts of hypertrophy and hyperplasia is smooth muscle hypertrophy/hyperplasia in the uterus in pregnancy.

XIV. Metaplasia

  A. **Metaplasia** is defined as the reversible replacement of one adult cell type by another adult cell type, usually as an adaptive process instigated by the host tissue as a response against chronic irritation (e.g., smoking, infection).

  B. Clinical examples include the presence of increased goblet cells in the terminal bronchioles of a smoker (normally not present in this location) and mucus-secreting glandular epithelium in the distal esophagus (normally squamous) as a reaction against acid injury from gastric reflux (called **Barrett's esophagus**).

  C. An example of mesenchymal metaplasia is the development of bone in an area of muscle trauma.

XV. Dysplasia (atypical hyperplasia)

  A. Dysplasia is a potentially reversible atypical hyperplasia that is characterized by a disorderly proliferation of cells with nuclear variation in size and shape and increased mitotic activity with normal mitotic spindles.

  B. Dysplasia arises from a metaplastic or hyperplastic process and may progress to cancer through a series of steps if the irritating stimulus is not removed.

    1. Using the bronchial mucosa in a smoker as an example, the following progression occurs: normal pseudostratified ciliated columnar epithelium → goblet cell hyperplasia and basal cell hyperplasia → squamous metaplasia → squamous dysplasia (mild, moderate, severe) → squamous carcinoma in situ (limited to the full thickness of the epithelium) → invasive squamous carcinoma (invades through the basement membrane and has the ability to metastasize).

    2. Up to a certain point in the cell, dysplasia is a reversible process if the irritant is removed (e.g., by cessation of smoking).

  C. Other clinical examples of dysplasia include cervical dysplasia associated with the human papillomavirus and atypical endometrial hyperplasia from unopposed estrogen stimulation.

QUESTIONS

DIRECTIONS. (ITEMS 1–5): Each of the numbered items or incomplete statements in this section is associated with a photograph and is followed by answers or by completions of the statement. Select the ONE lettered answer that is BEST in each case. Correct answers and explanations are given at the end of the chapter.

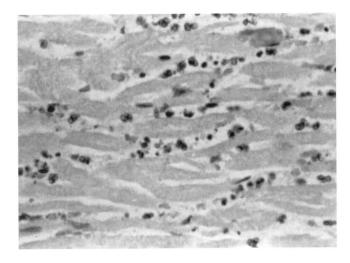

1. In the initial development of the histologic changes illustrated in this cardiac muscle, which of the following most likely occurred?

   (A) Reduction in phosphofructokinase activity
   (B) Decreased intracellular pH
   (C) Decreased anaerobic glycolysis
   (D) Reduced cytosolic concentration of calcium
   (E) Increased citrate concentration

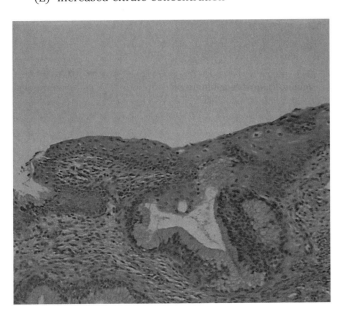

2. The growth alteration illustrated in this biopsy specimen of the transformation zone in the cervix is most similar to which one of the following growth alterations?

   (A) Mucosal changes that commonly occur in the bronchus of a smoker
   (B) Increased skeletal muscle mass in a weight lifter
   (C) Increase in myometrial tissue in a gravid uterus
   (D) Red blood cell proliferation in the bone marrow in hypoxemia
   (E) Reduction in brain mass in chronic ischemia

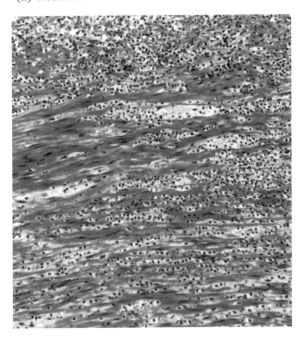

3. The pathologic process illustrated in this section of appendix is the same process that is primarily involved in

   (A) an acute myocardial infarction
   (B) immune vasculitis
   (C) dry gangrene
   (D) brain infarction
   (E) apoptosis

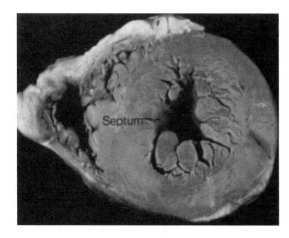

Septum

4. The growth alteration present in this heart is most closely related to which one of the following growth alterations?

(A) Lactation in breast tissue
(B) Regeneration of liver tissue after injury
(C) Denervation of skeletal muscle
(D) Reaction of esophageal squamous epithelium to acid injury
(E) Bladder smooth muscle reaction to urethral obstruction

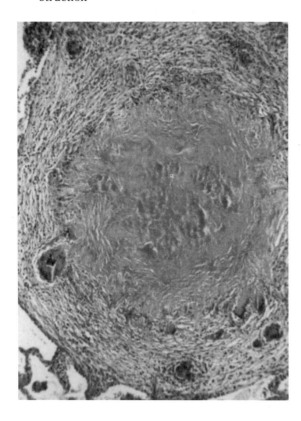

5. The pathologic process illustrated in this section of lung is most closely associated with

(A) apoptosis
(B) fibrinoid necrosis
(C) a cellular immune reaction
(D) enzymatic fat necrosis
(E) ischemic injury

Directions. (Items 6–17): Each of the numbered items or incomplete statements in this section is followed by answers or by completions of the statement. Select the ONE lettered answer that is BEST in each case.

6. Which of the following disorders is associated with hypoxemia?

(A) Carbon monoxide poisoning
(B) Methemoglobinemia
(C) Cyanide poisoning
(D) Pulmonary embolus
(E) Iron deficiency anemia

7. Free radical injury is primarily associated with

(A) acetaminophen hepatotoxicity
(B) necrosis in immune vasculitis
(C) fatty change in the liver in a patient with alcoholism
(D) granuloma formation in a patient with tuberculosis
(E) dystrophic calcification in acute pancreatitis

8. From the following list of alterations, select an early event in hypoxic cell injury that is directly related to adenosine triphosphate (ATP) deficiency.

(A) Lipid peroxidation
(B) Nuclear pyknosis
(C) Cellular swelling
(D) Formation of free radicals
(E) Cell membrane damage

9. Apoptosis rather than tissue necrosis is more likely involved in which of the following disorders or physiologic events?

(A) Involution of the thymus
(B) Abnormal mitochondrial structure
(C) Widespread tissue necrosis
(D) Inflammatory infiltrate
(E) Faint cytoplasmic staining

10. Fatty change in the liver in alcoholics is most likely associated with a/an

(A) reduced formation of acetyl-CoA
(B) reduction in lipolysis in adipose tissue
(C) increased β-oxidation of fatty acids
(D) increased formation of NAD^+
(E) increased synthesis of glycerol 3-phosphate

11. Assuming that the arterial blood supply to each of the following organs is occluded, which organ would have a gross appearance that is different from the others?

(A) Heart
(B) Lung
(C) Kidney
(D) Spleen
(E) Liver

12. A disorder that is associated with a black, nonmelanin pigment is

(A) Addison's disease
(B) a nevocellular nevus (mole)
(C) black lung disease
(D) a malignant melanoma
(E) the adrenogenital syndrome

13. Which of the following abnormalities is associated with a nonhemoglobin-derived pigment?

    (A) "Heart failure" cell in sputum
    (B) Brown atrophy of the heart in an elderly man
    (C) Jaundice in a patient with hepatitis
    (D) Kernicterus in a newborn baby with anemia
    (E) Pink-colored urine in a patient with hemolysis

14. Both hyperplasia and hypertrophy may occur with

    (A) skeletal muscle
    (B) smooth muscle
    (C) cardiac muscle
    (D) a lower motor neuron
    (E) a lens cell

15. Hyperplasia rather than metaplasia is best represented by

    (A) benign squamous epithelium lining the true vocal cord
    (B) bone in an area of previous muscle injury
    (C) increased goblet cells in the stomach mucosa
    (D) squamous epithelium in the bladder in schistosomiasis

    (E) increased goblet cells in the bronchus of a smoker

16. Which of the following is primarily an example of hypoplasia rather than atrophy?

    (A) Small left ventricle in a newborn with heart failure
    (B) Loss of skeletal muscle mass in a cast
    (C) Loss of renal mass in renal artery atherosclerosis
    (D) Loss of muscle mass in a 90-year-old man
    (E) Decreased thickness of the adrenal cortex in hypopituitarism

17. Metastatic rather than dystrophic calcification is primarily represented by

    (A) calcific aortic stenosis in a patient with a bicuspid aortic valve
    (B) calcifications in the left upper quadrant of the abdomen
    (C) calcification of the pineal gland in an elderly man
    (D) calcification of renal tubular basement membranes in primary hyperparathyroidism
    (E) calcified atherosclerotic plaques in the abdominal aorta

ANSWERS AND EXPLANATIONS

1. The answer is B: decreased intracellular pH. The photograph depicts coagulation necrosis of cardiac muscle with preservation of the cellular outlines, loss of nuclei, and an infiltrate of neutrophils. In hypoxic cell injury, there is enhanced anaerobic glycolysis due to allosteric activation of phosphofructokinase by increased AMP and low citrate levels. Lactic acid is the end product of anaerobic metabolism and, along with calcium, is responsible for denaturation of both structural and enzymatic proteins, which produces the histologic findings shown in the photograph. (Photomicrograph reproduced, with permission, from R. Virmani, J.B. Atkinson, and J.J. Fenoglio. *Cardiovascular Pathology.* Philadelphia, W.B. Saunders Co., 1991, p. 95.)

2. The answer is A: mucosal changes that commonly occur in the bronchus of a smoker. The cervical biopsy exhibits squamous metaplasia replacing the normal mucus-secreting glandular epithelium of the endocervix. This is similar to squamous metaplasia of pseudostratified ciliated columnar epithelium in the bronchial mucosa of smokers. Hypertrophy occurs in the skeletal muscle in a weight lifter. Both hypertrophy and hyperplasia are present in the smooth muscle in a gravid uterus. Hyperplasia of the red blood cell series occurs in hypoxemia owing to erythropoietin stimulation. Reduced brain mass in chronic ischemia is the result of atrophy. (Photomicrograph reproduced, with permission, from E. Hernandez and B. Atkinson (eds.). *Clinical Gynecologic Pathology.* Philadelphia, W.B. Saunders Co., 1995, p. 116.)

3. The answer is D: brain infarction. The section of appendix reveals a diffuse inflammatory infiltrate consisting primarily of neutrophils ("squiggly" nuclei), which is an example of liquefactive necrosis. Infarction of the brain, unlike infarction of other tissues, is associated with liquefactive necrosis, since the brain tissue is rich in

lysosomes and lacks firm structural support. An acute myocardial infarction is an example of coagulation necrosis. Immune vasculitis is most commonly associated with fibrinoid necrosis. Dry gangrene is primarily coagulation necrosis with mummification of tissue (diabetic foot). Apoptosis is individual cell necrosis without an inflammatory infiltrate. (Photomicrograph reproduced, with permission, from B.C. Morson. *Color Atlas of Gastrointestinal Pathology.* London, Harvey Miller Publishers, W.B. Saunders Co., 1988, p. 157.)

4. The answer is E: bladder smooth muscle reaction to urethral obstruction. The left ventricle and septum are thickened, which is an example of hypertrophy of cardiac muscle. Contraction of smooth muscle in the bladder wall against increased resistance from urethral obstruction would produce muscle hypertrophy. Lactation in breast tissue and regeneration of liver tissue after injury are examples of hyperplasia. Denervation of skeletal muscle produces atrophy. The reaction of esophageal squamous epithelium to acid injury is the development of mucus-secreting glandular tissue (Barrett's esophagus), which is an example of glandular metaplasia. (Photomicrograph reproduced, with permission, from R. Virmani, J.B. Atkinson, and J.J. Fenoglio. *Cardiovascular Pathology.* Philadelphia, W.B. Saunders Co., 1991, p. 280.)

5. The answer is C: cellular immune reaction. The section shows a well-circumscribed area with amorphous material in the center (caseous necrosis, in this case) surrounded by an inflammatory infiltrate within which are multinucleated giant cells and lymphocytes. This constellation of findings is consistent with a granuloma, which is an example of delayed-reaction hypersensitivity (cellular immunity) involving macrophages and CD4 helper T cells. Apoptosis refers to individual cell necrosis without inflammation. Fibrinoid necrosis is associ-

ated with immunologic injury. Enzymatic fat necrosis occurs in acute pancreatitis. Ischemia most commonly leads to atrophy or coagulation necrosis rather than granuloma formation. (Photomicrograph reproduced, with permission, from T.V. Colby, C. Lombard, S.A. Yousem, and M. Kitaichi. *Atlas of Pulmonary Surgical Pathology.* Philadelphia, W.B. Saunders Co., 1991, p. 186.)

6. The answer is D: pulmonary embolus. A pulmonary embolus produces a perfusion defect in the lungs that decreases oxygenation, thus producing hypoxemia, or a low PaO_2. In CO poisoning, CO competes with O_2 for binding to the heme group, hence lowering the SaO_2 without affecting the PaO_2. MetHb is iron in the $+3$ state, which cannot bind with O_2, hence decreasing the SaO_2 without affecting the PaO_2. Cyanide inhibits cytochrome oxidase in the oxidative pathway without altering the SaO_2 or the PaO_2. In iron deficiency anemia (or any anemia), the Hb concentration is decreased, which reduces the total O_2 content without altering the SaO_2 or PaO_2.

7. The answer is A: acetaminophen hepatotoxicity. Acetaminophen is converted by the hepatocyte cytochrome P-450 system into a free radical (FR), which is responsible for producing diffuse liver cell necrosis. Fibrinoid necrosis is associated with immune vasculitis, which may involve a small component of neutrophil-related FR injury. Fatty change in alcoholic liver disease is due to increased synthesis or reduced secretion of triacylglycerol (TG) from the liver. Tuberculous granuloma formation is a cellular immune response associated with the release of cytokines from macrophages and helper T cells. Dystrophic calcification in acute pancreatitis involves the deposition of calcium in damaged tissue.

8. The answer is C: cellular swelling. Owing to the loss of the ATP-dependent sodium pump, water enters the cell and produces cellular swelling, referred to as cloudy swelling. This is an *early*, reversible finding of hypoxic cell injury. Lipid peroxidation is primarily associated with FR injury of the cell membrane and membranes surrounding organelles. Nuclear pyknosis is a calcium mediated injury. The formation of FRs in hypoxic cell injury occurs in injured mitochondria. Cell membrane damage is a *late* finding that is associated with FR damage as well as calcium activation of cell membrane phospholipases.

9. The answer is A: involution of the thymus. Apoptosis refers to individual cell necrosis without an inflammatory infiltrate. Cellular organelles are intact, so abnormal mitochondrial structures are not expected. There is nuclear pyknosis and eosinophilic staining cytoplasm.

10. The answer is E: increased synthesis of glycerol 3-phosphate. In the metabolism of alcohol, NADH + H$^+$, acetate (simple fatty acid), and acetyl-CoA are end products that contribute to fatty change in the hepatocyte. Acetyl-CoA is used to synthesize fatty acids, which are added to glycerol 3-phosphate to form triacylglycerol (TG). Fatty acids also derive from increased lipolysis of adipose tissue, excess acetate from alcohol metabolism, and inhibition of β-oxidation of fatty acids by NADH. Increased NADH also increases the formation of dihydroxyacetone phosphate in the glycolytic cycle that is converted to glycerol 3-phosphate, the carbohydrate backbone of TG synthesis.

11. The answer is B: lung. Ischemic infarcts of tissue are either pale or hemorrhagic, depending on the texture of the tissue. Infarctions of solid organs, such as the heart, kidney, spleen, and liver, are pale, since red

blood cells (RBCs) are confined to the area of the damaged blood vessels. However, lung parenchyma is loosely textured, which facilitates the dispersal of RBCs throughout the infarcted tissue.

12. The answer is C: black lung disease. Black lungs are due to the deposition of anthracotic pigment, or coal dust (an environmental pollutant), in the alveolar macrophages (called "dust cells"), lung tissue, and hilar lymph nodes. In Addison's disease and the adrenogenital syndrome, hypocortisolism is present, the former from destruction of the adrenal glands and the latter from an enzyme deficiency in cortisol synthesis (21-hydroxylase). Loss of the negative feedback of cortisol on ACTH increases ACTH and its stimulatory effect on skin pigmentation. Nevocellular nevi and malignant melanomas are examples of benign and malignant disorders of the melanocyte, respectively.

13. The answer is B: brown atrophy of the heart in an elderly man. Brown atrophy is due to accumulation of lipofuscin, which is the leftover undigestible lipid material commonly seen in atrophic cells. Hemosiderin, bilirubin, and hematin are all derived from the breakdown of Hb. Heart failure cells are alveolar macrophages, with hemosiderin derived from the degradation of RBCs released from damaged capillaries in congested lungs. Kernicterus is the deposition of UCB (lipid-soluble bilirubin) in the brain of newborns with Rh hemolytic disease. Pink-colored urine in a patient with hemolysis of red blood cells is due to hemoglobin (hemoglobinuria).

14. The answer is B: smooth muscle. Smooth muscle is a stable cell that is normally in the G_0 phase of the cell cycle. It must be stimulated to enter the cycle to divide (e.g., estrogen stimulation in pregnancy). Stable cells undergo both hypertrophy and hyperplasia, since they have the capacity to divide. However, skeletal muscle, cardiac muscle, and specialized cells, such as lower motor neurons and cells in the lens of the eye, are permanent cells. These cells are terminally differentiated and are unable to divide. Skeletal and cardiac muscle are limited to hypertrophy in response to an increased workload.

15. The answer is E: increased goblet cells in the bronchus of a smoker. Goblet cells are normally present in the mainstem bronchus; therefore, an increase in these cells represents hyperplasia. Metaplasia is the replacement of one adult cell type by another adult cell type. Benign squamous epithelium lining the true vocal cord is an example of squamous metaplasia, since the true vocal cord is normally surfaced by pseudostratified ciliated columnar epithelium. Bone in an area of previous muscle injury represents osseous metaplasia. Increased numbers of goblet cells in the stomach mucosa is an example of glandular metaplasia, since goblet cells are normally located in the intestinal mucosa rather than the stomach. Squamous epithelium in the bladder in schistosomiasis is squamous metaplasia, since the bladder is normally lined by transitional epithelium.

16. The answer is A: small left ventricle in a newborn with heart failure. Hypoplasia refers to an incomplete or partial development of an organ or tissue, in this case, a hypoplastic left heart. It differs from atrophy in that atrophy begins with a normal-sized organ that subsequently becomes smaller as cell mass is lost. Atrophy is the primary growth alteration associated with the loss of skeletal muscle mass in a cast, loss of renal mass in renal artery atherosclerosis, loss of muscle mass in a 90-year-old man, and decreased thickness of the adrenal cortex in hypopituitarism.

17. The answer is D: calcification of renal tubular basement membranes in primary hyperparathyroidism. Metastatic calcification is the deposition of calcium into normal tissue due to the presence of hypercalcemia and/or hyperphosphatemia. Primary hyperparathyroidism is associated with hypercalcemia. An excess of calcium commonly deposits in renal tubular basement membranes, resulting in a condition called nephrocalcinosis. Dystrophic calcification refers to the calcification of previously damaged tissue in the presence of normal serum calcium and phosphorous concentrations. Examples include calcific aortic stenosis in a patient with a bicuspid aortic valve, calcifications in the left upper quadrant noted on a radiograph (enzymatic fat necrosis in pancreatitis), calcification of the pineal gland in an elderly man (a normal age-dependent finding), and calcified atherosclerotic plaques in the abdominal aorta.

CHAPTER THREE

INFLAMMATION AND

REPAIR

SYNOPSIS

OBJECTIVES

1. To understand the pathogenesis of acute inflammation, its morphologic expressions in tissue, and the process of organization and repair of damaged tissue.
2. To understand the pathogenesis of chronic inflammation and its morphologic appearances in tissue.
3. To understand the laboratory manifestations of inflammation including leukocyte alterations, anemia, and the erythrocyte sedimentation rate.

Objective 1: To understand the pathogenesis of acute inflammation, its morphologic expressions in tissue, and the process of organization and repair of damaged tissue.

I. Overview of acute inflammation
  A. Acute inflammation is a transient process that occurs within minutes of injury and may last for hours or days.
  B. The cardinal signs of acute inflammation are **rubor** (redness; histamine-mediated), **tumor** (swelling; histamine-mediated), **calor** (heat; histamine-mediated), **dolor** (pain; prostaglandins and bradykinin), and **functio laesa** (loss of function).
II. Vascular events in acute inflammation
  A. Blood flow into the microcirculation is primarily controlled by altering the smooth muscle tone (via vasodilation or vasoconstriction) in the arterioles by chemical mediators and neurogenic reflexes.
    1. **Anaphylatoxins** C3a and C5a stimulate the release of **histamine** from mast cells and basophils located in the area of injury.
    2. Histamine vasodilates the precapillary arterioles, leading to an increase in blood flow (calor and rubor), and also stimulates the contraction of endothelial cells in the postcapillary venules, leaving basement membrane exposed in the gaps between cells.
    3. Vessel permeability is increased owing to the combination of increased intravascular hydrostatic pressure (due to increased blood flow) and reduced oncotic pressure from the loss of protein into the interstitial space (tumor) through the endothelial gaps.
  B. Loss of intravascular fluid disrupts normal laminar flow and enhances the aggregation of RBCs into a "stack of coins" configuration (rouleaux).

III. Cellular events in acute inflammation
  A. Sequential neutrophil (leukocyte) events include margination, adhesion, emigration (diapedesis), directed movement (chemotaxis), and phagocytosis.
    1. **Margination** of neutrophils to the periphery of vessels is the result of mechanical displacement by the clumped RBCs and receptor-mediated chemotaxis by chemotactic agents.
    2. **Adhesion molecules** are synthesized by endothelial cells and leukocytes.
      a. Leukocyte adhesion molecule synthesis (CD11/CD18 complex composed of glycoproteins and β1- and β2-integrins) is enhanced by interleukin-1 (IL-1), tumor necrosis factor (TNF), C5a, and LTB₄.
      b. Synthesis of endothelial cell leukocyte adhesion molecule-1 (which adheres to neutrophil receptors) and intercellular adhesion molecule-1 (which attaches to neutrophils and lymphocytes) is enhanced by IL-1 and TNF.
      c. Corticosteroids inhibit adhesion molecule synthesis, thereby decreasing neutrophil adhesion and increasing the circulating absolute neutrophil count (neutrophilic leukocytosis).
      d. Endotoxins enhance neutrophil adhesion, leading to a reduction in the peripheral blood absolute neutrophil count (neutropenia).
    3. **Emigration (diapedesis)** of leukocytes is facilitated by focal dissolution of the exposed basement membranes by leukocyte-derived collagenases (i.e., type IV collagen).
      a. Emigration into the interstitial space produces a protein and cell-rich fluid called an **exudate**.
      b. Exudates dilute toxins (bacterial), supply antibodies, and promote an immunologic response in lymph nodes, draining an area of infection.
    4. **Directed movement (chemotaxis)** to the area of injury is facilitated by chemotactic agents such as C5a, LTB₄, IL-8, and bacterial products.
    5. **Phagocytosis** refers to leukocyte engulfment of microorganisms (also of foreign particles and cellular debris).
      a. **Opsonization** of bacteria (or foreign materi-

als) by IgG and C3b enhances the phagocytic process, since neutrophils and monocytes possess membrane receptors for IgG and C3b.

  b. Bacteria are engulfed by pseudopodia and trapped within **phagosomes**, which then fuse with lysosomes containing **myeloperoxidase** (MPO) to form **phagolysosomes**.

  c. In the **Chédiak-Higashi syndrome**, a defect in microtubule polymerization in leukocytes not only impairs leukocyte motility but also prevents the fusion of lysosomes with phagosomes to form phagolysosomes.

B. Neutrophils and monocytes are armed with both O_2-dependent (MPO system and O_2 free radicals) and O_2-independent mechanisms (lysosomal enzymes) for killing bacteria.

  1. The **O_2-dependent MPO system** is the most potent bactericidal mechanism available to neutrophils and monocytes (but not to macrophages).

    a. Following phagocytosis, **NADPH oxidase** (located in the leukocyte cell membrane) in association with NADPH, converts molecular O_2 into singlet oxygen.

    b. The release of energy from this reaction is called the **respiratory burst**, which can be detected by the nitroblue tetrazolium (NBT) dye test.

    c. Singlet oxygen is converted to hydrogen peroxide by superoxide dismutase (SOD).

    d. Catalyzed by MPO, peroxide is combined with chloride ions to form HOCl (hypochlorous acid, or bleach), which destroys bacteria.

  2. **Chronic granulomatous disease** (CGD) of childhood is an X-linked recessive disease characterized by the absence of NADPH oxidase.

    a. The respiratory burst mechanism is eliminated (negative NBT dye test), so peroxide is unavailable to generate HOCl.

    b. *Staphylococcus aureus* is catalase positive, so endogenously derived peroxide is quickly destroyed by its own catalase, thereby evading destruction.

    c. Streptococci are catalase negative, so when they generate peroxide, the missing ingredient is now available to form HOCl, and the organisms are destroyed.

C. In addition to neutrophils, other cells involved in acute inflammation include eosinophils, mast cells and basophils, lymphocytes, platelets, and endothelial cells.

  1. **Eosinophils** are the dominant cells in allergic reactions (e.g., bronchial asthma) and immune reactions against invasive helminthic infections (e.g., strongyloidiasis).

    a. They are attracted to the area of inflammation by eosinophil chemotactic factor and histamine released by mast cells and basophils.

    b. Their orange-red granules are refractile (cylindrical crystals that form **Charcot-Leyden crystals**) and contain a toxic cationic protein called major basic protein.

  2. **Mast cells** and **basophils** contain preformed primary mediators in their purple granules.

    a. The primary mediators are histamine, che-

motactic factors for neutrophils and eosinophils, and proteases.

    b. Primary mediators are released by IgE antibodies, anaphylatoxins C3a and C5a, and physical stimuli (e.g., heat).

    c. Following the initial release reaction, mast cells and basophils synthesize and release prostaglandins and leukotrienes to further enhance the inflammatory reaction.

  3. **Lymphocytes** are the primary effector cells in acute viral infections.

    a. When **B cells** are antigenically stimulated, they transform into plasma cells that produce antibodies which act as opsonins (IgG) and neutralizing agents against bacterial toxins and viruses.

    b. **T cells** secrete cytokines (lymphokines) that assist in the regulation of the immune response (e.g., type IV cellular immunity).

  4. **Platelets** have granules that release chemical mediators (e.g., histamine) as well as enzymes that synthesize **thromboxane A_2**, which is a potent vasoconstrictor and platelet aggregator.

  5. **Endothelial cells** contain **prostacyclin** (a vasodilator and platelet inhibitor) and **nitric oxide** (a potent vasodilator).

IV. Overview of chemical mediators in acute inflammation (Table 3–1)

  A. Some mediators are formed from proteins circulating in plasma (e.g., Hageman factor XII production of bradykinin), while others are derived from cells involved in the inflammatory response (e.g., histamine).

  B. Activated **Hageman factor XII** is responsible for producing a fibrin clot (which traps bacteria and plugs up leaky vessels), stimulating the **kinin system** to produce **bradykinin** (a vasodilator and pain stimulator), and interacting with the **fibrinolytic system**, which produces **plasmin** (which activates complement and removes exudate).

  C. Lysosomal enzymes are located in membrane-bound organelles in neutrophils and monocytes.

    1. In neutrophils, they are present within primary (azurophilic) and specific granules.

      a. **Primary granules** contain MPO (the key enzyme), proteases, hydrolases, cationic proteins, and bactericidal factors.

      b. **Specific granules** are found in the myelocyte stage up to the segmented neutrophil stage and contain lactoferrin, alkaline phosphatase (a marker of neutrophil maturity), lysozyme, adhesion molecules, and collagenase.

    2. Monocyte granules carry MPO, proteases, and hydrolases but lose MPO when they enter tissue and become macrophages.

  D. Activation of cellular phospholipases in the cell membranes of the cellular constituents within the inflammatory process results in the release of **arachidonic acid**, which is enzymatically converted to prostaglandins and leukotrienes.

    1. Corticosteroids inhibit phospholipase A_2, thereby blocking both prostaglandin and leukotriene synthesis.

    2. Aspirin and NSAIDs inhibit cyclooxygenase, which blocks prostaglandin synthesis.

  E. Cytokines are protein products emitted by T cells, macrophages, and other cell types.

    1. IL-1 and TNF are primarily secreted by macro-

TABLE 3–1. Important Chemical Mediators in Inflammation

Mediator	Derivation	VD/VC*	Vessel Permeability	Adhesion/ Chemotaxis	Opsonin	Pain
Histamine	Cells—mast cells and platelets	+/−	Increase	−/+ (for eosinophils)	No	No
Serotonin	Cells—mast cells and platelets	+/−	Increase	−/−	No	No
LTB$_4$	Cells—leukocytes	−/−	No effect	+/+	No	No
LTC$_4$-D$_4$-E$_4$	Cells—leukocytes	+(E4)/+	Increase	−/−	No	No
Prostaglandins	Cells—membranes of most cells	+/−	Increase	−/−	No	Yes
PAF†	Cells—leukocytes and mast cells	+/− or +	Increase	+/+	No	No
C3a	Cell	+/−	Increase	−/−	No	No
C5a	Cell	+/−	Increase	+/+	No	No
C3b	Cell	−/−	No effect	−/−	Yes	No
C567	Cell	−/−	No effect	−/+	No	No
Bradykinin	Plasma	+/−	Increase	−/−	No	Yes
Nitric oxide	Cells—endothelial and macrophages	+/−	Increase	−/−	No	No

* VD, vasodilator; VC, vasoconstrictor.
† PAF in low concentration vasodilates and in high concentration constricts.

phages and endothelial cells and stimulate **acute phase-reactant** (APR) **synthesis** by the liver.
  a. APRs include fibrinogen, complement, and C-reactive protein (complement activator and opsonin).
  b. The synthesis of binding proteins, such as transferrin and albumin, is decreased.
2. Additional functions of IL-1 and TNF include the production of fever (via stimulation of PGE$_2$ synthesis in the hypothalamus), release of neutrophils (postmitotic pool) from the bone marrow, and stimulation of B- and T-cell activity.
V. Macroscopic appearances of acute inflammation in tissue
  A. **Serous inflammation** is the elaboration of a thin, watery exudate with insufficient amounts of fibrinogen to form fibrin material (e.g., blister fluid).
  B. **Catarrhal (phlegmonous) inflammation** connotes the excessive production of mucous secretions (e.g., a runny nose).
  C. **Fibrinous inflammation** consists of a fibrinogen-rich exudate that forms excess fibrin which produces a "bread and butter" appearance on serosal surfaces (e.g., fibrinous pericarditis).
  D. **Suppurative (purulent) inflammation** refers to a localized collection of pus (liquefactive necrosis) with the formation of an abscess (e.g., lung abscess).
  E. **Cellulitis** signifies the presence of a thin, watery exudate (liquefactive necrosis) that spreads throughout subcutaneous tissue (e.g., **erysipelas** due to *Streptococcus pyogenes*, a hyaluronidase [spreading factor] producer).
  F. **Pseudomembranous inflammation** refers to toxin-induced superficial mucosal damage, with the formation of a necrotic membrane along a mucosal surface (e.g., pseudomembrane of diphtheria).
VI. Outcomes of acute inflammation
  A. The three potential outcomes of acute inflammation are resolution (healing), organization and repair with scar tissue formation, and progression to chronic inflammation.

B. **Resolution** refers to the restoration of damaged epithelium back to its original structure and function without scar tissue formation.
  1. It is dependent on the regenerative capacity of the parenchymal tissue involved and an intact connective tissue framework (scaffolding).
  2. **Labile tissues** (e.g., squamous epithelium) have stem cells for replication, and **stable tissues** (e.g., liver, smooth muscle) have resting cells that are able to enter the cell cycle when stimulated by hormones or growth factors.
  3. **Permanent tissues** (e.g., skeletal and cardiac muscle) have cells that are terminally differentiated (unable to divide), so repair is by scar tissue formation.
C. With more extensive damage, the process of **organization and repair** with scar formation is the primary mechanism of healing.
  1. **Granulation tissue** formation is paramount in this type of healing and consists of a richly vascularized stroma containing plump fibroblasts and inflammatory cells (macrophages, lymphocytes, and plasma cells).
    a. **Fibronectin** (derived from macrophages, fibroblasts, and endothelial cells) and various growth factors enhance granulation tissue formation.
    b. Growth factors, such as platelet-derived growth factor, have mitogenic (induce cell mitosis) properties that facilitate the proliferative phase of repair.
    c. **Fibroblasts** synthesize collagen and also synthesize additional actin and myosin filaments for motility as well as contraction to bring wound edges together (**via myofibroblasts**).
    d. **Angiogenesis** (formation of blood vessels) is enhanced by fibronectin and the secretion of **basic fibroblast growth factor** (BFGF) by activated macrophages.
  2. The healing of a surgical wound on the skin by **primary intention**, where the edges of the

wound are apposed by sutures, is an excellent model of wound repair.

  a. On the first day, the wound fills up with a blood clot and neutrophils appear at the margin of the wound.

  b. After 1–2 days, a single layer of epithelial cells derived from the apposed edges of the skin seal the wound.

  c. In 2–3 days, macrophages migrate into the tissue to remove fibrin and to replace neutrophils.

  d. On day 3, granulation tissue is present, and by day 5, it completely fills the incision defect.

  e. Fibroblasts in the granulation tissue begin synthesizing type III collagen.

  f. After 7–10 days, the tensile strength of the wound is only 10% of the tissue's original tensile strength.

  g. Type III collagen is eventually replaced by type I collagen with the aid of collagenases. (Zinc is a cofactor.)

  h. After 3 months, the wound has achieved a maximal tensile strength of 80%.

3. In healing by **secondary intention**, where the wound is left open, myofibroblasts contribute to wound contraction.

4. Factors that detract from normal wound healing include infection (most important), tissue hypoxia, and trace element deficiencies (e.g., copper, a cofactor for lysyl oxidase, which enhances cross-bridging between collagen fibrils).

  a. Vitamin C deficiency (scurvy) leads to defective collagen synthesis, since the vitamin is responsible for hydroxylation of proline and lysine residues.

  b. A **keloid** is a form of abnormal wound healing with the production of hypertrophic scar tissue (thick bands composed of type III collagen) resembling a tumor (common among African Americans).

  c. **Marfan syndrome** is an autosomal dominant disease with a defect in fibrillin, a glycoprotein secreted by fibroblasts that is important as a scaffolding for elastin in connective tissue.

  d. In the **Ehlers-Danlos syndrome**, there are defects in collagen structure, synthesis, secretion, or degradation.

Objective 2: To understand the pathogenesis of chronic inflammation and its morphologic appearances in tissue.

VII. Pathogenesis and morphologic appearances of chronic inflammation

  A. Chronic inflammation is the host's response to persistence of an injurious agent, leading to incomplete healing and the formation of scar tissue.

    1. It may arise from acute inflammation that has not responded adequately to therapy or to the host's immune response (e.g., acute viral hepatitis C progressing to chronic hepatitis in an intravenous drug abuser).

    2. It may occur in the absence of a prolonged phase of acute inflammation in such conditions as tuberculosis (TB; granulomatous inflammation), autoimmune disease (e.g., systemic lupus erythematosus [SLE]), or as a reaction of tissue to persistence of nondegradable material (e.g., silicone in a breast implant).

  B. Macrophages are the key effector cells in chronic inflammation.

    1. They derive from monocytes that migrate into tissue.

    2. They are scavenger cells that remove large, particulate matter by phagocytosis or small, soluble debris by pinocytosis (the macrophage membrane invaginates around the debris).

    3. Along with CD4 T helper cells, they are important in the formation of granulomas (type IV cellular immunity).

    4. They enhance host responses by secreting cytokines, such as IL-1, TNF, and B- and T-cell growth factors.

  C. The gross appearance of chronic inflammation is dependent on the type of chronic inflammation and the tissue involved.

    1. Granulomas may have a caseous (cheesy) appearance if they are secondary to TB or systemic fungal infection (e.g., histoplasmosis).

    2. Loss of the bicarbonate-rich mucous barrier coating the gastric mucosa (secondary to NSAID use or infection by *Helicobacter pylori*), may result in the formation of an **ulcer** (excavation of the mucosal surface) and the potential for perforation or bleeding.

    3. When hollow organs (e.g., bowel and bladder) that are acutely or chronically inflamed are closely approximated, there is a potential for pathologic communications to develop between the two structures that are called **fistulas** (e.g., a colovesical fistula developing between the colon and bladder).

Objective 3: To understand the laboratory manifestations of inflammation including leukocyte alterations, anemia, and the erythrocyte sedimentation rate.

VIII. Leukocyte and red blood cell alterations in inflammation

  A. In acute inflammation due to bacterial infections, there is an absolute neutrophilic leukocytosis, a left shift (band neutrophils >10%), toxic granulation (prominence of the azurophilic granules), cytoplasmic vacuoles (phagolysosomes), and Döhle's bodies (gray cytoplasmic inclusions representing dilated endoplasmic reticulum).

  B. In acute viral infections (e.g., infectious mononucleosis due to the Epstein Barr virus), antigenically stimulated lymphocytes (**atypical lymphocytes**) are present in the peripheral blood.

  C. **Eosinophilia** (increased numbers of eosinophils in the peripheral blood) is a characteristic finding in type I, IgE-mediated hypersensitivity reactions (e.g., bronchial asthma) and invasive helminthic infections (e.g., strongyloidiasis).

  D. In chronic inflammation associated with bacterial infections involving microorganisms with low inherent pathogenicity (e.g., TB), autoimmune disease (e.g., SLE), or malignancy, there is usually an absolute increase in peripheral blood monocytes (**monocytosis**).

E. In chronic infections, the **anemia of chronic disease** (ACD) is a potential complication.
   1. One host response to inflammation is to make iron less available to bacteria, since iron enhances the replication of certain strains of bacteria.
   2. ACD is due to a combination of an MPS iron blockade within macrophages, a reduction in the hepatic synthesis of the iron-binding protein called transferrin, and a mild hemolytic component.
F. The **erythrocyte sedimentation rate** (ESR) is deter-

mined by measuring the rate of settling of RBCs in a vertically oriented tube over 1 hour in millimeters/hour.
   1. When RBCs aggregate into clumps or rouleaux secondary to an increase in fibrinogen and/or γ-globulins, the resulting increase in weight of the RBCs favors increased settling.
   2. The ESR is increased in acute and chronic inflammation and in anemia.
   3. Abnormally shaped cells, such as sickle cells, or too many RBCs (polycythemia) reduce the ESR.

QUESTIONS

DIRECTIONS. (ITEMS 1–4): Each of the numbered items in this section is associated with a photograph and is followed by answers of the statement. Select the ONE lettered answer that is BEST in each case. Correct answers and explanations are given at the end of the chapter.

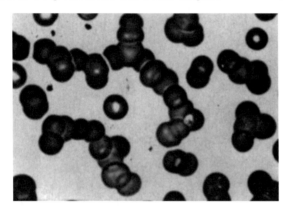

1. You would least expect the RBC findings depicted in this peripheral smear in which one of the following disorders?

   (A) Polycythemia rubra vera
   (B) Rheumatoid arthritis
   (C) Multiple myeloma
   (D) Crohn's disease
   (E) Tuberculosis

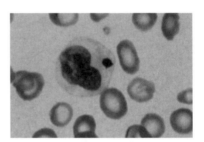

2. This lymphocyte is one of many leukocytes in the peripheral smear from a 3-year-old child with recurrent bacterial infections. His nitroblue tetrazolium (NBT) dye test is normal. The mechanism of this patient's disease is most likely related to

   (A) deficient NADPH oxidase
   (B) deficiency of glucose-6-phosphate dehydrogenase
   (C) a defect in adhesion molecules
   (D) deficiency of C3
   (E) a defect in microtubule polymerization

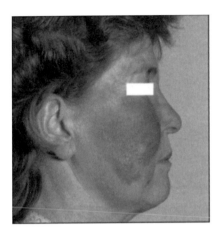

3. The facial lesion in this febrile, 27-year-old woman is painful, raised, and hot. This lesion is an example of which type of inflammation?

   (A) Suppurative inflammation
   (B) Fibrinous inflammation
   (C) Subcutaneous inflammation (cellulitis)
   (D) Catarrhal inflammation
   (E) Granulomatous inflammation

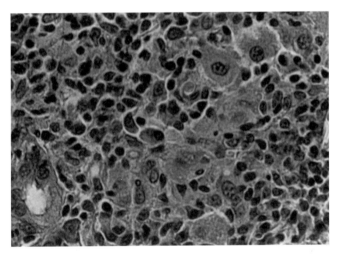

4. This photograph represents one of many portal triads in a liver biopsy performed on a 29-year-old intravenous drug abuser with jaundice. The histologic findings are most consistent with which one of the following types of inflammation?

   (A) Suppurative inflammation
   (B) Chronic inflammation
   (C) Granulomatous inflammation
   (D) Acute inflammation
   (E) Fibrinous inflammation

   DIRECTIONS. (ITEMS 5–11): Each of the numbered items in this section is followed by answers of the statement. Select the ONE lettered answer that is BEST in each case.

5. In which of the following groups of chemical mediators are both of the mediators vasodilators?

   (A) Histamine and tumor necrosis factor (TNF)
   (B) C3a and LTB$_4$
   (C) Prostacyclin (PGI$_2$) and C5a
   (D) Interleukin-1 and thromboxane A$_2$
   (E) C3b and bradykinin

6. A 5-year-old boy has recurrent *Staphylococcus aureus* infections. His peripheral blood leukocytes are normal in appearance. The nitroblue tetrazolium (NBT) dye test is abnormal. Which of the following best describes the pathogenesis of his disease?

   (A) Deficiency of NADPH oxidase
   (B) Defect in microtubule polymerization
   (C) Deficiency of C3
   (D) Deficiency of myeloperoxidase
   (E) Deficiency of immunoglobulins

7. Arrange the following vessel and leukocyte events in acute inflammation into the proper sequence.

   1. Leukocyte adhesion
   2. Arteriolar vasodilation
   3. Increased vessel permeability
   4. Neutrophil margination

   (A) 3-2-4-1
   (B) 2-3-4-1
   (C) 3-2-1-4
   (D) 3-4-2-1
   (E) 2-3-1-4

8. You would expect absolute neutrophilic leukocytosis in a patient with

   (A) endotoxic shock
   (B) viral pneumonia
   (C) bronchial asthma
   (D) Cushing's syndrome
   (E) systemic lupus erythematosus (SLE)

9. A report of "toxic granulation and left shift" on a peripheral smear best describes a patient with

   (A) allergic rhinitis
   (B) acute appendicitis
   (C) whooping cough
   (D) rheumatoid arthritis
   (E) a pinworm infestation

10. Arrange the following events in healing by primary intention into the proper sequence.

    1. Peak granulation tissue forms
    2. Macrophages replace neutrophils
    3. Tensile strength is 10%
    4. Continuous epithelial lining seals the wound

    (A) 2-3-4-1
    (B) 4-1-2-3
    (C) 2-4-3-1
    (D) 4-2-1-3
    (E) 2-4-1-3

11. In which of the following groups do both factors result in structurally abnormal collagen in a wound?

  (A) Copper deficiency and scurvy
  (B) Zinc deficiency and tissue hypoxia
  (C) Infection and obesity
  (D) Marfan's syndrome and anemia
  (E) Ehlers-Danlos syndrome and hypoxemia

DIRECTIONS. (ITEMS 12–13): For each numbered item se-

lect the ONE lettered option that is most closely associated with it.

  (A) Neutrophils   (F) Eosinophils
  (B) B lymphocytes   (G) Monocytes
  (C) T lymphocytes   (H) Mast cells
  (D) Killer cell   (I) Endothelial cells
  (E) Natural killer cell (J) Fibroblast

12. Contain Weibel-Palade bodies

13. Charcot-Leyden crystals develop from these cells

ANSWERS AND EXPLANATIONS

1. The answer is A: polycythemia rubra vera (PRV). The peripheral smear exhibits a "stack of coins" configuration of the RBCs consistent with a rouleau. Rouleaux are due to an increase in fibrinogen or γ-globulins and are responsible for an increase in the ESR. RBC crowding rather than rouleaux occurs in PRV. Chronic inflammatory disorders, such as rheumatoid arthritis, TB, and Crohn's disease show an increase in IgG and fibrinogen. Multiple myeloma, a malignant plasma cell disorder, is associated with a monoclonal (single clone of plasma cells) increase in γ-globulins, usually IgG. (Photomicrograph reproduced, with permission, from J.B. Henry. *Clinical Diagnosis and Management by Laboratory Methods,* 19th ed. Philadelphia, W.B. Saunders Co., 1996, p. 681.)

2. The answer is E: a defect in microtubule polymerization. The lymphocyte contains a giant lysosome consistent with Chédiak-Higashi syndrome. Defects in microtubule polymerization lead to abnormalities in chemotaxis (directed movement) and the emptying of lysosomal enzymes into phagosomes to produce phagolysosomes. Deficient NADPH oxidase is present in chronic granulomatous disease of childhood, which results in an absent respiratory burst (abnormal NBT dye test). Deficiency of glucose-6-phosphate dehydrogenase produces a hemolytic anemia. A defect in adhesion molecules leads to recurrent infections and the absence of a leukocyte response in inflamed tissue. A deficiency of C3 is associated with severe infections due to the absence of C3b, an opsonizing agent. (Photomicrograph reproduced, with permission, from J.B. Henry. *Clinical Diagnosis and Management by Laboratory Methods,* 19th ed. Philadelphia, W.B. Saunders Co., 1996, p. 681.)

3. The answer is C: subcutaneous inflammation (cellulitis). The facial lesion represents erysipelas, which is a cellulitis associated with group A streptococci (*S. pyogenes*), which elaborate hyaluronidase (spreading factor). Coagulase produced by *S. aureus* tends to trap bacteria in fibrin, thereby localizing infection in the form of an abscess (suppurative inflammation). Fibrinous inflammation is due to increased vessel permeability and the deposition of fibrin on serosal surfaces. Catarrhal inflammation refers to excessive mucus production (nasal secretions in the common cold). Granulomatous inflammation is chronic inflammation associated with granuloma formation. (Photograph reproduced, with permission, from M.A. Mir. *Atlas of Clinical Diagnosis.* Philadelphia, W.B. Saunders Co., 1995.)

4. The answer is B: chronic inflammation. The photograph

exhibits chronic inflammatory cells (lymphocytes and plasma cells) in the portal triad. In an intravenous drug abuser, it most likely represents chronic hepatitis due to hepatitis B. Suppurative inflammation (a variant of acute inflammation) is associated with a neutrophil-dominant exudate. Granulomatous inflammation (a variant of chronic inflammation) has epithelioid cells (activated macrophages) and multinucleated giant cells. Fibrinous inflammation does not exhibit a characteristic cellular infiltrate. (Photomicrograph reproduced, with permission, from N. Gitlin and R.M. Strauss. *Atlas of Clinical Hepatology.* Philadelphia, W.B. Saunders Co., 1995.)

5. The answer is C: prostacyclin (PGI_2) and C5a. Prostacyclin is produced by endothelial cells. It is a vasodilator and platelet aggregation inhibitor. C3a and C5a are anaphylatoxins that stimulate mast cell release of histamine, which is a potent vasodilator. IL-1 and TNF are produced by macrophages and endothelial cells and are important in the stimulation of APR synthesis in the liver. LTB_4 increases the synthesis of leukocyte adhesion molecules and is a chemotactic agent. Thromboxane A_2 is produced by platelets; it is a vasoconstrictor and platelet aggregator. C3b is an opsonizing agent. Bradykinin is a vasodilator and stimulates pain fibers.

6. The answer is A: deficiency of NADPH oxidase. The patient has chronic granulomatous disease, which is an X-linked recessive disease characterized by the absence of the respiratory burst (abnormal NBT dye test) and inability to generate hydrogen peroxide. *S. aureus* is catalase (which degrades peroxide) positive; therefore, any peroxide produced by the organism is neutralized. A defect in microtubule polymerization characterizes the Chédiak-Higashi syndrome (normal NBT dye test). A deficiency of C3, MPO, or immunoglobulins does not result in an abnormal NBT dye test.

7. The answer is B: 2-3-4-1. In acute inflammation, the order of vascular and leukocyte events is as follows: histamine-mediated precapillary vasodilation and contraction of venular endothelial cells → increased vessel permeability → neutrophil margination → leukocyte adhesion to endothelial cells → leukocyte emigration (diapedesis) → directed chemotaxis of leukocytes → phagocytosis.

8. The answer is D: Cushing's syndrome. Corticosteroids (and catecholamines) decrease adhesion molecule synthesis, resulting in an increase in circulating neutrophils. Endotoxins increase neutrophil adhesion and hence decrease the total leukocyte count. Viral pneu-

monia, bronchial asthma, and SLE are associated with lymphocyte-, eosinophil-, and monocyte-dominant smears, respectively.

9. The answer is B: acute appendicitis. A report of "toxic granulation and left shift" on a peripheral smear best describes a patient with a bacterial infection (e.g., acute appendicitis). Toxic granulation refers to the presence of increased azurophilic granules containing MPO, while left shift indicates that immature neutrophils (>10% bands) are present in the peripheral smear in response to the infection. Allergic rhinitis, whooping cough, rheumatoid arthritis, and pinworm infestation are associated with eosinophilia, lymphocytosis (*Bordetella pertussis*), monocytosis, and no abnormalities, respectively. Pinworms are not invasive helminthic infections and do not produce eosinophilia.

10. The answer is D: 4-2-1-3. The correct sequence for healing by primary intention is as follows: continuous epithelial lining seals the wound (1–2 days) → macrophages replace neutrophils (2–3 days) → peak granulation tissue forms (5 days) → tensile strength is 10% (7–10 days) → maximal tensile strength is 80% by 3 months.

11. The answer is A: copper deficiency and scurvy. Copper is a cofactor for lysyl oxidase, which is responsible for cross-linking of collagen fibrils. Scurvy is a deficiency of ascorbic acid (vitamin C), which hydroxylates proline and lysine in collagen. Zinc is a cofactor in collagenases, which replace normal type III collagen with normal type I collagen in remodeling of a wound. In Marfan's syndrome, there is a defect in fibrillin, which is important in elastic tissue. Tissue hypoxia (inadequate oxygenation of tissue), hypoxemia (low PaO_2), severe anemia, infection, and obesity impair the proper healing of a wound. Ehlers-Danlos syndrome is characterized by defects in collagen structure, synthesis, secretion, and degradation.

12. The answer is I: endothelial cells. Endothelial cells contain Weibel-Palade bodies, which store von Willebrand's platelet adhesion factor. They are an excellent marker on electron microscopy for the endothelial origin of a tumor.

13. The answer is F: eosinophils. Charcot-Leyden crystals develop from the crystalline material in the refractile granules of eosinophils. These spear-shaped crystals are frequently seen in the sputum of asthmatics.

CHAPTER FOUR

IMMUNOPATHOLOGY

SYNOPSIS

OBJECTIVES

1. To understand the pathophysiology, laboratory, and clinical aspects of the immunodeficiency disorders.
2. To understand the major histocompatibility complex and its relationship to transplantation and disease.
3. To understand the laboratory and clinical aspects of the hypersensitivity disorders.
4. To understand the laboratory and clinical aspects of autoimmune diseases.

Objective 1: To understand the pathophysiology, laboratory, and clinical aspects of the immunodeficiency disorders.

I. Overview of the immune system and B- and T-cell testing
   A. The immune system consists of B, T, natural killer (NK) and phagocytic cells, and the complement system.
   B. Factors predisposing to immune disorders include prematurity, autoimmune (AI) diseases, lymphoproliferative (LP) disorders, infections (AIDS), and immunosuppressive (IS) therapy.
   C. Flow cytometry is useful in identifying B- and T-cell markers (proteins) by means of fluorescent antibodies.
      1. B cells account for 10–20% of the total lymphocyte count and contain intracytoplasmic μ heavy chains (pre-B cell), surface μ heavy chains (mature B cell; antigen recognition site), and surface receptors (e.g., IgG Fc receptor).
      2. T cells account for 60–70% of the total lymphocyte count and possess markers for the following T cell subsets: CD3 (antigen receptor for all T cells), CD4 (helper cells), and CD8 (cytotoxic and suppressor cells).
   D. Quantitative measurement of serum immunoglobulins (Igs) and detection of isohemagglutinins against blood group antigens are used to evaluate B-cell function.
      1. Igs in decreasing order of concentration are IgG, IgA, IgM, IgD, and IgE.
         a. Since IgM synthesis begins at birth, the presence of IgM in the newborn indicates a fetal intrauterine infection (e.g., cytomegalovirus [CMV] infection).
         b. IgG synthesis begins at 2 months of age, hence the presence of IgG in cord blood is maternally derived.
      2. Isohemagglutinins are present in patients with blood group A (anti-B IgM), group B

(anti-A IgM), and group O (anti-A IgM, anti-B IgM, and anti-A, B IgG).
      3. Isohemagglutinins are absent in blood group AB individuals and in newborns.
   E. Functional assays are available for B and T cells.
      1. Mitogen assays involve the *in vitro* interaction of specific mitogens with patient lymphocytes (e.g., phytohemagglutinin for T cells and staphylococcus A for B cells), which are stimulated to divide (increased uptake of tritiated thymidine) if they are functional.
      2. Skin testing with common antigens (e.g., mumps) produces an inflammatory reaction in the presence of normal T-cell function (the absence of a response is called **anergy**).

II. B-cell immunodeficiency (ID) disorders
   A. **Bruton's agammaglobulinemia** is a sex-linked recessive (SXR) disease whose pathogenesis involves the failure of pre-B cells to differentiate into mature B cells.
      1. Maternally derived IgG protects the newborn for a few months before affected infants begin to develop sinopulmonary disease associated with *Streptococcus pneumoniae, Haemophilus influenzae,* and *Staphylococcus aureus.*
      2. Since cell-mediated immunity (CMI) is intact, there is an effective host defense against most viruses and fungi.
   B. **Common variable immune deficiency** (CVID) first presents between 15 and 35 years of age with recurrent sinopulmonary infections due to decreased Ig production.
      1. There is an intrinsic defect in the maturation of B cells into antibody-producing plasma cells.
      2. CVID patients are also prone to giardiasis, malabsorption (e.g., celiac sprue), and autoimmune disease (e.g., pernicious anemia).
   C. **Selective IgA deficiency**, the most common hereditary immunodeficiency, is due to an intrinsic defect in the differentiation of B cells committed to synthesizing IgA or to a defect in T cells that prevents B cells from synthesizing IgA.
      1. Symptomatic patients usually have recurrent problems with sinopulmonary infections (owing to lack of secretory IgA) and an increased incidence of giardiasis, autoimmune disease, and allergies.
      2. Both serum and secretory IgA levels are decreased.
   D. **Sex-linked lymphoproliferative** (LP) **syndrome** is an Epstein-Barr virus (EBV)–related disease associated with hypogammaglobulinemia and an increased incidence of malignant LP disorders.

III. T cell and combined B and T cell immunodeficiency disorders
   A. The **DiGeorge syndrome** (thymic hypoplasia) is marked by the failure of the third and fourth pharyngeal pouches to develop, with subsequent absence of all four parathyroid glands (causing hypocalcemia and tetany) and the thymus (absent thymic shadow on chest x-ray).
      1. Patients have abnormal facies and an increased incidence of truncus arteriosus, in which the aorta and pulmonary artery share a common trunk (causing cyanosis).
      2. Defective CMI results in chronic candidiasis and *Pneumocystis carinii* (PC) pneumonitis.
      3. As with all T-cell immunodeficiencies, blood transfusions containing immunocompetent donor cells may result in a graft-versus-host (GVH) reaction or transmission of CMV in lymphocytes, hence the importance of irradiating blood before transfusion.
   B. **Severe combined immunodeficiency** (SCID) is characterized by deficiencies in both B and T cells inherited in either an autosomal or an SXR pattern.
      1. Approximately 50% of children with the autosomal recessive (AR) pattern have a deficiency of adenosine deaminase, which leads to an accumulation of adenine that is toxic to both B and T lymphocytes.
      2. Children with SCID present with life-threatening infections often associated with pneumonia secondary to *P. carinii* pneumonitis.
      3. SCID is the first genetic disease for which gene therapy has been used to replace the missing enzyme—adenosine deaminase—in the host's DNA.
   C. **Wiskott-Aldrich syndrome** is an SXR disease with a triad of thrombocytopenia, eczema, and recurrent sinopulmonary infections complicated by an increased risk for development of malignant lymphomas.
      1. Laboratory studies reveal low IgM levels and increased concentrations of IgG, IgA, and IgE.
      2. Defects in CMI develop later in the course of the disease.
   D. **Ataxia telangiectasia** (AT) is an autosomal recessive disease consisting of cerebellar ataxia, prominent arteriolar telangiectasias (small collections of dilated blood vessels) around the eyes and on the skin, and severe sinopulmonary disease.
      1. Along with Bloom's disease and Fanconi's syndrome, AT is a **chromosome instability syndrome**.
      2. These syndromes carry an increased susceptibility for chromosomal mutations owing to DNA enzyme repair defects, leading to an increased risk for development of lymphomas or leukemias.
   E. The **acquired immunodeficiency syndrome** (AIDS), caused by the HIV-1 RNA retrovirus, is the most common acquired immunodeficiency in the United States.
      1. AIDS is currently the most common cause of death in black men and women from 25 to 44 years of age.
      2. The virus destroys CD4 T helper cells.
         a. HIV has been isolated in blood (the most infective body fluid), semen, breast milk (women should not breast-feed their infants), and other body fluids.
         b. Macrophages represent the primary reservoir for HIV as well as the vehicle for carrying HIV into the CNS.
      3. Adult transmission of AIDS is primarily via anal intercourse between homosexuals or vaginal intercourse in heterosexuals, particularly from male to female.
         a. The second most common route of exposure is through blood via the sharing of needles between intravenous (IV) drug abusers.
         b. Less commonly, transmission occurs via blood transfusion (1:676,000 risk) or by accidental needle sticks (0.3% risk).
      4. Children most frequently contract AIDS from an infected mother, who is usually an IV drug abuser.
         a. Transplacental (vertical) transmission accounts for approximately 30–50% of cases, while perinatal factors, such as breast-feeding (the most significant factor) and blood contamination during delivery, account for the remainder of cases.
         b. Treatment of asymptomatic pregnant women with azidothymidine (AZT) has reduced the rate of infants developing AIDS from 13–40% to less than 10%.
         c. All newborns of HIV-positive women are HIV positive owing to the transplacental passage of maternal IgG anti-HIV antibodies.
      5. The subsets of individuals that become HIV positive in decreasing order of frequency are homosexual or bisexual men, IV drug abusers, heterosexual contacts, and those individuals who receive blood or blood products (including hemophiliacs).
      6. The **acute phase** of HIV infection develops within 2–4 weeks of contracting the virus.
         a. It is characterized by a mononucleosis-like syndrome (fatigue, sore throat, and lymphadenopathy), normal to low CD4 counts, and an increase in the p24 antigen (a marker of disease activity).
         b. Antibodies against gp120 (the envelope protein that binds to the CD4 molecule) and other antibodies are not detected for approximately 4–12 weeks (window period).
         c. Positive ELISA screens (which detect gp120 antibodies) are confirmed by the Western blot analysis, which detects more than one HIV antibody (e.g., p24 and gp41).
      7. After the acute phase, patients enter an asymptomatic **latent phase**, in which the actively proliferating virus is present within dendritic cells located in the lymph nodes.
         a. After an average span of 4–10 years, patients enter the **late phase** of the disease, where the CD4 count drops to below 400 cells/μL, the p24 antigen resurfaces, and opportunistic infections develop.
         b. An opportunistic infection (usually *P. carinii* pneumonitis) or a CD4 count of ≤200 cells/μL is sufficient to diagnose AIDS.

c. The prophylactic use of trimethoprim and aerosolized pentamidine has significantly reduced *P. carinii* pneumonitis, so that it no longer is the most common cause of death in AIDS.

d. Currently, the wasting syndrome (release of tumor necrosis factor-α), disseminated CMV, and *Mycobacterium avium-intracellulare* (MAI) infections are the most frequent causes of death.

e. The average life span from the beginning of infection to death of the patient is 10 years.

8. AIDS is a multisystem disorder with the lungs representing the most frequently involved site.

9. Other laboratory abnormalities present in AIDS include reversal of the normal 2:1 CD4/CD8 suppressor T cell ratio to less than 1, absolute lymphopenia (decreased CD4 cells), hypergammaglobulinemia (polyclonal B-cell stimulation by EBV and CMV), decreased mitogen blastogenesis, anergy to skin testing, and decreased production of cytokines (interleukin-2, γ-interferon).

10. Azidothymidine (AZT) in combination with other dideoxynucleoside drugs is the initial treatment of choice (they block reverse transcription).

IV. Disorders of the complement system
 A. The complement system consists of proteins primarily synthesized by the liver as acute phase reactants (Figure 4–1).
  1. Complement components augment vascular and cellular events in acute inflammation, lyse cells (bacteria), and participate in cytotoxic immunity and immune complex hypersensitivity reactions.
  2. When activated, the classical and alternative pathways both converge on C3 and, along with C5 convertase, activate the membrane attack complex (MAC), which is cytolytic.
  3. **Decay accelerating factor** (DAF) located on cell membranes enhances the degradation of C3 and C5 convertase, thereby protecting the cell against MAC destruction.
  4. **C1 esterase inhibitor** exerts a negative control on the activation of C1 in the classical pathway.
 B. The concentration of C4 is used to evaluate the classical pathway, factor B the alternative pathway, and C3 either system.
  1. Activation decreases the concentration of intact complement components (e.g., C3) but

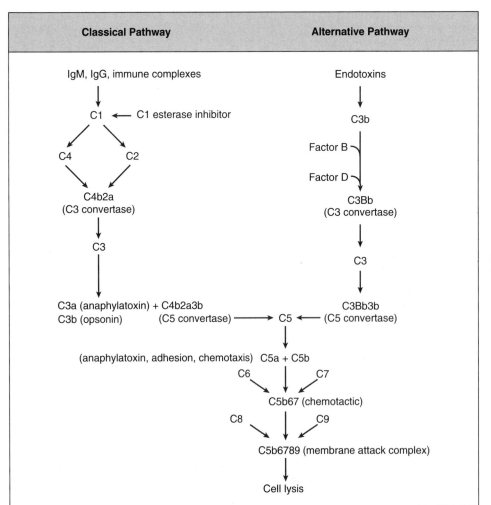

FIGURE 4–1. Classical and alternative complement pathways.

increases the concentration of split fragments (e.g., C3a).

2. Activation of the classical pathway produces a low C4, low C3, and normal factor B and the alternative pathway a low factor B, low C3, and normal C4.

3. Functional assessment of the complement system is obtained with the **total hemolytic complement assay** (CH_{50}).

C. Complement disorders are either acquired (more common) or inherited.

1. Low complement levels are most commonly due to their utilization in antibody-complement reactions (e.g., immune complex diseases).

2. **Paroxysmal nocturnal hemoglobinuria** (PNH) is an acquired stem cell disorder associated with a membrane defect involving the loss of DAF, which leaves the hematopoietic cells (neutrophils, RBCs, and platelets) susceptible to intravascular destruction (pancytopenia) by MAC.

3. **C1 esterase inhibitor deficiency** (e.g., hereditary angioedema) is an autosomal dominant disease that results in the excessive release of C2-derived kinins (causing increased vessel permeability), leading to swelling of the face and oropharynx (respiratory embarrassment).

4. C2 deficiency is the most common hereditary deficiency and is associated with an increased incidence of autoimmune disease (e.g., systemic lupus erythematosus [SLE]).

5. C5–C8 deficiency is associated with disseminated gonococcemia.

Objective 2: To understand the major histocompatibility complex and its relationship to transplantation and disease.

V. Overview of the major histocompatibility complex (MHC)

A. The MHC, known collectively as the HLA (human leukocyte antigen) system, is located on chromosome 6.

B. The gene products (class I and class II antigens) are membrane-associated glycoproteins that are located on all nucleated cells, where they serve as a marker of identity.

C. The HLA-A, -B, and -C gene loci code for class I antigens (recognized by CD8 cytotoxic T cells) that are located on all nucleated cells (not mature RBCs).

D. The HLA-D, -DR, -DP, -DQ, and -DO gene loci code for class II antigens (recognized by CD4 helper T cells) that are located on antigen-presenting cells (macrophages, Langerhans' cells in the skin, B cells, and activated T cells).

E. Individuals inherit one HLA haplotype from each parent in codominant fashion (both haplotypes are capable of expressing themselves), which when combined, become the HLA genotype of the individual.

VI. Laboratory assessment in transplantation

A. HLA testing is useful in transplantation workups, paternity suits, crossmatches for compatible platelets, and identification of patients who are at risk for certain disorders (e.g., the association between HLA B-27 and ankylosing spondylitis).

B. Successful transplantation requires compatibility of ABO blood groups, absence of preformed anti-HLA cytotoxic antibodies in the recipient's serum, and as close a match of HLA-A, -B, and -D loci between recipient and donor as possible.

1. A **lymphocyte crossmatch** screens for anti-HLA antibodies directed against donor lymphocytes.

2. The HLA-A and -B derived class I antigens on lymphocytes are identified by serologic testing using known test sera (e.g., anti-HLA-A3 antibodies) and reacting individual antibodies against recipient and donor lymphocytes (**lymphocyte microcytotoxicity test**).

3. Class II antigen (D loci) matching requires a **mixed lymphocyte reaction** (MLR) whereby functional lymphocytes from the recipient and previously irradiated (killed) donor lymphocytes are mixed together with tritiated thymidine to detect the degree of compatibility between their D loci (increased radioactivity indicates incompatibility).

4. To check for a **graft-versus-host reaction** (see ¶D, below), the recipient's lymphocytes are irradiated (killed) and functional donor lymphocytes are reacted against the host's HLA-D loci.

VII. Transplantation and transplantation rejection

A. An **autograft** is a transplant of tissue from self to self, a **syngeneic graft** (**isograft**) is between identical twins, an **allograft** is between unrelated individuals, and a **xenograft** is from one species to another (e.g., pig heart transplant).

B. The chance of a sibling having another sibling with a 0, 1, or 2 haplotype match is 25%, 50%, and 25%, respectively (parents are a one haplotype match).

C. The three types of transplant rejection of an allograft are designated hyperacute, acute, and chronic rejection.

1. **Hyperacute rejection** usually occurs within minutes of vascular attachment of the allograft (e.g., kidney) owing to the presence of ABO incompatibility or preformed cytotoxic antibodies directed against donor antigens, both of which produce vessel injury and thrombosis (type II hypersensitivity).

2. **Acute rejection** is the most common type and usually surfaces within the first 3 months following transplantation.

a. Both cell-mediated (more important) and antibody-mediated reactions occur in the graft.

b. The antibody (humoral) component produces a necrotizing vasculitis with subsequent vessel damage and intravascular thrombosis (type II antibody-mediated hypersensitivity reaction) or intimal thickening with obliteration of the vessel lumen if the graft is in place for a longer period of time.

c. The CMI component is an interaction between donor macrophages and host cytotoxic and helper T cells that results in an extensive interstitial infiltrate in the graft, edema, and cytokine damage to the tissue (type IV cell-mediated hypersensitivity reaction).

d. Acute rejection is potentially reversible with the use of immunosuppressive drugs such as cyclosporin A (which blocks CD4 helper cell release of interleukin-2 [IL-2]), corticosteroids (lymphotoxic), and OKT$_3$ (a monoclonal antibody directed against the CD3 antigen receptor).

3. **Chronic rejection** is irreversible and generally occurs over months to years.
   a. Extensive fibrosis and chronic ischemia due to vessel damage with intimal thickening and luminal obliteration mark the histologic findings.
   b. The pathogenesis is not well characterized but involves the release of growth factors from activated macrophages.

D. The GVH reaction is a potential complication in bone marrow and liver transplants and in blood transfusions administered to patients with T-cell immunodeficiency conditions.
   1. The reaction is initiated when donor lymphocytes produce IL-2, which activates host NK cells (designated lymphokine-activated NK cells, or LAKs), the primary effector cells in acute GVH reactions.
   2. LAKs produce extensive epithelial cell necrosis in the biliary tract (jaundice), the skin (maculopapular rash), and the gastrointestinal tract (diarrhea).

E. Immunosuppressive therapy has increased the incidence of cervical cancer, malignant lymphomas (immunoblastic), and basal and squamous cell carcinomas of the skin (most common overall malignancy).

VIII. Types of transplants
A. Corneal transplants have the best overall graft survival rate.
B. Living donor renal transplants with a two haplotype match have a >90% 5-year survival rate that drops to 80% with a one haplotype match.
C. Cadaver transplants between unrelated donors are the most common renal transplants and have a survival rate similar to a one haplotype match, particularly if the patient receives multiple blood transfusions prior to the surgery (which possibly induces tolerance to the allograft).
D. Bone marrow transplants are primarily used in the treatment of aplastic anemia, leukemia, and certain types of immunodeficiencies.
   1. Donor marrow contains pluripotential hematopoietic stem cells that repopulate the lymphoid, erythroid, myeloid, and megakaryocytic series in the recipient.
   2. The recipient assumes the ABO group of the donor.

IX. HLA haplotypes and disease relationships and risk
A. Patients with HLA-associated diseases have a familial predisposition to the disease, weak penetrance (it does not have to occur), and abnormalities in their immune system that predispose to autoimmune diseases.
B. Important HLA-disease relationships include hemochromatosis with HLA-A3 (risk 7%), celiac disease with HLA-B8 and -DR3 (risk 13%), ankylosing spondylitis with HLA-B27 (risk 80%), multiple sclerosis with HLA-DR2 (risk 3%), type I insulin-dependent diabetes mellitus with HLA-DR3 and -DR4

(risk 3%), and rheumatoid arthritis (RA) with HLA-DR4 (risk 6%).

Objective 3: To understand the laboratory and clinical aspects of the hypersensitivity disorders.

X. Type I immediate hypersensitivity disorders
A. These are IgE antibody-mediated reactions involving the activation of mast cells/basophils with release of preformed chemical mediators (e.g., histamine) that increase vessel permeability and alter smooth muscle tone.
   1. Sensitization to an allergen first requires antigen processing by macrophages, which later interact with CD4 T$_H$2 cells.
   2. CD4 T$_H$2 cells stimulate B-cell production of IgE antibodies that attach to the cell membrane of mast cells and basophils.
   3. When allergens (e.g., pollens) cross-link two subjacent IgE antibodies on the membrane, mast cells/basophils release preformed mediators including histamine, proteases, and chemotactic factors for neutrophils and eosinophils (Chapter 3).
   4. The release reaction is followed by the formation of arachidonic acid with subsequent production and release of prostaglandins (increase vessel permeability) and leukotrienes (bronchoconstrictors).

B. The term **atopy** refers to the familial predisposition for developing an allergic reaction.
   1. Atopy is often manifested by reactions involving the skin (eczema, hives), eyes (conjunctivitis), nose (rhinitis), respiratory tract (asthma, anaphylactic reactions), and gastrointestinal tract (diarrhea).
   2. Laboratory tests that evaluate atopy include the total IgE concentration (**paper-based radioimmunosorbent test** [PRIST] procedure), **prick (scratch) skin testing** of allergens (most sensitive test), measurement of specific IgE antibodies (**radioallergosorbent test** [RAST]), and nasal smears and peripheral blood evaluation for eosinophils.

XI. Type II cytotoxic hypersensitivity disorders
A. These reactions include antibody-mediated cytotoxic reactions that involve complement activation with subsequent cell lysis, recruitment of inflammatory cells or NK cells, and autoantibodies against receptors.
   1. Antibody (IgG or IgM)-complement–mediated lysis of cells involves attachment of the antibodies onto a target cell with subsequent MAC destruction of the cell (e.g., ABO mismatch and hyperacute transplant rejection).
   2. Antibodies attached to target tissue may activate the complement system, leading to chemotaxis of neutrophils that produce tissue damage (e.g., Goodpasture's syndrome with antiglomerular and pulmonary capillary basement membrane antibodies).
   3. Hematopoietic cells coated by antibodies (IgG) and/or complement (C3b) are rendered more susceptible to phagocytosis and destruction by fixed macrophages (e.g., IgG-mediated warm autoimmune hemolytic anemias, Rh and ABO hemolytic disease of the newborn).

4. In **antibody-dependent cell-mediated cytotoxicity** (ADCC), cells coated by specific IgG antibodies (without complement) are rendered susceptible to lysis by NK cells (or other cells), which have low-affinity IgG Fc receptors (e.g., NK destruction of tumor cells and eosinophil destruction of helminths coated by IgE antibodies).

5. Diseases characterized by autoantibodies against receptors include myasthenia gravis (anti–acetylcholine receptor antibodies) and Graves' disease (thyroid-stimulating Ig directed against the thyroid-stimulating hormone [TSH] receptor).

B. Laboratory assessment of some of these reactions includes the **direct Coombs test** (detects IgG and/or C3 on RBCs), the **indirect Coombs test** (identifies specific antibodies in the serum [anti-D]), and immunofluorescent studies that localize deposits of antibody or complement in tissue (e.g., immune complex vasculitis).

XII. Type III immune complex (IC) hypersensitivity disorders

A. These reactions involve the deposition of circulating complexes of antigen bound to IgG or IgM in target tissue with subsequent complement activation and recruitment of neutrophils and macrophages that damage the tissue.

1. First exposure to an antigen initiates the formation of antibodies, which on second exposure leads to the production of antigen-antibody immune complexes that deposit in tissue, activate complement, and recruit neutrophils and macrophages that produce tissue damage.

2. Vasculitis and glomerulonephritis (GN) are common manifestations of this reaction.

B. **Farmer's lung** is a classic example of a localized immune complex (Arthus) reaction secondary to exposure to thermophilic actinomycetes in the air (granulomas representing type IV cellular immunity form later).

C. **Serum sickness** (e.g., as a result of treatment of rattlesnake envenomation), the prototype of systemic immune complex disease, is characterized by fever, urticaria, generalized lymphadenopathy, arthritis, GN, and vasculitis.

D. Other examples of systemic immune complex disease are poststreptococcal GN (bacterial antigens plus antistreptococcal antibodies), SLE (DNA plus anti-DNA antibodies), rheumatoid arthritis (IgM antibody against IgG), and polyarteritis nodosa (hepatitis B surface antigen plus anti–surface antigen antibody).

XIII. Type IV T cell–mediated hypersensitivity disorders

A. This is an antibody-independent reaction that involves CD4 helper T cells (which release lymphokines) that participate in **delayed reaction hypersensitivity** (DRH) reactions and CD8 cytotoxic T cells (which release perforins) that are cytolytic to target cells.

B. DRH reactions include those associated with **allergic contact dermatitis** (e.g., poison ivy, nickel, soaps), various types of skin tests (e.g., tuberculin sensitivity), and CMI responses to intracellular pathogens with granuloma formation (e.g. histoplasmosis).

1. In allergic contact dermatitis, low-molecular-weight antigens are phagocytosed by Langerhans' cells, transported to regional lymph nodes, and presented to T lymphocytes, which become sensitized to the antigen.

2. Antigen reexposure leads to an inflammatory response owing to the release of cytokines from the previously sensitized T lymphocytes.

3. A patch test is the application of a suspected irritant onto a patch, which is then applied to the skin to see whether a reaction occurs.

4. Other examples of a DRH reaction are the purified protein derivative (PPD) skin test for *Mycobacterium tuberculosis* (TB) and granuloma formation.

a. After processing of the organisms by alveolar macrophages, the macrophages interact with CD4 T_H1 class cells, leading to the formation of a granuloma (Chapter 3).

b. After PPD is injected into the skin and phagocytosed by Langerhans' cells, the macrophage presents the processed antigen to the previously sensitized memory T_H1 helper cells, which release cytokines that produce erythema and induration.

C. Cytotoxic T cells interact with class I antigens on nucleated cells.

1. Alteration of class I antigens (in a neoplastic or virus-infected cell) or foreign antigens (in a transplant) on a cell membrane activates cytotoxic T cells, which destroy the cell.

2. Clinical examples of this type of CMI are acute transplant rejections and the destruction of hepatitis B–infected hepatocytes.

Objective 4: To understand the laboratory and clinical aspects of autoimmune diseases.

XIV. Pathogenesis of autoimmune disease

A. Autoimmune diseases are associated with the loss of self-tolerance and subsequent reactions against the host's own tissue.

B. The loss of self-tolerance may be due to emergence of a sequestered antigen (e.g., sperm), an imbalance favoring CD4 T helper cells over CD8 T suppressor cells, an alteration of self-antigens by a drug (e.g., α-methyldopa) or by a pathogen (e.g., coxsackievirus), cross-reactivity (mimicry) between self and foreign antigens (e.g., rheumatic fever), abnormal immune response genes on chromosome 6 (Ir genes), or polyclonal activation of B lymphocytes (e.g., EBV).

XV. Types of autoimmune disease and laboratory assessment

A. Autoimmune diseases are classified as either organ-specific or systemic.

1. Organ-specific diseases include Addison's disease (destruction of the adrenal glands) and pernicious anemia (destruction of parietal cells).

2. Systemic diseases include SLE, rheumatoid arthritis (RA), and progressive systemic sclerosis (PSS).

B. Laboratory testing for autoimmune diseases primarily involves the use of the serum antinuclear antibody (ANA) test as a screen for systemic diseases and specific antibody tests for organ-specific diseases.

1. The major groups of nuclear antibodies are directed against DNA (double-stranded [ds] and single-stranded [ss]), histones, acidic proteins (anti-Smith [Sm] and antiribonucleoprotein [RNP]) and nucleolar antigens.
2. The serum ANA provides a pattern of nuclear fluorescence (e.g., speckled, rim, homogeneous, and nucleolar) and an antibody titer.
3. Since the **lupus erythematosus (LE) cell** (neutrophil with phagocytosed DNA previously altered by IgG antibodies) is not specific for SLE, its usefulness is questionable.
4. Important autoantibodies are listed in Table 4–1.

XVI. Rheumatoid arthritis (RA)
   A. RA is a female predominant, chronic, systemic, inflammatory autoimmune disease occurring between 30 and 50 years of age.
      1. Microbial infections (?Epstein-Barr virus), host genetic factors (HLA-DR4), and immunoregulatory problems have been implicated in its pathogenesis.
      2. Injury (?origin) results in an influx of CD4 T cells and macrophages to the synovial tissue with local stimulation of B cells to produce IgM autoantibodies directed against the Fc receptor of IgG (rheumatoid factor [RF]).
         a. RF aggregates into immune complexes that activate the complement system, leading to chemotaxis of neutrophils into the joint space, phagocytosis of immune complexes (ragocytes), and release of inflammatory mediators.
         b. Macrophages release interleukin-1 (IL-1) and tumor necrosis factor (TNF-α), which induce synovial cells to release inflammatory mediators that destroy connective tissue, cartilage, and bone.
         c. Chronically inflamed synovial tissue containing numerous plasma cells begins to proliferate (**pannus** formation) and destroy the articular cartilage, leading to reactive fibrosis and fusion (ankylosis) of the joint.
   B. RA is insidious in onset and presents with multisystem disease.
      1. Joint disease is symmetric and involves the metacarpophalangeal (MCP) and proximal interphalangeal (PIP) joints of the hands as well as other joints (e.g., atlantoaxial joint with the potential for vertebrobasilar insufficiency).
         a. Morning stiffness is a classic feature of RA.
         b. Advanced disease in the hands and wrists produces ulnar deviation of the fingers owing to laxity of the soft tissue.
         c. Carpal tunnel syndrome (compression of the median nerve) is commonly present.
      2. Extra-articular features of RA are widespread.
         a. Subcutaneous (rheumatoid) nodules occur on extensor surfaces.
         b. Small to medium vessel vasculitis leads to skin ulcerations.
         c. Pulmonary disease is manifested by diffuse interstitial fibrosis (restrictive lung disease), rheumatoid nodules in the parenchyma, chronic pleuritis, pleural effusions, and an association with coal worker's pneumoconiosis and silicosis, which is called **Caplan's syndrome**.
         d. Anemia of chronic inflammation is the most common anemia, with iron deficiency and autoimmune hemolytic disease occurring less commonly.
         e. Reactive (secondary) amyloidosis occurs owing to increased hepatic synthesis of serum-associated amyloid (SAA) protein as an acute-phase reactant.
         f. Other syndromes include **Sjögren's syndrome** (RA plus dry eyes and dry mouth) and **Felty's syndrome** (RA plus autoimmune neutropenia and splenomegaly).
   C. Laboratory abnormalities associated with RA include a positive RF (70%), a normal to increased serum complement (C3), increased erythrocyte sedimentation rate (ESR), polyclonal gammopathy, and a positive serum ANA (30%).

XVII. Juvenile rheumatoid arthritis (JRA)
   A. JRA is a chronic synovial inflammatory condition that frequents patients under 16 years of age.
      1. It is more commonly observed in girls than in boys and has three variants: Still's disease (20%), polyarticular JRA (40%), and pauciarticular JRA (40%).
      2. Unlike adult RA patients, JRA patients are more likely to be RF negative (seronegative).
   B. Clinical findings are similar to adult RA with each variant emphasizing a particular component (systemic disease with fever and rash in Still's disease, disabling arthritis in the polyarticular variant, and

TABLE 4–1. Autoantibodies in Autoimmune Disease

Autoantibody	Disease
Antiacetylcholine receptor antibody (AChR)	Generalized myasthenia gravis (90%)
Anticentromere antibody	CREST syndrome (60%) and PSS (30%)
Antigliadin antibody	Celiac disease (95%)
Anti–glomerular basement membrane antibody	Goodpasture's syndrome (>90% sensitivity and specificity)
Anti-insulin and anti–islet cell antibodies	Anti-insulin antibodies: type I diabetes mellitus and in patients taking bovine or porcine insulin but not human insulin
	Anti–islet cell antibodies: type I diabetes mellitus (60–90%)
Antimicrosomal antibody	Hashimoto's autoimmune thyroiditis (97%) and autoimmune hepatitis (70%)
Antimitochondrial antibody	Primary biliary cirrhosis (90–100%)
Antineutrophil cytoplasmic antibody (ANCA)	C (cytoplasmic) ANCA: Wegener's granulomatosis (>90% sensitivity)
	P (perinuclear) ANCA: polyarteritis nodosa (>80%)
Anti–parietal cell and intrinsic factor antibodies	Parietal cell antibodies: pernicious anemia (90%)
	Intrinsic factor antibodies: type I (blocking antibody that prevents B_{12} from binding to IF; 50% sensitivity) and type II (binding antibody that binds to IF or the IF-B_{12} complex), the former having the greater specificity for diagnosing pernicious anemia
Anti–smooth muscle antibody	Autoimmune hepatitis (70%)
Antithyroglobulin antibody	Hashimoto's autoimmune thyroiditis (85%) and Graves' disease (30%)

uveitis with the potential for blindness in the pauciarticular variant).

XVIII. Systemic lupus erythematosus (SLE)
  A. SLE is a female predominant autoimmune disorder resulting from an interplay of disturbances in immune regulation (polyclonal activation of B cells) and genetic, hormonal (e.g., increased estrogen activity), and environmental triggers (e.g., sunlight, procainamide).
  B. SLE may be localized to the skin (discoid lupus) or involve multiple systems.
    1. Arthritis or arthralgias involving small joints (e.g., the hands) are the most common presenting symptom.
    2. Avascular (aseptic) necrosis of the femoral head often complicates long-term corticosteroid therapy.
    3. Cutaneous lesions involve immune complex deposition of anti-DNA antibodies along the basement membrane that is restricted to the area of the rash in discoid lupus but present in both normal and involved skin in SLE.
    4. The classic butterfly rash occurs in 50% of cases.
    5. Fibrinous pericarditis is the most common cardiovascular manifestation of SLE and often is accompanied by pericardial effusion (collection of fluid in the pericardial sac).
    6. Valvular disease (Libman-Sacks endocarditis) is characterized by warty, nonembolic vegetations (fibrinoid necrosis) scattered over the valve surfaces and endocardium.
    7. Pulmonary disease most frequently presents with pleuritis and a pleural effusion; however, chronic interstitial lung disease with a restrictive pattern similar to that seen in RA and PSS also occurs.
    8. Autoimmune hemolytic anemia, thrombocytopenia, and leukopenia are potential complications.
    9. Renal disease (50–60%), a common cause of death in SLE, is usually associated with diffuse proliferative GN and the presence of anti-dsDNA (increased anti-ssDNA) antibodies (Chapter 17).
    10. Antiphospholipid antibodies (lupus anticoagulant and anticardiolipin antibody) are frequently responsible for midtrimester fetal loss due to vessel thrombosis in the placenta.
    11. Patients with anti-SS-A (Ro) antibodies (IgG) frequently are delivered of newborns with complete heart block.
  C. Laboratory abnormalities associated with SLE include a positive serum ANA (99%), anti-dsDNA (70%), anti-Sm (30%), and anti-SS-A (Ro; 30%).
    1. Complement C3 levels are low in active disease.
    2. A biologic false-positive syphilis serology (positive RPR [rapid plasma reagin] and VDRL [Venereal Disease Research Laboratories] with a negative FTA-ABS [fluorescent treponema antibody absorption test]) occurs in 25% of patients owing to cross-reactivity of anticardiolipin antibodies with the cardiolipin in the test systems for the RPR and VDRL.
  D. Drug-induced SLE (most often due to procainamide) differs from SLE in a number of important parameters including abrupt rather than slow onset, a very low incidence of renal and CNS involvement, absent anti-dsDNA and anti-Sm antibodies, normal complement levels, and elevated antihistone (95%) antibodies.

XIX. Progressive systemic sclerosis (PSS)
  A. PSS (scleroderma) is a female predominant autoimmune disease that initially involves small vessels and later excessive deposition of normal collagen (?stimulus) in multiple organ systems.
    1. Skin changes are characterized by parchment-like appearance, swelling of the fingers and hands, tight facial features, multiple punctate blood vessel dilatations (telangiectasias), and Raynaud's phenomenon (color changes in the fingers due to vasospasm and digital vessel thickening), which is the most common initial sign of PSS.
    2. Other findings include polyarthritis, dysphagia for solids and liquids (lack of peristalsis), malabsorption, renal disease (GN, severe hypertension and renal failure), pulmonary disease (diffuse interstitial pneumonitis with fibrosis is the most common cause of death), and left ventricular dysfunction.
  B. A localized variant of PSS designated **CREST syndrome** refers to _c_alcinosis (fingertips) and anti-centromere antibodies, _R_aynaud's phenomenon, _e_sophageal motility dysfunction, _s_clerodactyly, and _t_elangiectasias.
  C. Laboratory abnormalities in PSS include positive tests for ANA (70–90%), anti-Scl-70 (70%), and anti-centromere antibodies (30%).

XX. Dermatomyositis/polymyositis
  A. Dermatomyositis (DM) and polymyositis (PM) are both associated with an inflammatory myopathy with or without involvement of the skin, the former representing DM and the latter PM.
  B. Clinical findings include muscle pain and atrophy, dysphagia, puffy eyelids with a purple-red discoloration (heliotrope eyelids), and an increased risk for malignant neoplasms (15–20%), particularly of the lung.
  C. Laboratory test abnormalities include an elevated serum creatine kinase and positive anti-JO-1 antibodies in 18–25% of cases.
  D. Confirmation is secured by a muscle biopsy exhibiting lymphocytic infiltration.

XXI. Mixed connective tissue disease (MCTD)
  A. MCTD shares features of SLE, PSS, and polymyositis; follows a more benign course than the other autoimmune diseases; and rarely involves the kidney.
  B. Antiribonucleoprotein (RNP) antibodies are present in most cases.

XXII. Sjögren's syndrome (SS)
  A. Sjögren's syndrome is female predominant disease associated with RA and complicated by immune system destruction of the lacrimal and salivary glands, resulting in dry eyes (keratoconjunctivitis), dry mouth (xerostomia), and an increased incidence of malignant lymphoma.
  B. Tubulointerstitial disease leads to distal renal tubular acidosis (type I).
  C. Laboratory abnormalities include positive serum tests for ANAs (50–80%), anti-SS-A/Ro (70–80%), and anti-SS-B/La (50–70%; more specific than anti-Ro) antibodies.
    1. A positive RF is noted in 75–90% of patients.
    2. The confirmatory test is lip biopsy of a minor salivary gland demonstrating lymphocytic destruction of the glands.

[handwritten margin note:] Antiphospholipid Syndrome
- Spontaneous Abortion
- thrombocytopenia
- thrombosis

QUESTIONS

Directions. (Items 1–11): Each of the numbered items or incomplete statements in this section is followed by answers or by completions of the statement. Select the ONE lettered answer or completion that is BEST in each case. Correct answers and explanations are given at the end of the chapter.

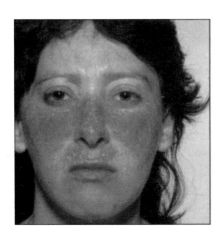

1. This 25-year-old woman also has laboratory findings of hematuria and RBC casts. Which of the following additional laboratory abnormalities would you expect this patient to have?

   (A) Low C1 esterase inhibitor levels
   (B) Low factor B concentration
   (C) Anergic skin panel
   (D) Positive anti–double-stranded DNA antibody
   (E) Elevated IgE antibody titer

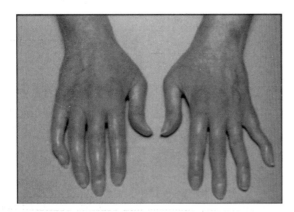

2. These are the hands of a 46-year-old woman with dysphagia for solids and liquids. Which of the following laboratory findings is most likely in this patient?

   (A) Positive anti-SS-A(Ro)
   (B) Positive anticentromere antibody
   (C) Positive anti-Smith antibody
   (D) Positive antiribonucleoprotein antibody
   (E) Positive anti–double-stranded DNA antibody

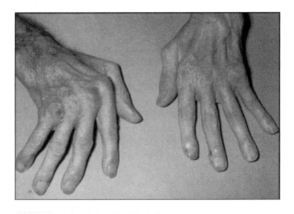

3. This photograph depicts the hands of a 45-year-old woman who complains of feeling "sand in my eyes" and "difficulty with swallowing dry crackers." You would expect the patient to have positive results for which of the following groups of tests?

   (A) Rheumatoid factor and anti-SS-B(La) antibody
   (B) Anti-Smith antibody and anti–double-stranded DNA antibody
   (C) Anticentromere antibody and rheumatoid factor
   (D) Rheumatoid factor and anti–double-stranded DNA antibody
   (E) Anti-Scl-70 antibody and anti-Smith antibody

4. Complement assumes a pivotal role in

   (A) antibody-dependent cellular cytotoxicity
   (B) mast cell degranulation
   (C) delayed-reaction hypersensitivity
   (D) paroxysmal nocturnal hemoglobinuria
   (E) cytolysis by cytotoxic CD8 T cells

5. Which of the following groups of diseases fall into the same hypersensitivity reaction classification?

   (A) Allergic rhinitis and poison ivy
   (B) ABO incompatibility and skin reaction to a bee sting
   (C) Hyperacute transplant rejection and serum sickness
   (D) Nickel contact dermatitis and atopic dermatitis
   (E) Graves' disease and Goodpasture's syndrome

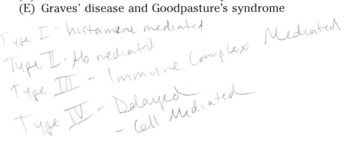

6. The following are the laboratory test results for a newborn boy, mother, and putative father in a paternity suit. Their RBCs are reacted against anti-A, anti-B, and anti-D antigen test sera for ABO and Rh phenotyping, and their sera are reacted against A and B test RBCs to check for isohemagglutinins. See table below.

RBCs reacted against:

	Anti-A	Anti-B
Mother	Positive	Negative
Putative father	Negative	Negative
Newborn	Negative	Negative

Serum reacted against:

Anti-D	A test cells	B test cells
Negative	Negative	Positive
Positive	Positive	Positive
Negative	Negative	Negative

You can conclude from the laboratory data that the

(A) newborn child is blood group A and Rh negative
(B) putative father is blood group AB and Rh positive
(C) mother is blood group B and Rh negative
(D) newborn child's serum reaction with A and B test cells is a laboratory error
(E) newborn child's ABO group and Rh findings are compatible with the mother and putative father

7. A newborn boy was cyanotic at birth and developed clinical signs of tetany within the first 24 hours. You would expect additional evaluation of the patient or the patient's mother to reveal

(A) absence of the thymic shadow on a chest x-ray of the newborn
(B) a sex-linked recessive disease in the newborn
(C) increased cord blood IgM in the newborn
(D) absence of maternal IgG antibodies in the newborn's serum
(E) combined B- and T-cell immunodeficiency in the newborn

8. Which of the following disorders has a pathogenesis involving the activation of complement with the production of chemotactic substances that result in neutrophil-related injury to tissue?

(A) Myasthenia gravis
(B) Tuberculous granuloma
(C) Poststreptococcal glomerulonephritis
(D) Destruction of invasive helminths
(E) Acute rejection of a kidney transplant

9. Which laboratory finding would a patient with the acquired immunodeficiency syndrome be least likely to demonstrate?

(A) Elevated p24 antigen
(B) Hypogammaglobulinemia
(C) Anergy
(D) Abnormal mitogen assay
(E) CD4 T helper count $\leq$200 cells/μL

10. A patient with aplastic anemia who recently underwent a bone marrow transplant developed a generalized maculopapular rash, jaundice, and diarrhea. The pathogenesis of this complication is most likely due to

(A) destruction of tissue by lymphokine-activated natural killer cells
(B) destruction of tissue by CD8 cytotoxic T cells
(C) vessel thrombosis secondary to damage by anti-HLA antibodies
(D) an interaction between CD4 T helper cells and macrophages
(E) immune complex deposition with subsequent activation of the complement system

11. Which of the following cells or chemical mediators is least likely to be involved in an acute rejection of a living donor kidney transplant?

(A) Donor CD4 helper T cells
(B) Host CD8 cytotoxic T cells
(C) Host natural killer cells
(D) Donor macrophages
(E) Interleukins 1 and 2

DIRECTIONS. ITEMS 12–13: For each of the following patients with recurrent infections, select the most likely diagnosis.

A. Bruton's agammaglobulinemia
B. Acquired immunodeficiency syndrome
C. Severe combined immunodeficiency
D. Common variable immune deficiency
E. Wiskott-Aldrich syndrome
F. Ataxia telangiectasia
G. Sex-linked lymphoproliferative syndrome
H. IgA deficiency

12. An 8-year-old boy has recurrent sinopulmonary infections, intermittent bouts of diarrhea, and a history of atopy. His CBC, platelet count, and peripheral smear examination are unremarkable. Sweat chloride tests have been routinely negative in the past. He has a normal total IgG and IgE concentration.

13. A 3-year-old boy has a history of recurrent sinopulmonary infections, epistaxis, and eczema. Scattered petechiae and ecchymoses are noted over his trunk and extremities. He has markedly elevated IgE levels.

ANSWERS AND EXPLANATIONS

1. The answer is D: positive anti–double-stranded DNA. The photograph exhibits the classic butterfly rash of SLE. The history of hematuria and RBC casts indicates renal disease (diffuse proliferative GN), which invariably is associated with anti-dsDNA antibodies. C1 esterase inhibitor deficiency (angioedema) is associated with excessive release of C2-derived kinins, which increase vessel permeability, leading to subcutaneous edema, most commonly involving the face and oropharynx. A low factor B concentration implies activation of the alternative complement pathway. SLE is associated with activation of the classical pathway (low C4 and C2). An anergic skin panel is present in patients with a defect in CMI. Elevated IgE antibody titers are a feature of type I hypersensitivity reactions. SLE is a type III immune complex disease. (Photomicrograph reproduced, with permission, from M.A. Mir. *Atlas of Clinical Diagnosis.* Philadelphia, W.B. Saunders Co., 1995.)

2. The answer is B: positive anticentromere antibody. The patient's hands depict sclerodactyly (tapered fingers), which along with a history of dysphagia for solids and liquids suggests CREST syndrome or PSS. Both autoimmune diseases have an elevation of anticentromere antibodies, Raynaud's phenomenon, dystrophic calcification of the fingertips, and telangiectasias (dilatation of small blood vessels). PSS involves other organs, such as the kidneys, lungs, and heart. A positive anti-SS-A(Ro) is present in Sjögren's syndrome and SLE, the latter also associated with anti-Smith and anti–double-stranded DNA antibodies as well. Antiribonucleoprotein antibodies are a feature of MCTD. (Photomicrograph reproduced, with permission, from M.A. Mir. *Atlas of Clinical Diagnosis.* Philadelphia, W.B. Saunders Co., 1995.)

3. The answer is A: rheumatoid factor and anti-SS-B(La) antibody. The photograph depicts symmetric ulnar deviation of the hands (rheumatoid arthritis), which along with the history of "sand in my eyes" (keratoconjunctivitis sicca—dry eyes) and "difficulty with swallowing dry crackers" (xerostomia—dry mouth) is the classic triad for Sjögren's syndrome (SS). Anti-SS-B(La) antibodies are more specific for Sjögren's syndrome than are anti-SS-A(Ro) antibodies. SS is characterized by autoimmune destruction of the minor salivary and lacrimal glands. Anti-Smith and anti–double-stranded DNA antibody are present in SLE, anticentromere antibodies in CREST syndrome and PSS, and anti-Scl-70 antibodies in PSS. (Photomicrograph reproduced, with permission, from M.A. Mir. *Atlas of Clinical Diagnosis.* Philadelphia, W.B. Saunders Co., 1995.)

4. The answer is D: paroxysmal nocturnal hemoglobinuria (PNH). PNH is an acquired stem cell disorder with absence of decay accelerating factor, which normally degrades C3 and C5 convertases on hematopoietic cell membranes, thereby preventing complement destruction. Complement is not involved in ADCC (a variant of type II hypersensitivity), mast cell degranulation (IgE antibodies), delayed-reaction hypersensitivity (CMI), and cytolysis by cytotoxic CD8 T cells (CMI).

5. The answer is E: Graves' disease and Goodpasture's syndrome. These two disorders are both examples of type II hypersensitivity, the former representing an autoantibody against a receptor (thyroid-stimulating Ig against the TSH receptor) and the latter antibodies against glomerular and pulmonary capillary basement membranes. Allergic rhinitis, atopic dermatitis, and the skin reaction to a bee sting are histamine-mediated type I hypersensitivity reactions. Poison ivy and nickel skin reactions are examples of contact dermatitis, which is a CMI (type IV hypersensitivity) reaction. ABO incompatibility and hyperacute transplant rejection are cytotoxic antibody-mediated reactions (type II hypersensitivity). Serum sickness is an immune complex–mediated type III hypersensitivity reaction.

6. The answer is E: newborn child's ABO group and Rh findings are compatible with the mother and putative father. The mother is blood group A (positive RBC reaction against anti-A test sera and a positive reaction of serum against B RBCs [indicating the presence of anti-B isohemagglutinins]), and she is Rh negative (D antigen negative). The putative father is blood group O (negative RBC reactions against anti-A and -B test sera but positive reactions against A and B RBC test cells [indicating the presence of anti-A and anti-B isohemagglutinins]), and he is Rh positive (D antigen positive). The newborn is blood group O and would not be expected to have isohemagglutinins at birth, since IgM synthesis begins at birth and IgG synthesis a few months later. The newborn is also Rh negative. If the mother is an AO phenotype rather than an AA phenotype, an O baby is possible (AO mother × OO father = AO and OO children). If the father is a heterozygote D (i.e., Dd) rather than a homozygote D (i.e., DD), it is possible for the newborn to be Rh negative (dd mother × Dd father = 25% chance of a dd child). HLA testing and DNA testing would be more definitive methods of determining parentage.

7. The answer is A: absence of the thymic shadow on a chest x-ray of the newborn. A newborn with cyanosis at birth and tetany most likely has the DiGeorge syndrome, which is a pure T-cell deficiency with failure of development of the third and fourth pharyngeal pouches (absent thymus and parathyroid glands [tetany due to hypocalcemia]). There is no distinct inheritance pattern. Truncus arteriosus (the aorta and pulmonary artery share a common trunk) is a cyanotic congenital heart disease commonly associated with the syndrome. An increased cord blood IgM in a newborn suggests an intrauterine infection (e.g., CMV), which would not be associated with cyanotic congenital heart disease and hypoparathyroidism. An absence of maternal IgG antibodies in the newborn's serum would imply hypogammaglobulinemia in the mother, which is unlikely and would not explain the findings in the newborn. None of the combined B- and T-cell immunodeficiencies (e.g., SCID) are associated with cyanotic heart disease and hypoparathyroidism.

8. The answer is C: poststreptococcal glomerulonephritis. Poststreptococcal GN is an immune complex–mediated (type III hypersensitivity) disease. The pathogenesis of immune complex disease involves the activation of complement with the production of C5a, a chemotactic agent that attracts neutrophils to the area of immune complex deposition. Myasthenia gravis is associated with an autoantibody against acetylcholine receptors (type II hypersensitivity). A tuberculous granuloma is a cell-mediated delayed-reaction hypersensitivity that does not utilize complement or neutrophils. Destruc-

tion of invasive helminths is by a variant of ADCC (type II hypersensitivity) involving eosinophil destruction of helminths. Acute rejection of a kidney transplant is primarily a type IV hypersensitivity reaction involving cytotoxic CD8 T cells, with a minor component of antibody-mediated damage.

9. The answer is B: hypogammaglobulinemia. Patients with the acquired immunodeficiency syndrome (AIDS) have hypergammaglobulinemia owing to polyclonal stimulation of B cells by EBV and CMV. The p24 antigen, a marker of disease activity, has a bimodal peak—one at the onset of HIV infection and the other at the onset of overt AIDS. Owing to destruction of CD4 T helper cells, T-cell function is impaired, leading to anergy (lack of skin response to common antigens), an abnormal mitogen assay (no response to T-cell mitogens), and a low CD4 T helper cell count ($\leq$200 cells/μL).

10. The answer is A: destruction of tissue by lymphokine-activated natural killer cells. Patients who undergo bone marrow transplants are at risk for the graft-versus-host reaction owing to the release of interleukin-2 by donor helper T cells with subsequent activation of lymphokine-activated NK cells. NK cells are responsible for producing a maculopapular rash and epithelial necrosis in the biliary tract (jaundice) and gastrointestinal tract (diarrhea). Destruction of tissue by CD8 cytotoxic T cells is seen in acute transplant rejection. Vessel thrombosis secondary to damage by anti-HLA antibodies is responsible for hyperacute transplant rejection. An interaction between CD4 T helper cells and macrophages is an example of delayed reaction hypersensitivity, which is a feature of granuloma formation and contact dermatitis. Immune complex deposition with subsequent activation of the complement system is the mechanism of injury in type III hypersensitivity reactions.

11. The answer is A: donor CD4 helper T cells. In an acute rejection of a living donor kidney transplant, donor macrophages interact with host CD8 cytotoxic T cells and host CD4 helper T cells, the latter releasing interleukin-2, which stimulates host antibody formation (the humoral component of graft rejection) and proliferation of additional CD8 cytotoxic T cells that destroy the graft. Host macrophages and NK cells also contribute to destruction of the graft. Interleukin-1 is released by the donor macrophages and host macrophages.

12. The answer is H: IgA deficiency. IgA deficiency is the most common hereditary immunodeficiency. When symptomatic, it presents with recurrent sinopulmonary infections (most common), intermittent bouts of diarrhea (malabsorption, giardiasis), a history of atopy, and an increased incidence of autoimmune disease (e.g., celiac disease). The CBC, platelet count, and peripheral smear examination are not diagnostic. A sweat chloride test for cystic fibrosis is negative. Both IgA and secretory IgA are deficient, while all other Igs are normal.

13. The answer is E: Wiskott-Aldrich syndrome. This syndrome is an SXR disease with a triad of recurrent sinopulmonary disease, eczema, and thrombocytopenia (epistaxis, petechiae, and ecchymoses). It is a combined B- and T-cell immunodeficiency with low IgM and elevated IgG, IgA, and IgE levels.

CHAPTER FIVE

FLUIDS AND

HEMODYNAMICS

SYNOPSIS

OBJECTIVES

1. To describe the pathogenesis of edema.
2. To demonstrate the morphologic and pathophysiologic effects of hyperemia (congestion) in various organs.
3. To review volume disorders secondary to alterations in sodium and/or water.
4. To review the hemodynamic alterations associated with hypovolemic, cardiogenic, and septic shock.
5. To understand the pathophysiology of acid-base disorders (respiratory and metabolic) in clinical medicine.
6. To review the hemostatic system and alterations in the vascular, platelet, coagulation, and fibrinolytic systems.
7. To understand the pathophysiology of the thrombotic and embolic disorders.

Objective 1: To describe the pathogenesis of edema.

I. Edema
   A. Edema is excessive fluid accumulation in the interstitial space or in body cavities (effusions) secondary to alterations in Starling's forces, acute inflammation, or lymphatic blockage (lymphedema).
      1. **Intravascular alterations in Starling's forces** resulting in edema include an **increase in hydrostatic pressure** and/or a **decrease in oncotic pressure**, the latter correlating with hypoalbuminemia.
         a. **Pitting edema** refers to pressure-induced indentation of the skin due to excess fluid in the interstitial space.
         b. In **dependent edema**, excess interstitial fluid accumulates in dependent areas of the body (e.g., feet).
      2. Acute inflammation produces edema secondary to an increase in vessel permeability.
      3. Lymphatic obstruction (e.g., postmastectomy irradiation, filariasis) produces a nonpitting edema **(lymphedema)**.
      4. **Hydrothorax** (pleural effusion), **hydropericardium** (pericardial effusion), and **ascites** (peritoneal effusion) are examples of noninflammatory edema in body cavities.
      5. Generalized edema with body cavity effusions is called **anasarca**.

   B. Starling's force alterations result in a cell-poor and protein-poor (< 3 g/dL) fluid called a **transudate**.
      1. Transudates secondary to an **increase in hydrostatic pressure** are dependent pitting edema (right heart failure), pulmonary edema (left heart failure), and ascites in cirrhosis (portal vein hypertension).
      2. Transudates derived from a **decrease in oncotic pressure** include pitting edema secondary to cirrhosis (reduced synthesis of albumin), the nephrotic syndrome (massive proteinuria), and kwashiorkor (reduced protein intake).
   C. Increased vessel permeability produces a cell-rich and protein-rich fluid (> 3 g/dL plus neutrophils) called an **exudate** (Chapter 3).

Objective 2: To demonstrate the morphologic and pathophysiologic effects of hyperemia (congestion) in various organs.

II. Hyperemia (congestion)
   A. **Active hyperemia (congestion)** refers to an increase in arterial or arteriolar blood flow secondary to neurogenic reflexes (e.g., blushing) or chemically induced vasodilatation (e.g., histamine; Chapter 3).
   B. **Passive hyperemia (congestion)** is brought about by a reduction in venous blood flow from an area (e.g., hepatic congestion in right heart failure).

Objective 3: To review volume disorders secondary to alterations in sodium and/or water.

III. Body fluid compartments
   A. **Total body water** (TBW) is approximately 60% of the body weight in kilograms.
      1. TBW is distributed between the **intracellular fluid** (ICF; 40%) and the **extracellular fluid** (ECF; 20%) **compartments**.
      2. The ECF is further subdivided into the **interstitial fluid** (ISF; 13% of ECF) and **vascular** (~7% of ECF) **compartments**.
   B. **Total body sodium** ($TBNa^+$) is primarily limited to the ECF compartment, whereas **total body po-**

tassium (TBK$^+$) primarily occupies the ICF compartment.

IV. Plasma osmolality

A. The plasma osmolality (Posm) represents the solute concentration (275–295 mOsm/kg) in plasma.

B. The formula to calculate Posm is as follows:

$$Posm = 2\,Na^+ + glucose\ (mg/dL)/18 \\ + blood\ urea\ nitrogen\ (mg/dL)/2.8$$

1. Sodium and glucose are **impermeant solutes**, which means that they are limited to the ECF compartment.

2. The interchange of water between the ECF and ICF compartments is primarily controlled by alterations in the serum Na$^+$ concentration that establish an osmotic gradient favoring water movement from a low- to a high-solute concentration.

   a. In **hyponatremia** (reduced Na$^+$ concentration), water is directed into the ICF compartment, producing ICF compartment expansion.

   b. In **hypernatremia** (increased Na$^+$ concentration), water moves into the ECF, which leads to contraction of the ICF compartment.

3. In **hyperglycemic conditions** (e.g., diabetic ketoacidosis), glucose overrides Na$^+$ as the primary osmotic force.

   a. Water moves from the ICF into the ECF compartment and produces **dilutional hyponatremia**.

   b. To correct for the dilutional effect of glucose on Na$^+$, the following formula is utilized:

$$Corrected\ serum\ Na^+ = serum\ Na^+ \\ + (glucose\ [mg/dL]/100 \times 1.6)$$

4. Urea and alcohol are **permeant solutes** that diffuse through cell membranes without establishing an osmotic gradient, hence increasing the Posm without producing water movements.

5. The calculation of **effective osmolality** (Eosm) provides a more accurate assessment of water homeostasis by excluding the blood urea nitrogen (BUN) from the equation:

$$Eosm = 2\,Na^+ + glucose/18$$

   a. A **normal Eosm** connotes the presence of an **isotonic** condition in the ECF compartment (no osmotic gradient).

   b. A **low Eosm** indicates the presence of a **hypotonic** condition (e.g., hyponatremia) and the presence of a gradient favoring ICF expansion.

   c. A **high Eosm** reflects a **hypertonic** state (e.g., hypernatremia or hyperglycemia), which leads to ICF contraction.

V. Volume regulation

A. Maintenance of the ECF volume involves the integration of factors that (1) control thirst, (2) activate the renin-angiotensin-aldosterone system, (3) reabsorb free water in the kidneys (antidiuretic hormone [ADH]), and (4) control the renal reabsorption of Na$^+$.

B. The **effective arterial blood volume** (EABV) represents the amount of total circulating volume required to stimulate volume receptors (baroreceptors).

1. The EABV usually parallels the existing ECF volume except in edema states.

2. Alterations in Starling's forces that produce edema trap large volumes of fluid in the interstitial space (increasing total ECF volume), which reduces venous return to the right heart, hence decreasing the EABV.

C. The **volume (stretch) receptors** include the **low-pressure baroreceptors** in the left atrium and major thoracic veins and the **high-pressure baroreceptors** in the carotid sinus and aortic arch (innervated by cranial nerves IX and X).

1. A reduction in the EABV stimulates the baroreceptor reflex.

   a. The reflex increases sympathetic outflow to the heart and blood vessels, with a subsequent increase in heart rate, cardiac contractility, peripheral vasoconstriction, systemic venoconstriction, and mean arterial blood pressure.

   b. The reflex stimulates the posterior pituitary release of ADH, which increases the reabsorption of free water (see ¶C.5, below) in the kidneys.

   c. The reflex directly stimulates the juxtaglomerular (JG) apparatus located in the afferent arterioles of the kidneys, with subsequent release of the enzyme renin.

2. A reduction in the EABV also activates the **renin-angiotensin-aldosterone** (RAA) **system** owing to reduced renal blood flow to the juxtaglomerular apparatus.

   a. Renin initiates the following reaction sequence: it cleaves renin substrate (angiotensinogen) into **angiotensin I** (ATI) → pulmonary **angiotensin converting enzyme** (ACE) converts ATI into angiotensin II (ATII) → ATII is converted into angiotensin III (ATIII).

   b. ATII functions include (1) peripheral vasoconstriction (which increases blood pressure), (2) stimulation of aldosterone release (which increases Na$^+$ reabsorption, hence increasing blood volume and cardiac output), and (3) direct stimulation of the thirst center (which increases blood volume).

3. **Atrial natriuretic peptide** (ANP) and **prostaglandin E$_2$ (PGE$_2$)** serve a counterregulatory role against ATII.

   a. ANP is released from the left atrium in response to atrial distention (e.g., left heart failure).

   b. ANP functions include (1) the inhibition of ADH release, the ATII effect on stimulating thirst, aldosterone secretion, renal reabsorption of Na$^+$ (direct effect), and renin release, and (2) vasodilatation of the peripheral resistance vessels.

   c. **PGE$_2$** functions consist of the inhibition of ADH and renal reabsorption of Na$^+$, and since PGE$_2$ is a potent intrarenal vasodilator, it offsets the intrarenal vasoconstrictive effects of ATII and the catecholamines.

D. The response of the kidneys to volume contraction or overload is integrally related to the above baroreceptor and RAA responses initiated by changes in the EABV.

1. The **proximal tubules** isosmotically (i.e., urine filtrate has the same osmolality after reabsorption) remove water and other solutes (e.g., 60% of Na^+).

    a. The glomerular **filtration fraction** (FF) (glomerular filtration rate/renal plasma flow) and **Starling's forces** in the peritubular capillaries (e.g., hydrostatic pressure [P_H] and oncotic pressure [P_O]) control the reabsorption or loss of solutes in the proximal tubule.

    b. **Decreased EABV** results in (1) an increase in the FF ($\uparrow$ FF $= \downarrow$ GFR/$\downarrow\downarrow$ RPF), (2) an increase in the filtered load of Na^+, and (3) $P_H < P_O$, hence favoring isosmotic reabsorption of Na^+ back into the ECF (random urine Na^+ (UNa^+) measurement is < 20 mEq/L).

    c. **Increased EABV** leads to (1) a decrease in the FF ($\downarrow$ FF $= \uparrow$ GFR/$\uparrow\uparrow$ RPF), (2) a decrease in the filtered load of Na^+, and (3) $P_H > P_O$, hence favoring the renal loss of Na^+ (random UNa^+ frequently > 20 mEq/L).

2. The **thin descending limb** is permeable only to water, hence the filtrate becomes hypertonic (maximum, 1200 mOsm/kg) by the time it reaches the loop of Henle.

3. The **thin ascending limb** is impermeable to water but permeable to Na^+ and Cl^-, hence reducing the osmolality of the filtrate.

4. The **distal tubule** subdivides into the **thick ascending limb** (diluting segment), the **macula densa** (which abuts the juxtaglomerular apparatus), and the **distal convoluted tubule**.

    a. In the thick ascending limb **(medullary segment)**, an active **$Na^+/K^+/2$ Cl^- cotransport pump** generates a hypotonic fluid (~150 mOsm/kg) consisting of **obligated water** (that must accompany solute) and **free water** (water left over after Na^+, K^+, and Cl^- are actively reabsorbed).

    b. In the **cortical segment** of the thick ascending limb, there is an Na^+/K^+ pump that may be blocked by thiazides.

    c. The **macula densa** is a modified chemoreceptor that senses volume and Na^+ alterations in the distal tubule that either stimulate or inhibit renin release by the juxtaglomerular apparatus.

    d. The **distal convoluted tubule** has an aldosterone-enhanced Na^+/K^+-ATPase exchange pump.

       (1) Na^+ is reabsorbed in exchange for K^+, which when depleted is replaced by H^+ exchange with Na^+.

       (2) Distal secretion of K^+ is enhanced by augmented Na^+ delivery to the distal tubule (e.g., loop or thiazide diuretics block Na^+ reabsorption more proximally), which often leads to hypokalemia.

       (3) Reduced K^+ secretion occurs when aldosterone is either blocked (e.g., by spironolactone) or is deficient (e.g., in Addison's disease), hence predisposing to hyperkalemia.

5. In the **late distal** and **collecting ducts**, the presence of ADH results in the reabsorption of free water (negative free water clearance, which concentrates the urine), while the absence of ADH results in the loss of free water (positive free water clearance, which dilutes the urine).

    a. ADH release is inhibited by a low Posm (hyponatremia) or an increase in the EABV (baroreceptor reflex) and is stimulated by an increased Posm (hypernatremia) or a decrease in the EABV.

    b. The **collecting duct** has an aldosterone-enhanced Na^+/K^+-ATPase pump and an aldosterone-dependent H^+ (proton)/K^+-ATPase pump (see below).

VI. Integrated response to alterations in the EABV

   A. A **low EABV** (e.g., hypovolemia) results in (1) the baroreceptor reflex stimulation of ADH release (reabsorption of free water), (2) increased proximal tubule reabsorption of Na^+ in isosmotic proportions ($P_O > P_H$), and (3) stimulation of aldosterone (which reabsorbs Na^+ in exchange for K^+ or H^+).

      1. The reabsorbed fluid is hypotonic (slightly more water is reabsorbed than Na^+).

      2. Distribution of the hypotonic fluid is dependent on whether it alters the serum Na^+ concentration (hence the osmotic gradient that results in water movement between the ECF and ICF) and on the status of Starling's forces, which determine whether the fluid will remain in the intravascular space or be redirected into the ISF.

   B. An **increased EABV** (e.g., hypervolemia) (1) blocks the release of ADH, (2) increases proximal tubule loss of Na^+ ($P_H > P_O$), and (3) inhibits the release of aldosterone.

VII. Fluid derangements involving sodium

   A. **Total body osmolality** reflects the electrolyte concentration in *all* body fluid compartments, i.e., the total exchangeable body Na^+ ($TBNa^+$) plus the total exchangeable body K^+ (TBK^+) divided by the total body water (TBW).

      1. The serum Na^+ does not always correlate with the $TBNa^+$, since serum Na^+ is only one component of the total body osmolality.

         a. The above relationship of $TBNa^+ + TBK^+$/TBW does correlate with the serum Na^+ such that alterations in $TBNa^+$, TBK^+, or TBW directly affect the final serum Na^+ concentration.

         b. To simplify the above concept, the following relationship of serum Na^+ concentration with total body osmolality is used here: **serum $Na^+ \cong TBNa^+$/TBW.**

      2. Fluids in the ECF that are either gained or lost when compared to the Posm are designated **isotonic** (having the same osmolality), **hypotonic** (having less osmolality), or **hypertonic** (having greater osmolality) (Table 5–1).

         a. The physical examination approximates the $TBNa^+$ status of the patient ($\downarrow TBNa^+ = $ volume depletion; $\uparrow TBNa^+ = $ pitting edema, body effusions; normal $TBNa^+ = $ normal examination), while a daily body weight reflects total fluid gains or losses in the body compartments.

         b. UNa^+ is > 20 mEq/L if there is renal loss of Na^+ (e.g., due to diuretics) and < 20 mEq/L with extrarenal loss of Na^+ (e.g., due to diarrhea or sweating).

   B. **Hyponatremia** is a decreased serum Na^+ concen-

TABLE 5–1. Sodium and Water Disorders

Fluid Disorder	TBNa$^+$/TBW Physical Examination	Clinical Associations	Compartment Relationships
Normonatremia Isotonic loss (loss of equal amounts of H_2O and Na^+)	↓ TBNa$^+$/↓ TBW Volume depletion	1. Adult diarrhea 2. Third space loss ("nonfunctional ECF"): edematous bowel wall in a bowel infarct/obstruction, peripancreatic fluid accumulation in acute pancreatitis, ascites, massive soft tissue injuries, burns	Normal ECF: ↓, EABV: ↓ ISF: ↓, ICF: N
Isotonic gain (gain of equal amounts of H_2O and Na^+)	↑ TBNa$^+$/↑ TBW Pitting edema	1. Excessive infusion of isotonic saline	Normal ECF: ↑, EABV: ↑ ISF: ↑, ICF: N
Hyponatremia Depletion (loss of more Na$^+$ than H_2O: hypertonic loss)	↓↓ TBNa$^+$/↓ TBW or if patient has access to water: ↓↓ TBNa$^+$/↑↑↑ TBW Volume depletion	1. Diuretic use: most common cause, particularly loop diuretics 2. Mineralocorticoid deficiency: Addison's disease, adrenogenital syndrome (21-hydroxylase) 3. Any loss or gain of fluid (isotonic, hypotonic, or hypertonic) in which the patient has access to water and increases the TBW in the denominator: e.g., sweating or diarrhea	ECF: ↓, EABV: ↓ ISF: ↓, ICF: ↑
Dilutional (gain of more H_2O than Na$^+$ but both are increased)	↑ TBNa$^+$/↑↑ TBW Pitting edema	1. Right heart failure 2. Cirrhosis of the liver 3. Nephrotic syndrome: minimal change disease (child), membranous glomerulonephritis (adult) 4. Malabsorption: celiac disease 5. Malnutrition: kwashiorkor (protein deprivation)	ECF: ↑, EABV: ↓ ISF: ↑, ICF: ↑

Table continued on following page

TABLE 5–1.   Sodium and Water Disorders *Continued*

Fluid Disorder	TBNa⁺/TBW Physical Examination	Clinical Associations	Compartment Relationships
Dilutional (gain of pure H_2O and no Na^+)	$\leftrightarrow$TBNa⁺/ $\uparrow\uparrow$ TBW Normal	1. Inappropriate ADH syndrome (SiADH): small-cell carcinoma of lung, use of chlorpropamide or alkylating agents, CNS infection or tumor 2. Psychogenic polydipsia 3. Hypothyroidism (loss of inhibitory effect of thyroid hormone on ADH activity) 4. Hypocortisolism (loss of inhibitory effect of cortisol on ADH activity)	ECF: ↑, EABV: ↑ ISF: ↑, ICF: ↑
Hypernatremia Mixed hypotonic loss (loss of more H_2O than Na^+ but both are lost)	$\downarrow$ TBNa⁺/ $\downarrow\downarrow$ TBW Volume depletion	1. Diarrhea in an infant 2. Osmotic diuresis (caused by glucosuria, mannitol, urea) 3. Sweating	ECF: ↓, EABV: ↓ ISF: ↓, ICF: ↓
Hypertonic gain (gain of more Na^+ than H_2O but both are increased)	$\uparrow\uparrow$ TBNa⁺/ $\uparrow$ TBW Pitting edema	1. Excessive $NaHCO_3$ infusion 2. Infusion of Na-containing antibiotics: penicillin, carbenicillin 3. Saline abortions	ECF: ↑, EABV: ↑ ISF: ↑, ICF: ↓
Pure water loss (hypotonic loss of pure H_2O and no Na^+)	$\leftrightarrow$TBNa⁺/ $\downarrow\downarrow$ TBW Normal	1. Insensible water loss (loss of H_2O without salt): fever, low humidity environment (desert), hypermetabolic state (hyperthyroidism), inadequately humidified respirator 2. Diabetes insipidus: central (lack of ADH due to stalk transection or tumor), nephrogenic (lithium use, severe hypokalemia)	ECF: ↓, EABV: ↓ ISF: ↓, ICF: ↓

tration (< 136 mEq/L) that produces a hypotonic state with a decrease in Eosm.

1. It represents a defect in the generation and excretion of free water, which corresponds to the exact amount of water that must be removed from plasma to restore a normal Eosm.
   a. To generate free water, the Na^+, K^+, and $2 Cl^-$ in the cotransport pump in the thick ascending limb must be actively reabsorbed without water, thereby leaving behind the free water necessary for dilution.
   b. ADH must be absent for free water to be excreted, hence there is an increased clearance of free water, which is called a positive free water clearance ($+CH_2O$).
2. Free water abnormalities may be the result of (1) inadequate delivery of Na^+ to the thick ascending limb diluting segment (e.g., de-

creased EABV), (2) inhibition of the thick ascending limb $Na^+/K^+/2\ Cl^-$ cotransport pump (e.g., from use of a loop diuretic), and (3) excessive free water reabsorption due to the presence of ADH (e.g., inappropriate ADH syndrome).

3. Clinical manifestations include changes in the central nervous system (CNS; e.g., mental status alterations, seizures) and neuromuscular system (e.g., muscle cramps).

4. Rapid intravenous fluid correction of hyponatremia with saline may result in **central pontine myelinolysis,** an irreversible demyelinating disorder.

C. **Hypernatremia** is a serum Na^+ concentration $>$ 145 mEq/L that produces a hypertonic state characterized by an increased Eosm.

1. The ICF compartment is contracted owing to an osmotic gradient favoring the movement of water into the ECF compartment.

2. Patients have CNS signs and symptoms (e.g., convulsions, increased reflexes) and commonly have hypernatremia owing to a lack of access to water (e.g., an elderly patient with a stroke), which limits their ability to replace TBW.

3. Rapid correction of fluid losses in hypernatremia may result in brain herniation and death.

Objective 4: To review the hemodynamic alterations associated with hypovolemic, cardiogenic, and septic shock.

VIII. Shock

A. Shock results in the hypoperfusion of tissue with subsequent impaired tissue oxygenation.

B. The four types are (1) hypovolemic shock (e.g., due to hemorrhage or excessive sweating), (2) cardiogenic shock (e.g., pump failure secondary to an acute myocardial infarction), (3) septic shock (gram-negative endotoxic shock), and (4) neurogenic shock (loss of vasomotor tone in venules and small veins as in fainting, spinal cord injury, or use of autonomic blocking agents).

1. Loss of 20% of the blood volume (about 1000 mL) results in **hypovolemic shock.**

a. In blood loss, the hemoglobin (Hb) and hematocrit (Hct) may remain normal for 1–3 days owing to the equal loss of plasma and RBCs and to vascular contraction around the reduced volume of blood.

b. Laboratory abnormalities include metabolic acidosis secondary to retention of lactate from tissue hypoxia and hyperglycemia due to glycogenolysis from the release of cortisol, glucagon, and catecholamines.

2. **Cardiogenic shock** can arise from an acute myocardial infarction, valvular disease, and cardiomyopathies (Chapter 10).

3. **Septic (endotoxic) shock** may be associated with endotoxin-containing gram-negative bacteria (e.g., *Escherichia coli*), exotoxin-producing gram-positive organisms, and fungi.

a. The acute phase is characterized by (1) peripheral arteriolar vasodilatation (warm skin, reduced oxygen exchange in tissue leading to tissue hypoxia and then to lactic acidosis and hypotension), (2) high-output cardiac failure (dilated arterioles shunt more blood through the microcirculation back to the heart), and (3) sinus tachycardia.

b. Endotoxins primarily bind to CD14 receptors on leukocytes, endothelial cells, and other cells, resulting in direct injury or the release of the following chemical mediators.

(1) **Interleukin-1** (IL-1) and **tumor necrosis factor** (TNF) are released from macrophage activation (the increased neutrophil adhesion to vessels leads to vessel damage).

(2) **Nitric oxide (endothelium-derived relaxing factor)** is a potent vasodilator derived from endothelial cells and activated macrophages.

(3) Anaphylatoxins **C3a** and **C5a** (vasodilators) are released from endotoxin activation of the alternative pathway.

(4) **Prostaglandins** (vasodilators), **leukotrienes** (vasoconstrictors), and **myocardial depressant factor** (which reduces ventricular contractility) are additional mediators involved in endotoxic shock.

c. Multiorgan dysfunction is the most common cause of death.

(1) Cardiac abnormalities consist of muscle necrosis (infarction, contraction band necrosis), decreased cardiac contractility (depressant factor), increased left ventricular end-diastolic volume (LVEDV), decreased ejection fraction (stroke volume/LVEDV), normal stroke volume, and increased cardiac output (increased venous return plus sinus tachycardia).

(2) Microvascular injury often precipitates disseminated intravascular coagulation (DIC).

(3) Neutrophil-related injury in the lungs predisposes to the adult respiratory distress syndrome.

(4) Hypotension and tissue hypoxia commonly produce ischemic acute tubular necrosis (the kidney is the organ most frequently affected in shock).

d. The mortality rate in septic shock is 20–80%.

4. Differences between endotoxic shock and cardiogenic/hypovolemic shock include warm skin (in the former) rather than cold, clammy skin (peripheral vasoconstriction) and an increased (in the former) rather than a decreased cardiac output.

Objective 5: To understand the pathophysiology of acid-base disorders (respiratory and metabolic) in clinical medicine.

IX. Overview of acid-base physiology

A. The normal arterial pH range is between 7.35 and 7.45.

1. An increase in pH ($>$ 7.45) produces **alkalemia** (fewer H ions), whereas a decrease in pH (pH $<$ 7.35) results in **acidemia** (more H ions).

2. In the Henderson-Hasselbalch equation (pH $=$ 6.1 $+$ log HCO_3^-/H_2CO_3), $H_2CO_3 = 0.03 \times PCO_2$ (40 mm Hg), or 1.2 mmol, and the normal HCO_3^- is 24 mEq/L, hence the ratio of base to acid is 20/1 (24/1.2), which maintains the pH at 7.40.

3. Alterations in arterial pH are counteracted by extracellular (e.g., the HCO_3^-/H_2CO_3 buffer pair)

and intracellular (e.g., reduced Hb) buffering systems in concert with respiratory and renal compensation (PCO_2 and HCO_3^- alterations, respectively).

   a. In acidosis (respiratory or metabolic), excess H ions are buffered by cells (e.g., RBCs) in exchange for K^+ (often resulting in hyperkalemia) to counterbalance the intracellular gain of positive charges.

   b. In alkalosis (respiratory or metabolic), cells provide H ions to the ECF in exchange for ICF uptake of K^+ (resulting in hypokalemia) to balance the loss of intracellular positive charges.

4. In respiratory disorders, which involve alterations in the arterial PCO_2 ($PaCO_2$, where a = arterial) nonrenal mechanisms may contribute or remove HCO_3^- in exchange for Cl^- as an initial step in compensation.

5. In metabolic disorders, which involve changes in HCO_3^- concentration, the respiratory system responds quickly (within 12–24 hours) to compensate by either retaining or clearing CO_2.

B. The kidney must reabsorb all the filtered HCO_3^- each day in order to prevent metabolic acidosis owing to the normal production of 1 mEq/kg of new acid per day.

1. **Bicarbonate reabsorption** occurs mainly via the processes of **reclamation** and **regeneration (new synthesis)**, both of which are closely linked to the secretion of H ions in the kidney tubules.

2. **Reclamation** of HCO_3^- occurs primarily in the proximal tubules (and to a lesser extent in the distal and collecting ducts) when H ions are secreted into the tubular lumen, resulting in the following sequence of reactions: H ions are secreted into the lumen → H ions combine with HCO_3^- to form H_2CO_3 → H_2CO_3 dissociates into H_2O and CO_2 (catalyzed by carbonic anhydrase) CO_2 reenters the tubular cell to form H_2CO_3 (catalyzed by intracytoplasmic carbonic anhydrase) → H_2CO_3 dissociates into H^+ and HCO_3^- → HCO_3^- is reabsorbed (reclaimed) without a net loss of H ions.

3. **Regeneration** of HCO_3^- coincides with the secretion of excess H^+ (acidosis) in the collecting tubules by the **aldosterone-enhanced H^+/K^+-ATPase pump** and their excretion as **titratable acid** ($H_2PO_4^-$) or as **NH_4Cl** ($NH_3 + H^+ + Cl^- → NH_4Cl$).

   a. CO_2 enters the tubules from the blood (not urine) and combines with H_2O to form H_2CO_3, which dissociates into H^+ and HCO_3^-.

   b. The H ions are secreted by the proton pump in exchange for K ions.

   c. H ions are excreted with phosphate or ammonia.

   d. The HCO_3^- is reabsorbed back into the ECF.

   e. H ions are lost, and a new HCO_3^- is synthesized.

X. Acid-base disorders

A. There are four primary acid-base disorders that present either as a single disorder (simple disorder) or in combinations (mixed disorder).

1. Primary alterations in the arterial PCO_2 include **respiratory acidosis** (increase in $PaCO_2$; ↓ pH ≅ ↑ HCO_3^-/↑↑ $PaCO_2$) and respiratory alkalosis (decrease in $PaCO_2$; ↑ pH ≅ ↓ HCO_3^-/↓↓ $PaCO_2$).

2. Primary alterations in HCO_3^- are designated **metabolic acidosis** (decrease in HCO_3^-; ↓ pH ≅ ↓↓ **HCO_3^-/↓ $PaCO_2$**) and **metabolic alkalosis** (increase in HCO_3^-; ↑ pH ≅ ↑↑ **HCO_3^-/↑ $PaCO_2$**).

B. **Compensation** is the homeostatic mechanism that brings the arterial pH close to but not usually into the normal range of 7.35–7.45, where the ratio of HCO_3^-/PCO_2 is 20/1.

1. Since arterial pH is proportionate to the ratio of HCO_3^-/$PaCO_2$ (20/1 = pH of 7.40), compensation *always moves in the same direction* as the primary disorder in order to bring the ratio of HCO_3^-/$PaCO_2$ as close to 20/1 as possible.

   a. Thus, compensation for a primary increase in HCO_3^- (metabolic alkalosis) requires an increase in the $PaCO_2$ (respiratory acidosis), while a reduced HCO_3^- concentration (metabolic acidosis) is counterbalanced by a decrease in the $PaCO_2$ (respiratory alkalosis).

   b. A primary increase in the $PaCO_2$ (respiratory acidosis) is compensated for by an increase in HCO_3^- (metabolic alkalosis), while a primary decrease in the $PaCO_2$ (respiratory alkalosis) requires a reduction in HCO_3^- (metabolic acidosis).

2. Compensation has different stages of development, hence the terms **uncompensated** (compensation for that disorder is still in the normal range), **partially compensated** (compensation is outside its normal range and the pH is moving toward but not into the normal range), and **fully compensated** (pH is in the normal range; this rarely occurs).

C. **Respiratory acidosis** represents **alveolar hypoventilation** (reduced ventilation resulting in hypercapnia), leading to a $PaCO_2$ > 44 mm Hg (33–44 mm Hg).

1. **Acute** respiratory acidosis is distinguished from **chronic** respiratory acidosis by a serum HCO_3^- concentration > 30 mEq/L, which indicates that renal compensation has occurred.

2. **Hypoventilation** is the inability of the lungs to excrete CO_2, which may be the result of the following:

   a. Depression of the medullary respiratory center in the brain (e.g., due to barbiturate or narcotic use).

   b. Upper airway obstruction (e.g., due to epiglottitis).

   c. Weakness or paralysis of the muscles of respiration (e.g., paralysis of the diaphragm).

   d. Primary lung disease (e.g., chronic obstructive pulmonary disease [COPD]).

   e. Factors that restrict the return of CO_2 from the tissues to the lungs (e.g., severe congestive heart failure).

3. Clinical manifestations include somnolence (CO_2 narcosis) and increased intracranial pressure (respiratory acidosis increases cerebral vessel dilatation and permeability), which may progress to papilledema (edema of the optic disk) and brain herniation.

4. Laboratory findings include the following:

   a. Arterial pH < 7.35.

b. $PaCO_2 > 44$ mm Hg.

c. Normal to increased serum HCO_3^- (metabolic alkalosis as compensation).

d. Hypoxemia (low PaO_2 resulting from a proportionate decrease in alveolar PO_2 as the alveolar PCO_2 increases).

e. Hypochloremia (owing to the exchange of Cl^- for HCO_3^- leaving cells).

f. Hypoxemic stimulation of erythropoietin release and increased synthesis of RBCs (**secondary polycythemia**; Chapter 12).

D. **Respiratory alkalosis** is defined as a $PaCO_2 < 33$ mm Hg (33–44 mm Hg; hypocapnia).

1. **Acute** and **chronic** respiratory alkalosis are distinguished on the basis of the serum HCO_3^- concentration with levels < 18 mEq/L indicating chronic disease, since renal compensation has occurred (metabolic acidosis), while values ≥ 18 mEq/L represent acute respiratory alkalosis.

2. Respiratory alkalosis is associated with hyperventilation secondary to one of the following:

   a. Respiratory center stimulation (e.g., normal pregnancy [progesterone effect], endotoxemia, salicylates, liver failure).

   b. Primary lung disease (e.g., pulmonary embolus, mild to moderate bronchial asthma).

3. Clinical associations include tetany (alkalosis increases negative charges on albumin, causing it to bind more ionized calcium), lightheadedness, and circumoral and digital paresthesias (numbness and tingling associated with tetany).

4. Laboratory abnormalities consist of the following:

   a. Arterial pH > 7.45.

   b. $PaCO_2 < 33$ mm Hg (33–44 mm Hg).

   c. Normal to decreased serum HCO_3^- (metabolic acidosis as compensation).

   d. Hyperchloremia (exchange of Cl^- for HCO_3^-).

   e. Hypophosphatemia (alkalosis stimulates glycolysis, leading to increased phosphorylation of glucose).

   f. A low ionized calcium concentration.

E. **Metabolic alkalosis** is defined as a serum HCO_3^- of > 28 mEq/L (22–28 mEq/L).

1. The first stage in the pathogenesis of metabolic alkalosis is generation of alkalosis by a **loss of H ions** (e.g., due to vomiting, diuretic use) or a **gain in HCO_3^-** (e.g., due to mineralocorticoid excess, antacid use).

   a. In **vomiting**, every milliequivalent of HCl lost is equivalent to a milliequivalent gain of HCO_3^- owing to parietal cell synthesis and secretion of H^+ into the stomach counterbalanced by the secretion of HCO_3 anions into the blood (alkaline tide).

      (1) The loss of HCl leaves large amounts of unneutralized HCO_3^- behind in the blood, increasing the filtered load of HCO_3^-, which surpasses the proximal renal tubule threshold for HCO_3^- (~24 mEq/L), leading to its excretion as $NaHCO_3$ (alkaline urine pH; $UNa^+ > 20$ mEq/L).

      (2) The loss of Cl ions as HCl reduces the amount of Cl ions filtered in the urine ($UCl^- \leq 20$ mEq/L).

      (3) The excessive renal loss of Na^+ and fluid loss associated with vomiting produces volume contraction, a reduction in the EABV, and increased proximal reabsorption of Na^+ and HCO_3^- (the urine pH becomes acid [**paradoxical aciduria**]) with a reduction in the loss of Na^+ ($UNa^+ < 20$ mEq/L) and HCO_3^- (raising the renal threshold for HCO_3^- reclamation).

      (4) Correction of the volume contraction with isotonic saline (which normalizes the EABV) with or without the administration of chloride corrects the metabolic alkalosis.

   b. **Diuretics** produce metabolic alkalosis by blocking Na^+ reabsorption, which increases the distal delivery of Na^+, hence augmenting the exchange of Na^+ for K^+ (**hypokalemia**) and Na^+ for H^+, the latter leading to HCO_3^- reclamation (**metabolic alkalosis**).

   c. **Primary aldosteronism (Conn's syndrome)** is caused by autonomous secretion of aldosterone (mineralocorticoid excess) from a benign adenoma arising in the zona glomerulosa of the adrenal cortex.

      (1) Aldosterone increases the distal reabsorption of Na^+ (**hypernatremia**) in exchange for K^+ (**hypokalemia**) and H^+ (**metabolic alkalosis**) and also enhances the distal H^+/K^+-ATPase pump with subsequent new synthesis of HCO_3^- (see ¶IX.B.3, above).

      (2) The increase in Na^+ reabsorption produces volume overload and an increase in plasma volume.

      (3) This increases the EABV, leading to decreased proximal tubule reabsorption of Na^+ ($P_H > P_O$), increased renal loss of Na^+ ($UNa^+ > 20$ mEq/L), and the **absence of pitting edema**, since the renal losses of Na^+ counterbalance the gain in Na^+.

      (4) In addition to **mild hypernatremia**, **severe hypokalemia**, and **metabolic alkalosis**, patients have a **low renin diastolic hypertension** owing to the increase in plasma volume (which increases cardiac output) and peripheral resistance (Na^+ opens up calcium channels in the resistance arterioles, leading to vasoconstriction).

   d. Metabolic alkalosis is also generated by a **gain in HCO_3^-** owing to excessive HCO_3^- intake from absorbable antacids or intravenous infusion or to oxidative metabolism, whereby acetate, lactate, and citrate ions are converted to HCO_3 ions on a milliequivalent to milliequivalent basis.

2. The second stage in the pathogenesis of metabolic alkalosis is **maintaining** an increase in serum HCO_3^-, primarily the result of volume contraction, which reduces the EABV, subsequently increasing the proximal reabsorption of Na^+ and reclamation of HCO_3^-.

3. Clinical abnormalities associated with metabolic alkalosis include an increased risk for ventricular arrhythmias owing to hypoxia in myocardial tissue from a left-shifted O_2 dissociation curve and hypoxemia due to compensation by respiratory acidosis, which automatically lowers the PaO_2.

F. **Metabolic acidosis** is defined as a serum HCO_3^- concentration < 22 mEq/L (22–28 mEq/L).

1. The first type, **increased anion gap** (AG) **metabolic acidosis**, implies that an acid with an anion other than Cl^- has been added to the ECF (e.g., lactate, acetoacetate, β-hydroxybu-

tyrate, salicylate, phosphate, sulfate, formate [due to metabolic conversion from methyl alcohol], or oxalate [due to metabolic conversion from ethylene glycol]).

  a. When the most common anions (Cl^- and HCO_3^-) are subtracted from the most common cation (Na^+), an apparent AG is present owing to the presence of anions (e.g., albumin, phosphate, sulfate, lactate) unaccounted for in the formula, which is as follows:

$$AG = Na^+ - (Cl^- + HCO_3^-)$$

  b. Using normal values, AG = 140 mEq/L − (104 mEq/L + 24 mEq/L) = 12 mEq/L ± 4 mEq/L (8–16 mEq/L).

  c. For example, if 10 mEq/L of H-lactate is buffered by HCO_3^-, the HCO_3^- drops from 24 to 14 mEq/L and 10 mEq/L of lactate anions is left over, hence maintaining electroneutrality:

10 H-lactate + 10 NaHCO$_3$
    → H$_2$CO$_3$ + **10 Na-lactate**
      H$_2$O + CO$_2$

AG = 140 mEq/L − (104 mEq/L + **14 mEq/L**) = 22 mEq/L, indicating the presence of 10 mEq/L of unaccounted for anions, representing the **10 mEq/L of Na-lactate ions**.

2. In **normal AG metabolic acidosis**, the second type, there is a loss of HCO_3^- anions, which are replaced milliequivalent for milliequivalent by an equal number of Cl^- anions, hence maintaining a normal AG and electroneutrality.

  a. For example, if 10 mEq/L of HCO_3^- is lost, the HCO_3^- concentration drops from 24 to 14 mEq/L and the Cl^- concentration increases (hyperchloremic metabolic acidosis) from 104 mEq/L to 114 mEq/L, hence maintaining a normal AG (AG = 140 − [114 + 14] = 12 mEq/L).

  b. Loss of HCO_3^- may occur in the gastrointestinal tract (e.g., due to diarrhea) or in the kidneys (e.g., from renal tubular acidosis).

  c. **Proximal renal tubular acidosis** (type II RTA) is distinguished by a low proximal tubule threshold for HCO_3^- reabsorption (the normal level of 24 mEq/L drops to 15–20 mEq/L), hence bicarbonaturia (urine pH > 5.5) occurs when the serum HCO_3^- is raised above the lower threshold.

    (1) When the serum HCO_3^- eventually drops to 15 mEq/L, HCO_3^- reabsorption can occur at the lower threshold for HCO_3^- in the proximal tubule, hence the urine pH becomes more acidic (< 5.5) and the metabolic acidosis reaches a steady state.

    (2) Most cases of type II RTA are acquired and include such disorders as primary hyperparathyroidism (parathormone blocks the proximal reabsorption of HCO_3^-) and heavy metal poisoning (e.g., lead).

  d. **Distal RTA** (type I) is the most common RTA.

    (1) Most cases are due to a defect in the aldosterone-enhanced H^+/K^+-ATPase pump in the collecting tubules.

    (2) Some cases reflect the inability of the kidneys

to maintain a steep urine-to-blood proton (H^+) gradient in the collecting duct, hence secreted protons recycle back into the blood.

    (3) Unlike in proximal RTA, the urine pH is consistently > 5.5 and severe hypokalemia is likely to occur, since the proton/K^+-ATPase pump is defective and K^+ is unable to exchange for H ions.

    (4) Na^+ and calcium losses are also increased, the latter predisposing to calcium phosphate stones (a common finding).

3. Clinical findings associated with metabolic acidosis include the following:

  a. Hyperventilation (Kussmaul's breathing—deep, rapid respirations).

  b. A negative inotropic effect on the myocardium (diminished responsiveness to catecholamines).

  c. Osteoporosis (bone buffers excess H ions).

  d. Warm shock (acidosis increases arteriolar vasodilatation, which reduces the total peripheral resistance, leading to high-output cardiac failure).

4. Laboratory abnormalities include the following:

  a. Arterial pH < 7.35.

  b. Serum HCO_3^- < 22 mEq/L (22–28 mEq/L).

  c. $PaCO_2$ < 33 mm Hg (respiratory alkalosis as compensation).

  d. Possible hyperkalemia (transcellular shift of H^+ into cells in exchange for K^+; see ¶IX.A.3.a, above).

  e. Hyperglycemia (acidosis inhibits glycolysis).

  f. Hyperuricemia (competition with uric acid for secretion in the proximal tubules).

G. Laboratory diagnosis of simple and mixed acid-base disorders

1. The history and physical examination coupled with procurement of arterial blood gases (ABGs) and serum electrolytes are necessary to distinguish simple from mixed disorders.

2. Simple acid-base disorders present with or without compensation.

3. Mixed disorders are a blend of two or more acid-base disorders occurring at the same time (e.g., in a patient with diabetic ketoacidosis [increased AG metabolic acidosis] who is vomiting [metabolic alkalosis]).

  a. The final pH, $PaCO_2$, and HCO_3^- concentration depends on which of the two or more disorders is most severe (in the above example, if both were of equal severity, the pH, $PaCO_2$, and HCO_3^- would all be normal).

  b. Clues suggestive of a mixed disorder include the following:

    (1) A normal pH in the presence of an abnormal $PaCO_2$ or HCO_3^- (e.g., primary metabolic acidosis + primary respiratory alkalosis [endotoxic shock, salicylate intoxication], primary respiratory acidosis + primary metabolic alkalosis [patient with COPD who is taking a loop diuretic]).

    (2) Extreme acidemia (e.g., primary metabolic acidosis + primary respiratory acidosis [cardiorespiratory arrest]), producing a very low pH.

    (3) Extreme alkalemia (e.g., primary respiratory alkalosis + primary metabolic alkalosis [e.g.,

in a pregnant woman who is vomiting]), producing a very high pH.

4. The distinction between simple and mixed disorders is further enhanced by the use of formulas that calculate the expected compensation for a simple acid-base disorder (Tables 5–2 and 5–3).

    a. When the calculated compensation is approximately the same as the measured concentration, a simple disorder is present.

    b. If there is significant disagreement between the calculated and measured value, the possibility of a mixed disorder should be considered.

H. Potassium (K^+) disorders

1. Potassium is maintained within a narrow range of 3.5–5.0 mEq/L.

2. It is the major ICF cation and serves to maintain cell volume and the resting membrane potential.

3. The serum concentration of K^+ is affected by variables such as the following:

    a. Factors that alter its secretion in the distal tubule (e.g., aldosterone, augmented Na^+-K^+ exchange; see ¶V.D.4.d.2, above).

    b. pH (transcellular shifts in alkalosis [hypokalemia] and acidosis [hyperkalemia]; see ¶IX.A.3, above).

    c. Insulin (hyperkalemia stimulates insulin release, whereas hypokalemia inhibits its release).

    d. β_2-Agonists (e.g., albuterol).

4. **Hypokalemia** is defined as a serum $K^+ < 3.5$ mEq/L.

    a. The pathophysiologic classification for hypokalemia encompasses problems such as the following:

      (1) Decreased intake (e.g., "tea and toast" diet).

      (2) Transcellular shift (e.g., alkalosis, insulin therapy, and use of β_2-agonists).

      (3) Gastrointestinal loss (e.g., due to diarrhea or vomiting).

      (4) Renal loss (e.g., due to use of diuretics [the most common cause], proximal and distal RTA).

    b. Hypokalemia has a negative impact on the neuromuscular system (owing to changes in the intracellular/extracellular membrane potential), skeletal and heart muscle (e.g., it produces U waves on an electrocardiogram), and kidneys (e.g., refractoriness to ADH, leading to nephrogenic diabetes insipidus).

5. **Hyperkalemia** is defined as a serum $K^+ > 5.5$ mEq/L.

    a. The pathophysiologic classification for hyperkalemia includes the following:

      (1) Increased release from damaged tissue (e.g., rhabdomyolysis [rupture of muscle]).

      (2) Transcellular shift (e.g., due to acidosis, digitalis toxicity [digitalis blocks the Na^+/K^+-ATPase pump], or use of a β-adrenergic antagonist [e.g., propranolol]).

      (3) Decreased renal excretion (e.g., due to renal failure [the most common cause] or hypoaldosteronism [Addison's disease]).

      (4) Pseudohyperkalemia (e.g., with hemolysis of blood secondary to phlebotomy).

    b. Hyperkalemia primarily affects the heart,

where it produces peaked T waves (as a result of accelerated repolarization of cardiac muscle) and cardiac standstill in diastole.

    c. In treating hyperkalemia, the heart is first protected by infusion of calcium gluconate, which antagonizes the cardiac conduction abnormalities.

I. Selected acid-base disorders

1. Hyponatremia associated with pitting edema often accompanies congestive heart failure, cirrhosis, malabsorption, nephrotic syndrome, and malnutrition.

    a. In **right heart failure**, the increase in hydrostatic pressure in the systemic venous system drives a transudate into the interstitial space, producing dependent pitting edema.

      (1) Venous return to the right heart is reduced, hence the cardiac output and EABV are reduced.

      (2) The reduced EABV stimulates the release of ADH (baroreceptors), aldosterone (RAA system activation), and increased proximal tubule reabsorption of Na^+ ($P_O > P_H$ in peritubular capillaries; $UNa^+ < 20$ mEq/L), resulting in reabsorption of a hypotonic fluid, which produces hyponatremia (serum $Na^+ \cong \uparrow TBNa^+ / \uparrow\uparrow TBW$).

      (3) The increased venous hydrostatic pressure redirects the reabsorbed fluid into the interstitial space, exacerbating the edema without increasing the EABV.

      (4) The $\uparrow TBNa^+$ distributes primarily in the ECF compartment (Na^+ is an impermeant solute) and in the interstitial space, whereas the $\uparrow\uparrow TBW$ is distributed primarily in the ICF compartment (via osmosis) and to a lesser extent in the ECF compartment.

    b. A reduction in oncotic pressure (e.g., due to hypoalbuminemia in cirrhosis, nephrotic syndrome, or malnutrition) producing pitting edema results in the same series of events noted above for right heart failure owing to reduced venous return to the heart.

2. The **inappropriate ADH syndrome** (SiADH) is due to excessive reabsorption of free water (not salt) that results in a dilutional hyponatremia (serum $Na^+ \cong TBNa^+ / \uparrow\uparrow$ **TBW**).

    a. Since the $TBNa^+$ is normal, there is neither volume depletion nor pitting edema (only an increase in $TBNa^+$ produces pitting edema) on physical examination.

    b. As free water continues to accumulate in the ECF compartment, the osmotic gradient favors movement into the more spacious ICF compartment, then the ISF, and finally the smaller vascular compartment, leading to an increase in the EABV.

      (1) Peritubular capillary $P_H > P_O$, hence decreasing proximal tubule reabsorption of Na^+, urea, uric acid, etc.

      (2) Suppressed RAA.

    c. Causes of SiADH include the following:

      (1) Ectopic secretion from a small-cell carcinoma in the lung.

      (2) Lung infection (e.g., tuberculosis).

      (3) Stimulation of ADH release by drugs (e.g., chlorpropamide, morphine, oxytocin).

      (4) CNS disorders (e.g., tumor, infection).

TABLE 5–2.   Expected Compensatory Responses for Simple Acid-Base Disorders*

Disorder	Expected Compensation
Metabolic acidosis: pH <7.35, HCO_3^- <22 mEq/L Limits of compensation: If the measured $PaCO_2$ is <10 mm Hg, consider a mixed disorder with an additional component of primary respiratory alkalosis. Arrows indicate magnitude. pH PCO_2 HCO_3^- Metabolic acidosis ↓ ↓ ↓↓ ↓PCO_2 = respiratory alkalosis as compensation.	$\Delta PCO_2 = 1.2 \times \Delta HCO_3^- \pm 2$ *Subtract* ΔPCO_2 from 40 mm Hg $\pm$ 2 mm Hg. A measured PCO_2 < calculated PCO_2 indicates an additional primary respiratory alkalosis (blowing off more CO_2 than required for normal compensation). A measured PCO_2 > calculated PCO_2 indicates an additional primary respiratory acidosis (retaining more CO_2 than required for compensation).
Metabolic alkalosis: pH >7.45, HCO_3^- >28 mEq/L Limits of compensation: If the measured $PaCO_2$ is >55 mm Hg, consider a mixed disorder with an additional component of primary respiratory acidosis. pH PCO_2 HCO_3^- Metabolic alkalosis ↑ ↑ ↑↑ ↑PCO_2 = respiratory acidosis as compensation.	$\Delta PaCO_2 = 0.7 \times \Delta HCO_3^- \pm 2$ mm Hg *Add* ΔPCO_2 to 40 mm Hg $\pm$ 2 mm Hg. A measured PCO_2 < calculated PCO_2 indicates an additional primary respiratory alkalosis (blowing off more CO_2 than is required for compensation). A measured PCO_2 > calculated PCO_2 indicates an additional primary respiratory acidosis (retaining more CO_2 than is required for compensation).
Acute respiratory acidosis: pH <7.35, $PaCO_2$ >44 mm Hg, HCO_3^- ≤30 mEq/L Limits of compensation: If the measured HCO_3^- is >45 mEq/L, consider a mixed disorder with an additional component of primary metabolic alkalosis. If the measured HCO_3^- is <23 mEq/L, consider a mixed disorder with an additional component of primary metabolic acidosis. pH PCO_2 HCO_3^- Respiratory acidosis ↓ ↑↑ ↑ ↑HCO_3^- = metabolic alkalosis as compensation.	$\Delta HCO_3^- = 0.10 \times \Delta PaCO_2$ *Add* ΔHCO_3^- to the normal of 24 mEq/L. A measured HCO_3^- < calculated HCO_3^- indicates an additional primary metabolic acidosis (HCO_3^- is lower than it should be for normal compensation). A measured HCO_3^- > calculated HCO_3^- indicates an additional primary metabolic alkalosis (HCO_3^- is higher than it should be for normal compensation).
Chronic respiratory acidosis: pH <7.35, $PaCO_2$ >44 mm Hg, HCO_3^- >30 mEq/L Limits of compensation: See acute respiratory acidosis. pH PCO_2 HCO_3^- Respiratory acidosis ↓ ↑↑ ↑* ↑*HCO_3^- = greater degree of metabolic alkalosis as compensation than in acute respiratory acidosis owing to renal compensation; the pH would be closer to the normal range than in acute disease.	$\Delta HCO_3^- = 0.40 \times \Delta PCO_2$ *Add* ΔHCO_3^- to the normal of 24 mEq/L. A measured HCO_3^- < calculated HCO_3^- indicates an additional primary metabolic acidosis (HCO_3^- is lower than it should be for normal compensation). A measured HCO_3^- > calculated HCO_3^- indicates an additional primary metabolic alkalosis (HCO_3^- is higher than it should be for normal compensation).
Acute respiratory alkalosis: pH >7.45, $PaCO_2$ <33 mm Hg, HCO_3^- ≥18 mEq/L Limits of compensation: If the measured HCO_3^- is <12 mEq/L, consider an additional component of primary metabolic acidosis. pH PCO_2 HCO_3^- Respiratory alkalosis ↑ ↓↓ ↓ ↓HCO_3^- = metabolic acidosis as compensation.	$\Delta HCO_3^- = 0.20 \times \Delta PCO_2$ *Subtract* ΔHCO_3^- from the normal of 24 mEq/L. A measured HCO_3^- < calculated HCO_3^- indicates an additional primary metabolic acidosis (HCO_3^- is lower than it should be for normal compensation). A measured HCO_3^- > calculated HCO_3^- indicates an additional primary metabolic alkalosis (HCO_3^- is higher than it should be for normal compensation).
Chronic respiratory alkalosis: pH >7.45, $PaCO_2$ <33 mm Hg, HCO_3^- <18 mEq/L but >12 mEq/L. Limits of compensation: See acute respiratory alkalosis. pH PCO_2 HCO_3^- Respiratory alkalosis ↑ ↓↓ ↓* ↓*HCO_3^- = greater degree of metabolic acidosis as compensation than in the acute disorder owing to renal loss of HCO_3^-; the pH would be closer to normal.	$\Delta HCO_3^- = 0.50 \times \Delta PCO_2$ *Subtract* ΔHCO_3^- from the normal of 24 mEq/L. A measured HCO_3^- < calculated HCO_3^- indicates an additional primary metabolic acidosis (HCO_3^- is lower than it should be for normal compensation). A measured HCO_3^- > calculated HCO_3^- indicates an additional primary metabolic alkalosis (HCO_3^- is higher than it should be for normal compensation).

* Reference intervals are as follows: pH, 7.35–7.45; $PaCO_2$, 33–44 mm Hg; HCO_3^-, 22–28 mEq/L; ΔHCO_3^-, change from the normal of 24.0 mEq/L; $\Delta PaCO_2$, change from the normal of 40 mm Hg. Serum electrolytes: serum Na^+, 136–145 mEq/L; serum K^+, 3.5–5.0 mEq/L; serum Cl^-, 95–105 mEq/L; serum HCO_3^-, 22–28 mEq/L; anion gap (AG = Na^+ − [Cl^- + HCO_3^-]), 12 mEq/L $\pm$ 4 mEq/L. The limits of compensation are based on experiments on volunteers.

TABLE 5–3. Clinical Examples of Acid-Base Disorders

Case Presentation	Provisional Diagnosis Based on Arterial Blood Gas and Serum Electrolyte Results	Definitive Diagnosis Based on Calculation of Expected Compensation
The patient is a 40-year-old male with severe diarrhea for 1 week. He has been eating ice chips. He is volume depleted and hypotensive. pH PCO₂ HCO₃⁻ 7.28 28 13 Na⁺ K⁺ Cl⁻ HCO₃⁻ AG 134 2.6 109 13 12	pH, 7.28; acidemia (<7.35). PCO₂, 28; respiratory alkalosis (<33 mm Hg). HCO₃⁻, 13; metabolic acidosis (<22 mEq/L). Provisional diagnosis: metabolic acidosis with partially compensated respiratory alkalosis (PCO₂ is outside the normal range, but the pH is not in the normal range). The patient's access to ice chips has led to a slight hyponatremia ($\downarrow$ TBNa⁺/$\uparrow\uparrow$ **TBW**) rather than a normal Na⁺, as expected with isotonic loss of fluid in adult diarrhea. The AG is 12 mEq/L (134 − [109 + 13] = 12), which is consistent with a normal AG metabolic acidosis (HCO₃⁻ loss in stool).	Use the metabolic acidosis formula: Δ PCO₂ = 1.2 × Δ HCO₃⁻ ± 2 = 1.2 × (24 − 13) = ~13 mm Hg. Expected PCO₂ = 40 − 13 = 27 mm Hg ± 2 (25–29). Measured PCO₂ = 28 mm Hg. Definitive diagnosis: diarrhea leading to a normal AG metabolic acidosis with partially compensated respiratory alkalosis. It is complicated by hypovolemia secondary to fluid losses plus an additional component of hyponatremia and hypokalemia.
The patient is an 18-year-old woman with an acute anxiety reaction. Carpopedal spasm is present on examination. pH PCO₂ HCO₃⁻ 7.56 24 21 Na⁺ K⁺ Cl⁻ HCO₃⁻ AG 138 3.4 102 21 15	pH, 7.56; alkalemia (>7.45). PCO₂, 24; respiratory alkalosis (<33 mm Hg). HCO₃⁻, 21; metabolic acidosis (<22 mEq/L). Provisional diagnosis: acute respiratory alkalosis with partially compensated metabolic acidosis (HCO₃⁻ is outside the normal range, but the pH is not normal). K⁺ is slightly decreased owing to movement into cells in exchange for H⁺ ions coming out of cells as nonrenal compensation. The AG is slightly increased, since alkalosis enhances glycolysis and the production of lactate.	Use the acute respiratory alkalosis formula: Δ HCO₃⁻ = 0.20 × Δ PCO₂ = 0.20 × (40 − 24) = 3.2 mEq/L. Expected HCO₃⁻ = 24 − 3.2 = 20.8 mEq/L. Measured HCO₃⁻ = 21 mEq/L. Definitive diagnosis: acute respiratory alkalosis with partially compensated metabolic acidosis. It is complicated by tetany owing to the effect of alkalosis on increasing negative charges on albumin, hence lowering the ionized calcium.
The patient is a 52-year-old African American man with essential hypertension for which he is taking hydrochlorothiazide. He complains of weakness. Vital signs include a BP of 142/92 mm Hg and an HR of 100 beats/minute. His mucous membranes are dry. pH PCO₂ HCO₃⁻ 7.50 47 35 Na⁺ K⁺ Cl⁻ HCO₃⁻ AG 132 2.7 80 35 15	pH, 7.50; alkalemia (>7.45). PCO₂, 47; respiratory acidosis (>44 mm Hg). HCO₃⁻, 35; metabolic alkalosis (>28 mEq/L). Provisional diagnosis: metabolic alkalosis with partially compensated respiratory acidosis (PCO₂ is outside the normal range, and the pH is not in the normal range). The mild hyponatremia is due to the distal tubule block in Na⁺ reabsorption and hypertonic loss of fluid (more Na⁺ than H₂O). Hypokalemia is secondary to an augmented exchange of K⁺ with Na⁺ in the late distal tubule and collecting ducts. The AG is slightly increased owing to alkalosis-enhanced glycolysis and increased formation of lactate.	Use the metabolic alkalosis formula: Δ PaCO₂ = 0.7 × Δ HCO₃⁻ ± 2 mm Hg = 0.7 × (35 − 24) = ~8 mm Hg. Expected PaCO₂ = 40 + 8 = 48 ± 2 mm Hg (46–50). Measured PaCO₂ = 47 mm Hg. Definitive diagnosis: metabolic alkalosis with partially compensated respiratory acidosis secondary to use of a thiazide diuretic. His condition is complicated by hyponatremia and hypokalemia, the latter producing muscle weakness.
The patient is an afebrile 48-year-old man with a 20-pack-year history of smoking. He has had a productive cough in the morning for 9 months of the year for the last 5 years. Physical examination reveals an increased anteroposterior (AP) diameter and sibilant rhonchi throughout both lung fields that clear with coughing. pH PCO₂ HCO₃⁻ 7.33 60 31 Na⁺ K⁺ Cl⁻ HCO₃⁻ AG 137 4.8 93 31 13	pH, 7.33; acidemia (<7.35). PCO₂, 60; respiratory acidosis (>44 mm Hg). HCO₃⁻, 31; metabolic alkalosis (>28 mEq/L). Provisional diagnosis: chronic respiratory acidosis (HCO₃⁻ >30 mEq/L indicates renal compensation) with a partially compensated metabolic alkalosis.	Use the chronic respiratory acidosis formula: Δ HCO₃⁻ = 0.40 × Δ PCO₂ = 0.40 × (60 − 40) = 8 mEq/L. Expected HCO₃⁻ = 24 + 8 mEq/L = 32 mEq/L. Measured HCO₃⁻ = 31 mEq/L (close enough to 32 mEq/L). Definitive diagnosis: chronic respiratory acidosis with partially compensated metabolic alkalosis. There is clinical evidence of chronic bronchitis (productive cough for more than 3 consecutive months for 2 consecutive years) and emphysema ($\uparrow$ anteroposterior diameter).
The patient is a 25-year-old woman with a suspected barbiturate overdose. She is semicomatose. pH PCO₂ HCO₃⁻ 7.20 74 28 Na⁺ K⁺ Cl⁻ HCO₃⁻ AG 140 4.0 100 28 12	pH, 7.20; acidemia (<7.35). PCO₂, 74; respiratory acidosis (>44 mm Hg). HCO₃⁻, 28; normal. Provisional diagnosis: acute respiratory acidosis, uncompensated (HCO₃⁻ is not outside the normal range).	Use the acute respiratory acidosis formula: Δ HCO₃⁻ = 0.10 × Δ PaCO₂ = 0.10 × (74 − 40) = 3.4 mEq/L. Expected HCO₃⁻ = 24.0 + 3.4 = 27.4 mEq/L. Measured HCO₃⁻ = 28 mEq/L (close enough). Definitive diagnosis: uncompensated acute respiratory acidosis, possibly due to a drug overdose pending laboratory drug screening.

Table continued on following page

TABLE 5–3. Clinical Examples of Acid-Base Disorders *Continued*

Case Presentation	Provisional Diagnosis Based on Arterial Blood Gas and Serum Electrolyte Results	Definitive Diagnosis Based on Calculation of Expected Compensation
The patient is a 39-year-old man with alcoholism. He has dependent pitting edema and ascites. His BP and HR are normal. pH PCO$_2$ HCO$_3^-$ 7.48 20 14 Na$^+$ K$^+$ Cl$^-$ HCO$_3^-$ AG 130 2.8 100 14 16	pH, 7.48; alkalemia (>7.45). PCO$_2$, 20; respiratory alkalosis (<33 mm Hg). HCO$_3^-$, 14; metabolic acidosis (<22 mEq/L). Provisional diagnosis: chronic respiratory alkalosis (HCO$_3^-$ <18 but >12 mEq/L) with partially compensated metabolic acidosis. There is a possible additional component of primary metabolic acidosis owing to the presence of an increased AG.	Use the chronic respiratory alkalosis formula: Δ HCO$_3^-$ = 0.50 × Δ PaCO$_2$ = 0.50 × (40 − 20) = 10 mEq/L. Expected HCO$_3^-$ = 24 − 10 = 14 mEq/L. Measured HCO$_3^-$ = 14 mEq/L. Definitive diagnosis: chronic respiratory alkalosis with partially compensated metabolic acidosis. The increased AG may be due to alkalosis-enhanced glycolysis and/or a slight increase in lactic acid/keto acids but not high enough to produce a mixed disorder.
The patient is a 48-year-old woman with rheumatoid arthritis. She is taking aspirin for her arthritis and is complaining of ringing in her ears. The respiratory rate is increased. pH PCO$_2$ HCO$_3^-$ 7.42 16 10 Na$^+$ K$^+$ Cl$^-$ HCO$_3^-$ AG 137 5.2 105 10 22	pH, 7.42; normal (7.35–7.45). PCO$_2$, 16; respiratory alkalosis (<33 mm Hg). HCO$_3^-$, 10; metabolic acidosis (<22 mEq/L). Provisional diagnosis: since acid-base disorders do not have full compensation (normal pH), the patient most likely has a mixed primary metabolic acidosis (due to salicylic acid) and primary respiratory alkalosis (salicylates overstimulate the CNS respiratory center).	In this case, either the metabolic acidosis or the chronic respiratory alkalosis formula may be used. (Note: the HCO$_3^-$ is actually below the limit of compensation for chronic respiratory alkalosis, which is 12 mEq/L; therefore, primary metabolic acidosis must be present, since the HCO$_3$ is <12 mEq/L.) Δ PCO$_2$ = 1.2 × Δ HCO$_3^-$ ± 2 = 1.2 × (24 − 10) = 17 mm Hg. Expected PCO$_2$ = 40 − 17 = 23 mm Hg ± 2 (21–25 mm Hg). Measured PCO$_2$ = 10 mm Hg, which is much lower than it should be for compensation; therefore, a primary respiratory alkalosis must also be present. Since primary metabolic acidosis and primary respiratory alkalosis have an additive effect on lowering the HCO$_3^-$, its level went below the limits of compensation and the pH normalized.
The patient is a 57-year-old man with chronic renal failure who presents with dyspnea. Bilateral inspiratory rales are noted on auscultation. There is dependent pitting edema in the lower extremities. He is cyanotic. His BP is 100/70 mm Hg, HR 130 beats/minute, and respiratory rate 24 breaths/minute. pH PCO$_2$ HCO$_3^-$ 7.28 38 17 Na$^+$ K$^+$ Cl$^-$ HCO$_3^-$ AG 132 5.8 89 17 26	pH, 7.28; acidemia (<7.35). PCO$_2$, 38; normal (33–44 mm Hg). HCO$_3^-$, 17; metabolic acidosis (<22 mEq/L). Provisional diagnosis: primary metabolic acidosis, uncompensated (PCO$_2$ is in the normal range). Since respiratory compensation is usually rapid, an underlying respiratory acidosis has not been excluded, especially since the patient is in heart failure (inspiratory rales). The electrolytes reveal a mild hyponatremia (↑ TBNa$^+$/↑↑ TBW) most likely associated with a hypotonic gain of more water than salt (TBNa$^+$ is increased, since pitting edema is present). Hyperkalemia is noted owing to a combination of reduced renal excretion and movement of K$^+$ ions out of cells in response to intracellular buffering of H$^+$ ions.	Use the metabolic acidosis formula: Δ PCO$_2$ = 1.2 × Δ HCO$_3^-$ ± 2 = 1.2 × (24 − 17) = ~8 mm Hg. Expected PCO$_2$ = 40 − 8 = 32 mm Hg ± 2 (30–34 mm Hg). Measured PCO$_2$ = 38 mm Hg, which is higher than it should be for compensation. Hence, there is a primary component of respiratory acidosis, which is keeping with the patient's clinical presentation.

d. Laboratory abnormalities include the following:
   (1) Severe hyponatremia.
   (2) UNa$^+$ > 20 mEq/L (effect of increased EABV on the proximal tubule; see ¶V.D.1.c, above).
   (3) Urine osmolality (Uosm) > Posm (ADH concentrates the urine, plus increased loss of solutes from the proximal tubule).
   (4) A low serum BUN and uric acid (which are lost in the urine with Na$^+$ from decreased proximal reabsorption).
e. The treatment of SiADH requires water restriction.
3. **Addison's disease** occurs when >90% of the functional capacity of the adrenal glands has been destroyed.
   a. Autoimmune destruction accounts for most cases (Chapter 19).
   b. The absence of aldosterone activity in the distal and collecting tubules results in a hypertonic loss of Na$^+$ (**hyponatremia**; ↓ serum Na$^+$ ≅ ↓↓ **TBNa$^+$**/↓ TBW; UNa$^+$ > 20 mEq/L) and the retention of K$^+$ (**hyperkalemia**) and H ions (**normal AG metabolic acidosis**, since retained H ions bind with Cl ions).
   c. Na$^+$ loss results in hypovolemic shock, and hyperkalemia poses a serious threat for conduction disturbances in the heart.
   d. The absence of cortisol produces the following:
      (1) An additional component of **SiADH**, since cortisol normally inhibits ADH activity, which is now left unopposed.
      (2) **Fasting hypoglycemia** resulting from loss of the gluconeogenic properties of cortisol.
      (3) **Hyperpigmentation** of the skin owing to loss of the inhibitory effect of cortisol on adrenocorticotropic hormone (ACTH).

Objective 6: To review the hemostatic system and alterations in the vascular, platelet, coagulation, and fibrinolytic systems.

XI. Normal hemostasis
  A. **Endothelial cells** provide an anticoagulant function in the uninjured state and a procoagulant role when injured.
    1. They synthesize anticoagulants such as **tissue plasminogen activator** (tPA), which activates plasminogen to produce plasmin, a fibrinolytic agent, and **prostacyclin** (PGI$_2$; a vasodilator and inhibitor of platelet aggregation), which derives from the action of cyclooxygenase on arachidonic acid.
    2. They synthesize **von Willebrand's factor** (VIII:vWF), a procoagulant that binds to glycoprotein receptor Ib (GPIb) on the platelet membrane, producing **platelet adhesion** in areas of endothelial injury.
    3. Exposure of subendothelial tissue after injury not only produces platelet adhesion but also leads to activation of factors XII and XI (by exposure of collagen) in the intrinsic coagulation system and factor VII in the extrinsic system by **tissue thromboplastin** released by the injured endothelial cells.
  B. **Platelets** derived from cytoplasmic fragmentation of megakaryocytes are released into the circulation (150,000–400,000 cells/μL), where they live for 9–10 days.
    1. One third of the total platelet pool is stored in the spleen and exchanges freely with the circulating pool.
    2. GPIb and fibrinogen (GPIIb/IIIa) receptors are present on the platelet surface.
    3. The platelet membrane contains **platelet factor 3** (PF3), which is the phospholipid substrate upon which the clotting sequence must occur.
    4. Platelet adhesion is a stimulus for the conversion of arachidonic acid to **thromboxane A$_2$** (TXA$_2$; a platelet aggregator and vasoconstrictor) and the release of chemicals (**release reaction**) from **alpha granules** (e.g., VIII:vWF, fibrinogen) and from **dense bodies** (e.g., ADP, calcium).
    5. **Platelet cyclooxygenase** is more susceptible to inactivation by aspirin (irreversible) and NSAIDs (reversible) than is endothelial cell cyclooxygenase, underscoring the role of the former in inhibiting platelet aggregation.
    6. After platelets aggregate in the vessel lumen (induced by TXA$_2$ and ADP), fibrinogen molecules attach to GPIIb/IIIa, leading to the formation of a **primary hemostatic plug**, which stops small vessel bleeding.
  C. The **coagulation system** produces the **stable fibrin clot**, which requires the following:
    1. Synthesis of serine proteases in the liver (e.g., most of the coagulation factors).
    2. Activation of factors XII and VII.
    3. Production of thrombin.
    4. Conversion of fibrinogen into a fibrin clot by thrombin.
  D. The **coagulation cascade system** consists of an extrinsic and intrinsic system.
    1. The **extrinsic system** rapidly generates small quantities of thrombin once factor VII is activated by tissue thromboplastin.
    2. The **intrinsic system** begins with the activation of the **contact factors**, which include factors XII and XI as well as high-molecular-weight kininogen (HMWK) and prekallikrein.
      a. Subendothelial collagen and kallikrein activate factor XII (Hageman factor) to form XIIa, which subsequently activates XI to form XIa, whose reaction is enhanced by HMWK.
      b. Factor XIa activates factor IX to form IXa, which participates in a four-component system consisting of IXa, VIII:C (coagulant factor VIII), PF3, and calcium ions, all of which convert factor X to Xa.
    3. Both the extrinsic and intrinsic systems utilize the same **final common pathway** beginning with the activation of factor X to Xa.
      a. Factor Xa participates in a four-component system consisting of Xa, V, PF3, and calcium (**prothrombin complex**), which cleaves prothrombin (factor II) into the enzyme thrombin.
      b. Thrombin cleaves fibrinogen into **fibrin monomer** plus **fibrinopeptides A** and **B** (which are excellent markers of fibrinogen activation).
      c. Fibrin monomers undergo further alteration to soluble fibrin, which is acted upon factor XIII (which produces covalent protein-protein cross-linking) to form **insoluble fibrin**.
    4. The **kinin system** is important in the inflammatory response (Chapter 3) as well as activation of the fibrinolytic system and factor XII.
    5. The **vitamin K–dependent factors** consist of factors II, VII, IX, X, protein C, and protein S.
      a. They are synthesized in the liver as precursors that become functional once they are **γ-carboxylated** by vitamin K$_1$.
      b. γ-Carboxylation of glutamic acid residues provides each factor with binding sites for calcium and PF3, both of which are essential for proper functioning of the cascade sequence.
  E. **Plasma proteins** provide procoagulants (coagulation factors, tissue thromboplastin), anticoagulants (antithrombin III, proteins C and S), fibrinolytic proteins (plasmin), and complement.
    1. Anticoagulants include **antithrombin III** (ATIII), **protein C**, and **protein S**.
    2. **Heparin** markedly enhances **ATIII** activity, which has an inhibitory effect on serine proteases (particularly thrombin and factor X).
    3. **Proteins C** and **S** inactivate factors V and VIII and enhance fibrinolytic activity.
  F. The **fibrinolytic system** breaks down the stable clot in order to restore blood flow.
    1. It is activated primarily by the action of tPA on plasminogen to form the enzyme plasmin.
    2. Plasmin acts on clot-associated fibrin monomers as well as circulating fibrinogen and clot-associated fibrinogen to produce **fibrin(ogen) degradation products** (FDPs) **X, Y, D,** and **E.**
  G. In summary, the general sequence of reactions with small vessel injury includes vascular (vasoconstriction), platelet (adhesion and aggregation),

coagulation (stable clot), and fibrinolytic (dissolution of the clot) phases.

XII. Laboratory evaluation of hemostasis

A. Platelet tests are quantitative (e.g., platelet count) or test platelet function (e.g., bleeding time).

1. The **platelet count** is the most cost-effective test.

2. The **bleeding time** (BT; < 10 minutes) evaluates vessel integrity and platelet function up to the formation of the primary hemostatic plug, which coincides with the cessation of bleeding in the test.

   a. It is normal in coagulation factor deficiencies (e.g., hemophilia A), since the coagulation system is most responsible for the stable clot.

   b. It is prolonged in the following disorders:

      (1) Vascular disease (e.g., scurvy).

      (2) Thrombocytopenia (fewer platelets available for aggregation).

      (3) Von Willebrand's disease (VWD) (absence of VIII:vWF for platelet adhesion).

      (4) In patients taking aspirin or other NSAIDs (which inhibit TXA_2 formation), this being the main cause of a prolonged BT.

3. **Platelet aggregation studies** evaluate the *in vitro* response of platelet-rich plasma to aggregating agents (e.g., ADP).

   a. The **ristocetin aggregation test** evaluates the interaction of circulating VIII:vWF (derived from endothelial cells) with the antibiotic ristocetin, which facilitates binding of the factor to platelets, leading to aggregation, hence providing documentation of an intact VIII:vWF/GPIb receptor system.

   b. The **ristocetin cofactor assay** is the single best test for diagnosing von Willebrand's disease.

B. Coagulation system tests

1. The **prothrombin time** (PT; 11–15 seconds) evaluates the integrity of the extrinsic system down to the formation of a clot (**VII → X → V → II → I →** clot).

   a. A deficiency of one or more of the above factors prolongs the PT.

   b. The **international normalized ratio** (INR) is employed to standardize the reporting of PT results in patients taking warfarin owing to the different reagents used.

   c. The PT is the most sensitive test for the following measurements:

      (1) Detecting final common pathway deficiencies (factor X → clot).

      (2) Confirming factor VII deficiency.

      (3) Following patients on warfarin therapy (use the INR results).

      (4) Evaluating the severity of liver disease.

2. The **activated partial thromboplastin time** (aPTT; 25–35 seconds) evaluates the intrinsic system down to the formation of a clot (**XII → XI → IX → VIII → X → V → II → I →** clot) and is also the test of choice for monitoring heparin therapy.

3. **Factor assays** are available for most coagulation factors.

   a. In addition to VIII:vWF, other factor VIII assays are available to help distinguish von Willebrand's disease and hemophilia A.

   b. Immunologic assays measure the concentration of **VIII:antigen** (VIII:Ag), which is a carrier protein for circulating VIII:vWF, and VIII:coagulant (VIII:C) in the intrinsic system.

   c. **Factor VIII:C assays** measure the percent concentration of factor VIII in the intrinsic system.

4. **Mixing studies** differentiate true factor deficiencies from factor deficiencies secondary to destruction by antibodies (inhibitors).

   a. Using hemophilia A as an example, in hereditary deficiency of VIII:C, the prolonged aPTT (XII → XI → IX → **VIII** → X → V → II → I → clot) is corrected by mixing 0.5 mL of normal plasma (contains VIII:C) with 0.5 mL of patient plasma (deficient in VIII:C), since enough VIII:C has been added to correct the aPTT.

   b. Plasma containing antibodies (circulating anticoagulants) against factor VIII:C will not correct the prolonged aPTT after being mixed with normal plasma, owing to the destruction of factor VIII:C in the normal plasma.

C. Fibrinolytic system tests

1. **Degradation products** (FDPs) X, Y, D, and E of plasmin-mediated cleavage of fibrinogen, clot-associated fibrinogen, or clot-associated fibrin monomers are detected by agglutination slide tests.

2. The **D-dimer assay** (agglutination test) specifically detects **clot-associated fibrin** degradation products that have been **cross-linked (D-dimers)** by factor XIII, hence distinguishing them from the X, Y, D, and E fragments, which derive from breakdown of circulating fibrinogen, fibrinogen associated with a clot, and fibrin clots.

XIII. Physical findings in hemostasis disorders

A. Vascular and platelet abnormalities are characterized by the following signs:

1. Epistaxis (nosebleeds; the most common manifestation).

2. Easy bruising.

3. Cutaneous bleeding.

   a. Petechiae (1- to 3-mm pinpoint hemorrhages).

   b. Ecchymoses (purpuric lesions about the size of a quarter).

4. Prolonged bleeding from superficial scratches (no primary hemostatic plug).

B. Coagulopathies are associated with the following conditions:

1. Bleeding after molar extractions (only a primary plug prevents bleeding).

2. Delayed bleeding after surgery (only a primary plug prevents bleeding).

3. Hematuria or gastrointestinal bleeding.

4. Bleeding into tissues (muscle) or spaces (joints).

XIV. Vascular disorders

A. **Hereditary hemorrhagic telangiectasia (Osler-Weber-Rendu disease)** is an autosomal dominant disease that presents with epistaxis and telangiectasias (dilated vascular channels) in the mouth and gastrointestinal tract (bleeding with iron deficiency).

B. Acquired vascular disorders include the following:
1. **Scurvy** (Chapter 6), with defects in collagen synthesis.
2. **Hypercortisol states** (Chapter 19), with defective collagen synthesis.
3. **Senile purpura** (atrophy of perivascular support).
4. **Henoch-Schönlein purpura** (Chapter 10), an immune complex vasculitis with palpable purpura (due to inflammation).

XV. Platelet disorders
A. Platelet disorders are **quantitative** abnormalities (e.g., thrombocytopenia, thrombocytosis) or **qualitative** (functional) abnormalities (e.g., aspirin inhibition of platelet aggregation).
B. **Thrombocytopenia** (too few platelets) may result from decreased production, increased destruction, or abnormal distribution (e.g., splenomegaly).
1. **Production disorders** are those which interfere with thrombopoiesis (e.g., aplastic anemia due to a drug, leukemia).
2. **Destruction disorders** are broadly subclassified as immune or nonimmune.
   a. **Idiopathic thrombocytopenic purpura** (ITP) is an autoimmune disease characterized by the development of IgG antibodies against the GPIIb/IIIa receptor on platelets with subsequent removal of the sensitized platelets by splenic macrophages (a type II hypersensitivity reaction).
      (1) It is the most common cause of thrombocytopenia in children and presents with an abrupt onset of epistaxis associated with development of petechiae and ecchymoses.
      (2) Megakaryocytes are present in the marrow, but the platelets are peripherally destroyed by the spleen (which usually is normal in size).
      (3) High-dose corticosteroids are used to treat symptomatic patients, and recovery is the rule within 4–6 weeks.
   b. **Autoimmune thrombocytopenias** associated with **systemic IgG-mediated immune diseases** (e.g., systemic lupus erythematosus) are insidious in onset and tend to persist in spite of corticosteroid therapy, splenectomy, or immunosuppressive therapy.
   c. **Virus-associated immune thrombocytopenias** (immunocomplex or antibody destruction of platelets) may accompany cytomegalovirus, infectious mononucleosis, and HIV infection.
   d. **Drug-induced autoimmune thrombocytopenia** (most commonly due to drug-dependent IgG antibodies) may occur with exposure to quinidine, sulfa compounds, penicillin, heparin, and thiazides.
   e. **Alloimmune thrombocytopenias** are a group of disorders in which the host develops IgG antibodies after exposure to foreign antigens (e.g., platelet HLA or PL^A1 antigens) from another individual (e.g., a fetus or blood product).
   f. **Thrombotic thrombocytopenic purpura** (TTP), a nonimmune thrombocytopenia, occurs mainly in young women and is characterized by the following pentad: severe thrombocytopenia; microangiopathic hemolytic anemia, in which schistocytes (fragmented RBCs) are present; neurologic abnormalities (often severe); renal failure (usually mild); and fever.
      (1) It is secondary to endothelial damage of small vessels by an unknown circulating factor in plasma, leading to widespread platelet thrombus formation (not a fibrin clot as in DIC) and thrombocytopenia (platelet consumption).
      (2) Obstruction of the microvasculature by platelet thrombi damages RBCs (intravascular hemolysis) and produces widespread organ injury.
   g. The **hemolytic uremic syndrome** (HUS), a nonimmune thrombocytopenia, occurs primarily in infants and young children and is clinically similar to TTP except for milder neurologic abnormalities, more severe renal disease, and in some cases a history of exposure to a toxin produced by *E. coli* serotype 0157:H7 consumed in raw ground beef.
C. **Thrombocytosis** (too many platelets; > 400,000 cells/μL) may be associated with chronic iron deficiency anemia, splenectomy, tuberculosis, or an underlying malignancy.
D. **Qualitative** (**functional**) **platelet disorders** can be hereditary or acquired (more common).
1. The BT is prolonged regardless of the platelet count.
2. Drugs that inhibit platelet function (e.g., aspirin) are the most common cause of platelet dysfunction.
3. Platelet dysfunction (prolonged BT) is the most common acquired defect in **uremia** and frequently complicates liver failure, DIC (FDPs inhibit platelet aggregation), multiple myeloma (excessive immunoglobulins inhibit platelet aggregation), VWD (see ¶XVI.C, below), and the myeloproliferative diseases (e.g., polycythemia rubra vera).
4. Hereditary disorders affect either platelet adhesion (e.g., VWD) or platelet aggregation (e.g. storage pool defects, with deficiency of ADP).

XVI. Coagulation disorders
A. Coagulation disorders can be either hereditary (usually single deficiencies) or acquired (e.g., defective production, pathologic inhibition, or consumption).
B. **Hemophilia A** is a sex-linked recessive (SXR) disease transferred to males from female carriers, who transmit the disease to 50% of their sons and to 50% of their daughters (who will be carriers).

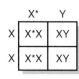 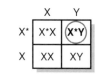

	XY Normal male
	XX Normal female
	X*Y Hemophilia A
	X*X Carrier female

1. The abnormal site on the X chromosome can be detected prenatally using restriction fragment length polymorphism (RFLP).
2. Laboratory findings include the following:
   a. Deficiency of factor VIII:C (coagulant factor).
   b. Normal VIII:Ag and VIII:vWF levels.
   c. Prolonged aPTT (XII → XI → IX → **VIII** → X → V → II → I → clot).
   d. Normal PT (VII → X → V → II → I → clot).

e. Normal BT (no platelet defects).

f. Immediate increase in the synthesis of new VIII:C after infusion of products containing factor VIII that is not in excess of the amount of factor VIII infused.

3. Female carriers are best detected by DNA techniques; however, a ratio of VIII:C/VIII:Ag < 0.75 is highly suggestive of a carrier state.

4. Clinical abnormalities relate to the degree of factor deficiency, with patients having < 1% VIII:C activity experiencing spontaneous hemarthroses and bleeding from the circumcision site at birth and those with > 25% to < 50% VIII:C activity remaining asymptomatic or subject to late rebleeding after surgery or trauma.

5. Depending on the severity of disease, treatment includes replacement therapy (lyophilized factor VIII concentrate, which has a small risk of transmitting HIV infection; recombinant factor VIII, which carries no risk of HIV infection; or desmopressin in mild cases to increase the synthesis of all the factor VIII components).

C. **VWD** is the most common hereditary bleeding disorder.

1. Classical type I VWD (75–80% of cases) is inherited as an autosomal dominant disease.

2. VWD presents with signs related to a platelet adhesion defect (epistaxis, increased bruising, menorrhagia) or coagulation deficiency (gastrointestinal bleeding often associated with angiodysplasia).

3. Laboratory findings include the following:

a. Prolonged BT.

b. Prolonged aPTT with a normal PT.

c. Low percent activity for factors VIII:vWF, VIII:C (< 40% of normal), and VIII:Ag.

d. Slow but sustained increase in new factor VIII synthesis that is greater than the amount of factor VIII infused.

4. Other variants of VWD differ in their inheritance patterns, BT results, platelet response to ristocetin, multimeric patterns (polymers of increasing molecular weight and size that are detected by electrophoretic techniques), and concentrations of VIII:vWF, VIII:Ag, VIII:C, and ristocetin cofactor.

5. Cryoprecipitate (a single-donor component containing factors VIII:C and VIII:vWF) is the mainstay of treatment, while desmopressin and estrogen/progestin compounds are useful in mild cases (estrogen increases factor VIII synthesis).

D. **Hemophilia B** (factor IX deficiency; Christmas disease) has an SXR inheritance pattern, a prolonged aPTT (XII → XI → **IX** → VIII → X → V → II → I → clot), and a similar clinical presentation to hemophilia A.

E. **Circulating anticoagulants** are antibodies (inhibitors) against certain coagulation factors that render those factors inactive, hence the confusion with a coagulation deficiency.

1. **Factor VIII inhibitors** are the most common inhibitors and are associated with the postpartum state, chlorpromazine therapy, and factor VIII treatment of hemophilia A patients.

2. **Factor V inhibitors** are encountered with streptomycin or aminoglycoside therapy, while **factor XIII inhibitors** are sometimes noted in patients taking isoniazid.

3. Mixing studies do not correct the prolonged PT or aPTT.

4. The **lupus anticoagulant** (LA) and **anticardiolipin antibodies** (ACA) are associated with the **antiphospholipid** (APL) **syndrome**.

a. They belong to a family of antibodies that react to phospholipids bound to plasma proteins (e.g., coagulation factors).

b. APLs occur in ~25% patients with SLE, but they are also present in AIDS, other autoimmune diseases, malignancy, old age, and patients who take drugs such as chlorpromazine and procainamide.

c. APLs damage endothelial cells, predisposing the patient to vessel thrombosis (e.g., placental bed thrombosis with fetal wastage, strokes, myocardial infarction).

d. LA acts against PF3 in the prothrombin complex, causing a prolongation of the aPTT (90%) and PT (20%).

e. ACA reacts against the cardiolipin in the RPR and VDRL test system, producing a **biologic false-positive syphilis serology** (FTA-ABS is negative).

F. **Vitamin K deficiency** produces a hemorrhagic diathesis as a result of multiple coagulation defects.

1. Vitamin K is a fat-soluble vitamin that converts the precursor **vitamin K–dependent factors II, VII, IX, X, protein C,** and **protein S** into functional coagulation factors by posttranslational γ-carboxylation of glutamyl residues in the N-terminal portion of the proteins.

a. **Epoxide reductase** catalyzes the conversion of the relatively inactive vitamin K_2 to the more active vitamin K_1, which is responsible for the γ-carboxylation process.

b. The activated factors have the following biological half-lives: factor VII and protein C, 6 hours; factors IX and X, 24 hours; and factor II (prothrombin), 60 hours.

2. Vitamin K is obtained from the diet and also synthesized by colonic bacteria.

3. Causes of vitamin K deficiency include the following:

a. Fat malabsorption (e.g., due to celiac disease, bile salt deficiency, or pancreatic disease).

b. Use of broad-spectrum antibiotics, which destroy colonic bacteria.

c. The newborn state (bacterial colonization is lacking at birth, and there is a danger of hemorrhagic disease unless the newborn is treated with intramuscular vitamin K).

d. Coumarin derivatives, which inhibit epoxide reductase.

G. **Disseminated intravascular coagulation** (DIC) is an intravascular thrombohemorrhagic disorder characterized by laboratory evidence of activation of the procoagulant and fibrinolytic systems, resulting in end-organ damage or failure.

1. Precipitating factors include the following:

a. Septicemia (e.g., due to endotoxins, which is the most common cause).

b. Obstetrical problems (e.g., amniotic fluid embolism causing thromboplastin release).

c. Hemolytic transfusion reactions (e.g., in a

blood group A patient who receives group B blood).

d. Massive trauma (e.g., release of tissue thromboplastin).

e. Malignancy (e.g., acute progranulocytic leukemia, metastatic carcinoma).

2. The pathophysiology of DIC initially involves activation of the coagulation and fibrinolytic systems by one of the above precipitating factors.

   a. The coagulation system is responsible for the following:

   (1) Activating the kinin system (to increase vessel permeability and vessel dilation, leading to shock).

   (2) Generating massive quantities of thrombin to form fibrin clots (thrombin deposits in the microcirculation and consumes platelets and coagulation factors).

   (3) Activating the fibrinolytic system (factor XII, kinins), leading to the formation of plasmin.

   b. Plasmin does the following:

   (1) Activates the complement system (anaphylatoxins C3a and C5a cause mast cell release of vasoactive amines that produce increased vessel permeability and vasodilatation, leading to shock).

   (2) Cleaves fibrinogen and fibrin clot into X, Y, D, and E degradation products (which interfere with normal clot formation and platelet function).

   (3) Degrades clotting factors (causing multiple factor deficiencies).

   (4) Cleaves fibrin clots to form D-dimers.

   c. The result of all these interacting events is a combination of thrombosis and bleeding.

3. Patients present with the following signs:

   a. Widespread oozing of blood from wounds and venipuncture sites.

   b. Subcutaneous bleeds and ecchymoses.

   c. Anemia secondary to damage of circulating RBCs by fibrin clots (microangiopathic hemolytic anemia with schistocytes) and blood loss.

   d. Widespread organ dysfunction involving the kidneys (renal failure), lungs (adult respiratory distress syndrome), and CNS (stroke).

4. Laboratory abnormalities include the following:

   a. Prolonged PT and aPTT (due to clot consumption of fibrinogen, V, VIII, and prothrombin).

   b. Elevation of fibrinopeptide A (a cleavage product of fibrinogen).

   c. Increased PF4 (an indicator of platelet activation).

   d. Presence of D-dimers and fibrin(ogen) degradation products (the best overall test to document DIC).

   e. Decreased ATIII concentration (ATIII is used up in the neutralization of serine proteases).

   f. Thrombocytopenia (due to platelets consumed in the clots).

5. The *sine qua non* for the **treatment of DIC** is to treat the underlying disease in conjunction with ancillary treatment consisting of the following:

   a. Subcutaneous low-dose heparin, which blocks thrombin and other serine proteases, hence reducing clot formation.

   b. Blood component therapy (packed RBCs, platelets, fresh-frozen plasma, cryoprecipitate).

H. **Severe liver disease** (e.g., cirrhosis, fulminant hepatic failure) produces multiple coagulation deficiencies, since the liver is the primary site of coagulation factor synthesis.

1. Prolongation of the PT without normalization after intramuscular vitamin K administration indicates severe liver disease.

2. Fresh-frozen plasma is given when significant bleeding occurs and the PT is prolonged.

I. Primary **fibrinolytic disorders** (e.g., due to excess plasminogen activation in open heart surgery, radical prostatectomy) are uncommon and involve the action of plasmin on fibrinogen and clotting factors without the formation of clots (hence, FDPs are increased but D-dimers are absent).

Objective 7: To understand the pathophysiology of the thrombotic and embolic disorders.

XVII. Thrombosis disorders

A. A **thrombus** is an adherent intravascular mass composed of varying proportions of coagulation factors, RBCs, and platelets.

1. In vessels having a rapid blood flow (e.g., **arteries**), thrombi are composed of platelets with some fibrin and appear firm and pale **(pale thrombus)** owing to the relative absence of entrapped RBCs.

2. In sluggish circulation (e.g., **veins**), thrombi are primarily composed of a dark red mass of fibrin **(red thrombus)** within which are entrapped RBCs, white blood cells, and a few platelets.

3. **Postmortem clots** are not attached to the vessel wall, have a "currant jelly" appearance if composed of RBCs (when clotting occurs rapidly), or a "chicken fat" appearance when composed of congealed plasma (when clotting occurs slowly and RBCs separate from plasma).

B. **Risk factors for venous thrombosis** include (1) surgery (general and orthopedic), (2) immobility (postoperative state), (3) obesity, (4) congestive heart failure, (5) malignancy, and (6) use of oral contraceptives.

C. **Risk factors for arterial thrombosis** consist of (1) atherosclerosis (most common), (2) smoking, (3) hypertension, (4) diabetes mellitus, (5) LDL $\geq$ 160 mg/dL, (6) HDL $\leq$ 35 mg/dL, and (6) a family history of premature acute myocardial infarction or stroke.

D. **Thrombogenesis** is enhanced by (1) endothelial injury, (2) altered blood flow (e.g., stasis or turbulence), and (3) hypercoagulable states.

1. **Endothelial injury** and **turbulent blood flow** are associated with pale thrombi in the heart and arteries (particularly at bifurcation sites and overlying atherosclerotic plaques).

2. **Stasis of blood flow** is associated with red thrombi in the venous system (particularly the deep saphenous veins in the calf).

3. **Hypercoagulable states** usually predispose to red thrombi in venous thrombosis.

   a. They may be hereditary (uncommon) or acquired.

b. Acquired conditions include the following:
   (1) Disseminated cancer, which causes thrombocytosis and elevation of coagulation factors, such as fibrinogen, V, and VIII.
   (2) Oral contraceptive use (estrogen increases the concentration of coagulation factors and decreases ATIII concentration).
   (3) Hyperviscosity of blood secondary to polycythemia (in which there is an excess number of RBCs) or hypergammaglobulinemia, particularly an increase in IgM (Waldenström's macroglobulinemia).

c. **Hereditary ATIII deficiency** has an autosomal dominant inheritance pattern.
   (1) Patients present at a young age with a history of recurrent deep venous thrombosis with or without recurrent pulmonary emboli.
   (2) Both functional (does ATIII work?) and immunologic (is ATIII present?) assays are available to secure the diagnosis.
   (3) The treatment during active thrombosis is with very high doses of heparin, while coumarin derivatives (e.g., warfarin) are used for prophylaxis.

d. **Hereditary deficiencies of either protein C or protein S** follow an autosomal dominant inheritance pattern.
   (1) Patients present at a young age with recurrent deep venous thrombosis and pulmonary emboli.
   (2) **Hemorrhagic skin necrosis** may occur in heterozygotes, who have 50% levels of protein C that reduce to 0% levels when the patient is given the initial loading dose of warfarin, which produces widespread thrombosis of vessels in the skin.
   (3) Heparin is employed in acute thrombosis, and coumarin derivatives are used for long-term maintenance (started at low levels to prevent skin necrosis).

E. Possible sequelae of thrombus formation include the following:
   1. Thromboembolization (see below) with the potential for infarction.
   2. Dissolution of the clot by the fibrinolytic system.
   3. Organization and possible recanalization of the clot with restoration of blood flow.
   4. Infection of the thrombus with the potential for septic embolization and "metastatic" abscess formation.

XVIII. Embolism
A. **Embolism** is occlusion of a vessel by a mass (solid, liquid, or gaseous), with subsequent transportation of that mass by the blood stream to a distant site.
B. Most **pulmonary emboli** originate from the femoral veins in the upper thigh, whereas most arterial emboli arise from the left heart (Chapter 11).
C. **Paradoxical emboli** arise in the venous system and pass through an atrial septal defect (ASD) into the systemic circulation.

D. **Fat embolization** occurs when there are traumatic fractures of the long bones (particularly the shaft of the femur) and pelvis.
   1. Microglobules of fat from the bone marrow or surrounding adipose tissue enter the circulation and lodge in the microvasculature throughout the body.
   2. Fatty acids damage vessel endothelium, resulting in thrombosis.
   3. The symptoms and signs of fat embolism are usually delayed 24–72 hours, after which patients may experience (a) CNS dysfunction (ischemia, hemorrhage, and necrosis), (b) respiratory failure (hypoxemia and severe dyspnea), and (c) thrombocytopenia (platelets adhere to fat; there are petechiae over the upper half of the body and conjunctiva).
   4. The diagnosis is made on clinical grounds, since laboratory tests are not diagnostic.
   5. Mortality is < 10% and is usually related to the CNS abnormalities.

E. **Amniotic fluid embolization** is a potential complication of a difficult labor and delivery.
   1. It presents with a sudden onset of respiratory distress, cardiovascular collapse, and bleeding secondary to DIC (the amniotic fluid is rich in thromboplastin).
   2. The presence of lanugo hair or fetal skin in the right side of the heart on pulmonary artery catheterization or autopsy (the mortality rate is 80%) confirms the diagnosis.

F. **Air embolism** may complicate surgery around the head and neck or catheter insertion into the jugular or subclavian veins.
   1. Air is suctioned into the venous system owing to the negative intrathoracic pressure on inspiration.
   2. Approximately 100 mL of air in the circulation can be fatal, since it mixes with blood in the right heart and produces a frothy material that blocks pulmonary blood flow.

G. **Decompression sickness (caisson disease)** occurs when inert gases dissolved in tissues come out of physical solution when environmental pressure falls too rapidly.
   1. It most commonly occurs in diving, since the atmospheric pressure increases by 1 for every 33 feet of descent into the water, hence increasing the dissolution of nitrogen into the tissues.
   2. Rapid ascent from the water allows nitrogen gas bubbles to come out of tissue like bubbles in a soda bottle.
   3. The bubbles lodge in the blood vessels of muscles and joints, the latter area predisposing to the "bends," which is the most common manifestation.
   4. Treatment involves the administration of oxygen and prompt recompression in a hyperbaric chamber with 100% oxygen.

QUESTIONS

DIRECTIONS. (ITEMS 1–15): Each of the numbered items or incomplete statements in this section is followed by answers or completions of the statement. Select the ONE lettered answer or completion that is BEST in each case. Correct answers and explanations are given at the end of the chapter.

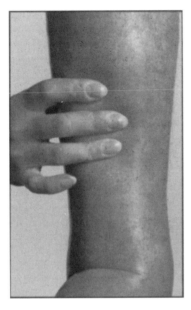

1. The photograph is of the lower extremity of a 45-year-old man who has a long history of untreated ischemic heart disease. Additional findings include tender hepatomegaly, neck vein distention, and scattered wet rales at both lung bases. You would expect this patient to have

(A) normal effective arterial blood volume (EABV)
(B) normal total body sodium (TBNa⁺)
(C) inhibition of antidiuretic hormone (ADH)
(D) reduced plasma oncotic pressure
(E) peritubular capillary oncotic pressure greater than hydrostatic pressure

2. Which of the following represents an exudate rather than a transudate associated with a Starling's force alteration?

(A) Pleural effusion in a patient with fever and a consolidation in the lung
(B) Bibasilar inspiratory rales 2 days following acute myocardial infarction
(C) Ascites in a child with protein malnutrition
(D) Pleural effusion (hydrothorax) in a patient with left heart failure
(E) Presacral pitting edema in a patient with congestive heart failure

3. Which of the following is more characteristic of arterial thrombi than of venous thrombi?

(A) They develop in areas of stasis.
(B) Coumarin derivatives rather than aspirin are preventative.

(C) They are primarily composed of fibrin, RBCs, and platelets.
(D) They are red thrombi that adhere to areas of injury.
(E) They develop in areas of turbulence around vessel bifurcations.

4. A construction worker fell off a two-story building and had massive crush injuries associated with multiple fractures of his pelvis and a comminuted fracture of the right femur. On the second hospital day, he developed mental status abnormalities, petechial lesions over his upper torso, severe dyspnea, and hypoxemia. The patient has most likely developed

(A) disseminated intravascular coagulation (DIC)
(B) fat embolism
(C) endotoxic shock
(D) thrombotic thrombocytopenic purpura (TTP)
(E) a pulmonary embolus

5. Which of the following is representative of hemophilia A rather than von Willebrand's disease (VWD)?

(A) Low factor VIII:Ag
(B) Low factor VIII:C
(C) Abnormal ristocetin cofactor assay
(D) Normal bleeding time
(E) Platelet adhesion defect

6. Which of the following groups of signs is indicative of a coagulation disorder rather than a platelet disorder?

(A) Epistaxis and easy bruisability
(B) Late rebleeding and hemarthroses
(C) Bleeding from superficial scratches and epistaxis
(D) Ecchymoses and intramuscular hematoma
(E) Petechiae and spontaneous bruising

7. An elderly man with urinary retention secondary to urethral obstruction by prostatic hyperplasia suddenly develops fever, hypotension, oozing of blood from intravenous and multiple venipuncture sites, and large areas of subcutaneous bleeding. The CBC exhibits absolute neutropenia, thrombocytopenia, and a normocytic anemia. Schistocytes are noted in the peripheral blood smear. You would expect additional laboratory studies to reveal

(A) an increase in fibrin(ogen) degradation products
(B) a normal D-dimer assay
(C) increased antithrombin III levels
(D) a serial increase in fibrinogen
(E) absence of fibrinopeptide A

8. A 32-year-old woman with a recent history of a viral illness abruptly develops fever, neurologic abnormalities, renal failure, thrombocytopenia, and a normocytic anemia with schistocytes noted in the peripheral blood. The mechanism for this patient's disease most closely relates to

(A) absence of the PL^A1 antigen on her platelets
(B) IgG antibodies against the GPIIb/IIIa receptor on her platelets

(C) absent GPIIb/IIIa receptors on her platelets

(D) endothelial cell injury with widespread platelet thrombosis

(E) absence of factor VIII:vWF

9. A patient with a $PaCO_2$ of 20 mm Hg (33–44 mm Hg) as compensation would most likely have a primary disorder arising from which of the following clinical disorders?

(A) Renal failure

(B) Gastritis with vomiting

(C) Pulmonary embolus

(D) Paralysis of the diaphragm

(E) Volume depletion secondary to diuretic use

10. A 42-year-old woman presents with extreme muscle weakness. The physical examination reveals a normal blood pressure and pulse, generalized muscle weakness, nonreactive deep tendon reflexes, and occasional premature ventricular contractions (PVCs). An electrocardiogram confirms the presence of PVCs and also exhibits sagging of the ST segment, depression of the T waves, and the presence of U waves. The following laboratory studies are available:

Serum sodium	136 mEq/L	(normal, 136–145 mEq/L)
Serum potassium	2.5 mEq/L	(normal, 3.5–5.0 mEq/L)
Serum chloride	109 mEq/L	(normal, 95–105 mEq/L)
Serum bicarbonate	15 mEq/L	(normal, 22–28 mEq/L)
Urine pH	6.0	

The mechanism for this patient's clinical and laboratory abnormalities most closely relates to

(A) inhibition of the $Na^+/K^+/2\ Cl^-$ cotransport pump in the thick ascending limb

(B) destruction of the juxtaglomerular apparatus

(C) a defect in the collecting tubule proton/K^+-ATPase pump

(D) mineralocorticoid excess secondary to an adrenal tumor

(E) surreptitious intake of a thiazide diuretic

11. A febrile 56-year-old smoker with long-standing chronic bronchitis presents with a spiking fever and a cough that is productive of a mucoid, greenish-yellow sputum interspersed with flecks of blood. A Gram stain reveals fat gram-negative rods with capsules in close proximity to neutrophils. Physical examination reveals inspiratory rales in the right posterior lower lobe, with decreased percussion and a positive E to A sign. Sibilant rales are scattered throughout both lung fields. Prior to his chest x-ray, he is inadvertently given 100% oxygen by Venturi mask, following which he lapses into a semicomatose state. The mechanism for this last event most closely relates to

(A) a right posterior lobe pneumonia

(B) sepsis secondary to *Klebsiella pneumoniae*

(C) cerebral edema secondary to respiratory acidosis

(D) loss of the hypoxemic stimulus for breathing

(E) acute bronchitis superimposed on chronic respiratory acidosis

Items 12–15

Match the following sets of electrolytes and random urine sodium (Na) measurements with the appropriate clinical description.

	Serum Na$^+$ (136–145 mEq/L)	Serum Cl$^-$ (95–105 mEq/L)	Serum K$^+$ (3.5–5.0 mEq/L)	Serum HCO$_3^-$ (22–28 mEq/L)	Random UNa$^+$ (<20 mEq/L)
A.	132	86	2.6	30	>20
B.	150	107	2.0	34	>20
C.	128	96	5.5	20	>20
D.	120	86	3.4	22	>20
E.	132	94	5.8	18	>20
F.	139	94	3.0	18	>20

12. The patient is a thin, 34-year-old woman with weakness, polyuria, diastolic hypertension, and tetany. There is no evidence of pitting edema or volume depletion. An ECG reveals prominent U waves and a random urine potassium is > 20 mEq/L.

13. The patient is a 58-year-old smoker with cough, weight loss, a left hilar mass on a chest x-ray, and mental status abnormalities. A computerized tomographic (CT) scan of the brain is negative for metastatic disease. There is no evidence of pitting edema or volume depletion.

14. The patient is a 38-year-old woman with increased mucosal pigmentation, weakness, and an ECG exhibiting peaked T waves. The physical examination reveals hypotension and dry mucous membranes.

15. The patient is a 62-year-old woman with chronic congestive heart failure who is taking a diuretic. She feels very weak and has dry mucous membranes on physical examination.

Items 16–19

Match the following sets of arterial blood gases with the appropriate clinical description.

	pH (7.35–7.45)	PaCO$_2$ (33–44 mm Hg)	HCO$_3^-$ (22–28 mEq/L)
A.	7.12	50	16
B.	7.23	68	27
C.	7.30	30	14
D.	7.33	60	31
E.	7.37	72	40
F.	7.38	14	8
G.	7.40	40	24
H.	7.48	20	14
I.	7.52	49	39
J.	7.52	25	20

16. A 58-year-old smoker has an increased anteroposterior diameter, flattened diaphragms, and productive cough for most months of the year for the last 8 years.

17. A 32-year-old man with chronic peptic ulcer disease has pyloric obstruction and incomplete emptying of his stomach after eating. He has received continual nasogastric suctioning for the last 24 hours without adequate fluid replacement.

18. A 45-year-old woman 2 days postcholecystectomy has a sudden onset of pleuritic chest pain and tachypnea.

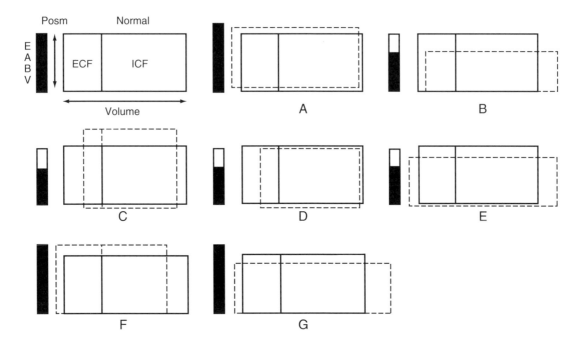

The right calf is swollen, hot, and tender on dorsiflexion of the foot.

19. A 39-year-old homeless man presents in a stuporous state and is noted to have retinal abnormalities on examination. The serum blood urea nitrogen (BUN) and creatinine are normal. An increased anion gap is noted on his electrolyte measurements. The calculated osmolality is 285 mOsm/kg (275–295 mOsm/kg), but the measured osmolality is 385 mOsm/kg.

Items 20–23

Match the following diagrams of the extracellular and intracellular fluid compartments with the appropriate clinical description. The height of the compartment (y-axis) correlates with the plasma osmolality (Posm), while the width of the compartment (x-axis) indicates volume changes. The small bar graph to the left of the ECF compartment indicates the effective arterial blood volume (EABV).

20. An obese, 48-year-old man presents with excessive sweating and a history of inadequate fluid intake while working outdoors on a hot, humid day. Physical examination reveals hypotension and poor skin turgor.

21. A 52-year-old woman with a history of type II diabetes mellitus controlled by chlorpropamide presents with mental status abnormalities. She has a normal physical examination with normal skin turgor. The random UNa^+ is 80 mEq/L.

22. A 45-year-old man has generalized pitting edema, hypertension, and a +4 dipstick test for protein. The 24-hour urine measurement for protein is 9 g.

23. A 45-year-old man with acute pancreatitis is inadvertently given 8 L of isotonic saline instead of 3 L as prescribed. He has mild dependent pitting edema.

Items 24–27

Match the following sets of hemostasis test results with the appropriate clinical description.

	Bleeding Time	Platelet Count	Prothrombin Time (PT)	Partial Thromboplastin Time (PTT)
A.	Prolonged	Decreased	Normal	Normal
B.	Prolonged	Normal	Normal	Normal
C.	Prolonged	Decreased	Prolonged	Prolonged
D.	Prolonged	Normal	Prolonged	Prolonged
E.	Normal	Normal	Prolonged	Normal
F.	Normal	Normal	Normal	Prolonged
G.	Prolonged	Normal	Normal	Prolonged
H.	Normal	Normal	Prolonged	Prolonged

24. A 23-year-old woman has menorrhagia, easy bruisability, and an abnormal ristocetin cofactor assay.

25. A 42-year-old man with a strong family history of coronary artery disease has been advised to take aspirin every other day.

26. An afebrile 7-year-old boy presents with epistaxis, petechiae, and ecchymoses 2 weeks following a viral infection. Physical examination is otherwise unremarkable. He has a normal hemoglobin. His condition improves with corticosteroid treatment.

27. A 6-year-old child develops neurologic abnormalities, hemolytic anemia, and renal failure shortly after attending a picnic at which hamburgers were served. The peripheral smear reveals numerous schistocytes.

ANSWERS AND EXPLANATIONS

1. The answer is E: peritubular capillary oncotic pressure greater than hydrostatic pressure. The photograph depicts a patient with dependent pitting edema of the lower extremity. He has a history of ischemic heart disease, and the physical findings indicate left heart failure (wet rales at the lung bases) that has progressed to right heart failure (pitting edema, neck vein distention, and congestive hepatomegaly). The EABV is decreased in either left or right heart failure. This activates the baroreceptor reflex, which stimulates the hypothalamic release of ADH. Reduced renal blood flow activates the RAA system, with subsequent release of aldosterone. The peritubular capillary hydrostatic pressure is decreased, hence increasing the oncotic pressure, leading to enhanced proximal tubular reabsorption of Na^+ and a random UNa^+ to < 20 mEq/L. A hypotonic fluid (more water than salt) is the final tonicity of the reabsorbed fluid, which would produce hyponatremia ($\downarrow$ serum $Na^+ \cong \uparrow TBNa^+/\uparrow\uparrow TBW$). Owing to an increase in systemic venous hydrostatic pressure from right heart failure, the reabsorbed fluid is redirected into the interstitial space, thereby exacerbating the pitting edema without contributing to an increase in the EABV. The excess in $TBNa^+$, which is limited to the ECF compartment, along with the increased venous hydrostatic pressure is primarily responsible for producing pitting edema in this patient. (Photograph reproduced, with permission, from M.A. Mir. *Atlas of Clinical Diagnosis.* Philadelphia, W.B. Saunders Co., 1995, p. 237).

2. The answer is A: pleural effusion in a patient with fever and a consolidation in the lung. The latter represents an exudate (increased cells and protein) secondary to pneumonia in the lung, with subsequent increase in vessel permeability along the pleural surface. Pus in the pleural cavity is called empyema. The remaining choices are all examples of transudates (low protein and very few cells) that are due to an alteration in Starling's forces. Bibasilar inspiratory rales 2 days following acute myocardial infarction indicates pulmonary edema (increased pulmonary venous hydrostatic pressure) secondary to left heart failure. A pleural effusion (hydrothorax) in a patient with left heart failure has a similar mechanism. Ascites in a child with protein malnutrition (kwashiorkor) is secondary to a reduction in oncotic pressure related to hypoalbuminemia. Presacral pitting edema in a patient with congestive heart failure is dependent edema associated with an increase in hydrostatic pressure.

3. The answer is E: they develop in areas of turbulence around vessel bifurcations. Arterial thrombi, or pale thrombi, are primarily composed of platelets held together by loose fibrin strands. They develop in areas of turbulence (over an atherosclerotic plaque or at vessel bifurcations). Venous clots, or red thrombi, are composed of fibrin, RBCs, and platelets. They develop in areas of stasis (e.g., deep saphenous veins in a postsurgical patient lying in bed) and in hypercoagulable states (e.g., ATIII deficiency). Both arterial and venous thrombi have lines of Zahn (alternating layers with varying amounts of platelets, RBCs, platelets, etc.). Couma-

rin derivatives prevent the formation of a fibrin clot and so are useful in treating venous thrombi rather than arterial thrombi. Aspirin irreversibly inhibits platelet cyclooxygenase, thereby preventing the synthesis of TXA_2 and inhibiting platelet aggregation associated with arterial thrombi.

4. The answer is B: fat embolism. The patient has fat embolism secondary to multiple fractures of his pelvic bones and femur, resulting in the escape of fat microglobules into the microcirculation. CNS signs (e.g., mental status abnormalities), dyspnea (perfusion defects in the pulmonary capillaries leading to hypoxemia), and petechial lesions over the upper torso are usually delayed in onset until 24–48 hours after the injury. Fat emboli locally release fatty acids that damage the endothelium, hence favoring the development of platelet thrombi that consume platelets (thrombocytopenia). Fat embolism should not be confused with DIC (thrombohemorrhagic signs and symptoms), TTP (fever, renal failure, CNS signs, hemolytic anemia, and thrombocytopenia), endotoxic shock (warm shock with high-output failure), or a pulmonary embolus (sudden onset of pleuritic chest pain and right ventricular strain). Corticosteroids are sometimes used with varying success.

5. The answer is D: normal bleeding time. Hemophilia A is an SXR disease with a deficiency of factor VIII:C and normal concentrations of VIII:Ag and VIII:vWF (normal ristocetin cofactor assay and ristocetin aggregation test). Since there is not a platelet adhesion defect, the bleeding time is normal. Classical VWD is an autosomal dominant disease characterized by deficiencies of all the factor VIII components. The platelet adhesion defect is due to a deficiency of VIII:vWF synthesized by endothelial cells. It binds to the GPIb receptor on platelets, which sets off platelet synthesis of TXA_2 and the release of aggregating agents (ADP) from the dense bodies. Without platelet adhesion, the primary hemostatic plug cannot develop, so the bleeding time is prolonged.

6. The answer is B: late rebleeding and hemarthroses. These signs are associated with coagulation rather than platelet disorders. Since a stable clot does not form in a coagulation deficiency, only a primary hemostatic plug prevents bleeding from small blood vessels. The plugs are frequently dislodged with movement of the patient, resulting in late rebleeding. Hemarthroses (bleeding into joints) and intramuscular hematomas are primarily seen in severe cases ($< 1\%$ factor levels) of hemophilia A and B (factor IX deficiency). Platelet disorders are characterized by epistaxis (most common), easy bruisability or spontaneous bruising, petechiae, ecchymoses, and bleeding from superficial scratches (no primary hemostatic plug).

7. The answer is A: an increase in fibrin(ogen) degradation products. The patient has endotoxic shock arising from gram-negative sepsis secondary to urinary retention, which became the catalyst for the development of DIC. Activation of factor XII results in a three-pronged sequence of events including (1) the generation of thrombin to form fibrin clots in the microcirculation (causing an increase in fibrinopeptide A and RBC damage in the

form of schistocytes); (2) activation of the kinin system, which increases vessel permeability and produces vasodilatation leading to shock; and (3) activation of the fibrinolytic system with the release of plasmin. Plasmin, in turn, (1) degrades clotting factors; (2) degrades fibrin clots to form degradation products (X, Y, D, and E) and cross-linked fibrin monomers (D-dimers), which inhibit platelet aggregation; and (3) activates the complement system with the release of C3a and C5a (anaphylatoxins) that further enhance vasodilatation and shock. The consumption of clotting factors (fibrinogen, V, VIII, prothrombin) and platelets causes anticoagulation in the patient, resulting in bleeding into the skin and oozing from venipuncture sites. ATIII levels are reduced owing to its consumption in the neutralization of thrombin and other serine proteases.

8. The answer is D: endothelial cell injury with widespread platelet thrombosis. The patient has thrombotic thrombocytopenic purpura (TTP), which consists of a pentad of fever, neurologic abnormalities, renal failure (mild), microangiopathic hemolytic anemia (schistocytes present), and thrombocytopenia. An unknown plasma factor damages the endothelium, resulting in platelet adhesion and thrombus formation. The thrombi block blood flow in multiple organ systems and damage RBCs. Plasmapheresis removes the plasma factor. TTP is not DIC, since coagulation factors are not consumed. Absence of the PL^{A1} antigen may be associated with isoimmune neonatal thrombocytopenia (analogous to Rh sensitization, except that the fetus is positive for PL^{A1} antigen) and posttransfusion purpura (in which patients develop anti-PL^{A1} antibodies from a previous transfusion and subsequent exposure to PL^{A1}-positive platelets destroys the transfused platelets as well as their own platelets). Antibodies (IgG) against the GPIIb/IIIa receptor (fibrinogen receptor) on platelets are the mechanism for autoimmune thrombocytopenia. Absent GPIIb/IIIa receptors (plus a deficiency of thrombosthenin, a platelet contractile protein) is the abnormality in Glanzmann's disease, which is an autosomal recessive disease associated with severe bleeding. Absence of factor VIII:vWF is seen in VWD and is responsible for the platelet adhesion defect and prolonged bleeding time.

9. The answer is A: renal failure. The patient has a low PaCO$_2$ (respiratory alkalosis), which must be compensation for metabolic acidosis as a primary disorder, which in this case is renal failure (increased anion gap metabolic acidosis). Vomiting and diuretics both produce primary metabolic alkalosis having respiratory acidosis as compensation. A pulmonary embolus is associated with tachypnea, which produces a primary respiratory alkalosis, whose compensation is metabolic acidosis. Paralysis of the diaphragm results in primary respiratory acidosis, which has metabolic alkalosis as compensation.

10. The answer is C: a defect in the collecting tubule proton/K$^+$-ATPase pump. The patient has a type I distal RTA. Dysfunction of the proton/K$^+$-ATPase pump reduces H$^+$ secretion, which in turn decreases the new synthesis of bicarbonate. The excess H ions combine with Cl ions to form HCl, hence producing a normal AG metabolic acidosis (in this case, AG = 136 mEq/L − [109 mEq/L + 15 mEq/L] = 12 mEq/L). Reduction in the exchange of H ions for K ions results in massive K$^+$ wasting, which produces muscle weakness, nonreactive deep tendon reflexes, ventricular arrhythmias, and prominent U waves on an ECG. Inability to secrete excess H ions in the urine results in a urine pH that is consistently > 5.5. Destruction of the juxtaglomerular apparatus produces type IV RTA, which consists of low plasma renin activity (synthesized in the juxtaglomerular apparatus), hypoaldosteronism (no ATII to stimulate its release), and retention of H ions (normal AG metabolic acidosis) and K$^+$ (hyperkalemia). Inhibition of the Na$^+$/K$^+$/2 Cl$^-$ cotransport pump in the thick ascending limb is noted with use of loop diuretics. Augmented distal delivery of excess Na$^+$ results in hyponatremia (hypertonic loss of Na$^+$), hypokalemia (augmented exchange with Na$^+$), and metabolic alkalosis (H ions exchange with Na$^+$ and increase bicarbonate reclamation). Mineralocorticoid excess secondary to an adrenal tumor represents primary aldosteronism, or Conn's syndrome. Diastolic hypertension, hypernatremia, hypokalemia, and metabolic alkalosis are the key abnormalities. Surreptitious intake of a thiazide diuretic produces the same findings as for a loop diuretic.

11. The answer is D: loss of the hypoxemic stimulus for breathing. The patient has a right posterior lobe lobar pneumonia secondary to *Klebsiella pneumoniae* with an added component of acute respiratory acidosis in addition to his already existing chronic respiratory acidosis from COPD. This mixed acid-base disorder further increases the PaCO$_2$, which further drops the PaO$_2$. Central chemoreceptors in the medulla are responsive to the pH of the cerebrospinal fluid (CSF). As CO$_2$ diffuses into the CSF, it combines with H$_2$O to form H$_2$CO$_3$, which dissociates into H ions and HCO$_3$ anions. Hydrogen ions act directly on the central chemoreceptors that stimulate breathing. Hence, increases in PaCO$_2$ and H ions are the stimuli for breathing, leading to elimination of excess CO$_2$, whereas a decrease in PaCO$_2$ and H ions inhibits breathing, with subsequent retention of CO$_2$. The peripheral chemoreceptors are stimulated by hypoxemia (a decrease in PaO$_2$), an increase in PaCO$_2$ (a less sensitive stimulus than noted in the central chemoreceptors), and an increase in H ions (in the carotid bodies only). Unlike the central chemoreceptors, the peripheral chemoreceptors are primarily responsible for the stimulation of respiration in response to hypoxemia, which is further potentiated by the presence of an increased PaCO$_2$ (which automatically decreases the PaO$_2$) and a reduction in arterial pH. Oxygen therapy must be approached with extreme caution, since some patients with chronic respiratory acidosis depend on hypoxemia as the primary stimulus for breathing. These patients have correction of the CSF pH back into the normal range despite increased PaCO$_2$ levels. Hence, H ions no longer stimulate the central chemoreceptors, and since they are insensitive to hypoxemia, the peripheral O$_2$-sensitive chemoreceptors (the carotid body in particular) assume responsibility for breathing. The administration of high-flow O$_2$ (> 28% O$_2$) may halt respiration in these patients by removing their stimulus for breathing.

12. The answer is B: serum Na$^+$, 150 mEq/L; serum Cl$^-$, 107 mEq/L; serum K$^+$, 2.0 mEq/L; serum bicarbonate, 34 mEq/L; UNa$^+$ > 20. The patient has primary aldosteronism, or Conn's syndrome. An unregulated increase in aldosterone leads to excess Na$^+$ retention (hypernatremia, diastolic hypertension) and augmented exchange of Na$^+$ for K$^+$ and H$^+$ in the distal and collecting ducts (hypokalemia—muscle weakness and metabolic alkalosis from increased reclamation of bicarbonate). In addition, there is an increased EABV, resulting in a

peritubular capillary $P_H > P_O$ and proximal tubule loss of Na^+ ($UNa^+ > 20$ mEq/L). The net renal loss of Na^+ counterbalances the excessive renal reabsorption of Na^+ by aldosterone, hence pitting edema is not seen in primary aldosteronism. Polyuria is due to the effect of chronic hypokalemia on renal tubules, which become refractory to ADH (acquired nephrogenic diabetes insipidus). Tetany is secondary to the effect of alkalosis, which increases negative charges on albumin. This causes albumin to bind more calcium than normal (it normally binds only 40% of circulating Ca^{2+}), and so additional calcium is removed from the ionized calcium pool, leading to tetany.

13. The answer is D: serum Na^+, 120 mEq/L; serum Cl^-, 86 mEq/L; serum K^+, 3.4 mEq/L; serum bicarbonate, 22 mEq/L; $UNa^+ > 20$. The patient has SiADH, most likely from a primary small-cell carcinoma of the lung with ectopic secretion of ADH. Excess ADH produces an unrestrained increase in the reabsorption of free water. This dilutes the serum Na^+ in the ECF compartment, producing a severe hyponatremia and osmotic shift of water into the ICF compartment. The EABV increases with subsequent suppression of aldosterone secretion. The peritubular capillary hydrostatic pressure is increased, leading to proximal tubule loss of Na^+ ($UNa^+ > 20$ mEq/L). The combination of Na^+ loss and concentration of the urine by ADH produces a Uosm that is greater than the Posm. Since the $TBNa^+$ is normal in SiADH, there is no evidence of pitting edema.

14. The answer is C: serum Na^+, 128 mEq/L; serum Cl^-, 96 mEq/L; serum K^+, 5.5 mEq/L; serum bicarbonate, 20 mEq/L; $UNa^+ > 20$. The patient has Addison's disease with destruction of the adrenal glands and loss of mineralocorticoids and cortisol. Hypoaldosteronism results in a hypertonic loss of Na^+ in the urine (hyponatremia with dehydration, increased UNa^+), retention of K^+ (hyperkalemia with peaked T waves), and retention of H ions (normal AG metabolic acidosis). Hypocortisolism leaves ACTH unopposed, hence producing increased skin pigmentation, most noticeable in the oral mucosa.

15. The answer is A: serum Na^+, 132 mEq/L; serum Cl^-, 86 mEq/L; serum K^+, 2.6 mEq/L; serum bicarbonate, 30 mEq/L; $UNa^+ > 20$. The patient is taking a diuretic, which predisposes to metabolic alkalosis. There is a hypertonic loss of fluid (hyponatremia, increased UNa^+, volume depletion) and augmented exchange of Na^+ for K^+ (hypokalemia, muscle weakness) and H^+ (increased bicarbonate reclamation leads to metabolic alkalosis) in the late distal and collecting tubules.

16. The answer is D: pH, 7.33 (7.35–7.45); $PaCO_2$, 60 mm Hg (33–44 mm Hg); HCO_3^-, 31 mEq/L (22–28 mEq/L). The patient has COPD secondary to smoking. The productive cough is secondary to chronic bronchitis. Chronic respiratory acidosis would be the expected ABG abnormality. A $PaCO_2$ of 60 mm Hg is respiratory acidosis ($PaCO_2 > 44$ mm Hg), an HCO_3^- of 31 mEq/L is metabolic alkalosis ($HCO_3^- > 28$ mEq/L), and the pH of 7.33 (< 7.35) is indicative of acidemia. This represents a primary respiratory acidosis with a partially compensated metabolic alkalosis (HCO_3^- is outside the normal range, and the pH is not in the normal range). Since the HCO_3^- is > 30 mEq/L, chronic rather than acute respiratory acidosis is present. Using the formula for chronic respiratory acidosis, the expected and calculated compensation are similar.

$$\Delta HCO_3^- = 0.40 \times \Delta PaCO_2; \text{ therefore, } \Delta HCO_3^- = 0.40 \times (60 - 40) = 8 \text{ mEq/L.}$$

$\Delta HCO_3^- = 24 + 8 = 32$ mEq/L, which is close enough to the measured HCO_3^- of 31 mEq/L; therefore, it is a simple rather than a mixed disorder.

17. The answer is I: pH, 7.52 (7.35–7.45); $PaCO_2$, 49 mm Hg (33–44 mm Hg); HCO_3^-, 39 mEq/L (22–28 mEq/L). The patient has metabolic alkalosis secondary to nasogastric suctioning of gastric acid from the stomach. A $PaCO_2$ of 49 mm Hg is respiratory acidosis ($PaCO_2 > 44$ mm Hg), an HCO_3^- of 39 mEq/L is metabolic alkalosis ($HCO_3^- > 28$ mEq/L), and the pH of 7.52 (> 7.45) is indicative of alkalemia. Therefore, the patient has a primary metabolic alkalosis with a partially compensated respiratory acidosis ($PaCO_2$ is outside the normal range, and the pH is not in the normal range). Using the formula for metabolic alkalosis, the expected and calculated compensation are similar.

$$\Delta PaCO_2 = 0.7 \times \Delta HCO_3^- \pm 2 \text{ mEq/L; therefore, } \Delta PaCO_2 = 0.7 \times (39 - 24) = 10.5 \text{ mEq/L.}$$

$$\Delta PaCO_2 = 40 + 10.5 = 50.5 \text{ mm Hg with } a \pm 2 \text{ range of 48.5–52.5 mm Hg.}$$

Since the measured $PaCO_2$ of 49 mm Hg is within the expected range of compensation, this is a simple rather than a mixed disorder.

18. The answer is J: pH, 7.52 (7.35–7.45); $PaCO_2$, 25 mm Hg (33–44 mm Hg); HCO_3^-, 20 mEq/L (22–28 mEq/L). The patient has a pulmonary embolus with infarction (pleuritic chest pain), which produces a perfusion defect in the lungs and hypoxemia. Pleuritic chest pain and stimulation of the J receptors in the lung interstitium produces tachypnea (rapid shallow breathing) and dyspnea (difficulty with breathing), leading to a respiratory alkalosis. A $PaCO_2$ of 25 mm Hg is respiratory alkalosis ($PaCO_2 < 33$ mm Hg), an HCO_3^- of 20 mEq/L is metabolic acidosis ($HCO_3^- < 22$ mEq/L), and the pH of 7.52 (> 7.45) is indicative of alkalemia. Hence, the patient has a primary respiratory alkalosis with a partially compensated metabolic acidosis (HCO_3^- is outside the normal range, and the pH is not in the normal range). Since the HCO_3^- is ≥ 18 mEq/L, it is an acute rather than a chronic respiratory alkalosis (< 18 mEq/L but > 12 mEq/L). Using the formula for acute respiratory alkalosis to calculate the expected compensation, the patient has a simple disorder.

$$\Delta HCO_3^- = 0.20 \times \Delta PaCO_2; \text{ therefore, } \Delta HCO_3^- = 0.20 \times (40 - 25) = 3.$$

$$\Delta HCO_3^- = 24 - 3 = 21 \text{ mEq/L, which is close enough to the measured } HCO_3^- \text{ of 20 mEq/L.}$$

Postsurgical patients are particularly prone to developing deep saphenous vein thrombosis in the lower extremities and embolization to the lungs from the femoral vein as the thrombus propagates proximally. The pain in the calf associated with dorsiflexion of the foot is called Homan's sign.

19. The answer is C: pH, 7.30 (7.35–7.45); $PaCO_2$, 30 mm Hg (33–44 mm Hg); HCO_3^-, 14 mEq/L (22–28 mEq/L). The patient has ingested methyl alcohol (methanol), which is first converted to formaldehyde and then to formic acid. Formic acid irritates the optic nerve, producing blurry vision and possible permanent blindness. Furthermore, the addition of formic acid to the ECF pro-

duces an increased anion gap metabolic acidosis. A $PaCO_2$ of 30 mm Hg is respiratory alkalosis ($PaCO_2 <$ 33 mm Hg), an HCO_3^- of 14 mEq/L is metabolic acidosis ($HCO_3^- < 22$ mEq/L), and the pH of 7.30 (< 7.35) is indicative of acidemia. Therefore, the patient has a primary metabolic acidosis with a partially compensated respiratory alkalosis ($PaCO_2$ is outside the normal range, and the pH is not in the normal range). The metabolic acidosis formula used to calculate the expected compensation indicates the presence of a simple acid-base disorder.

$$\Delta\ PaCO_2 = 1.2 \times \Delta\ HCO_3^- \pm 2 \text{ mm Hg; therefore,}$$
$$\Delta\ PaCO_2 = 1.2 \times (24 - 14) = 12 \text{ mm Hg.}$$

$$\Delta\ PaCO_2 = 40 - 12 = 28 \text{ mm Hg, with a}$$
$$\pm\ 2 \text{ range of } 26\text{--}30 \text{ mm Hg.}$$

The calculated $PaCO_2$ is within range of the measured $PaCO_2$; therefore, the disorder is a simple rather than a mixed disorder. A disparity between the calculated osmolality and the measured osmolality of >10 mOsm/kg indicates the presence of unmeasured osmoles (e.g., ethyl alcohol, ethylene glycol, methanol); given the history of visual abnormalities, methyl alcohol is the prime suspect. Infusion of ethyl alcohol is the treatment of choice, since both alcohols compete with alcohol dehydrogenase for metabolic breakdown. Unmetabolized methyl alcohol is then removed from the plasma by dialysis.

20. The answer is C. Excessive sweating produces a hypotonic loss of fluid (more water than salt), hence the patient should have hypernatremia ($\uparrow$ serum $\uparrow Na^+ \cong \downarrow TBNa^+/\downarrow\downarrow TBW$) and volume depletion (low $TBNa^+$). The Posm is increased, and the EABV is decreased (hypovolemia). Hypernatremia leads to an osmotic shift of water out of the ICF (contracted) into the ECF; however, owing to fluid loss from sweating, it does not replenish the ECF volume.

21. The answer is G. The patient has SiADH due to stimulation of ADH release by chlorpropamide, a first-generation oral sulfonylurea drug. Increased ADH leads to increased reabsorption of free water and a dilutional hyponatremia ($\downarrow$ serum $Na^+ \cong TBNa^+/\uparrow\uparrow TBW$). The osmotic gradient favors water movement into the ICF compartment (mental status abnormalities are related to cerebral edema). Eventually, the plasma volume increases as well as the EABV, which inhibits the RAA system (increasing renal blood flow) and reduces the proximal tubule reabsorption of Na^+, since the peritubular capillary hydrostatic pressure is greater than the oncotic pressure. This increases the random UNa^+ to > 20 mEq/L ($UNa^+ = 80$ mEq/L in this patient). Discontinuation of the drug and water restriction would correct the fluid overload.

22. The answer is E. The patient has the nephrotic syndrome (24-hour urine protein > 3.5 g). The loss of albumin is responsible for a reduction in oncotic pressure, leading to generalized edema (anasarca). Diffuse membranous glomerulonephritis is the most common cause of the adult nephrotic syndrome. Since a considerable amount of ECF volume is in the interstitial space, the venous return to the right heart is decreased, thereby producing a decreased EABV. The baroreceptor reflex stimulates the hypothalamic release of ADH, and the reduced renal blood flow activates the RAA system with subsequent release of aldosterone. The peritubular hydrostatic pressure is reduced, favoring the proximal tubule reabsorption of Na^+. The final tonicity of the reabsorbed fluid is hypotonic (more water than salt), which produces hyponatremia ($\downarrow$ serum $Na^+ \uparrow \cong TBNa^+/\uparrow\uparrow TBW$), pitting edema ($\uparrow TBNa^+$), and movement of water into the ICF. Unfortunately, the hypotonic fluid is driven into the interstitial space by the reduced plasma oncotic pressure without restoring the EABV. Note that schematics E and G are similar except for the EABV. Schematic E represents the patient with SiADH, with an increase in the EABV, whereas the patient with nephrotic syndrome had a decrease in the EABV owing to the alteration in Starling's forces.

23. The answer is A. Overzealous administration of isotonic saline will result in a fluid overload with no alteration in the serum Na^+, since the fluid is isotonic ($\leftrightarrow$ serum $Na^+ \cong \uparrow TBNa^+/\uparrow TBW$). Because the $TBNa^+$ is increased, the patient has pitting edema. The absence of an osmotic gradient leaves the ICF compartment volume the same, while the ECF compartment is expanded. The plasma volume is increased, hence increasing the EABV.

24. The answer is G: bleeding time, prolonged; platelet count, normal; prothrombin time (PT), normal; partial thromboplastin time (PTT), prolonged. The history and laboratory findings are consistent with VWD. All the factor components are decreased (VIII:vWF, VIII:Ag, VIII:C) in classical autosomal dominant VWD. The decreased VIII:vWF is responsible for the prolonged bleeding time (platelet adhesion defect) and the abnormal ristocetin platelet aggregation test (ristocetin enhances platelet aggregation if circulating VIII:vWF is present). Low VIII:C produces a prolonged aPTT, which is a measure of the intrinsic system (XII $\rightarrow$ XI $\rightarrow$ IX $\rightarrow$ **VIII** $\rightarrow$ X $\rightarrow$ V $\rightarrow$ II $\rightarrow$ I $\rightarrow$ clot). The PT is normal, since it evaluates the extrinsic system down to the formation of a clot (VII $\rightarrow$ X $\rightarrow$ V $\rightarrow$ II $\rightarrow$ I $\rightarrow$ clot). Menorrhagia is a common complication of VWD. Easy bruisability is a feature of a platelet abnormality, in this case, a defect in platelet adhesion.

25. The answer is B: bleeding time, prolonged; platelet count, normal; prothrombin time (PT), normal; partial thromboplastin time (PTT), normal. Aspirin irreversibly acetylates platelet cyclooxygenase, leading to inhibition of TXA_2 synthesis and subsequent inhibition of platelet aggregation. This prolongs the bleeding time but has no effect on the platelet count or coagulation studies, the latter not being affected by platelet abnormalities. Since arterial thrombi are primarily composed of platelets, aspirin prevents the formation of a thrombus overlying atherosclerotic plaque in the coronary vessels.

26. The answer is A: bleeding time, prolonged; platelet count, decreased; prothrombin time (PT), normal; partial thromboplastin time (PTT), normal. The patient has idiopathic (autoimmune) thrombocytopenia (ITP), which is produced by an IgG antibody against the fibrinogen receptor on platelets (GPIIb:IIIa), with subsequent removal of the sensitized platelets by macrophages in the spleen (type II hypersensitivity). Megakaryocytes are present in the bone marrow, indicating the absence of a production defect. Thrombocytopenia prolongs the bleeding time, since fewer platelets are available to form a primary hemostatic plug. Splenomegaly is not a feature of ITP. The condition resolves with corticosteroid therapy.

27. The answer is A: bleeding time, prolonged; platelet count, decreased; prothrombin time (PT), normal; partial thromboplastin time (PTT), normal. The patient has the hemolytic uremic syndrome (HUS) secondary to

ingestion of the toxin produced by *E. coli* serotype O157:H7 in improperly cooked ground beef. The toxin damages endothelial cells, resulting in the deposition of platelet thrombi that block the microvasculature (leading to CNS signs, renal failure, and thrombocytopenia) and injure RBCs, producing a microangiopathic hemolytic anemia characterized by numerous schistocytes (fragmented RBCs). Since the coagulation factors are not consumed (as they would be in DIC), the coagulation studies are normal. Thrombocytopenia prolongs the bleeding time.

CHAPTER SIX

DISORDERS OF NUTRITION

SYNOPSIS

OBJECTIVES

1. To understand how to assess the nutritional status of a patient.
2. To describe the clinical and laboratory aspects of the eating disorders including anorexia nervosa, bulimia nervosa, and obesity.
3. To review the clinical and laboratory aspects of protein-energy malnutrition (PEM) with particular reference to kwashiorkor and marasmus.
4. To understand the clinical disorders associated with micronutrient deficiency (vitamins and trace elements).
5. To describe the role of dietary fiber in disease.
6. To discuss the role of diet in preventing cancer.
7. To review the nutritional changes associated with aging.
8. To understand the significance of special diets.

Objective 1: To understand how to assess the nutritional status of a patient.

I. Nutritional assessment
   A. Dietary factors (high-fat, low-fiber diets) are associated with heart disease (36%), cancer (22%), and stroke (7%), accounting for two-thirds of all deaths in the United States.
   B. **Macronutrient deficiencies** (protein, fat, and carbohydrates) are assessed by measuring body weight (total body composition), measuring body fat composition in skin folds with calipers, and performing tests that evaluate immunocompetence (e.g., cutaneous sensitivity to common antigens) and protein concentration (e.g., albumin, transferrin, prealbumin, retinol-binding protein).
   C. **Micronutrient deficiencies** (vitamins and trace elements) are evaluated with "static" tests of nutritional status at a point in time (e.g., serum folate) or with functional tests that determine how the nutrient performs a specific biochemical event or physiologic function (e.g., the effect on transketolase activity after thiamine pyrophosphate is added).

Objective 2: To describe the clinical and laboratory aspects of the eating disorders including anorexia nervosa, bulimia nervosa, and obesity.

II. Eating disorders
   A. Anorexia nervosa and bulimia nervosa most commonly afflict young women and sometimes men.
      1. In **anorexia nervosa**, the patient has a distorted body image, resulting in significant weight loss.
         a. A loss of body weight below 15% of normal in women reduces the secretion of gonadotropin-releasing hormone (GnRH), thereby reducing gonadotropin secretion, with subsequent development of secondary amenorrhea (causing significant potential for osteoporosis).
         b. Stress hormones such as cortisol, adrenocorticotropic hormone (ACTH), and growth hormone are increased.
         c. Ventricular arrhythmias are the most common cause of death.
      2. **Bulimia nervosa** is the voluntary vomiting of food, usually after "bingeing" on massive amounts of food.
         a. The body weight is usually normal, and the body image is not as distorted as in anorexia nervosa.
         b. Physical signs include acid injury to tooth enamel, bruising of the knuckles, and swelling of the salivary glands.
         c. Serious complications related to vomiting include the Mallory-Weiss syndrome (laceration of esophageal or stomach mucosa), Boerhaave's syndrome (rupture of the stomach or distal esophagus), and electrolyte disturbances (hypokalemic metabolic alkalosis).
   B. **Obesity** is defined as a body weight >20% above the ideal body weight or a body mass index (BMI; the weight in kilograms divided by the height in meters squared) >30 kg/m^2.
      1. Its pathogenesis is multifactorial and includes hereditary factors (e.g., abnormality in the feeding and satiety center), ethnicity (e.g., increased prevalence in Native American, Hispanic, and African American populations), psychological factors (e.g., depression), and biological factors (e.g., hypothyroidism).
      2. In abdominal obesity (waist-to-hip ratio approaching 1), there is an increased incidence of coronary artery disease, hypertension, stroke, diabetes mellitus, cholesterol stones, and cancers of the breast and endometrium.

Objective 3: To review the clinical and laboratory aspects of protein-energy malnutrition (PEM) with particular reference to kwashiorkor and marasmus.

III. Protein-energy malnutrition (PEM)
   A. PEM occurs when the supply of protein and/or calories is inadequate for the demands of the body.
      1. The four phases of malnutrition are the following:

a. Inadequate availability of nutrients (e.g., poor diet, increased demand [as in pregnancy]) leading to a negative nitrogen balance.

b. Depletion of nutrient stores (water-soluble vitamins are more affected than fat-soluble vitamins).

c. Alteration in biochemical and physiological processes ("static" and functional tests are abnormal).

d. Symptomatic malnutrition (signs and symptoms of the deficiency are present).

2. Complications of malnutrition include the following:

a. Reduction in body mass and fat stores.

b. Organ atrophy.

c. Endocrine abnormalities (similar to those seen in anorexia nervosa).

d. Alterations in the immune system, such as anergy (no cutaneous reaction to antigens), reduced numbers of CD4 T helper cells, a low total lymphocyte count, defects in the complement system, and abnormal phagocytic function.

B. **Kwashiorkor** refers to protein deficiency in the presence of a normal caloric intake (primarily carbohydrates), whereas **marasmus** is a total calorie deprivation.

1. Abnormalities common to both subsets of PEM include anemia and growth failure.

2. Clinical findings more commonly associated with kwashiorkor include pitting edema (hypoalbuminemia), flaky-paint dermatitis, apathy, protuberant abdomen (a fatty liver due to excess carbohydrate intake and decreased apolipoprotein synthesis), diarrhea (loss of brush border enzymes), normal muscle mass and subcutaneous fat, and a depressed immune response.

3. Clinical findings more commonly noted in marasmus consist of loss of muscle mass and subcutaneous fat, alertness, and "broomstick" extremities.

Objective 4: To understand the clinical disorders associated with micronutrient deficiency (vitamins and trace elements).

IV. Vitamin overview

A. Vitamins are either fat soluble (vitamins A, D, E, and K) or water soluble (e.g., B_1, B_2, B_3, B_6).

B. Both types of vitamins are reabsorbed in the proximal small intestine with the exception of vitamin B_{12}, which is reabsorbed in the terminal ileum.

C. Vitamins are micronutrients that may serve as cofactors in biochemical reactions (water-soluble vitamins), as substrates in biochemical reactions (water-soluble vitamins), in cell growth and differentiation (A, folate, and B_{12}), as antioxidants (β-carotene, E, selenium), or as hormones (D).

V. Fat-soluble vitamin disorders

A. **Vitamin A (retinol)** functions in vision and promotes cell growth and differentiation.

1. Retinol normally maintains the light-sensitive pigment rhodopsin in the rods for night vision and iodopsin in the cones for daytime vision, prevents squamous metaplasia of epithelial cells, and serves as an antioxidant that traps free radicals (β-carotene effect).

2. Thyroxine enhances the conversion of β-carotene to retinol in the intestinal cell, following which retinol either circulates in association with retinol-binding protein (RBP) or is stored as retinol esters in the liver (esters are converted to retinol and then bound to RBP before entering the circulation).

3. Vitamin A **deficiency** is most commonly due to malabsorption, liver disease, or diets lacking β-carotene (e.g., due to decreased intake of green vegetables).

a. Ophthalmologic problems include night blindness (nyctalopia), squamous metaplasia of the corneal epithelium (Bitot's spots) and the lacrimal duct (xerosis, or drying of the eyes), softening of the cornea (keratomalacia), corneal ulcers, infection, and blindness.

b. Respiratory disorders consist of bronchitis and pneumonia (squamous metaplasia of the normally ciliated pseudostratified columnar epithelium) and possibly lung cancer.

c. Growth retardation is present in children owing to decreased epiphyseal bone formation.

d. Follicular hyperkeratosis (which looks like "goose bumps") occurs secondary to squamous metaplasia in the hair follicles.

4. Vitamin A **toxicity** is associated with an increase in intracranial pressure (which produces papilledema, bulging fontanelles, and convulsions), bone pain (periostitis), hypercalcemia (synergism with vitamin D and parathormone), and a yellowish discoloration of the skin (the sclera remains white).

B. **Vitamin D** is obtained from sunlight and dietary sources.

1. Skin-derived 7-dehydrocholesterol is converted to vitamin D_3 (cholecalciferol; effect of ultraviolet B light), and both skin- and diet-derived vitamin D are hydroxylated in the liver to form 25-(OH)-D_3 cholecalciferol (calcidiol).

a. 25-(OH)-D_3 may remain in the liver for storage, circulate in the blood bound to a protein (the main circulating form of non–renal-derived vitamin D), or undergo a second hydroxylation step in the kidneys via the enzyme 1α-hydroxylase, which converts 25-(OH)-D_3 to 1,25-(OH)$_2$-D_3 (calcitriol).

b. Enhancers of enzyme synthesis include parathormone (PTH) and hypophosphatemia, while inhibitors of enzyme synthesis consist of 1,25-(OH)$_2$-D_3 and hyperphosphatemia (when inhibition occurs, 25-(OH)-D_3 is converted to an inactive metabolite designated 24,25-(OH)$_2$-D_3).

c. Receptors for vitamin D are located in the duodenum (where they reabsorb calcium and phosphorus) and on osteoblasts (where they initiate the mineralization of bone and cartilage).

d. When PTH attaches to its receptors on osteoblasts, interleukin-1 is released, which activates osteoclasts, with the subsequent release of calcium into the blood (vitamin D assists in this function as well).

e. Both PTH and calcitriol directly stimulate macrophage precursors in the bone marrow to differentiate into osteoclasts, further enhancing bone resorption.

f. Approximately 40% of the total calcium in plasma is bound to albumin (hypoalbuminemia decreases the total calcium concentration), 13% is complexed with citrate and phosphate, and the remaining 47% represents physiologically active ionized calcium.

g. Osteoclasts have receptors for calcitonin, which normally inhibits their activity.

h. A decrease in $1,25\text{-}(OH)_2\text{-}D_3$ concentration in plasma leads to the following series of biochemical reactions: hypocalcemia and hypophosphatemia (decreased reabsorption) → increased PTH (stimulus of hypocalcemia; secondary hyperparathyroidism) → an unfavorable solubility product (calcium × phosphorus) for bone mineralization → increased bone resorption by osteoclasts (increased PTH) → a bone disease called rickets in children and osteomalacia in adults.

i. An increase in $1,25\text{-}(OH)_2\text{-}D_3$ concentration in plasma produces the following series of reactions: hypercalcemia and hyperphosphatemia → suppression of PTH release (hypercalcemia and increased $1,25\text{-}(OH_2)\text{-}D_3$) → excess bone resorption ($1,25\text{-}(OH)_2\text{-}D_3$ increases osteoclast synthesis) → increased solubility product that drives calcium into soft tissue (metastatic calcification).

j. Either an increase or a decrease in vitamin D results in excess bone resorption.

2. Vitamin D **deficiency** results from poor diet (in people with alcoholism or the elderly), malabsorption of fat (celiac disease), liver disease (cirrhosis), renal failure (the most common cause; due to reduced quantities of 1α-hydroxylase), hypoparathyroidism or hyperphosphatemia (owing to decreased enzyme synthesis), or genetic diseases characterized by either enzyme deficiency (type I vitamin D–dependent rickets) or a deficiency of vitamin D receptors in target tissue (type II vitamin D–dependent rickets).

a. Clinical findings common to both rickets and osteomalacia are a loss of bone density (osteopenia), Looser's lines (blood vessels in the metaphysis push aside the soft osteoid, producing linear lines resembling a fracture), and bowed legs (the soft osteoid yields under stress).

b. Clinical findings predominating in rickets rather than osteomalacia consist of defective mineralization of cartilage in the epiphyseal growth plates as well as abnormal calcification of osteoid at the bone-osteoid interface (adults have only defective mineralization of the diaphysis), skeletal deformities, widening of the osteoid seams in the epiphyses (rachitic rosary), and craniotabes (excess osteoid in the skull produces an increased elastic recoil on palpation).

c. Measurement of the serum $25\text{-}(OH)\text{-}D_3$, representing vitamin D generated from diet and photoformation (nonrenal sources of vitamin D), best represents vitamin D status owing to its circulating half-life of 3 weeks.

d. Because of the short half-life of $1,25\text{-}(OH)_2\text{-}D_3$ (4–6 hours), its measurement is most useful in differentiating type I from type II vitamin D–dependent rickets (decreased and increased, respectively).

e. Hypocalcemia is present in all the diseases associated with vitamin D deficiency previously listed.

f. Hypophosphatemia occurs in deficiency of nonrenal origin (e.g., malabsorption, poor diet) and in types I and II vitamin D–dependent rickets.

g. Defective mineralization of bone leading to rickets and osteomalacia may also occur with hypophosphatemia, since phosphorus is the driving force for depositing calcium in bone once the solubility product is favorable for mineralization.

h. Hyperphosphatemia is noted in deficiency of renal origin (decreased excretion) and in hypoparathyroidism (retention of phosphate; PTH is normally phosphaturic).

i. PTH levels are generally increased in all the deficiencies (except hypoparathyroidism).

j. $25\text{-}(OH)\text{-}D_3$ levels are normal in all the deficiencies (except for deficiency of nonrenal origin, in which it is decreased).

3. **Hypervitaminosis D** is associated with metastatic calcification to multiple organ systems, most notably the kidneys (nephrocalcinosis) and laboratory abnormalities consisting of hypercalcemia, hyperphosphatemia, hypercalcinuria (which predisposes to stone formation), and low PTH levels (effect of hypercalcemia).

C. **α-Tocopherol** is the most active form of **vitamin E**.

1. The primary function of α-tocopherol is as an antioxidant that prevents free radical catalyzed–lipid peroxidation of polyunsaturated fatty acids in cell membranes throughout the body.

2. Vitamin E **deficiency** is uncommon and is associated with neurologic problems (ataxia, peripheral neuropathy), muscle degeneration, and hemolytic anemia, the last most commonly in premature infants.

D. **Vitamin K_1** is produced in plants and is converted by bacteria in the large bowel to the less active vitamin K_2.

1. Vitamin K_1 is a coenzyme for protein activation of the liver-derived vitamin K–dependent factors (II [prothrombin], VII, IX, X, proteins C and S) by posttranslational γ-carboxylation of their glutamic acid residues (Chapter 5).

2. Vitamin K **deficiency** produces a hemorrhagic disorder (Chapter 5) and may be secondary to breast milk feeding in newborns (decreased vitamin K in breast milk plus decreased bacterial flora in the newborn bowel), fat malabsorption (e.g., bile salt deficiency), drugs interfering with vitamin K metabolism (e.g., warfarin), and antibiotic therapy (which destroys the vitamin-producing bacteria).

VI. Water-soluble vitamin disorders

A. Water-soluble vitamins are important primarily in biochemical reactions where they may act as reducing agents (vitamin C); as cofactors in oxidative decarboxylation (thiamine, pyridoxine), oxidative phosphorylation (riboflavin, niacin), carboxylase (biotin), and transamination (pyridoxine) reactions; as components of coenzyme A (pantothenic acid); and in DNA synthesis (folate and B_{12}).

B. **Vitamin C (ascorbic acid)** is present in citrus fruits, green vegetables, and other fruits and vegetables.

1. Ascorbic acid (AA) primarily acts as a reducing agent (e.g., in posttranslational modification of proline and lysine in collagen synthesis, in reduction of iron from the ferric to the ferrous state), and as an antioxidant (e.g., it traps free radicals).

2. **Deficiency** of ascorbic acid produces a condition called scurvy.

   a. Owing to a lack of hydroxylation, which interferes with the cross-linking of collagen fibers with each other, the tensile strength of collagen is impaired, hence disrupting normal wound healing, vascular stability (causing cutaneous and subperiosteal hemorrhage, hemarthroses, perifollicular hemorrhage), and bone formation (structurally abnormal osteoid leads to a scorbutic rosary of the ribs in children).

   b. Additional findings include corkscrew hairs, gum hyperplasia with periodontitis and loss of teeth, glossitis (inflammation of the tongue), anemia (iron or folate deficiency), and an increased bleeding time (Chapter 5).

3. **Excess** ascorbic acid produces false-negative reactions for blood, glucose, bilirubin, nitrites, and leukocyte esterase in urine tests that utilize dipstick reagents.

C. **Thiamine** is present in high concentration in meats (pork), grains (wheat), and legumes.

1. **Thiamine pyrophosphate** (TPP) is a cofactor in the oxidative decarboxylation and RBC transketolase enzyme reactions (two-carbon transfer reactions) in the pentose phosphate pathway.

   a. Owing to its important role as a cofactor in the pyruvate dehydrogenase complex, which converts pyruvate into acetyl-CoA (acetyl-CoA then combines with oxaloacetate to produce citrate in the tricarboxylic acid cycle), a deficiency of thiamine has a direct effect on reducing ATP synthesis, hence producing major alterations in the nervous and cardiovascular systems.

   b. In branched-chain amino acid metabolism, branched chain α-keto acid dehydrogenase complex requires TPP as a cofactor (absence of this enzyme results in maple syrup urine disease).

2. Thiamine **deficiency** results in the classic findings of beriberi (dry or wet).

   a. In Asia, deficiency is due to removal of the vitamin from the outer portion of rice, while in the United States, it is most commonly the result of a poor diet in alcoholism.

   b. Neurologic disturbances (dry beriberi; Chapter 22) include peripheral neuropathy (distal sensorimotor neuropathy), Wernicke's encephalopathy (confusion, ataxia, ophthalmoplegia [eye muscle palsies] and nystagmus), and Korsakoff's psychosis (inability to remember new and old information and confabulation).

   c. Beriberi heart disease (wet beriberi; Chapter 10) is primarily of the congestive (dilated) type and presents with both left and right heart failure.

   d. The laboratory diagnosis is secured by performing a functional assay that compares the basal and stimulated RBC transketolase activity before and after administration of TPP (transketolase activity is decreased in the basal state and increased after TPP infusion, indicating thiamine deficiency).

D. **Riboflavin (B_2)** is present in dairy products, liver, and green leafy vegetables and is also synthesized by bacteria in the bowel.

1. It is an essential component of flavin mononucleotide (FMN) and flavin adenine dinucleotide (FAD), which are important in oxidative phosphorylation reactions in the mitochondria, and it is an important component of glutathione reductase in the pentose phosphate shunt (reduced glutathione is a potent antioxidant).

2. Riboflavin **deficiency** is characterized by corneal neovascularization (the most common sign), a greasy appearing facial rash (seborrheic dermatitis), fissuring and dry scaling of the vermilion borders of the lips (cheilosis) and the angles of the mouth (angular cheilosis/stomatitis), and a magenta-colored tongue.

E. **Niacin (B_3)**, or **nicotinic acid**, is present in meats, fish, vegetables, nuts, and yeast; is synthesized by bacteria in the bowel; and is endogenously synthesized from tryptophan.

1. Both niacin and nicotinamide (derived from the diet and converted to nicotinic acid in the body) are required for the formation of nicotinamide adenine dinucleotide (NAD^+) and nicotinamide adenine dinucleotide phosphate ($NADP^+$), which are cofactors for most of the oxidation reduction reactions in the body.

2. Key reactions include the following:

$$\text{Glyceraldehyde 3-phosphate} \xrightleftharpoons{NAD^+/NADH\ +\ H^+} 1,3$$

diphosphoglycerate in glycolysis.

$$\text{Lactate} \xrightleftharpoons{NAD^+/NADH\ +\ H^+} \text{pyruvate in glycolysis.}$$

$$\text{Acetoacetate} \xrightleftharpoons{NADH/NAD^+} \beta\text{-hydroxybutyrate}$$

in ketone body synthesis.

$$\text{Malate} \xrightleftharpoons{NAD^+/NADH\ +\ H^+} \text{oxaloacetate in gluconeogenesis}$$

$$\text{Glucose 6-phosphate} \xrightarrow{NADP^+/NADPH\ +\ H^+} \text{6-phospho-}$$

gluconate in the pentose phosphate pathway.

3. Niacin **deficiency**, or **pellagra**, is common where corn is the primary source of energy (corn is deficient in tryptophan, hence the relationship with niacin deficiency).

   a. It is characterized by a triad of diarrhea, dementia, and dermatitis (increased skin pigmentation in sun-exposed areas, e.g., Casal's necklace).

   b. Tryptophan (an essential amino acid) deficiency also produces pellagra, hence the relationship with Hartnup disease (defective intestinal and renal uptake of neutral and essential amino acids) and the carcinoid syndrome (owing to increased synthesis of serotonin from tryptophan).

4. Niacin is used therapeutically in lowering LDL and VLDL owing to its inhibition of lipolysis in adipose tissue, hence reducing the release of fatty acids and lipid synthesis.

F. **Pyridoxine (B₆)** is abundant in most foods (but not in unfortified goat's milk).

1. It functions as a cofactor in the form of **pyridoxal phosphate**, which is involved in heme synthesis (conversion of glycine and succinyl-CoA to δ-aminolevulinic acid), transamination reactions (transfer of the amino group from an amino acid to an α-keto acid, e.g., alanine to α-ketoglutarate), deamination reactions (serine conversion to pyruvate and ammonia), decarboxylation reactions (histidine conversion to histamine and CO_2), niacin synthesis from tryptophan, and neurotransmitter synthesis (γ-aminobutyric acid, serotonin, and norepinephrine).

2. Pyridoxine **deficiency** is most commonly associated with use of certain drugs (e.g., isoniazid) and is associated with gastrointestinal (cheilosis/stomatitis and glossitis), hematologic (sideroblastic anemia with ringed sideroblasts; Chapter 12), and neurologic (abnormal electroencephalogram) abnormalities (convulsions).

G. **Pantothenic acid** is a component of coenzyme A (which transfers acyl groups) and fatty acid synthase (a key enzyme in fatty acid synthesis).

H. **Biotin** is involved in carboxylation reactions (e.g., the pyruvate carboxylase reaction in which pyruvate is converted into oxaloacetate) and may be deficient owing to the presence of avidin in raw egg whites, which prevents its absorption in the small bowel.

I. **Vitamin B₁₂** and **folate** (Chapter 12) are involved in DNA synthesis (deficiency of either vitamin results in a macrocytic anemia), and B₁₂ is active in propionate metabolism:

$$\text{Propionyl-CoA} \rightarrow \text{methylmalonyl-CoA}$$
$$\xrightarrow{B_{12}} \text{succinyl-CoA}$$

1. B₁₂ is a cobalamin compound (it contains cobalt in the center) that is primarily obtained from animal products in the diet and requires intrinsic factor, synthesized in the parietal cells of the stomach, for reabsorption in the terminal ileum (there is a potential problem with reabsorption if Crohn's disease is present).

2. B₁₂ removes the methyl group from methyltetrahydrofolate (circulating form of folate) to produce tetrahydrofolate (THF), which is a cofactor in purine and pyrimidine metabolism and in one-carbon transfers to other intermediates for the synthesis of amino acids, purines, and pyrimidines.

3. Deficiency of B₁₂ results in a build-up of propionates, which produces neurologic abnormalities.

4. Pernicious anemia is the most common cause of B₁₂ deficiency.

5. Folate is present in green leafy vegetables and whole grains in the polyglutamate form, which must be converted to a monoglutamate by intestinal conjugase (which is inhibited by phenytoin) in order to be reabsorbed in the jejunum.

6. Liver stores of folate last only 3–4 months, so dietary deficiency is common, particularly in non–beer-drinking people with alcoholism (beer is rich in folates).

VII. Trace element disorders

A. Trace elements are micronutrients that most commonly serve as cofactors in enzymes or are components of prosthetic groups.

B. Atomic absorption spectrophotometry is the gold standard in measuring trace elements.

C. Trace element deficiencies arise from decreased intake (e.g., due to total parenteral nutrition), decreased absorption (e.g., due to malabsorption, phytates in the diet), increased excretion (e.g., due to chelation therapy), and increased requirement (e.g., due to old age, diabetes mellitus).

1. **Chromium** potentiates insulin activity, hence its deficiency results in glucose intolerance.

2. **Copper** is involved in oxidation-reduction reactions and is bound in the circulation to ceruloplasmin, which is synthesized in the liver.

   a. It is a cofactor for the following enzymes:

   (1) Lysyl oxidase (it cross-links collagen to increase tensile strength).

   (2) Cytochrome *c* oxidase (it functions in the electron transport system).

   (3) Superoxide dismutase (SOD; an antioxidant that neutralizes superoxide free radicals).

   (4) Ferroxidase (it converts ferrous to ferric iron for binding to transferrin).

   (5) Tyrosinase (it converts tyrosine to dopa in melanin synthesis).

   b. Deficiency results in poor wound healing, dissecting aortic aneurysms, skin depigmentation, microcytic anemia (iron deficiency), and osteoporosis.

   c. Wilson's disease is an autosomal recessive disease characterized by a defect in the excretion of copper into bile that results in chronic liver disease, reduction in ceruloplasmin synthesis (low copper levels), and an increase in free copper, which deposits in the eye (Kayser-Fleischer ring) and the lenticular nuclei (Chapter 16).

3. **Fluorine** is incorporated into bone and tooth enamel.

   a. Deficiency leads to dental caries.

   b. Toxicity produces mottled teeth and calcification of ligaments and tendons.

4. **Manganese** is a cofactor for SOD and glycosyltransferases, which are involved in the synthesis of mucopolysaccharides.

5. **Molybdenum** is a cofactor in xanthine oxidase, which is important in uric acid synthesis in purine metabolism.

6. **Selenium** is a cofactor in glutathione peroxidase (which is important in the synthesis of glutathione, a potent antioxidant against peroxides) and iodinases that are involved in the peripheral conversion of thyroxine (T₄) to triiodothyronine (T₃).

   a. It serves its antioxidant role in the cytosol, whereas vitamin E primarily acts as an antioxidant in the cell membrane.

   b. Its deficiency results in muscle pain and weakness and cardiomyopathy.

7. **Zinc** is a cofactor in enzyme reactions.
   a. It is a cofactor for:
      (1) Carbonic anhydrase (for bicarbonate reabsorption in the kidneys).
      (2) SOD (it neutralizes superoxide free radicals).
      (3) Alkaline phosphatase (for bone mineralization).
      (4) Collagenases (it replaces type III collagen in a wound by type I collagen).
   b. Zinc deficiency is common in people with diabetes or alcoholism with cirrhosis.
   c. Zinc deficiency is associated with growth retardation, hypogonadism, dysgeusia (decreased taste sensation), poor wound healing, and a rash around the eyes and mouth.

Objective 5: To describe the role of dietary fiber in disease.

VIII. Dietary fiber
   A. Dietary fiber consists of endogenous components of plant materials that are resistant to human digestive enzymes (e.g., cellulose, lignin).
   B. The **insoluble**, or **nonfermentable**, part of fiber (e.g., wheat bran, wheat germ), absorbs water, binds potential carcinogens (e.g., lithocholic acid), and reduces stool transit time, thus protecting against constipation and diverticulosis.
   C. The **soluble**, or **fermentable**, portion of fiber (e.g., oat bran) lowers serum cholesterol, increases fecal bacterial mass, and has a hypoglycemic effect that improves carbohydrate metabolism in people with diabetes.
   D. Increased fiber reduces stool pH, which keeps secondary bile acids such as lithocholic acid (a carcinogen) in a protonated state, hence facilitating their excretion.
   E. Fiber reduces deconjugation of estrogen delivered in bile, so less hormone is reabsorbed back into the circulation (this may have a protective effect against breast, endometrial, and ovarian cancers).
   F. It is recommended that the daily diet contain 20–30 grams of fiber.

Objective 6: To discuss the role of diet in preventing cancer.

IX. Diet and cancer
   A. Evidence suggests that an increased intake of fiber and decreased intake in saturated fats and ω-6 polyunsaturated lipids has a protective effect against cancer.
   B. Evidence also suggests that increased dietary intake of cruciferous vegetables (e.g., broccoli and cauliflower) and fruits and vegetables containing β-carotenoids, vitamin C, and vitamin E reduces the risk for oral, esophageal, stomach, and lung cancers.
   C. Both an increase in dietary fat and a decrease in fiber enhance the carcinogenicity of lithocholic acid in producing colon cancer, the former by increasing the amount of lithocholic acid and the latter by increasing the exposure time of colonic epithelium to lithocholic acid.

D. Patients on a high-fat diet have an increase in free estrogen and estrogen metabolites that produce hormone imbalances which may predispose to an increased risk for breast, endometrial, ovarian, and prostate cancers.
   1. Monounsaturated oils such as olive oil and ω-3 polyunsaturated lipids (e.g., fish oils, canola oil) have a protective effect on hormone metabolism.
   2. Cereal fiber and pectin inhibit the recycling of hormones (e.g., estrogen).
   E. Foods contaminated with aflatoxins increase the risk for hepatocellular carcinoma.
   F. Free radicals and reactive oxygen molecules have been implicated in the initiation (irreversible mutation), promotion (clonal expansion of the initiated cell), and progression (later stages) of carcinogenesis.
      1. Reactive oxygen molecules (e.g., superoxide) are involved in all three stages owing to their ability to be directly mutagenic to DNA or to activate chemical procarcinogens into their active form.
      2. Dietary free-radical scavengers (antioxidants) such as β-carotene, vitamin C, and vitamin E inhibit all three stages.
      3. Selenium and vitamin E potentiate each other as antioxidants in chemical carcinogenesis.
   G. The following dietary recommendations have been advocated for cancer prevention:
      1. Avoid obesity.
      2. Decrease total fat intake to 30% of total calories (ideally <25%).
      3. Decrease saturated fat intake to <10% of the calories (ideally <7%).
      4. Increase the intake of whole-grain foods.
      5. Increase the intake of dark green, deep yellow, and orange vegetables rich in β-carotene and vitamin C.
      6. Increase the intake of cruciferous vegetables (e.g., broccoli, cauliflower).
      7. Reduce the amount of salt-cured and smoked meats as well as nitrite-cured foods.
      8. Either avoid or reduce alcohol intake.

Objective 7: To review the nutritional changes associated with aging.

X. Nutrition and aging
   A. The following nutritional changes are associated with aging:
      1. A decrease in body weight.
      2. A decrease in lean body mass (loss in skeletal muscle mass) and a relative increase in fat.
      3. A decline in energy requirements.
      4. A slight decline in basal calorie expenditure.
      5. A decline in the need for calories.
   B. Variables that contribute to dietary problems include drug interactions with nutrients, reduced renal function, and malabsorption of nutrients related to problems with gastric acidity.
   C. Dietary inadequacies are common for pyridoxine (B$_6$), vitamin D, folate, calcium, and zinc.
   D. Calcium and vitamin D supplementation slows the rate of bone loss in postmenopausal women with average diets.

Objective 8: To understand the significance of special diets.

XI. Special diets
   A. Restriction of sodium usually reduces the blood pressure and is a nonpharmacologic treatment for the edema states (e.g., congestive heart failure, chronic renal disease, cirrhosis).
   B. Protein-restricted diets are used to reduce the formation of urea and ammonia in patients with chronic renal disease and chronic liver disease.
   C. The Ornish diet is a vegan diet low in saturated fats and high in fiber that has been used to reverse calcified atherosclerotic plaques in coronary vessels.
      1. Pure vegan diets that are rich in soybean products provide an excellent source of proteins, calcium (hard tofu), and bioavailable iron.
      2. Concerns about B_{12} deficiency have been addressed by adding B_{12} to soybean products.

QUESTIONS

DIRECTIONS. (ITEMS 1–8): Each of the numbered items or incomplete statements in this section is followed by answers or completions of the statement. Select the ONE lettered answer or completion that is BEST in each case. Correct answers and explanations are given at the end of the chapter.

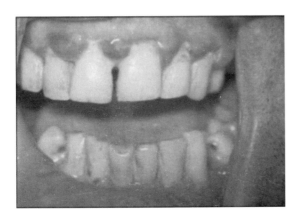

1. The patient in this photograph complains of a sore mouth, gums that bleed easily when brushed, and bone pain. Scattered ecchymoses are present over his arms and legs. The most likely diagnosis is a deficiency of

   (A) riboflavin
   (B) niacin
   (C) ascorbic acid
   (D) copper
   (E) vitamin K

2. Which of the following is more often associated with bulimia nervosa than with anorexia nervosa?

   (A) Significant weight loss
   (B) Metabolic alkalosis
   (C) Distorted body image
   (D) Secondary amenorrhea
   (E) Osteoporosis

3. Morbid obesity is least likely associated with

   (A) essential hypertension
   (B) left ventricular hypertrophy
   (C) increased risk of breast and endometrial cancer
   (D) rheumatoid arthritis
   (E) type II diabetes mellitus

4. A clinical or laboratory finding that is more frequently associated with marasmus than with kwashiorkor is

   (A) decreased muscle mass and subcutaneous fat
   (B) pitting edema
   (C) fatty liver
   (D) hypoalbuminemia
   (E) diarrhea

5. Which of the following clinical or laboratory abnormalities represents a water-soluble vitamin deficiency rather than a fat-soluble vitamin deficiency?

   (A) Nyctalopia
   (B) Squamous metaplasia
   (C) Hypocalcemia
   (D) Prolonged prothrombin time
   (E) Ringed sideroblasts

6. Hypovitaminosis D is least likely secondary to

   (A) chronic renal failure
   (B) cirrhosis of the liver
   (C) steatorrhea
   (D) a high-fat, low-fiber diet
   (E) hypoparathyroidism

7. Which of the following best describes the role of dietary fiber in preventing colon cancer?

   (A) It increases stool transit time.
   (B) It reduces the incidence of diverticulosis.
   (C) It increases the bulk of stool.
   (D) It enhances excretion of lithocholic acid.
   (E) It decreases the reabsorption of estrogen.

8. Which of the following represents a clinical finding in a water-soluble vitamin deficiency?

   (A) Osteomalacia
   (B) Follicular hyperkeratosis
   (C) Congestive cardiomyopathy
   (D) Mottled teeth
   (E) Dysgeusia

ANSWERS AND EXPLANATIONS

1. **The answer is C: ascorbic acid.** The patient has a history of a sore mouth, bleeding gums, bone pain, and evidence of vessel instability in the form of ecchymoses (subcutaneous bleeding), all of which are consistent with a diagnosis of scurvy. The photograph exhibits gingivitis and numerous dental caries. Ascorbic acid (AA) is responsible for the posttranslational hydroxylation of proline and lysine in collagen synthesis, hence its deficiency results in defective collagen, leading to vessel instability (bleeding gums, ecchymoses, subperiosteal bleeding). Riboflavin deficiency produces angular stomatitis, corneal neovascularization, and a magenta tongue. Niacin deficiency results in diarrhea, dementia, and dermatitis. Copper is a cofactor in lysyl oxidase (for cross-linking of collagen), cytochrome *c* oxidase (for electron transport), SOD (an antioxidant), ferroxidase (to promote binding of iron to transferrin), and tyrosinase (which is important in melanin synthesis). Vitamin K deficiency results in a hemorrhagic diathesis owing to a reduction in γ-carboxylation of glutamic acid residues in the precursor coagulation factors II, VII, IX, and X. (Photograph reproduced, with permission, from M. Mir. *Atlas of Clinical Diagnosis.* Philadelphia, W.B. Saunders Co., 1995, p. 74.)

2. **The answer is B: metabolic alkalosis.** Bulimia nervosa is defined as the voluntary vomiting of food (which produces metabolic alkalosis and hypokalemia), usually after "bingeing" on massive amounts of food. Unlike in anorexia nervosa, the body weight is usually normal to slightly decreased, body image is normal, and secondary amenorrhea with the risk of developing osteoporosis is not usually present. Physical signs related to vomiting include acid injury to tooth enamel, bruising of the knuckles, and swelling of the salivary glands. Additional complications include the Mallory-Weiss syndrome (laceration of the esophageal or stomach mucosa) and Boerhaave's syndrome (rupture of the stomach or distal esophagus).

3. **The answer is D: rheumatoid arthritis.** Morbid obesity is more commonly associated with osteoarthritis (wearing down of the articular cartilage) rather than with rheumatoid arthritis (autoimmune destruction of the articular cartilage). Complications of obesity include essential hypertension, left ventricular hypertrophy, an increased risk of cancer (breast, endometrial, ovarian, colorectal, pancreas, and biliary tract), coronary artery disease, stroke, and cholesterol gallstones.

4. **The answer is A: decreased muscle mass and subcutaneous fat.** Marasmus is defined as total calorie deprivation. Kwashiorkor refers to a normal caloric intake of predominantly carbohydrates and inadequate intake of protein. Hypoalbuminemia predisposes the patient to pitting edema (reduced oncotic pressure) and a fatty liver (reduced apolipoprotein synthesis). The muscle mass and subcutaneous fat are normal. Diarrhea, flaky-paint dermatitis, apathy, and impaired cellular immunity are also noted in kwashiorkor but not in marasmus. Both conditions are associated with growth failure and anemia.

5. **The answer is E: ringed sideroblasts.** Ringed sideroblasts are a feature of pyridoxine deficiency (B_6). Pyridoxine deficiency is most commonly associated with use of certain drugs (e.g., isoniazid). It functions as a cofactor in the form of pyridoxal phosphate, which is involved in heme synthesis, more specifically, the conversion of glycine and succinyl-CoA to δ-aminolevulinic acid within the mitochondria of a developing normoblast in the bone marrow. This reduces the amount of protoporphyrin available to combine with iron to form heme. Since iron is trapped in the mitochondria once it enters, it accumulates in the mitochondria (located around the nucleus of the RBC), hence producing the classic ringed sideroblast. Nyctalopia, or night blindness, is present in vitamin A (retinol) deficiency because of the vitamin's role in maintaining the light-sensitive pigment rhodopsin in the rods of the retina for adequate night vision. Vitamin A also prevents squamous metaplasia. Hypocalcemia occurs in vitamin D deficiency. A prolonged prothrombin time is associated with vitamin K deficiency owing to the vitamin's role in maintaining functional coagulation factors.

6. **The answer is D: a high-fat, low-fiber diet.** This type of diet has no effect on the reabsorption of the fat-soluble vitamin D. Defects in vitamin D metabolism produce deficiencies of the vitamin. Both skin- and diet-derived vitamin D are hydroxylated in the liver to form 25-(OH)-D_3 cholecalciferol (calcidiol), which may remain in the liver for storage, circulate in the blood bound to a protein (the main circulating form of non–renal-derived vitamin D), or undergo a second hydroxylation step in the kidneys via 1α-hydroxylase, which converts 25-(OH)-D_3 to 1,25-(OH)$_2$-D_3 (calcitriol). Enhancers of enzyme synthesis include parathormone (PTH) and hypophosphatemia. Hence, chronic renal failure (decreased enzyme), cirrhosis of the liver (decreased stores and defective first hydroxylation), steatorrhea (a sign in the stool of fat malabsorption), and hypoparathyroidism (decreased synthesis of the enzyme) are potential causes of hypovitaminosis D.

7. **The answer is D: it enhances excretion of lithocholic acid.** Increased fiber in the diet decreases stool transit time (less contact time for lithocholic acid with the colorectal epithelium), increases stool bulk (acts like a sponge, drawing water and other solutes into the fiber), reduces stool pH (increases the excretion of lithocholic acid), and reduces the reabsorption of cholesterol and estrogen (has a possible role in preventing breast, endometrial, and ovarian cancers). Diverticulosis does not predispose to colon cancer.

8. **The answer is C: congestive cardiomyopathy.** This is a sign of thiamine (B_1) deficiency, which is most commonly seen in people with alcoholism. Owing to thiamine's important role as a cofactor in the pyruvate dehydrogenase complex, which converts pyruvate to acetyl-CoA (acetyl-CoA then combines with oxaloacetate to produce citrate in the tricarboxylic acid cycle), a deficiency of thiamine reduces ATP synthesis, hence producing major alterations in the cardiovascular system. (It also affects the neurologic system, producing peripheral neuropathy, Wernicke's encephalopathy, and Korsakoff's psychosis.) A reduction in ATP in cardiac muscle results in poor contractility, hence predisposing to both left and right heart failure (wet beriberi). Follicular hyperkeratosis (squamous metaplasia in the hair follicles) is noted in vitamin A deficiency. Dysgeusia, or a lack of taste sensation, is present in patients with zinc deficiency.

CHAPTER SEVEN

GENETIC, CONGENITAL, AND DEVELOPMENTAL DISORDERS AND AGING

SYNOPSIS

OBJECTIVES

1. To be familiar with chromosome disorders associated with abnormalities in chromosome number and microdeletions.
2. To review mendelian inheritance disorders, disorders involving multifactorial inheritance, and disorders associated with mitochondrial DNA.
3. To describe disorders involving sex differentiation in both males and females.
4. To be able to calculate the prevalence of disease when given the carrier rate.
5. To discuss developmental disorders secondary to deformations and malformations.
6. To distinguish between stillbirths and spontaneous abortions.
7. To understand disorders associated with prematurity and the neonatal period of life.
8. To be aware of the differences between age-dependent and age-related disorders.

Objective 1: To be familiar with chromosome disorders associated with abnormalities in chromosome number and microdeletions.

I. Chromosome disorders
   A. Humans have **46 chromosomes** consisting of 22 pairs of autosomes (somatic chromosomes) and two sex chromosomes (XX = female and XY = male).
      1. **Meiosis** occurs in germ cells, hence the gametes contain the haploid number of chromosomes (23).
      2. According to **Lyon's hypothesis**, one of the two X chromosomes in a female is randomly inactivated (50% female and 50% maternally derived) and becomes a **Barr body** (a projection from the nucleus counted in squamous cells obtained by scrapings from the buccal mucosa).
         a. Normal females have one Barr body and normal males none.

   b. A male with Klinefelter's syndrome and an XXY genotype has one Barr body.
3. **Aneuploidy** refers to an uneven multiple of 23 chromosomes (e.g., Down syndrome with 47 chromosomes).
   a. It is most frequently due to **nondisjunction**, in which one set of homologous chromosomes fails to separate during the first meiotic division (one gamete has 22 chromosomes and the other 24 chromosomes).
   b. When nondisjunction occurs in mitosis of autosomal cells, the result is **mosaicism**, or the presence of two or more genetically different cell populations in the same patient (a common occurrence in Turner's syndrome).
4. A chromosome **translocation** is the transfer of one broken segment from one chromosome to another nonhomologous (different) chromosome.
5. The three important trisomy (47 chromosome) syndromes are summarized in Table 7–1.
6. **Turner's syndrome** and **Klinefelter's syndrome** are summarized in Table 7–2.
7. A partial **deletion of chromosome 5** produces a disease called the **cri du chat syndrome** (mental retardation, a cat-like cry, ventricular septal defects).
8. **Microdeletion syndromes** have been identified that exhibit **genomic imprinting**.
   a. Two examples are the **Prader-Willi** and **Angelman's syndromes**.
   b. Both of these diseases have a microdeletion on chromosome 15 in the same location; however, they produce entirely different diseases, since the chromosome derives from the father in Prader-Willi syndrome and from the mother in Angelman's syndrome.
9. A few **chromosome/disease associations** include chromosome 1 (neuroblastoma), chromosome 4 (Huntington's chorea), chromosome 7 (cystic fibrosis), chromosome 11 (Wilms' tumor), chromosome 13 (retinoblastoma), and chromosome 17 (neurofibromatosis).

TABLE 7–1.   Trisomy Syndromes

Trisomy Disorder	Pathogenesis	Physical Findings	Comment
Trisomy 21 (Down syndrome)	Trisomy 21 (95% of cases). Most common genetic cause of mental retardation.	Epicanthal folds with upward slanting of the eyes, simian palmar crease, flat facial profile. Congenital heart defects (40%; endocardial cushion defects; major survival factor in early childhood). GI problems: duodenal atresia and Hirschsprung's disease. Increased incidence of acute leukemia. Increased incidence of Alzheimer's disease (chromosome 21 codes for β-proteins, which are converted to amyloid [toxic to neurons]; major factor for longevity in older patients).	Prenatal findings in the mother: low AFP and unconjugated estriol and high β-hCG. Risk for Down syndrome in future pregnancies increases with maternal age.
Trisomy 18 (Edwards' syndrome)	Similar to Down syndrome. ~90% die in first month.	Severe mental retardation, overlapping fingers, ventricular septal defect (VSD), rocker-bottom feet.	
Trisomy 13 (Patau's syndrome)	Similar to Down syndrome. 100% lethal by 6 months of age.	Midline facial defect, severe mental retardation, cleft lip and palate, polydactyly, VSD.	

Objective 2: To review mendelian inheritance disorders, disorders involving multifactorial inheritance, and disorders associated with mitochondrial DNA.

II. mendelian disorders

A. Alternative forms of the same gene are called **alleles**.

1. If a gene on an autosome has two alleles, one that is normal (A) and one that is abnormal (a), the following combinations are possible: AA, Aa, and aa.
   a. Genes with the same alleles are called **homozygous** (e.g., AA or aa), while those with different alleles are called **heterozygous** (e.g., Aa).
   b. In **autosomal dominant** (AD) disorders, only one abnormal allele is necessary to express the disease (e.g., aa or Aa).
   c. In **autosomal recessive** (AR) diseases, both abnormal alleles must be present (e.g., aa, homozygous state) to express the disease.

B. AD diseases exhibit penetrance, variable expressivity, and in some cases, late onset of the disease (e.g., familial polyposis, Huntington's chorea).

1. When the frequency of expression of an AD trait is below 100% (i.e., a patient may have the abnormal gene but never expresses the disease), the trait is said to exhibit reduced **penetrance.**

2. If patients with an AD trait express the disease but at different levels of severity, this is called **variable expressivity** (e.g., neurofibromatosis).

C. Table 7–3 summarizes the characteristics of AD, AR, sex-linked recessive (SXR), and sex-linked dominant (SXD) disease (pedigrees are reviewed in the questions and answers).

1. **Examples of AD disorders,** in order of decreasing prevalence, are von Willebrand's disease, familial hypercholesterolemia, adult polycystic kidney disease, Huntington's chorea, neurofibromatosis, congenital spherocytosis, familial polyposis, and Marfan syndrome.
   a. **Neurofibromatosis** is associated with neurofibromas, iris hamartomas (Lisch nodules), café-au-lait spots, skeletal lesions (scoliosis), and an increased incidence of other tumors

TABLE 7–2.   Non-mendelian Sex Chromosome Disorders

Disorder	Pathogenesis	Clinical Findings	Laboratory Findings
Turner's syndrome	~50–60% are XO genotypes (45 chromosomes, no Barr body in buccal smear). Y chromosome (mosaic XO/46,XY) increases risk for ovarian cancer (dysgerminoma and gonadoblastoma). Ovaries devoid of follicles and oocytes (streak ovaries).	Newborns: cystic hygromas in neck (dilated lymphatic channels), preductal coarctation (20%), lymphedema of hands and feet. Adults: most common genetic cause of primary amenorrhea, webbed neck (50%), poor secondary sex characteristics, normal IQ.	Decreased estradiol, increased gonadotropins.
Klinefelter's syndrome	XXY genotype (47 chromosomes, Barr body present in buccal smear).	Eunuchoid proportions, hypogonadism with atrophic testicles (fibrosed seminiferous tubules [no sperm], hyperplastic Leydig's cells), gynecomastia (25%), increased learning disabilities (>60%).	Low testosterone, high FSH (loss of negative feedback from inhibin in Sertoli's cells, stimulates aromatase conversion of androgens into estrogen), high LH (loss of testosterone negative feedback), high estradiol.

TABLE 7–3.   Characteristics of Mendelian Disorders

Characteristic	Autosomal Dominant	Autosomal Recessive	Sex-linked Recessive	Sex-linked Dominant
Transmission	Males and females transmit disease. Only one parent has to have disease. 50% of children affected and 50% normal.	Both parents must be carriers (heterozygotes or homozygotes). 25% of children symptomatic, 50% carriers, 25% normal.	Males express disease. Affected male transmits abnormal gene to 100% of daughters (asymptomatic carriers), who then transmit disease to 50% of their sons.	Males and females express disease. Affected females transmit disease to 50% of sons and daughters. Affected males transmit disease to 100% of daughters.
Prevalence	70%	25%	4%	1%
Penetrance/variable expressivity/delayed onset of symptoms	Yes	No	No	No

(acoustic neuromas, meningiomas, optic nerve gliomas, pheochromocytoma).

   b. **Marfan's syndrome**, due to a defect in fibrillin, primarily affects the skeleton (eunuchoid proportions, arachnodactyly), eyes (dislocated lens), and cardiovascular system (mitral valve prolapse, dissecting aortic aneurysm).

  2. **Examples of AR diseases**, in order of decreasing prevalence, are hemochromatosis, sickle cell anemia, cystic fibrosis, Tay-Sachs disease, phenylketonuria, 21-hydroxylase deficiency, albinism, most of the mucopolysaccharidoses (but not Hunter's syndrome), the glycogenoses, and galactosemia.

   a. **Lysosomal storage diseases** are a group of diseases in which the absence of degrading enzymes leads to an accumulation of complex substrates (e.g., sphingolipids and mucopolysaccharides) in the lysosome.

   b. **Glycogenoses** involve an accumulation of glycogen in tissue owing to a problem with increased synthesis or decreased degradation of glycogen.

   c. Table 7–4 summarizes selected AR disorders.

  3. **Examples of SXR disorders** are Lesch-Nyhan syndrome (hyperuricemia and self-mutilation due to deficiency of HGPRT), fragile X syndrome (mental retardation, macroorchidism at puberty), hemophilia A and B, glucose-6-phosphate dehydrogenase deficiency, testicular feminization, chronic granulomatous disease of childhood, and Wiskott-Aldrich syndrome.

  4. An example of an SXD is vitamin D–resistant rickets (hypophosphatemia).

III. Multifactorial inheritance

  A. Multifactorial (polygenic) inheritance disorders are due to multiple small mutations plus the effect of environment.

  B. **Examples** include cleft lip or palate, congenital heart disease, coronary artery disease, gout, type II diabetes mellitus, hypertension, open neural tube defects, and congenital pyloric stenosis.

IV. Mitochondrial DNA disorders

  A. Mitochondrial DNA (mtDNA) disorders are secondary to a mutation in a mitochondrial gene, which primarily codes for enzymes involved in oxidative phosphorylation.

  B. The disorders are unique to females, since ova have more mitochondria than sperm (which lose their mitochondria during fertilization), and a woman with an mtDNA defect transmits it to all her children.

Objective 3: To describe disorders involving sex differentiation in both males and females.

V. Sex differentiation disorders

  A. An **XY karyotype** leads to medullary differentiation of the primitive gonadal tissue into sex cords (seminiferous tubules) and Leydig's cells, while an **XX karyotype** leads to preferential development of the germinal cortex into primordial follicles.

  B. A **true hermaphrodite** has both male and female gonads (ovary and testis).

  C. A **pseudohermaphrodite** is a person whose **phenotype** (appearance) is not in agreement with the **genotype** (true gonadal sex).

   1. A **male pseudohermaphrodite** is a genotypic male (XY with testes) who has genitalia and other changes that resemble a female's (e.g., testicular feminization).

   2. A **female pseudohermaphrodite** is a genotypic female (XX with ovaries) who phenotypically resembles a male (e.g., virilization in congenital adrenal hyperplasia).

  D. **Testicular feminization** is due to deficiency of androgen receptors.

   1. Testosterone is unable to effect development of the seminal vesicles, epididymis, and vas deferens (testicles are present, usually in the inguinal canal).

   2. Dihydrotestosterone is unable to produce male external genitalia or a prostate gland, hence the external genitalia remain female.

   3. Testosterone and follicle-stimulating hormone (FSH) levels are normal, but luteinizing hormone (LH) levels are increased, since LH is not responsive to the negative feedback of testosterone stimulation.

  E. **Congenital adrenal hyperplasia** (CAH, adrenogenital syndrome) is the most common adrenal disorder in children.

   1. Owing to a deficiency of 21-, 11-, or 17-hydroxylase enzymes, there is a deficiency of cortisol (hypocortisolism) with a subsequent increase in ACTH (Figure 7–1).

TABLE 7–4.   Summary Chart of Selected Autosomal Recessive Diseases

Disease	Pathogenesis	Clinical Findings
Phenylketonuria (PKU)	Phenylalanine hydroxylase, which converts phenylalanine to tyrosine, is deficient. Rising phenylalanine levels impair development of the brain, leading to severe mental retardation.	Babies are normal at birth since they need to be exposed to milk containing phenylalanine before the defect is uncovered. There is a mousy odor to the sweat (due to buildup of minor pathway products).
Galactosemia	Galactose comes from the metabolism of lactose (glucose + galactose). In galactosemia, there is a total lack of galactose-1-phosphate uridyltransferase (GALT) leading to a buildup of glucose 1-phosphate and galactose. Glucose 1-phosphate is converted to glucose 6-phosphate, which may be utilized as a substrate for glycolysis or gluconeogenesis.	Galactose 1-phosphate is toxic and damages tissue, resulting in neonatal cholestasis (may progress to cirrhosis), CNS damage (mental retardation), and renal damage (aminoaciduria). Excess galactose may be converted into the polyol (alcohol sugar) galactitol, which produces osmotic damage in the lens, nerve tissue, liver, and CNS. Neonatal hypoglycemia occurs owing to a lack of glucose 6-phosphate.
Essential fructosuria and hereditary fructose intolerance	Fructose derives from sucrose (glucose + fructose). Essential fructosuria is due to a deficiency of fructokinase (buildup of fructose, leading to benign fructosuria), while hereditary fructose intolerance is due to a deficiency of aldolase B, leading to an accumulation of fructose 1-phosphate (normally converted to glyceraldehyde and DHAP intermediates that may be used as a substrate for glycolysis or gluconeogenesis).	**Hereditary fructose intolerance** is characterized by hypophosphatemia (used to trap fructose in cells), leading to ATP depletion and the toxic effects of fructose 1-phosphate (neonatal cholestasis leading to liver failure). Fasting hypoglycemia is commonly observed.
Homocystinuria	Homocystinuria is due to a deficiency of cystathionine synthetase.	It resembles Marfan syndrome (arachnodactyly and a dislocated lens). Differentiating features from Marfan syndrome include mental retardation, thromboembolic phenomenon (homocysteine damages endothelial cells), and osteoporosis.
Alcaptonuria	Alcaptonuria (ochronosis) is secondary to a lack of homogentisate oxidase in the metabolism of phenylalanine.	There is an increase in homogentisic acid in urine, which is colorless at first but after oxidation upon exposure to light turns black. Homogentisic acid binds to collagen in connective tissue, tendons, and cartilage (causing crippling joint disease and intervertebral disk disease) and imparts a black color to all these tissues.
Glycogenoses		
Von Gierke's, Pompe's, and McArdle's diseases	**Von Gierke's disease** is due to deficiency of the gluconeogenic enzyme glucose-6-phosphatase.	Hypoglycemia, glycogen deposition in the liver and kidneys, no increase in glucose with glucagon stimulation.
	Pompe's disease is secondary to a deficiency of a lysosomal enzyme acid maltase.	Glycogen accumulation in the heart with death at an early age.
	McArdle's disease is due to a deficiency of muscle phosphorylase.	Muscle fatigue with exercise, no increase in lactic acid with exercise.
Sphingolipidoses		
Tay-Sachs disease: GM$_2$ gangliosidosis	Enzyme deficiency: hexosaminidase (α-subunit). Metabolite accumulation: GM$_2$ ganglioside. It is primarily seen in Ashkenazi Jews.	Patients are normal at birth but develop signs of severe mental retardation within 6 months. There is blindness, a cherry-red spot in the macula, muscle weakness, and flaccidity. Electron microscopy exhibits whorled configurations in the lysosomes.
Niemann-Pick disease	Enzyme deficiency: sphingomyelinase. Metabolite accumulation: sphingomyelin. The accumulation of sphingomyelin is primarily in macrophages (bubbly appearance) and in neurons.	There is severe mental retardation, massive hepatosplenomegaly, and deterioration of psychomotor function. The disease is fatal in early life. Zebra bodies are noted in lysosomes on electron microscopy.
Gaucher's disease	Enzyme deficiency: glucocerebrosidase. Metabolite accumulation: glucocerebroside. It is primarily noted in Ashkenazi Jews.	The adult type has an accumulation of glucocerebroside in macrophages (it has a fibrillary appearance) in the liver and spleen (massive hepatosplenomegaly) and in the bone marrow (produces pancytopenia). There is no CNS involvement.
Metachromatic leukodystrophy	Enzyme deficiency: arylsulfatase A. Metabolite accumulation: sulfatide. The myelin that is synthesized is abnormal, hence affecting the CNS and peripheral nerves.	There is mental retardation, peripheral neuropathy, and visceral organ abnormalities. The urine arylsulfatase activity is decreased or absent. The sulfatides stain positive with metachromatic stains.
Krabbe's disease	Enzyme deficiency: galactosylceramidase. Metabolite accumulation: galactocerebroside. Similar to metachromatic leukodystrophy, there is synthesis of an abnormal myelin.	There is progressive psychomotor retardation. The brain at autopsy reveals multinucleated globoid cells within which is located the galactocerebroside material.

TABLE 7–4. Summary Chart of Selected Autosomal Recessive Diseases *Continued*

Disease	Pathogenesis	Clinical Findings
Fabry's disease	Enzyme deficiency: α-galactocerebrosidase A. Metabolite accumulation: ceramide trihexoside.	It is characterized by angiokeratomas on the skin, hypertension, and renal failure. SXR disease.
Mucopolysaccharidoses		
Hurler's syndrome	Enzyme deficiency: α-1-iduronidase. Metabolite accumulation: dermatan sulfate and heparan sulfate.	Patients have severe mental retardation, coarse facial features, massive hepatosplenomegaly, clouding of the cornea, a high incidence of CAD owing to accumulation of the metabolites in the coronary vessels, joint stiffness, and vacuoles in leukocytes in the peripheral blood.
Hunter's syndrome	Enzyme deficiency: L-Iduronosulfate sulfatase. Metabolite accumulation: dermatan sulfate and heparan sulfate.	It is a milder disease than Hurler's syndrome. SXR disease.

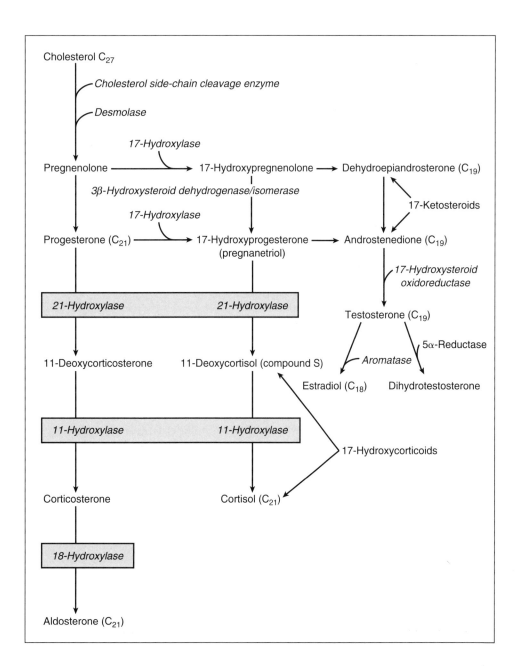

FIGURE 7–1. Adrenal gland biosynthetic pathways.

2. ACTH enhances melanin synthesis, stimulates hyperplasia of the adrenal cortex, and increases the production of products proximal to the enzyme block.
   a. Synthesis of the **17-ketosteroids** (C_{19} compounds; weak androgens), **dehydroepiandrosterone** (DHEA), and **androstenedione** require the 17-hydroxylase enzyme (testosterone is not a 17-ketosteroid).
      (1) Females deficient in 21- or 11-hydroxylase usually have ambiguous genitalia (female pseudohermaphrodites).
      (2) Males may develop precocious puberty.
   b. The urine metabolite of 17-hydroxyprogesterone (C_{21} compound) is **pregnanetriol**, which is often used as a screen (elevated value) for 21- or 11-hydroxylase deficiency.
   c. Deoxycortisol (compound S; C_{21} compound) and cortisol (C_{21} compound) plus their metabolites are called the **17-hydroxycorticoids**.
3. The zona glomerulosa primarily produces mineralocorticoids and has an 18-hydroxylase enzyme for conversion of corticosterone into aldosterone (C_{21} compound).
4. Deficiency of 21-hydroxylase accounts for ~95% of cases of CAH.
   a. Urinary 17-ketosteroids are increased (since they are proximal to the block), and 17-hydroxycorticoids are decreased.
   b. The weak mineralocorticoids (e.g., deoxycorticosterone) are decreased, hence the patients are salt losers (hyponatremia, hyperkalemia).
5. Deficiency of 11-hydroxylase shows an increase in urinary 17-hydroxycorticoids (deoxycortisol is proximal to the block), 17-ketosteroids, and deoxycorticosterone (leading to salt retention and hypertension).

Objective 4: To be able to calculate the prevalence of disease when given the carrier rate.

VI. Calculation of the prevalence of disease
   A. Using cystic fibrosis as an example, if the carrier rate of cystic fibrosis is 1/25, the prevalence of CF may be calculated as follows.
      1. The number of couples at risk is equal to the carrier rate in males × the carrier rate in females, or 1/25 × 1/25, hence 1/625 couples are at risk.
      2. The risk of having a child with CF is 1/4, hence 1/625 × 1/4 is equal to a prevalence of ~1/2500.
   B. The carrier rate of a disease can be calculated by the **Hardy-Weinberg equation**, which reflects the distribution of a mutant gene in the population.

TABLE 7–5. Noninfectious Teratogens Producing Malformations

Teratogen	Comments	Teratogen	Comments
Cocaine	Mother: abruptio placentae, premature labor. Newborn: CNS infarcts, intraventricular hemorrhage, genitourinary and gastrointestinal abnormalities.	Isotretinoin	Newborn: craniofacial abnormalities (small ears, micrognathia, cleft palate), cardiac defects, CNS malformations (microcephaly). Isotretinoin is used to treat acne. All female patients should have a pregnancy test before using drug and use contraception.
Diabetes mellitus	Newborn: increased birth weight (macrosomia), open neural tube defects, cleft lip/palate, respiratory distress syndrome, transposition of great vessels.	Lithium	Cardiac abnormalities (Ebstein's anomaly).
Diethylstilbestrol (DES)	Exposed newborn female: abnormalities in müllerian structures: vaginal adenosis (most common abnormality; precursor of clear cell adenocarcinoma of vagina), cervical incompetence, uterine and fallopian tube abnormalities.	Phenylketonuria	Pregnant mother with PKU not on a phenylalanine free diet: 25% chance of bearing child with congenital abnormalities and 90% chance of microcephaly and severe mental retardation.
Fetal alcohol syndrome	Fetal alcohol syndrome occurs in 2:1000 live births. It occurs in 30–45% of the offspring of women who have more than 4–6 drinks per day. It results in intrauterine growth retardation, maxillary hypoplasia, mental retardation (average IQ is 63; a key finding), microcephaly, atrial septal defects (least common finding), and hypoglycemia at birth.	Phenytoin	Newborn: hypoplasia of the distal phalanges (nail hypoplasia), CNS abnormalities, cleft lip/palate.
		Smoking	Newborn: low birth weight.
		Systemic lupus erythematosus	Pregnant mother with SLE who has anti-Ro IgG antibodies may have newborns with complete heart block.
Heroin	Newborn: SGA, high-pitched cry, excessive hunger/salivation/sweating/tremors, fist sucking, seizures, increased incidence of congenital infections (HIV, HBV).	Thalidomide	Newborn: limb abnormalities (amelia [absent limbs], phocomelia [seal-like limbs]).
		Valproate	Newborn: open neural tube defects.
		Warfarin	Newborn: 33% risk for CNS defects and nasal hypoplasia.

Objective 5: To discuss developmental disorders secondary to deformations and malformations.

VII. Deformations and malformations
- A. **Deformations** are anatomical defects resulting from mechanical factors (extrinsic forces) that usually occur during the last two trimesters after organs have developed (e.g., oligohydramnios producing facial and limb abnormalities).
- B. A **malformation** is a disturbance (e.g., drug use, infection) that occurs in the first trimester in the morphogenesis of an organ.
  1. **Hypospadias,** in which the urethra opens on the ventral surface of the penis, is the most common congenital malformation, followed by club foot and a ventricular septal defect.
  2. **Teratogens** are most detrimental during the embryonic period, which is the first 9 weeks of life.
  3. Table 7–5 summarizes noninfectious causes of malformations and Table 7–6 congenital infections that produce malformations.
     a. The TORCH syndrome is a group of congenital or perinatal infections.
     b. TORCH stands for *t*oxoplasmosis, *o*ther (HBV, AIDS, parvovirus, syphilis, etc.), *r*ubella, *c*ytomegalovirus, and *h*erpes.

Objective 6: To distinguish between stillbirths and spontaneous abortions.

VIII. Stillbirths and spontaneous abortions
- A. A **stillbirth** is delivery of a dead child, which is most often the result of antepartum hemorrhage (e.g., premature separation of the placenta).
- B. A **spontaneous abortion** is a pregnancy that terminates before the fetus is able to remain alive outside the uterus (22 weeks of gestation); 50% have a fetal karyotypic abnormality, usually trisomy 16.

Objective 7: To understand disorders associated with prematurity and the neonatal period of life.

IX. Disorders of prematurity and the neonatal period
- A. Newborns may be classified as **appropriate for gestational age** (AGA), **small for gestational age** (SGA), or **large for gestational age** (LGA).
- B. **Term newborns** are born between 37 and 42 weeks; preterm newborns, before 37 weeks; and postterm newborns, after 42 weeks.
- C. Mortality is highest in the SGA bracket.
- D. The majority of deaths in childhood occur during the neonatal period (first 4 weeks of life) and are most commonly due to the respiratory distress syndrome (RDS) and congenital anomalies.
- E. Major problems confronting **preterm infants** in-

TABLE 7–6. Congenital Infections Associated with Malformations

Infection	Comments	Clinical Findings	Laboratory Findings
Cytomegalovirus (CMV)	Most common *in utero* viral infection. Most cases asymptomatic (85–90%). Primarily transplacental transmission.	Symptomatic disease: hearing loss (most frequent sequela), periventricular calcification, neonatal cholestasis, anemia and thrombocytopenia, chorioretinitis (blindness), microcephaly.	Urine culture gold standard diagnostic test. Basophilic intranuclear inclusions ("owl's eyes") in renal tubular cells.
Rubella	Worse disease the earlier infection occurs in pregnancy. Primarily transplacental transmission.	Nerve deafness (most common defect), congenital heart disease (patent ductus arteriosus), cataract, mental retardation.	Positive serologic test (TO*R*CH)
Toxoplasmosis	Maternal infection secondary to exposure to oocysts in cat litter. Primarily transplacental transmission.	Chorioretinitis (blindness), periventricular calcifications, microcephaly, mental retardation, neonatal cholestasis.	Positive serologic test (*T*ORCH)
Herpes simplex	Primarily perinatal transmission while passing through birth canal (~3–10%) with active shedding of herpes genitalis, HSV-2. Baby should be delivered by cesarean section if viral shedding present.	Permanent neurologic sequelae common.	Positive serologic test (TORC*H*)
Syphilis	Primarily transplacental transmission later in pregnancy.	Symptoms and signs in first 1–2 months such as mucocutaneous lesions, pneumonia alba (lobar pneumonia), persistent rhinitis (snuffles), osteochondritis, hepatomegaly. Late manifestations include bone abnormalities (saber shins), rhagades (perioral linear scars), and Hutchinson's triad (malformed teeth [notched upper central incisors called Hutchinson teeth], eyes [interstitial keratitis; blindness], and ears [nerve deafness]).	Rising RPR/VDRL titer. Positive FTA-ABS-IgM.
Varicella-zoster virus		Newborns have limb hypoplasia, cortical atrophy in the brain, and skin lesions.	

volve organ immaturity (e.g., preterm lungs lack surfactant, which predisposes to RDS).

Objective 8: To be aware of the differences between age-dependent and age-related disorders.

X. Age-dependent and age-related disorders
   A. **Age-dependent disorders** (inevitable with age) include loss of elasticity of the aorta, osteoarthritis, decreased glomerular filtration rate, an obstructive pattern of lung disease (e.g., decreased FEV_{1sec}), prostate hyperplasia/cancer, autoantibodies, cataract, otosclerosis (conductive hearing loss), and presbycusis (nerve deafness).
   B. **Age-related disorders** (more prevalent in old age) include atherosclerosis, Alzheimer's disease, acute myocardial infarction, osteoporosis, Parkinson's disease, increased incidence of monoclonal antibodies, and increased incidence of ultraviolet light–induced skin cancers (basal cell carcinoma and squamous cell carcinoma).

QUESTIONS

DIRECTIONS. (ITEMS 1–9): Each of the numbered items or incomplete statements in this section is followed by answers or by completions of the statement. Select the ONE lettered answer or completion that is BEST in each case. Correct answers and explanations are given at the end of the chapter.

Items 1–6 involve the interpretation of pedigrees.

- ■ Affected male
- □ Normal male
- ● Affected female
- ○ Normal female

1. Which of the following genetic diseases best describes the pedigree depicted below?

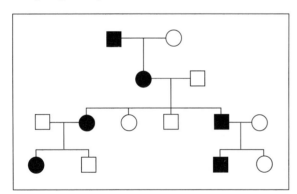

(A) Phenylketonuria AR
(B) Glucose-6-phosphate dehydrogenase deficiency SxR
(C) Neurofibromatosis AD
(D) Tay-Sachs disease AR
(E) Lesch-Nyhan syndrome SxR

2. Which of the following genetic diseases best describes the pedigree depicted below?

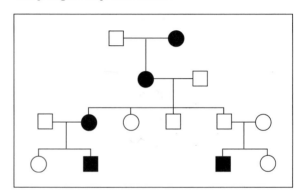

(A) Huntington's chorea AD
(B) Wiskott-Aldrich syndrome SxR
(C) Galactosemia AR
(D) Vitamin D–resistant rickets SxD
(E) Von Gierke's disease AR

3. The following pedigree is most consistent with which one of the following genetic disorders?

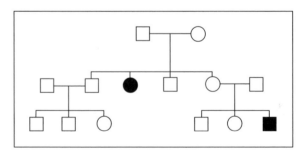

(A) Congenital spherocytosis AD
(B) Chronic granulomatous disease of childhood SxR
(C) Familial hypercholesterolemia AD
(D) Hemophilia A SxR
(E) Hemochromatosis AR

4. Which of the following genetic disorders is best represented by the following pedigree?

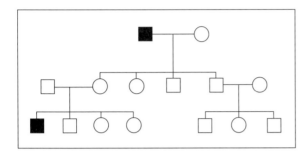

(A) Down syndrome
(B) Fragile X syndrome
(C) Cri du chat syndrome
(D) Hurler's syndrome
(E) Gaucher's disease

5. The following pedigree best describes which of the following genetic disorders?

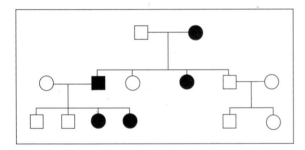

(A) Vitamin D–resistant rickets
(B) Hunter's syndrome
(C) Niemann-Pick disease
(D) Prader-Willi syndrome
(E) Klinefelter's syndrome

6. Which of the following disorders best describes the following pedigree?

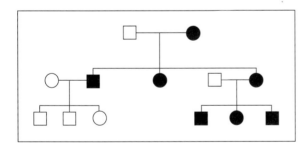

(A) Duchenne's muscular dystrophy
(B) Mitochondrial DNA disorder
(C) Triplet repeat disorder
(D) Galactosemia
(E) Testicular feminization

7. A newborn female with ambiguous genitalia is noted to have hypotension, hyponatremia, and hyperkalemia. You would least expect the patient to have

(A) an autosomal recessive disease
(B) hypocortisolism
(C) increased urine pregnanetriol
(D) elevation of the urine 17-hydroxycorticoids
(E) elevation of the urine 17-ketosteroids

8. A 40-year-old woman in her prenatal testing is noted to have a low serum α-fetoprotein and unconjugated estriol and an elevated β-hGG. You would expect her newborn child to have

(A) trisomy 13
(B) trisomy 18
(C) trisomy 21
(D) partial deletion of chromosome 5
(E) microdeletion of chromosome 15

9. Homocystinuria and Marfan syndrome both exhibit arachnodactyly and dislocated lenses. This is an example of

(A) pleiotropy
(B) variable expressivity
(C) genetic heterogeneity
(D) penetrance
(E) nondisjunction

DIRECTIONS. (ITEMS 10–13): Each set of matching questions in this section consists of a list of lettered options followed by several numbered items. For each numbered item, select the ONE option that is most closely associated with it. Each lettered option may be selected once, more than once, or not at all.

(A) Phenylketonuria
(B) Galactosemia
(C) Hereditary fructose intolerance
(D) Tay-Sachs disease
(E) Gaucher's disease
(F) Hurler's syndrome
(G) Von Gierke's disease
(H) Fetal alcohol syndrome
(I) Diethylstilbestrol
(J) Maternal smoking
(K) Isotretinoin
(L) Congenital cytomegalovirus
(M) Congenital toxoplasmosis
(N) Congenital rubella
(O) Congenital herpes
(P) Congenital syphilis

10. Mental retardation, microcephaly, and atrial septal defect

11. Newborn with hepatomegaly and fasting hypoglycemia who does not exhibit a rise in glucose with a glucagon or fructose challenge

12. Newborn with microcephaly, hepatosplenomegaly, periventricular calcifications, and abnormal intranuclear inclusions in renal tubular cells

13. Teenaged girl with acne has a baby with craniofacial, cardiac, and CNS malformations

ANSWERS AND EXPLANATIONS

1. The answer is C: neurofibromatosis. The pedigree depicts disease in both males and females,, ~50% of the children are involved, and one parent can pass on the disease. These findings best describe an AD inheritance pattern (neurofibromatosis). Phenylketonuria is an AR disease, glucose-6-phosphate dehydrogenase deficiency and Lesch-Nyhan syndrome are SXR diseases, and Tay-Sachs is an AR lysosomal storage disease.

2. The answer is A: Huntington's chorea. The pedigree exhibits both males and females with the disease, which excludes an SXR disease. Only one parent is necessary to transmit the abnormal gene. Approximately 50% of the children express the disorder except for one of the males who did not express the disease but did pass it on to his son. This is an example of 50% penetrance in an AD disease, since two first-generation children have the abnormal gene but only one expresses the disease. Huntington's chorea is an AD disease, Wiskott-Aldrich syndrome is an SXR disorder, galactosemia is AR, vitamin D–resistant rickets is SXD, and von Gierke's disease is AR.

3. The answer is E: hemochromatosis. The pedigree exhibits disease in both males and females, hence excluding an SXR disease. None of the parents express the disease but have transmitted the disease to their children, hence they must be asymptomatic carriers. Therefore, the pedigree best describes an AR disease (hemochromatosis). Congenital spherocytosis and familial hypercholesterolemia are both AD disorders, and chronic granulomatous disease of childhood and hemophilia A are both SXR disorders.

4. The answer is B: fragile X syndrome. The pedigree exhibits a male-dominant disorder, parents who do not express the disease, and a skipped generation before the males express the disease. This is compatible with an SXR disorder (fragile X syndrome), in which the affected male transmits the abnormal gene to his daughters (asymptomatic carriers), who then transmit it to 50% of their sons (symptomatic) and daughters (asymptomatic carriers). Down syndrome is a trisomy 21 syndrome, cri du chat is a partial deletion of chromosome 5, and both Hurler's and Gaucher's are AR diseases, the former a mucopolysaccharidosis and the latter a sphingolipidosis.

5. The answer is A: vitamin D–resistant rickets. The pedigree shows that both males and females express the disease and only one parent is necessary to transmit the abnormal gene to offspring. Note that the affected male always transmits the abnormal gene to all his daughters, while the affected female always transmits it to 50% of her sons and daughters. These findings are characteristic of an SXD disorder (vitamin D–resistant rickets). Hunter's syndrome is an SXR mucopolysaccharidosis, Niemann-Pick disease is an AR sphingolipidosis, Prader-Willi syndrome is an example of a microdeletion syndrome with genomic imprinting, and Klinefelter's syndrome is a 47,XXY chromosome disorder.

6. The answer is B: mitochondrial DNA disorder. The pedigree is unusual in that only the affected female transmits the disease and all her children are affected, while affected males do not transmit the disease to their children. This is a characteristic of mitochondrial DNA (mtDNA) disorders. Mitochondrial genes usually code for oxidative phosphorylation enzymes. The ovum contains mtDNA genes, but the sperm loses its mtDNA after fertilization, since the genes are located in the tail of the sperm. Hence, females transmit the disease to all their children, while affected males do not pass on the gene. Duchenne's muscular dystrophy and testicular feminization are both SXR disorders. Fragile X syndrome is an SXR disorder that is also an example of a triplet repeat disorder, in which there is a long repeating sequence of three nucleotides (CGG). Galactosemia is an AR disease.

7. The answer is D: elevation of the urine 17-hydroxycorticoids. The patient has congenital adrenal hyperplasia (an AR disease) secondary to 21-hydroxylase enzyme deficiency. The 17-ketosteroid compounds DHEA and androstenedione are proximal to the block and are responsible for her ambiguous genitalia (female pseudohermaphrodite). Pregnanetriol is the urine metabolite of 17-hydroxyprogesterone, which is also proximal to the block. Deoxycortisol and cortisol, representing the 17-hydroxycorticoids, are distal to the block, hence they would be decreased. The electrolyte abnormalities are due to the loss of weak mineralocorticoids distal to the block (deoxycorticosterone). The plasma ACTH would be elevated owing to reduced synthesis of cortisol.

8. The answer is C: trisomy 21. The triad of low AFP, low unconjugated estriol, and high β-hCG is characteristic of Down syndrome (trisomy 21). In addition, the patient is over 35 years of age, which imposes an additional risk for a trisomy condition. Trisomy 13 is called Patau's syndrome and trisomy 18 is Edwards' syndrome, neither one of which has the prenatal laboratory findings noted in this patient. Cri du chat syndrome is a partial deletion of chromosome 5, and a microdeletion of chromosome 15 is noted in Prader-Willi and Angelman's syndromes, which are examples of genomic imprinting.

9. The answer is C: genetic heterogeneity. Homocystinuria is an AR disease, and Marfan syndrome is an AD disease. When two or more diseases have similar findings but an entirely different pathogenesis, they exhibit genetic heterogeneity. Pleiotropy occurs when a disease affects multiple organ systems (e.g., sickle cell disease). Variable expressivity is noted in AD diseases and is characterized by different levels of severity of expression of a disease. For example, neurofibromatosis may present with a few café-au-lait spots or with extensive involvement of the skin causing gross disfigurement. Penetrance is also a feature of AD diseases and describes what percentage of people with the abnormal gene will actually express the disease. For example, if one of two people with the abnormal gene expresses the disease, there is a 50% penetrance. Nondisjunction refers to abnormal separation of homologous chromosomes during the first division in meiosis. It is the most common cause of monosomy and trisomy syndromes.

10. The answer is H: fetal alcohol syndrome. This syndrome occurs in 2:1000 live births. Mental retardation is the most common abnormality and atrial septal defect the least common defect. Maxillary hypoplasia is another finding.

11. The answer is G: von Gierke's disease. This is an AR disease with a deficiency of the gluconeogenic enzyme

glucose-6-phosphatase, which converts glucose 6-phosphate to glucose. Hence, glucose will not increase with stimulation of gluconeogenesis (glucagon, cortisol, fructose). Excess glucose 6-phosphate is converted to glycogen in the liver and kidneys, which are the locations of the gluconeogenic enzymes.

12. The answer is L: congenital cytomegalovirus. CMV is the most common congenital infection and is part of the TORCH syndrome. Urine culture is the gold standard for confirming the diagnosis. Cytology of the urine sediment frequently reveals the classic basophilic intranuclear inclusions.

13. The answer is K: isotretinoin. All women who are candidates for isotretinoin for treatment of acne should have a pregnancy test and, if it is negative, should be offered a contraceptive in order to avoid these complications.

CHAPTER EIGHT

ENVIRONMENTAL PATHOLOGY

SYNOPSIS

OBJECTIVES

1. To describe key abnormalities associated with mechanical, thermal, electrical, radiation, and high-altitude injury.
2. To review the important findings in the sudden infant death syndrome.
3. To be familiar with key chemical and drug injuries.

Objective 1: To describe key abnormalities associated with mechanical, thermal, electrical, radiation, and high-altitude injury.

I. Mechanical injuries
  A. **Fractures** are breaks in the continuity of previously normal bone (e.g., a comminuted fracture with more than three bone fragments) or diseased bone (e.g., pathologic fracture due to a metastatic lesion).
  B. **Contusions (bruises)** are a blunt-force injury to the skin with subsequent escape of blood into tissue.
  C. **Abrasions** are superficial excoriations of the epidermis that are inflicted by a direct or tangential blow to the skin.
  D. A **laceration** is a blunt-force injury that overstretches the skin, resulting in a tear that is bridged by vessels, nerves, and connective tissue.
  E. **Incisions** are wounds with sharp margins (e.g., a surgical wound) that do not have vessels, nerves, or connective tissue bridging the defect.
  F. **Gunshot wounds** are either penetrating (which do not exit the body) or perforating (which do exit the body).
    1. **Contact wounds** contain soot and gunpowder in the wound (called fouling).
    2. **Intermediate wounds** (inflicted from 1.5–3 feet away with a handgun) have powder tattooing (stippling) of the skin around the entrance site but no fouling.
    3. **Distant wounds** do not have powder tattooing.
    4. **Exit wounds** are typically larger and more irregular than entrance wounds.
  G. **Motor vehicle accidents** (MVAs) are the most common cause of accidental death between 1 and 24 years of age (exception: homicide in black men between 15 and 24 years of age).
    1. They are commonly alcohol related, particularly among teenagers.
    2. Seat belts and air bags have significantly reduced morbidity and mortality.
  H. **Drowning** is the third most common cause of death in children from 1 to 14 years of age.
    1. **Near drowning** is defined as survival following asphyxia secondary to submersion.

2. In **wet drowning** (90% of cases), there is an initial laryngospasm on contact with water, followed by relaxation and aspiration of water.
3. In **dry drowning** (10%), there is intense laryngospasm without significant relaxation.
4. Water (fresh or salt water) in the lungs destroys surfactant (produces atelectasis with intrapulmonary shunting), causes diffuse alveolar damage, and initiates spasm in the bronchioles.
5. The immediate cause of death in drowning is cardiac arrhythmia.

II. Thermal injuries
  A. **First-degree burns** are painful partial thickness burns (e.g., sunburn) that primarily produce cell necrosis limited to the epidermis and heal without scarring.
  B. **Second-degree burns** are painful partial thickness burns that involve the entire epidermis, form blisters within the epidermis, and heal without scarring.
  C. **Third-degree burns** are painless full thickness burns with extensive necrosis of the epidermis and adnexa and commonly heal with extensive scarring complicated by keloid formation.
  D. Infection is the most common overall cause of death (*Pseudomonas aeruginosa* is the most frequent cause).
  E. **Hyperthermia** is defined as a core body temperature that is >37.2°C.
    1. **Heat cramps** are seen in untrained athletes or laborers who become volume depleted, lose excessive amounts of salt and water, and develop muscle spasms a few hours later (no fever).
    2. **Heat exhaustion** is noted in athletes who are training in a hot and humid environment and who develop severe volume depletion with mild elevation in core body temperature (≤39°C).
    3. **Heat stroke** is characterized by core body temperatures ≥41°C with associated CNS depression and hypohidrosis (lack of sweating).
    4. **Malignant hyperthermia** is an AD disease with a defect in calcium release channels in the muscle sarcoplasmic reticulum that produces massive muscle contractions and extremely high temperatures after induction of anesthesia by halothane and succinylcholine.
  F. **Frostbite** is a form of localized tissue injury secondary to both direct (ice crystallization in cells) and indirect (vasodilatation and thrombosis) damage.
  G. **Generalized hypothermia** (core body temperature <35°C) occurs when the whole body is exposed to freezing temperatures for a prolonged period of time and may progress to circulatory failure and death.

III. Electrical injuries
  A. **Ohm's law** states that the current (I, expressed in amps) is equal to the voltage (E) divided by the resistance (R, expressed in ohms) to the flow of current: I (amps) = E (volts)/R (ohms).
  B. Current is the most important factor in electrocution.
    1. AC is more dangerous than DC.
    2. Dry skin has higher tissue resistance to current (particularly the hands and feet).
    3. Wet skin lowers the resistance to current (voltage is constant), hence increasing current, which may produce cardiorespiratory arrest.
IV. Radiation injuries
  A. γ-Rays, x-rays, and particulate radiation emitted by radioactive substances (e.g., α- and β-particles) are examples of **ionizing radiation**, since they produce transient ionization after tissue absorption.
    1. The shorter the wavelength of radiation, the greater the penetration (e.g., α- and β-particles have low penetration, whereas γ-rays have high penetration).
    2. Radiation effect on tissue is determined by the type of radiation, its cumulative dose, and the surface area of tissue exposed to that dose.
    3. Radiation produces both direct and indirect injury to DNA (most susceptible protein), the latter type by producing free radicals (e.g., hydroxyl radicals) from hydrolysis of water in the tissue.
    4. Tissue susceptibility to radiation is directly related to the degree of mitotic activity and indirectly to the degree of specialization of the tissue.
    5. The peak sensitivity of proliferating cells to radiation is in G_2 (synthesis of the mitotic spindle) and mitosis.
    6. Tissues with a high radiosensitivity are hematopoietic cells (e.g., lymphocytes) and germinal cells; tissues with low radiosensitivity include bone, mature cartilage, and muscle.
    7. **Total body irradiation** has its greatest effect on the hematopoietic system, resulting in lymphopenia, thrombocytopenia, and bone marrow hypoplasia.
  B. Nonionizing radiation injuries are due to ultraviolet (UV) light, lasers, microwaves, or infrared.
    1. The **UVB portion of ultraviolet light** is most responsible for sunburn (first- and second-degree burns) and skin cancer (e.g., basal cell carcinoma [most common], squamous cell carcinoma, and malignant melanoma).
    2. **Laser radiation** produces an intense area of localized heat that is equivalent to a third-degree burn.
V. High-altitude injuries
  A. The oxygen concentration is the same at high altitude (21%) as at sea level; however, the barometric pressure is decreased.
    1. Hyperventilation is a useful response to **high-altitude sickness**, since lowering alveolar CO_2 (respiratory alkalosis) automatically increases PAO_2, which leads to an increase in arterial PO_2.
    2. **Acute mountain sickness** occurs within the first 24–36 hours of an ascent above 8000–10,000 feet (2400–3000 m) and may be prevented or ameliorated by taking acetazolamide (carbonic anhydrase inhibitor) a few days before and during ascent.

Objective 2: To review the important findings in the sudden infant death syndrome.

VI. Sudden infant death syndrome (SIDS)
  A. SIDS, or crib death, is the sudden death of an infant under 1 year of age that remains unexplained after a complete postmortem examination.
  B. The peak incidence is between 2 and 3 months after birth.
  C. Sleeping in a supine position is most responsible for the decline in deaths due to SIDS.
  D. Maternal risk factors include low socioeconomic status, smoking, and drug abuse, while infant risk factors consist of prematurity and a history of previous SIDS victims in the family.
  E. The apnea hypothesis (respiratory center abnormality and/or obstruction to air flow) is favored as the terminal event in SIDS.
  F. Autopsy findings primarily exhibit signs of hypoxia (e.g., thickened pulmonary arteries, petechiae on the pleura and epicardium) and mild inflammation in the lungs.

Objective 3: To be familiar with key chemical and drug injuries.

VII. Chemical and drug injuries
  A. The major **drugs of abuse** are **sedatives** (e.g., barbiturates), **stimulants** (e.g., cocaine), and **hallucinogens** (e.g., lysergic acid diethylamide) with some overlap with certain drugs.
    1. **Heroin** is an addicting opiate (depressant derived from the poppy plant) that is administered by intravenous or subcutaneous ("skin popping") injection.
      a. **Skin abscesses** due to *Staphylococcus aureus* and granulomatous reactions against the cutting agents are the most common types of local infection.
      b. **HBV hepatitis** and *S. aureus* sepsis leading to infective endocarditis (tricuspid or aortic valve) are the most common systemic complications.
      c. Intravenous (IV) drug abuse accounts for 22% of cases of AIDS.
      d. Overdose is associated with noncardiogenic pulmonary edema and frothing of edema fluid from the mouth and nose.
      e. Naloxone is a specific opiate antagonist.
    2. **Barbiturates** are common sedatives, hypnotics, and anticonvulsants; overdose leads to respiratory acidosis and death.
    3. **Tricyclic antidepressants** are the most common cause of death due to a prescription drug in the United States; they primarily target the central nervous system (causing seizures and coma) and the cardiovascular system (leading to myocarditis and cardiomyopathy).
    4. **Cocaine** is the most common cause of death from an illicit drug in the United States and produces sympathomimetic (stimulant) and euphoric effects by blocking the reuptake of the neurotransmitters dopamine and norepinephrine by the presynaptic axon.
    5. **Marihuana** contains a psychoactive stimulant called Δ^9-tetrahydrocannabinol (THC) that may be associated with lung disease (e.g., COPD, cancer), fetal abnormalities (e.g., low birth weight),

psychomotor impairment (delayed reaction time, inability to judge speed and distance), conjunctival redness and gynecomastia.

6. Blood levels of **alcohol** (**ethanol**) ≥100 mg/dL, or 0.1%, are generally accepted as legal drunkenness.
   a. Alcohol is a CNS depressant that may be associated with Wernicke's encephalopathy (e.g., confusion, agitation, nystagmus) and Korsakoff's psychosis (e.g., memory problems).
   b. It adversely affects the liver (e.g., cirrhosis), pancreas (e.g., pancreatitis), hematopoietic system (e.g., folate deficiency), gastrointestinal system (e.g., esophageal varices), and lungs (e.g., *Klebsiella pneumoniae* pneumonia).

B. **Drug injuries** may be dose related or idiosyncratic (hypersensitivity reactions) and are summarized in Table 8–1.

C. **Chemical injuries** are summarized in Table 8–2.

D. **Smoking** is the most important cause of premature death in the United States.
   1. Cigarette smoke contains carbon monoxide, carcinogens (e.g., polycyclic hydrocarbons), cell irritants and toxins, and nicotine (addicting agent).
   2. The respiratory system is the primary target (e.g., COPD and primary lung cancer).

E. Arthropod envenomations include those due to centipedes, spiders, scorpions, Hymenoptera (e.g., bees), mites, lice, and fly larva.
   1. **Black widow spider** envenomation produces a momentary sharp pain at the envenomation site (venom is a neurotoxin), followed by localized cramping pain, intense abdominal contractions, and rigidity that simulate an acute abdomen.
   2. **Brown recluse spider** (violin spider) envenomation (necrotoxic venom) is less painful than that of the black widow and produces a bulla or pustule that progresses to extensive ulceration.
   3. **Bees, wasps, hornets,** and **fire ants** produce local or systemic IgE-mediated type I hypersensitivity reactions.
   4. **Poisonous snake** envenomations in the United States may be due to **pit vipers** (e.g., **rattlesnakes** [most common], **water moccasins**, and **copperheads**) or **coral snakes** (neurotoxin).
      a. The key to treatment of poisonous snake bites is to prevent victims from moving around and get them to a hospital as soon as possible.
      b. Application of tight tourniquets or ice and cutting and suctioning at the envenomation site are not recommended.

TABLE 8–1. Drug Injuries

Drug or Drug Effect	Comments
Acetaminophen	Hepatotoxicity due to the formation of free radicals that are neutralized by glutathione. N-Acetylcysteine restores glutathione levels.
Alkylating agents	Nitrogen mustards, chlorambucil, busulfan, cyclophosphamide, and mitomycin C induce marrow suppression, second malignancies (non-Hodgkin's lymphoma). Cyclophosphamide is associated with transitional cell carcinoma of the bladder and hemorrhagic cystitis.
Chloramphenicol	Aplastic anemia in adults and "gray baby syndrome" in newborns (hypothermia, bradycardia, diarrhea, cyanosis [gray skin], and hypotension).
Estrogen	**Increased estrogens:** They increase liver synthesis of proteins—coagulation factors (fibrinogen, V, VIII; increases venous thrombosis), angiotensinogen (produces hypertension), sex hormone–binding globulin (lowers free testosterone). They decrease antithrombin III (produces venous thrombosis). They increase the incidence of stroke (arterial thrombosis), pulmonary embolism (venous thrombosis from legs), and myocardial infarction (especially in those who smoke or are hypertensive). They stimulate tryptophan metabolism, hence lowering serotonin and producing depression. They are associated with an increased incidence of endometrial, ovarian, and breast carcinoma. Diethylstilbestrol in pregnant women predisposes their daughters to vaginal adenosis and clear-cell carcinoma of the vagina, cervical stenosis, and uterine and tubal abnormalities. Gynecomastia may occur in men. They may produce intrahepatic cholestasis and gallbladder disease. **Decreased estrogens:** They are associated with osteoporosis and CAD.
Interstitial pulmonary fibrosis	Interstitial pulmonary fibrosis is associated with exposure to amiodarone, bleomycin, busulfan, nitrofurantoin, methysergide (also retroperitoneal fibrosis and Raynaud's phenomenon).
Iron	Iron has a corrosive effect on the stomach (gastritis), produces hepatic necrosis and liver failure, and causes shock and metabolic acidosis. X-rays reveal radiopaque pills in the GI tract. Deferoxamine is used for chelation therapy.
Methotrexate	Methotrexate inhibits dihydrofolate reductase (causing megaloblastic anemia) and produces hepatic fibrosis.
Oral contraceptives	Ethinyl estradiol produces most of the complications. Estrogen in birth control pills has similar effects to unopposed estrogen; however, unlike unopposed estrogen, it does predispose to liver abnormalities (liver adenoma, hepatocellular carcinoma). Estrogen is protective for fibrocystic change in the breast, endometrial and ovarian cancer, pelvic inflammatory disease, acne, and rheumatoid arthritis.
Salicylates	Salicylates uncouple oxidative phosphorylation. They occur in high concentration in oil of wintergreen. They directly stimulate the respiratory center, producing a primary respiratory alkalosis. Lactic acidosis may occur from uncoupling of oxidative phosphorylation, and the addition of salicylic acid produces an increased anion gap metabolic acidosis. Children quickly pass through the respiratory alkalosis phase and present with profound metabolic acidosis. Adults commonly present with a mixed disorder including primary respiratory alkalosis and primary metabolic acidosis (pH is normal). They are associated with renal papillary necrosis (blocks vasodilator effect of renal prostaglandin), triad asthma (aspirin sensitivity + asthma + nasal polyps), acute gastritis, peptic ulcers (decreases prostaglandins), fulminant hepatitis, bleeding (platelet dysfunction, gastritis), vertigo and tinnitus, hyperpyrexia, convulsions, and coma. The urine is alkalinized to increase excretion.

TABLE 8–2. Summary of Chemical and Toxin Injuries

Chemical/Toxin	Comments
Alcohols	**Isopropyl alcohol (rubbing alcohol):** it produces deep coma and hyporeflexia. The metabolic end product in the liver is acetone, not acid (not metabolic acidosis). It increases the osmolal gap (difference between calculated and measured serum osmolality >10). **Methyl alcohol (wood alcohol):** It is present in windshield wiper fluid. It produces abdominal pain and optic nerve irritation (potential for blindness) by liver conversion into formic acid (increased AG metabolic acidosis). It increases the osmolal gap. It may produce necrosis/infarction of the putamen. Ethanol infusion competes with methyl alcohol for metabolism by alcohol dehydrogenase, so it can be removed by dialysis. **Ethylene glycol (antifreeze):** The liver converts it into glycolic and oxalic acids (increased AG metabolic acidosis). Oxalic acid forms calcium oxalate crystals in the renal tubules, producing renal failure. It increases the osmolal gap. Treatment is the same as for methyl alcohol. Diethylene glycol is twice as toxic as ethylene glycol and has an additional component of liver toxicity.
Benzene	Benzene may produce aplastic anemia and acute myelogenous leukemia.
Bromide	Bromides may depress the CNS and produce an acneiform, warty-appearing rash.
Carbon monoxide (CO)	CO is the most common cause of death due to poisoning in the United States. It is a common accidental injury or method of suicide. Sources include automobile exhaust, domestic gas, natural gas, smoke in fires, cigarette smoke (8–10%), methylene chloride (converted into CO), and wood stoves with a blocked vent. CO has 200–240 times higher affinity for Hb than O_2. Carboxyhemoglobin shifts the ODC to the left, hence reducing O_2 release to tissue. It also blocks cytochrome oxidase in the oxidative pathway. CO is odorless. The brain (globus pallidus and substantia nigra in particular) and heart are primarily affected, but changes also occur in the liver (fatty change) and other organs. CO accelerates atherosclerosis (endothelial injury). **Clinical:** Patients have a cherry red color to the skin and blood. The first sign is headache (~30% concentration). Concentrations above 60% generally result in death. **Laboratory:** There is a normal PaO_2, decreased oxygen saturation (occupies the heme group rather than O_2), and decreased oxygen content. Treatment is inhalation of 100% oxygen or placement in a hyperbaric chamber.
Carbon tetrachloride (CCl_4)	The liver converts CCl_4 to a CCl_3 free radical, which damages the liver (fulminant hepatitis, fatty change).
Chlorinated hydrocarbons	Chlorinated hydrocarbons are present in insecticides such as DDT. They produce toxic neuronal injury, resulting in hyperexcitability, convulsions, delirium, and coma.
Corrosives	Corrosives are usually strong acids or alkalis. Ingested alkalis (85% of cases) penetrate tissue owing to liquefactive necrosis. Acids (15% of cases) produce coagulation necrosis (less penetration). Swallowing lye (sodium hydroxide) produces severe corrosive esophagitis with subsequent stricture formation and a tendency for esophageal cancer. Endoscopy is recommended early to assess damage.
Cyanide	Cyanide is a systemic asphyxiant that blocks cytochrome oxidase in the oxidative phosphorylation system. Exposure occurs from combustion of polyurethane products during fires. It produces hypoxic cell injury in the brain, kidneys, liver, heart, etc. The breath has a bitter almond smell. Treatment consists of using nitrites (amyl and sodium nitrite) followed by thiosulfate. Nitrites create methemoglobin, which competes with cytochrome oxidase for cyanide. Thiosulfate combines with cyanide from cyanmethemoglobin to form a nontoxic thiocyanate.
Heavy metals	Heavy metals produce acute or chronic intoxication. They include lead (most common cause of chronic intoxication), arsenic (most common cause of acute intoxication), and mercury. Blood and/or urine tests are useful for screening. **Lead** (Chapter 12): It binds to disulfide groups and denatures enzymes (ribonuclease and ferrochelatase [most important] and ALA dehydrase in heme synthesis). The source in children is eating chips of old lead-based paints. Adult sources include exposure to lead in a battery factory (inhalation of dust or fumes), mining, glazed pottery, moonshine whiskey (from old lead radiators), and welding. Children absorb lead more readily than adults do. **Clinical:** In children, the brain is the target organ. Lead poisoning produces cerebral edema, demyelination, and necrosis. There is permanent CNS damage. Behavioral, motor, and cognitive dysfunctions all occur even at low levels. Children are prone to lead deposition in bone and developing teeth. It deposits in the epiphyses and produces a dense line visible on x-ray (the only heavy metal with this finding). Sideroblastic anemias may occur (microcytic, with coarse basophilic stippling). Lead colic may occur in both children and adults. A lead line in the gums is more common in adults with poor dentition (lead attaches to sulfides along the gingiva). Peripheral neuropathy, particularly wristdrop, is more common in adults. Renal abnormalities occur in both children and adults and include nephrotoxic acute tubular necrosis (coagulation necrosis of proteins in the proximal tubule leading to aminoaciduria, glucosuria, and proximal renal tubular acidosis, acid-fast inclusions in renal tubular cells) and interstitial nephritis associated with hyperuricemia (saturnine gout). **Laboratory:** blood levels are the best screen. RBC zinc protoporphyrin level is increased as well as urine δ-aminolevulinic acid. **Treatment:** dimercaprol (British antilewisite [BAL]), EDTA, and penicillamine. **Mercury:** It is toxic in the elemental form (dental amalgams), as an inorganic salt (GI and renal disease [similar to lead]), and in the organic form (CNS disease [cerebral and cerebellar neuron loss, constricted visual fields, called Minamata disease]). It is present in pesticides, neon lights, contaminated fish in polluted water (Japan). **Treatment:** Dimercaprol, penicillamine. **Arsenic:** Elemental arsenic is nontoxic. Toxic compounds include pentavalent salts, trivalent salts, and arsine gas. It is present in pesticides, animal dips, and Fowler's solution. **Clinical:** It produces a garlic odor to the breath. Other abnormalities include arsenic melanosis (gray skin with dark macules), CNS findings (headache, convulsions/coma [most common cause of death]), polyneuropathy, nephrotoxic acute tubular necrosis, hemolytic anemia, patchy alopecia, and watery diarrhea. Nails have transverse bands (Aldrich-Mees lines). It concentrates in keratin, hair, and nails. It is carcinogenic (causing squamous cell carcinoma of the skin, lung cancer, and liver angiosarcoma). **Treatment:** Dimercaprol.

Table continued on following page

TABLE 8–2. Summary of Chemical and Toxin Injuries *Continued*

Chemical/Toxin	Comments
Irritant gases	Irritant gases such as chlorine, fluorine, phosgene, sulfur dioxide, and nitric oxide dissolve in tissue to form acids that damage tissue, particularly the bronchioles (chemical bronchiolitis) and alveoli (edema and hyaline membranes).
Mushroom poisoning (*Amanita*)	Mushroom poisoning is due to ingestion of the mushrooms of *Amanita* species. The toxin inhibits RNA polymerase. **Clinical:** It produces abdominal pain, vomiting, bloody diarrhea, and jaundice from extensive fatty change in the liver. Fatty change also occurs in the heart, kidneys, and muscles. CNS abnormalities.
Organophosphates	Organophosphates are potent insecticides. They are readily absorbed through the skin, respiratory tract, and gastrointestinal tract. They produce an irreversible block of acetylcholinesterase with subsequent accumulation of acetylcholine at synapses and myoneural junctions. **Clinical:** There is initial excessive autonomic system activity (excessive lacrimation and salivation), fecal incontinence, and constricted pupils. Later findings consist of nicotinic effects such as muscle weakness/paralysis and muscle fasciculations. **Laboratory:** Serum and RBC cholinesterase (pseudocholinesterase) levels are decreased. Atropine is the treatment of choice. Pralidoxime (2-PAM) is also used.
Oxygen	Oxygen is toxic to the lungs when administered at 100% concentration for 24 hours. It forms superoxide free radicals that damage respiratory epithelium (diffuse alveolar damage, bronchopulmonary dysplasia) and retinal tissue (retrolental fibroplasia in newborns).
Petroleum products	Gasoline and kerosene cause euphoria (similar to drunkenness) when inhaled (or ingested). They are addictive. In toxic doses, CNS changes occur (drowsiness, convulsions) and tinnitus. In the lungs, they produce pulmonary edema and predispose to pneumonia by secondary bacterial colonization.
Strychnine	Strychnine is a powerful CNS stimulant. It inhibits postsynaptic inhibition, hence leading to tetanic convulsions, opisthotonus, risus sardonicus, and death.
Yellow (white) phosphorus	Yellow phosphorus initially produces gastrointestinal irritation and a garlic smell to the breath. Phosphorus uncouples oxidative phosphorylation. Injury is most severe in the liver (zone 1; periportal coagulation necrosis and fatty change) and kidneys (acute tubular necrosis).

QUESTIONS

DIRECTIONS. (ITEMS 1–6): Each of the numbered items or incomplete statements in this section is followed by answers or by completions of the statement. Select the ONE lettered answer or completion that is BEST in each case. Correct answers and explanations are given at the end of the chapter.

1. Which of the following drug or chemical injury relationships is correctly matched?

    (A) Acetaminophen: predisposition to hepatocellular carcinoma
    (B) Methyl alcohol: renal failure
    (C) Cocaine: excessive lacrimation and salivation
    (D) Ethanol: CNS stimulant
    (E) Carbon monoxide: necrosis of the globus pallidus

2. Which of the following drug or chemical injury relationships is correctly matched?

    (A) Benzene: liver cell necrosis
    (B) Lead: encephalopathy in children
    (C) Ethylene glycol: conversion to acetone
    (D) Unopposed estrogen: liver cell adenoma
    (E) Organophosphates: mydriasis

3. Which of following system/injury relationships associated with alcohol abuse is correctly matched?

    (A) CNS: necrosis of the putamen
    (B) Gastrointestinal: esophageal stricture
    (C) Hepatobiliary: hemochromatosis
    (D) Gastrointestinal: malabsorption
    (E) Hematologic: pernicious anemia

4. Which of the following system/injury relationships related to long-term cigarette smoking is correctly matched?

    (A) Respiratory: bronchiectasis
    (B) Gastrointestinal: Curling's ulcers
    (C) Hematologic: secondary polycythemia
    (D) Pancreas: acute pancreatitis
    (E) Reproductive: endometrial carcinoma

5. Which of the following physical injury relationships is correctly matched?

    (A) Fire: smoke inhalation is the most common cause of death
    (B) Heat cramps: temperature ≥41°C
    (C) Acute mountain sickness: respiratory acidosis
    (D) Electrical injury: voltage is the most important variable
    (E) Ionizing radiation injury: greatest effect is on RNA and protein synthesis

6. Which of the following injury relationships is correctly matched?

   (A) Near drowning: most commonly due to intense laryngospasm leading to asphyxia
   (B) Laceration: skin tear bridged by vessels, nerves, and connective tissue
   (C) Intermediate gunshot wound: fouling at the wound site
   (D) Sudden infant death syndrome: most common in newborns <1 month old
   (E) Pathologic fracture: hip fracture due to a motorcycle accident

   DIRECTIONS. (ITEMS 7–8): Each set of matching questions in this section consists of a list of lettered options followed by several numbered items. For each numbered item, select the ONE option that is most closely associated with it. Each lettered option may be selected once, more than once, or not at all.

   (A) Black widow spider envenomation
   (B) Brown recluse spider envenomation
   (C) Bee, wasp, hornet envenomation
   (D) Fire ant envenomation
   (E) Rattlesnake envenomation

7. Painful bite associated with board-like rigidity of the abdominal muscles

8. Painful bite associated with a wheal-and-flare reaction, vesiculation, and necrosis of the skin

---

ANSWERS AND EXPLANATIONS

1. The answer is E: carbon monoxide: necrosis of the globus pallidus. The hypoxic effect of chronic exposure to carbon monoxide is necrosis of the globus pallidus, leading to parkinsonism. Acetaminophen produces dose-dependent liver cell necrosis. Methyl alcohol is converted to formic acid (increased anion gap metabolic acidosis) and damages the optic nerve, leading to blindness. Cocaine blocks the uptake of dopamine and norepinephrine, hence producing sympathomimetic signs (e.g., mydriasis) rather than cholinergic signs of excessive lacrimation and salivation. Ethanol is a CNS depressant.

2. The answer is B: lead: encephalopathy in children. The CNS is primarily targeted in lead poisoning in children (not adults) owing to increased vessel permeability, leading to cerebral edema, demyelination, and necrosis. Benzene is associated with aplastic anemia and acute myelogenous leukemia. Ethylene glycol is converted to oxalic acid, which forms calcium oxalate crystals in the renal tubules, leading to renal failure. Unopposed estrogen is associated with endometrial and breast cancer, while oral contraceptives predispose to liver cell adenomas and hepatocellular carcinoma. Organophosphates irreversibly block acetylcholinesterase with subsequent accumulation of acetylcholine, leading to cholinergic signs and symptoms (e.g., miosis rather than mydriasis).

3. The answer is D: gastrointestinal: malabsorption. Alcohol abuse is the most common cause of chronic pancreatitis, which produces a deficiency of enzymes, leading to malabsorption. Necrosis of the putamen is noted with methyl alcohol poisoning. Esophageal varices (not esophageal strictures) are most commonly associated with portal hypertension secondary to alcoholic cirrhosis. People with alcoholism more commonly have acquired iron overload (hemosiderosis) involving the liver. Hemochromatosis is an AR iron overload disease. Pernicious anemia is an autoimmune disease producing macrocytic anemia. People with alcoholism most commonly have folate deficiency as a cause of macrocytic anemia.

4. The answer is C: hematologic: secondary polycythemia. Hypoxemia induced by COPD is a stimulus for erythropoietin release and secondary polycythemia. Bronchiectasis is most commonly caused by cystic fibrosis and tuberculosis. Curling's ulcers are associated with severe burns. Pancreatic carcinoma (not pancreatitis) is increased in smokers. Cervical cancer (not endometrial) is increased in smokers.

5. The answer is A: fire: smoke inhalation is the most common cause of death. Smoke inhalation (CO, cyanide gases) rather than direct burn injuries is the most common cause of death in fires. Heat stroke (not cramps) is associated with temperature $\geq 41°C$. Acute mountain sickness is associated with respiratory alkalosis as compensation for a low PaO_2. The amount of current is more important than voltage in electrical injuries. Ionizing radiation injury, either direct or indirect (free radicals from hydrolysis of water), has its greatest effect on DNA.

6. The answer is B: laceration: skin tear bridged by vessels, nerves, and connective tissue. Lacerations are a blunt-force injury producing overstretching of skin, leading to a tear. They are often confused with incisions created by a sharp object (not bridged by vessels, nerves, and connective tissue). Near drowning is most commonly due to wet drowning, where an initial laryngospasm is followed by relaxation and movement of water into the lungs. Contact wounds are associated with gunpowder and soot in the wound site (fouling), whereas intermediate gunshot wounds demonstrate powder tattooing. SIDS most often occurs between the second and third months of age and is uncommon in infants <1 month or >9 months. Pathologic fractures occur in bones with preexisting disease, hence a hip fracture due to a motorcycle accident does not qualify as a pathologic fracture.

7. The answer is A: black widow spider envenomation. The black widow injects a neurotoxin that produces muscle cramping simulating an acute abdomen.

8. The answer is D: fire ant envenomation. Fire ants, like bees, wasps, and hornets, produce a type I hypersensitivity reaction; however, the fire ant lesions are more likely to be vesiculated and associated with necrosis.

CHAPTER NINE

NEOPLASIA

SYNOPSIS

OBJECTIVES

1. To review the nomenclature of tumors and tumor-like conditions.
2. To discuss the properties of malignant cells.
3. To understand the role of oncogenes in cancer.
4. To be familiar with the grade and stage of cancer.
5. To review host-tumor and tumor-host relationships.
6. To discuss the role of tumor markers in oncology.
7. To understand the epidemiology of cancer.

Objective 1: To review the nomenclature of tumors and tumor-like conditions.

I. Nomenclature of tumors and tumor-like conditions
   A. Both benign and malignant tumors are composed of parenchyma consisting of proliferating cells and supporting connective tissue stroma.
      1. The parenchymal component of a tumor determines its biologic behavior.
      2. Most tumors are of epithelial origin (ecto-, endo-, mesoderm), while the remainder are of connective tissue origin.
   B. Benign tumors are named by adding the suffix "oma" to the cell type (e.g., lipoma).
      1. Those arising from glands are designated **adenomas** (e.g., tubular adenoma), while those from epithelial surfaces are called **polyps** (stalked or sessile) or papillomas (which have a branching pattern).
      2. Benign tumors commonly have capsules, grow slowly, do not invade (dermatofibroma is an exception), have minimal mitotic activity (normal spindles), and resemble the parent tissue.
      3. The suffix "oma" does not always indicate a benign tumor; e.g., melanoma, lymphoma, astrocytoma, and hepatoma are malignant tumors.
   C. Malignant tumors of epithelial origin are called **carcinomas**.
      1. Those arising from squamous epithelium (e.g., oral pharynx, esophagus, larynx, lung) are called **squamous cell carcinomas**.
      2. Those arising from glandular epithelium (e.g., stomach, colon, pancreas) are called **adenocarcinomas**.
      3. Those arising from transitional epithelium in the urinary system (e.g., bladder, renal pelvis) are designated **transitional cell carcinomas**.

4. **APUD** (*amine precursor uptake and decarboxylation*) **tumors** are neuroendocrine tumors (having dense-core neurosecretory granules on electron microscopy) that most commonly develop from neural crest and neural ectoderm (e.g., small-cell carcinoma of lung, carcinoid tumors).
5. Malignant tumors lack capsules, grow rapidly, have atypical mitotic spindles (tripolar), invade, can metastasize (exception is a basal cell carcinoma), and prefer lymphatic spread (exceptions are renal adenocarcinoma and hepatocellular carcinoma, which often invade vessels).
   D. **Sarcomas** are malignant tumors of connective tissue origin (e.g., fibrosarcoma, rhabdomyosarcoma [skeletal muscle], leiomyosarcoma [smooth muscle]).
      1. They are derived from mesenchymal tissue.
      2. They tend to be large, bulky, vascular, and necrotic and prefer hematogenous dissemination (exception is rhabdomyosarcoma, which prefers lymphatic spread).
   E. **Mixed tumors** have two different morphologic patterns that are derived from the same germ cell layer (e.g., mixed tumor of salivary gland).
   F. **Teratomas** derive from all three germ cell layers (e.g., teratoma of the ovary or testis).
      1. They commonly have teeth and bone, which are visible on x-ray.
      2. They are the most common germ cell tumors, which are totipotential tumors that may differentiate in any direction.
   G. The key distinction between benign and malignant tumors is the capacity of malignant tumors to invade and metastasize.
   H. **Hamartomas** are nonneoplastic lesions associated with an overgrowth of tissue that is normally present in the organ (e.g., bronchial hamartoma of lung, Peutz-Jeghers polyp, hyperplastic polyp).
   I. **Choristomas**, or heterotopic rests, are nonneoplastic and represent normal tissue in a foreign location (e.g., pancreatic tissue in the stomach).

Objective 2: To discuss the properties of malignant cells.

II. Properties of malignant cells
   A. Malignant tumor growth is primarily due to cell accumulation resulting from an increase in number of cells in the proliferative compartment.

B. Malignant cells have characteristic nuclear features (e.g., increased nuclear/cytoplasmic ratio, atypical mitotic spindles).

C. They possess simple biochemical systems (anaerobic metabolism), lack cohesiveness, are not contact inhibited, are transplantable, and are immortal in culture.

D. They have the capacity to invade and metastasize.
1. They have receptors for integrin molecules (laminin, fibronectin), which help them adhere to extracellular matrix; type IV collagenases, which dissolve basement membranes; and proteases.
2. They secrete transforming growth factor (TGF) α and β to promote angiogenesis and collagen deposition.
3. They disseminate by lymphatic spread (usually carcinomas), hematogenous spread (usually sarcomas), or by seeding within a body cavity (ovarian and colon cancer).
4. Metastasis is more common than a primary cancer in certain organs (e.g., lung, liver, brain, bone [most commonly the vertebral column], adrenals, lymph nodes).
    a. A primary lung cancer is the most common metastasis to the brain, liver, and adrenal glands.
    b. Breast and prostate cancer are the most common metastasis to the vertebral column via the Batson vertebral venous plexus.

Objective 3: To understand the role of oncogenes in cancer.

III. Oncogenesis
A. Cancer is a multistep process involving **initiation** (irreversible mutations involving protooncogenes), **promotion** (growth enhancement to pass on the mutations to other cells), and **progression** (development of tumor heterogeneity for metastasis, drug resistance, etc.).
B. **Protooncogenes** are precursors of oncogenes, or genes that produce cancer.
1. Protooncogenes are normally regulatory genes that code for proteins involved in growth and repair processes in the body.
2. The major classes of oncogene products involved in the normal growth process of cells are as follows:
    a. Growth factors (e.g., *sis* oncogene)
    b. Growth factor receptors (*erb*B2/*neu* [*HER*-2] oncogene)
    c. Membrane-associated protein kinases (e.g., *src* oncogene)
    d. Membrane-related guanine triphosphate (GTP)–binding proteins (e.g., *ras* oncogenes)
    e. Cytoplasmic protein kinases (e.g., *raf* oncogene)
    f. Transcription regulators located in the nucleus (e.g., c-*myc* oncogene)
3. **Tumor suppressor genes** (antioncogenes) are guardians of unregulated cell growth (e.g., *p53*, Rb oncogenes).
C. Activation of protooncogenes (e.g., *ras*) that are involved in the growth process or inactivation of suppressor genes (e.g., *p53*) is responsible for neoplastic transformation of a cell.
1. Point mutations, translocations (e.g., t8;142 in Burkitt's lymphoma), and gene amplification (multiple copies of the gene with overexpression of products) are mechanisms of activation.
    a. Overexpression of the *erb*B2 oncogene is noted in 20–30% of invasive ductal cancers of the breast and predicts poor survival.
    b. Activation of the *ras* protooncogene (point mutation) is associated with 30% of all human cancers including cancers of the lung, colon, and pancreas as well as leukemia (20–25% of acute myelogenous leukemia).
    c. Translocation of the *abl* protooncogene from chromosome 9 to chromosome 22 with formation of a large *bcr-abl* hybrid gene on chromosome 22 (Philadelphia chromosome) results in chronic myelogenous leukemia.
    d. Inactivation of suppressor genes (point mutation) leads to unrestricted cell division.
        (1) Inactivation of each of the *Rb1* suppressor genes on chromosome 13 is associated with malignant retinoblastoma in children.
        (2) Inactivation of the *p53* suppressor gene on chromosome 17 accounts for ~25–50% of all malignancies involving the colon, breast, lung, and central nervous system.
        (3) Inactivation of the APC suppressor gene (APC = *a*denomatous *p*olyposis *c*oli) on chromosome 5 is associated with the autosomal dominant familial polyposis syndrome and Gardner's syndrome.
        (4) Inactivation of the *NF1* and *NF2* suppressor oncogenes (NF = *n*euro*f*ibromatosis) on chromosomes 17 and 22, respectively, is associated with tumors (e.g., acoustic neuromas, meningiomas) present in types 1 and 2 neurofibromatosis, respectively.
2. **Chemicals** (Table 9–1), **viruses** (Table 9–2), **irradiation** (Table 9–3), and **physical agents** (e.g., burn scars) may initiate the above mutational events.
    a. Most chemical carcinogens are inactive in their native states and must be activated by enzymes in the cytochrome P-450 or other enzyme system (bacterial enzymes or enzymes induced by alcohol).
    b. Nonpermissive cells that prevent an oncogenic RNA or DNA virus from completing its replication cycle often produce changes in the genome that result in activation of protooncogenes or inactivation of suppressor genes.
    c. In radiation carcinogenesis, ionizing particles (e.g., α- and β-particles), γ-rays, and x-rays hydrolyze water into free radicals, which are mutagenic to DNA by activating protooncogenes.
    d. Ultraviolet light (particularly UVB) induces the formation of thymidine dimers, which distort the DNA molecule, leading to skin cancer (e.g., basal cell carcinoma [most common], squamous cell carcinoma, and malignant melanoma).

TABLE 9–1. Chemical Carcinogens

Carcinogen	Tumor
Aniline dyes	Transitional cell carcinoma of bladder, ureters, renal pelvis
Benzidine	Transitional cell carcinoma of bladder, ureters, renal pelvis
Cyclophosphamide	Transitional cell carcinoma of bladder, ureters, renal pelvis
Phenacetin	Transitional cell carcinoma of bladder, ureters, renal pelvis
Vinyl chloride	Angiosarcoma of liver
Thorotrast	Angiosarcoma of liver, hepatocellular carcinoma
Arsenic	Angiosarcoma of liver, squamous cell carcinoma of skin, lung cancer
Asbestos	Primary lung cancer if a smoker (cocarcinogen with smoking), mesothelioma if a nonsmoker (no relation to smoking)
Oral contraceptives	Liver cell adenomas, hepatocellular carcinoma
Aflatoxins (*Aspergillus flavus*; cocarcinogen with HBV)	Hepatocellular carcinoma
Cadmium	Prostate cancer, lung cancer
Polycyclic hydrocarbons (tobacco smoke); alcohol (cocarcinogen for oral, esophageal and laryngeal cancers)	Small cell carcinoma of lung; squamous cancers of oral cavity, esophagus, larynx, lung, cervix; transitional carcinoma of bladder; adenocarcinoma of pancreas
Chromium	Lung cancer
Nickel	Lung, nasal cavity cancer
Uranium (radon gas)	Lung cancer
Woodworking	Nasal cavity cancer
Chewing tobacco	Verrucous carcinoma in mouth
Alkylating agents	Acute leukemia, malignant lymphoma
Benzene	Acute leukemia
Diethylstilbestrol	Clear cell adenocarcinoma of cervix and vagina
Nitrosamines (inhibited by ascorbic acid and refrigeration)	Esophageal and gastric cancers
Tars, soots, oils	Squamous cell carcinoma of skin (or scrotum in chimney sweeps)

TABLE 9–2. Putative Oncogenic Viruses in Humans

Oncogenic Virus	Tumor
Human T-cell lymphotropic virus–1 (HTLV-1)	Adult T-cell leukemia/lymphoma
HTLV-2	Hairy cell leukemia
Human immunodeficiency virus (HIV)	CNS malignant lymphoma
Hepatitis C virus (HCV)	Hepatocellular carcinoma
Hepatitis B virus (HBV)	Hepatocellular carcinoma (aflatoxin B is a cocarcinogen)
Epstein-Barr virus	Burkitt's lymphoma, nasopharyngeal carcinoma, polyclonal malignant lymphoma
Human papillomavirus (Herpesvirus may act as a cocarcinogen)	Squamous cell carcinoma of the cervix, vagina, vulva, and anus; laryngeal papillomas (may progress to cancer)
Herpesvirus 8	Kaposi's sarcoma

TABLE 9–3. Ionizing Radiation–Induced Cancers

Cancer	Comments
Leukemia	Most common radiation-induced cancer. Seen in radiologists and those exposed to radiation emitted from atomic bomb (most developed chronic granulocytic leukemia).
Papillary carcinoma of thyroid	Radiation therapy to head and neck area (e.g., for acne).
Lung cancer	Exposure of uranium miners to radon gas.
Breast cancer	Unlikely to occur with current mammography instruments. May occur with exposure to radiation from nuclear plants and atomic bombs.
Osteogenic sarcoma	May occur in radiologists. Formerly seen in women who painted radium onto watch dials owing to its fluorescent properties.
Angiosarcoma	Thorotrast exposure.
Squamous and basal cell carcinomas of skin	β-Irradiation of skin.

Objective 4: To be familiar with the grade and stage of cancer.

IV. Grade and stage of cancer
  A. The grade of a cancer is based primarily on the histologic appearance of the tumor with regard to its degree of differentiation (e.g., low grade, high grade), mitotic activity, cellular atypia, and invasiveness.
  B. Tumor stage (the most important prognostic factor) is based on the size of the primary tumor and the presence or absence of lymph node or hematogenous dissemination to other sites.

Objective 5: To review host-tumor and tumor-host relationships.

V. Host defense against tumors
  A. Host defense against tumors is both humoral (via antibodies or complement) and cellular (e.g., cytotoxic T cells), the latter representing the more efficient killing mechanism.
  B. Tumors frequently produce tumor-specific antigens (TSAs) to which the host may develop antibodies; virus-induced cancers are the most antigenic and chemical-induced cancers the least antigenic.
VI. Tumor-host relationships
  A. **Cachexia** is the progressive wasting away of a patient and is due to the release of tumor necrosis factor-α (cachectin) from macrophages and from tumor cells.
  B. The **anemia of chronic disease** is the most common anemia in malignancy.
  C. Most cancer patients are in a **hypercoagulable state**, which predisposes them to thrombosis.
  D. Infections (especially gram-negatives) commonly complicate malignancy and are the most common cause of death in cancer.
  E. Benign and malignant tumors may produce **paraneoplastic syndromes** having distant effects by humoral mechanisms that do not involve either direct invasion or metastasis.
    1. **Hypercalcemia** secondary to secretion of a **parathormone-like peptide** (e.g., primary squamous cell carcinoma of lung and renal adenocarcinoma) is the most common paraneoplastic syndrome.
    2. **Eaton-Lambert syndrome** has myasthenia gravis–like features and is associated with small-cell carcinoma of the lung.
    3. **Cerebellar degeneration** (with ataxia, dysarthria, and nystagmus) is associated with cancers of the breast, lung, and lymph nodes.
    4. **Acanthosis nigricans** (a pigmented lesion usually located in the axilla) may be a phenotypic marker for gastric carcinoma.
    5. **Dermatomyositis** is the most common connective tissue disease associated with cancer (e.g., lung and breast carcinomas).
    6. Crops of **seborrheic keratoses** that develop suddenly (the Leser-Trélat sign) suggest an underlying gastrointestinal cancer.
    7. **Pulmonary osteoarthropathy** (clubbing of the nails, synovitis, and periosteal inflammation) may accompany primary lung cancers.
    8. Superficial migratory thrombophlebitis (**Trousseau's sign**) suggests carcinoma of the pancreas.
    9. Patients may present with the **nephrotic syndrome** owing to tumor antigens forming immunocomplexes in the glomerulus.
    10. Table 9–4 summarizes **ectopic hormone syndromes**.

TABLE 9–4.   Ectopic Hormone Syndromes

Ectopic Hormone	Tumor	Syndrome
Adrenocorticotropic hormone (ACTH)	Small-cell carcinoma of lung, medullary carcinoma of thyroid.	Cushing's syndrome (hyperpigmentation)
Antidiuretic hormone (ADH)	Small-cell carcinoma of lung.	Dilutional hyponatremia
β-Human chorionic gonadotropin (β-hCG)	Trophoblastic tumors: benign (hydatidiform mole and invasive mole), malignant (choriocarcinoma). Germ cell tumors of ovary and testis.	Gynecomastia (β-hCG is an LH analogue), hyperthyroidism (similar to TSH), precocious puberty in children.
Calcitonin	Medullary carcinoma of thyroid.	Hypocalcemia.
Erythropoietin	Renal adenocarcinoma, Wilms' tumor, hepatocellular carcinoma, Lindau–von Hippel disease (cerebellar hemangioblastoma, **renal adenocarcinoma**), kidney lesions (cysts, hydronephrosis), large uterine leiomyomas producing hydronephrosis.	Secondary polycythemia (normal PaO_2, ↑RBC mass, normal plasma volume).
Insulin-like growth factor	Hepatocellular carcinoma, retroperitoneal tumors.	Hypoglycemia.
Parathormone-like peptide	Squamous cell carcinoma of lung, renal adenocarcinoma, breast cancer, ovarian cancer.	Hypercalcemia (low PTH).
Serotonin	Carcinoid syndrome due to metastatic small bowel carcinoid to liver, small-cell carcinoma of lung, bronchial carcinoid, medullary carcinoma of thyroid.	Carcinoid syndrome: flushing, diarrhea, valvular lesions: tricuspid insufficiency and pulmonic stenosis.

Objective 6: To discuss the role of tumor markers in oncology.

VII. Tumor markers
  A. A tumor marker (e.g., hormone, enzyme) is a biochemical indicator of the presence of a neoplastic process.
  B. Markers may be used to screen for cancer but are more commonly used to follow the disease for recurrence or determine the degree of tumor burden in the patient (Table 9–5).

Objective 7: To understand the epidemiology of cancer.

VIII. Cancer epidemiology
  A. Smoking is responsible for a third of cancers.
  B. Other risk factors for cancer include a high-fat, low-fiber diet, obesity, and sedentary life-style.
  C. Men more commonly have cancer than women except for gallbladder and endocrine cancers.
  D. There is a 20% greater prevalence of cancer (e.g., prostate, lung, multiple myeloma) in African Americans than whites.
  E. The three most common cancers in men, in order of decreasing frequency, are prostate, lung, and colorectal, whereas in women they are breast, lung, and colorectal.
  F. The three most common cancers leading to death in men, in descending order, are lung, prostate, and colorectal, whereas in women, they are lung, breast, and colorectal.
  G. Cancer is second only to accidents as the most common cause of death in children, who are affected by, in descending order of incidence, acute lymphoblastic leukemia, tumors of the CNS, malignant lymphoma, neuroblastoma, Wilms' tumor, and embryonal rhabdomyosarcoma.
  H. Cancers that are decreasing in incidence include cancers of the stomach, cervix (owing to screening with the Pap test), and endometrium.
  I. Cancers that are increasing in incidence include cancers of the lung, breast (owing to mammography), prostate, and pancreas, multiple myeloma, malignant melanoma, and Hodgkin's disease.
  J. Certain genetic diseases are associated with an increased incidence of cancer; for example, xeroderma pigmentosum (AR) has a defect in DNA repair enzymes predisposing the patient to early development of UV light–induced skin cancers.
  K. Some precancerous conditions progress through a series of growth alterations before becoming cancerous.
    1. Cervical cancer progresses as follows: squamous metaplasia, squamous dysplasia (mild, moderate, severe), carcinoma in situ (full thickness but with preservation of the basement membrane), invasive cancer.
    2. Endometrial cancer has the following sequential steps: endometrial hyperplasia, atypical (dysplastic) endometrial hyperplasia, carcinoma in situ, invasive cancer.

TABLE 9–5.   Tumor Markers

Tumor Marker	Product and Cancer Association
α-Fetoprotein (AFP)	Gene product (oncofetal antigen). Hepatocellular carcinoma, germ cell tumors: yolk sac or endodermal sinus tumors of testicle or ovary. Testicular/ovarian cancer
α₁-Antitrypsin (AAT)	Enzyme. Hepatocellular carcinoma; yolk sac or endodermal sinus tumors of testicle or ovary.
β-hCG	Hormone. Trophoblastic tumor in germ cell tumors of ovary/testis and placenta: benign (hydatidiform and invasive moles), malignant (choriocarcinoma).
β₂-Microglobulin	Protein. Multiple myeloma (excellent prognostic factor). Light chains in urine (Bence Jones protein).
Bombesin	Peptide. Small-cell carcinoma of lung, neuroblastoma.
CA15-3	Glycoprotein (cancer *antigen*). Breast cancer.
CA19-9	Glycoprotein (cancer *antigen*). Pancreatic cancer (excellent marker).
CA125	Glycoprotein (cancer *antigen*). Surface-derived ovarian cancer (not very sensitive or specific).
Carcinoembryonic antigen (CEA)	Gene product (oncofetal antigen). Colorectal, pancreatic, breast, and small-cell cancer of lung. Bad prognostic sign if elevated preoperatively (greater incidence of undetected metastasis).
Lactate dehydrogenase (LDH)	Enzyme. Marker of Hodgkin's disease, cystic teratoma. Nonspecific general tumor marker.
Neuron-specific enolase (NSE)	Enzyme. Small-cell carcinoma of lung, neuroblastoma.
Prostate-specific antigen (PSA)	Glycoprotein. Prostate adenocarcinoma. Excellent sensitivity but poor specificity (increased in prostate hyperplasia). Excellent indicator of tumor burden. Not increased after rectal examination.

QUESTIONS

DIRECTIONS. (ITEMS 1–13): Each of the numbered items or incomplete statements in this section is followed by answers or by completions of the statement. Select the ONE lettered answer or completion that is BEST in each case. Correct answers and explanations are given at the end of the chapter.

1. The microscopic section is representative of a malignant tumor removed from a heavy smoker. Based on the histology of the tumor, it would least likely have arisen from which one of the following locations?

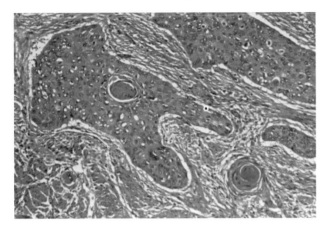

(A) Oral pharynx
(B) Pancreas
(C) Esophagus
(D) Cervix
(E) Larynx

2. This microscopic section is representative of a malignant tumor removed from a nonsmoking 55-year-old post-menopausal woman. The most likely location, based on the histology of the tumor, would be the

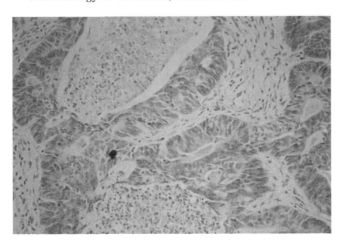

(A) oral pharynx
(B) skin
(C) urinary bladder
(D) vulva
(E) endometrium

3. The gross photograph represents a tumor that was removed from the pelvic cavity of a 17-year-old girl who presented with abdominal pain. An abnormality noted on an x-ray prompted its surgical removal. This tumor is best classified as a

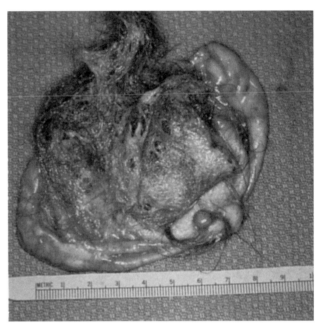

(A) mixed tumor
(B) teratoma
(C) hamartoma
(D) carcinoma
(E) sarcoma

4. The photograph represents a CT scan of a lumbar vertebra from a nonsmoking 58-year-old woman with severe low back pain. Based on the location of the lesion, you would expect the patient to have

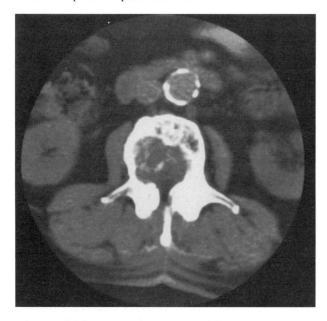

   (A) an abnormal mammogram
   (B) a primary lesion in the lung
   (C) a primary cancer of bone
   (D) an abnormal cervical Pap test
   (E) a history of postmenopausal bleeding

5. A malignancy with the potential for producing either secondary polycythemia or hypercalcemia would most likely be located in the

   (A) lung
   (B) liver
   (C) kidney
   (D) thyroid
   (E) breast

6. Metastatic cancer in the brain, adrenals, and liver would most likely have a primary cancer located in the

   (A) rectosigmoid
   (B) stomach
   (C) esophagus
   (D) breast
   (E) lung

7. In which one of the following oncogene groupings are both oncogenes activated by translocation?

   (A) *ras* and *erb*B2
   (B) *sis* and N-*myc*
   (C) *erb*B2 and *abl*
   (D) *abl* and c-*myc*
   (E) c-*myc* and *ras*

8. Which of the following groupings of tumors and etiologic agents are correctly matched?

   (A) Lung cancer: asbestos, alkylating agents, polycyclic hydrocarbons
   (B) Angiosarcoma: vinyl chloride, hepatitis B virus, Thorotrast
   (C) Acute leukemia: Down syndrome, benzene, ionizing radiation
   (D) Bladder cancer: cyclophosphamide, aniline dyes, arsenic
   (E) Nasal cavity cancer: woodworking, Epstein-Barr virus, alcohol

9. Which of the following tumor/electron microscope findings is correctly matched?

   (A) Small-cell carcinoma of the lung: dense-core neurosecretory granules
   (B) Angiosarcoma: tonofilaments
   (C) Rhabdomyosarcoma: Birbeck granules
   (D) Neuroblastoma: melanosomes
   (E) Histiocytosis X: Weibel-Palade bodies

10. Which of the following groupings of cancers, tumor markers, and pathogenic factors is correctly matched?

   (A) Hepatocellular carcinoma: β_2-microglobulin, aflatoxin
   (B) Breast cancer: CA125, ionizing radiation
   (C) Pancreatic carcinoma: bombesin, polycyclic hydrocarbons
   (D) Transitional cell carcinoma of the bladder: carcinoembryonic antigen, phenacetin
   (E) Choriocarcinoma: β-hCG, severe α-thalassemia

11. In which of the following locations would cancer most likely be associated with an increase in β-hCG and/or α-fetoprotein?

   (A) Liver
   (B) Testicle
   (C) Kidney
   (D) Lung
   (E) Adrenal medulla

12. Low back pain, an elevated alkaline phosphatase, and multiple radiodense lesions in the lumbar vertebrae in a 69-year-old male with a 20-year history of smoking would most likely be associated with a primary tumor located in the

   (A) lung
   (B) liver
   (C) colon
   (D) prostate
   (E) kidney

13. Inactivation of a suppressor gene is least likely associated with

   (A) Li-Fraumeni multicancer syndrome
   (B) human papillomavirus–induced cancers
   (C) retinoblastoma
   (D) familial polyposis
   (E) B-cell follicular lymphoma

ANSWERS AND EXPLANATIONS

1. The answer is B: pancreas. The section of tumor exhibits squamous features owing to the presence of well-circumscribed keratin pearls in the center of one of the sheets of tumor and in other areas. Squamous cancers in smokers would most likely be located in the oral pharynx, esophagus, cervix, and larynx. Cancers of the pancreas are glandular, hence are adenocarcinomas. (Photomicrograph reproduced, with permission, from B.C. Morson. *Color Atlas of Gastrointestinal Pathology.* London, W.B. Saunders Co., 1988, p. 280. © Harvey Miller, Ltd.)

2. The answer is E: endometrium. The microscopic section exhibits well-differentiated glands with necrotic material in the gland lumens consistent with adenocarcinoma. The most common primary cancer in the endometrium is adenocarcinoma, most commonly occurring in the postmenopausal woman. Squamous cell carcinoma is the most common primary cancer in the oral pharynx, skin, and vulva, while transitional cell carcinomas of the bladder frequent the urinary bladder. (Photomicrograph reproduced, with permission, from E. Hernandez and B.F. Atkinson. *Clinical Gynecologic Pathology.* Philadelphia, W.B. Saunders Co., 1995, p. 300.)

3. The answer is B: teratoma. The tumor represents a teratoma of the ovary. It exhibits hair and sebaceous material. Although not visible in the photograph, a tooth was present in the raised nodular area at the lower-right edge of the tumor. This localized area is called a Rokitansky tubercle and often contains other teratomatous elements derived from ecto-, endo-, and mesoderm. Mixed tumors have two types of tissue derived from only one germ layer. Hamartomas are non-neoplastic tumor-like masses representing an overgrowth of normal tissue in the tissue involved (e.g., bronchial hamartoma containing mature cartilage). Carcinomas are malignancies of epithelial tissue, which would be an uncommon pelvic mass in a young woman. Sarcomas are malignancies of mesenchymal tissue, which would be even rarer than carcinomas in this area. (Photograph reproduced, with permission, from E. Hernandez and B.F. Atkinson. *Clinical Gynecologic Pathology.* Philadelphia, W.B. Saunders Co., 1995, p. 478.)

4. The answer is A: an abnormal mammogram. The lumbar vertebra reveals lytic areas in the bone surrounded by sclerotic bone. Breast cancer is the most common metastatic cancer of bone in women, and the vertebral column is the most common location for metastasis owing to the Batson vertebral venous plexus. This plexus surrounds the vertebral column from the cranial cavity to the end of the spine. It is valveless and communicates with the caval system. Increased pressure in the caval system can drive tumor emboli into the Batson plexus, which sends tributaries deep into the vertebra and around the spinal cord. Hence, this patient would most likely have had an abnormal mammogram. Although lung cancer metastasizes to bone, the patient is a nonsmoker. Cervical cancer is uncommon owing to cervical Pap tests, so this choice would be unlikely. Multiple myeloma is the most common primary bone cancer and could present in this manner, but it is not as common as metastatic breast cancer. A history of postmenopausal bleeding suggests the possibility of an endometrial carcinoma as the primary site, but the lung is more commonly the site of metastasis than bone is. (Photomicrograph reproduced, with permission, from L.E. Wold, R.A. McLeod, F.H. Sim, and K.K. Unni. *Atlas of Orthopedic Pathology.* Philadelphia, W.B. Saunders Co., 1990, p. 268.)

5. The answer is C: kidney. Ectopic secretion of erythropoietin (secondary polycythemia) or a parathormone (PTH)-like peptide (hypercalcemia) would most likely be associated with a renal adenocarcinoma. Hepatocellular carcinoma may produce an insulin-like factor (hypoglycemia) or erythropoietin; squamous cell carcinoma of the lung, a PTH-like peptide; small-cell carcinoma of the lung, antidiuretic hormone (hyponatremia) and ACTH (hypercortisolism); medullary carcinoma of the thyroid, ACTH or calcitonin (hypocalcemia); and breast carcinoma, secretion of a PTH-like peptide.

6. The answer is E: lung. Metastatic disease is more common than a primary cancer in the lungs, liver, brain, lymph nodes, bone, and adrenals. Primary lung cancer is the most common primary site for metastatic lesions to the brain, adrenals, and liver. Cancer arising from the rectosigmoid most commonly metastasizes to the liver; stomach cancer to the liver; esophageal cancer to the liver; and breast cancer to the brain, lung, and bone.

7. The answer is D: *abl* and c-*myc*. Translocation of the *abl* oncogene (associated with nonreceptor tyrosine kinase activity) on chromosome 9 to chromosome 22 with subsequent fusion with the *bcr* gene to form a hybrid gene results in chronic myelogenous leukemia. Translocation of the c-*myc* oncogene (a transcription activator located in the nucleus) from chromosome 8 to chromosome 14 is associated with Burkitt's lymphoma. The *ras* oncogene is activated by a point mutation and is important in coding for the membrane-related guanine triphosphate (GTP)–binding proteins. The *sis* oncogene is involved with coding for growth factors and when activated is associated with overexpression of the growth factor. The *erb*B2 oncogene codes for a growth factor receptor with tyrosine kinase activity and is activated by gene amplification. The N-*myc* oncogene is activated by amplification.

8. The answer is C: acute leukemia: Down syndrome, benzene, ionizing radiation. Trisomy 21 (Down syndrome) shows an increased incidence of both acute myelogenous and lymphocytic leukemia in childhood. Benzene is associated with aplastic anemia and acute leukemia. Leukemia is the most common cancer associated with ionizing radiation. Lung cancer is associated with asbestos and polycyclic hydrocarbons (cigarette smoke); however, alkylating agents most often produce leukemias or malignant lymphomas. Angiosarcoma is associated with exposure to vinyl chloride and Thorotrast, but hepatitis B virus is implicated as the most common cause of hepatocellular carcinoma. Bladder cancer may be secondary to cyclophosphamide and aniline dyes; however, arsenic most commonly produces skin cancer, angiosarcomas of the liver, and lung cancer. Nasal cavity cancer is increased in people who work with wood, and the Epstein-Barr virus has been implicated in nasopharyngeal cancer. However, alcohol is most commonly associated with oral pharyngeal cancer and esophageal cancer.

9. The answer is A: small-cell carcinoma of the lung: dense-core neurosecretory granules. A small-cell carcinoma of the lung is an APUD tumor derived from neural ectoderm, which characteristically has dense-core neurosecretory granules. Other examples are carcinoid tumors and neuroblastoma. Angiosarcomas are associated with Weibel-Palade bodies, which contain von Willebrand's factor. Tonofilaments are a characteristic finding in carcinomas. Rhabdomyosarcomas have thick and thin myofilaments. Birbeck granules are noted in true histiocytes (Langerhans' cells), hence they are present in histiocytosis X. Melanosomes are characteristic of malignant melanoma.

10. The answer is E: choriocarcinoma: β-hCG, severe α-thalassemia. Choriocarcinoma is common in the Far East owing to the high incidence of α-thalassemia and spontaneous abortions secondary to Hb Bart's disease (absence of all four α-globulin chains). Spontaneous abortions predispose to choriocarcinoma. Hepatocellular carcinoma is associated with exposure to aflatoxins, particularly in unison with HBV postnecrotic cirrhosis. β_2-Microglobulin is a marker for multiple myeloma. Breast cancer is increased with exposure to ionizing radiation. Carcinoembryonic antigen and CA15-3 are tumor markers that are used to follow breast cancer for recurrence. CA125 is a tumor marker for ovarian cancer. Pancreatic carcinoma is associated with smoking (polycyclic hydrocarbons) and chronic pancreatitis. CA19-9 is a tumor marker for pancreatic cancer. Bombesin is a peptide marker for APUD tumors such as small-cell carcinoma of the lung and neuroblastoma. Transitional cell carcinoma of the bladder has no specific tumor marker. Predisposing factors include exposure to phenacetin, aniline dyes, cyclophosphamide, and polycyclic hydrocarbons. Carcinoembryonic antigen (CEA) is a tumor marker for colorectal cancer, pancreatic cancer, breast cancer, and small-cell carcinoma of the lung.

11. The answer is B: testicle. Testicular cancers are most commonly germ cell tumors, which are totipotential tumors having the capacity to differentiate into any tissue. Yolk sac tumors (endodermal sinus tumors) and nongestationally derived choriocarcinomas in a male are germ cell tumors that commonly secrete α-fetoprotein and β-hCG, respectively. Hepatocellular carcinoma of the liver can ectopically secrete α-fetoprotein. No malignant tumors in the kidney, lung, or adrenal medulla commonly secrete β-hCG.

12. The answer is D: prostate. The history of low back pain, an elevated alkaline phosphatase (from activated osteoblasts), and multiple radiodense lesions in the lumbar vertebrae indicates osteoblastic metastases, which in a male is most commonly secondary to prostate cancer. Lung and renal cancers most commonly produce osteolytic metastases. Colon and liver cancers may produce mixed types of metastases.

13. The answer is E: B-cell follicular lymphoma. The translocation of the B-cell immunoglobulin heavy-chain gene site located on chromosome 14 to a location in proximity to the *bcl*2 oncogene site on chromosome 18 causes overexpression of the bcl2 gene protein product. This product, for unknown reasons, inactivates the apoptosis gene responsible for programmed cell death of the B cell, hence the cells do not die. This translocation is associated with a follicular lymphoma. Inactivation of suppressor genes leads to unrestricted cell division. Examples of suppressor genes are *Rb1*, *p53*, and *APC*. *Rb1* is located on chromosome 13 and produces a product that suppresses E2F, a transcription factor in the retinal cells of the eye. Inactivation of *Rb1* on both chromosome 13's produces an unregulated growth of retinal cells, which is called a retinoblastoma. The *p53* suppressor gene located on chromosome 17 enhances expression of p21/CIP1, which normally suppresses a cell cycle regulatory kinase. Hence, inactivation or loss of *p53* (point mutation) leads to a faster movement of cells through the different phases of the cell cycle. The above alterations in the *p53* gene account for ~25–50% of all malignancies involving the colon, breast, lung, and central nervous system. Inactivation of *p53* is also involved in the autosomal dominant Li-Fraumeni multicancer syndrome (increased incidence of breast cancer, sarcomas, leukemia, and brain tumors). The APC suppressor gene (APC = *a*denomatous *p*olyposis *c*oli) on chromosome 5 is associated with the autosomal dominant familial polyposis syndrome and Gardner's syndrome.

SECTION III

SYSTEMIC PATHOLOGY

DISORDERS OF THE VASCULAR

SYSTEM AND HEART

AND PERICARDIUM

SYNOPSIS

OBJECTIVES

1. To outline normal and abnormal lipid metabolism.
2. To define and discuss diseases of the arterial system.
3. To define and review disorders involving the venous system.
4. To review disorders involving the lymphatic system.
5. To be familiar with the vasculitis syndromes and their pathogenesis.
6. To understand the pathogenesis of essential hypertension and causes of secondary hypertension.
7. To be familiar with the types of cardiac hypertrophy.
8. To discuss the similarities and differences between left, right, and high-output cardiac failure.
9. To outline the pathogenesis of the common acyanotic and cyanotic congenital heart diseases.
10. To review the pathogenesis of ischemic heart disease.
11. To understand the pathogenesis of congenital and acquired valvular disorders.
12. To outline the pathogenesis of diseases involving the myocardium.
13. To be familiar with disorders involving the pericardium.

Objective 1: To outline normal and abnormal lipid metabolism.

I. Lipid disorders
   A. **Lipoproteins** are composed of varying proportions of cholesterol (CH), triglyceride (TG), and phospholipids.
      1. **Chylomicrons** carry diet-derived triglyceride (TG), while **very low density lipoproteins** (VLDLs) transport liver-derived TG.
      2. **Intermediate-density lipoprotein** (IDL) and **low-density lipoprotein** (LDL), the primary vehicles for carrying cholesterol (CH), are derived from the degradation of VLDL in the peripheral blood by capillary lipoprotein lipase.
      3. **High-density lipoproteins** (HDLs; "good CH") carry apolipoprotein (apo) and remove CH from fatty streaks.
   B. The plasma concentration of CH and TG represent the total of each component in the various lipoprotein fractions.
      1. **Lipid profiles** include a measurement of CH, TG, and HDL-CH (HDL associated with CH) and a calculation of LDL using the following formula: **LDL = serum CH − serum HDL − (TG/5).**
      2. Patients must **fast** for 9–12 hours before the sample is collected in order to negate a false elevation of TG from the diet.
      3. **Variables that affect lipids** include **medications** (e.g., progesterone increases LDL, CH, and TG and decreases HDL) and **disease** (e.g., people with diabetes frequently have increased CH and TG and decreased HDL).
      4. **CH and HDL-CH** are used as the **initial screen for primary prevention of coronary artery disease** (CAD) in adults (no previous evidence of CAD), while **LDL is used for secondary prevention** (previous history of CAD).
      5. A **desirable CH level** is < 200 mg/dL; borderline-high, 200–239 mg/dL; and high, ≥ 240 mg/dL.
      6. A **desirable LDL level** is < 130 mg/dL; borderline-high, 130–160 mg/dL; and high, ≥ 160 mg/dL.
      7. **Factors that increase HDL** include exercise, weight loss, mild to moderate alcohol intake, and estrogen.
         a. Low (high-risk) HDL levels are < 35 mg/dL.
         b. A negative risk factor for CAD is a 60 mg/dL or greater HDL concentration.
      8. A **normal TG** is < 200 mg/dL; borderline-high, 200–400 mg/dL; high, 400–1000 mg/dL; and very high, > 1000 mg/dL.
      9. **Chylomicrons** form a supranate (layer of lipid settling on top of plasma), while **VLDL** forms an infranate (plasma turbidity throughout the sample) in plasma left in a refrigerator at 40C overnight (**standing chylomicron test**).
   C. The **major risk factors for CAD** were redefined by the National Cholesterol Education Program Expert Panel in 1993.

1. **Age** is the most important overall risk factor (male ≥ 45 years or female ≥ 55 years old).
2. A **family history** of premature CAD (i.e., AMI before age 55 in a father or before age 65 in a mother) is a major risk factor.
3. Current **cigarette smoking, hypertension** (i.e., blood pressure ≥ 140/90 mm Hg), **diabetes mellitus, HDL < 35 mg/dL** (≥ 60 mg/dL is a negative risk factor), and **LDL ≥ 160 mg/dL** are also major risk factors.
4. "**Soft**" **risk factors** include obesity (> 20% overweight), sedentary life-style, increased ferritin and lipoprotein(a) [Lp(a)], which is a lipoprotein that combines LDL with an inhibitor of plasminogen.

D. **Genetic hyperlipidemias** are less common than secondary, or acquired, hyperlipidemias.
   1. **Fredrickson's original classification of hyperlipidemias** was based on five types (I through V), which correlated with seven categories of genetic disorder.

   ↓apo C-II
   ↑chylomicrons

   a. **Type I** (familial lipoprotein lipase deficiency and cofactor [apo-C-II] deficiency) is due to a deficiency of apo-C-II or capillary lipoprotein lipase, leading to an increase in chylomicrons.
   b. **Type II** (polygenic hypercholesterolemia [most common], familial combined hypercholesterolemia, familial hypercholesterolemia) is caused by absent or defective LDL receptors or defective internalization of the LDL complex.

   IIa - ↑LDL
   ↑CH

   IIb - ↑LDL
   ↑CH
   ↑TG

      (1) **Type IIa** demonstrates an increase in LDL (often > 260 mg/dL) and CH, but a normal TG; **type IIb** is similar to IIa except that the TG is increased.
      (2) **Familial hypercholesterolemia** has an AD inheritance and is associated with **tendon xanthomas**, which are pathognomonic for the disease.

   ↓apo E

   c. **Type III** (familial dysbetalipoproteinemia, "remnant disease") is due to absent or defective apo-E, hence chylomicron and IDL remnants are not properly metabolized in the liver.

   ↑VLDL

   d. **Type IV** (familial hypertriglyceridemia), the **most common hyperlipidemia**, is secondary to decreased catabolism of VLDL.
   e. **Type V** is generally seen in a patient with familial hypertriglyceridemia who has exacerbating factors such as diabetic ketoacidosis or alcoholism leading to an increase in chylomicrons (type I) and VLDL (type IV).
   2. **Apo-B deficiency** (**abetalipoproteinemia**) is an AD inherited disease resulting in very low TG, CH, and LDL levels and clinical manifestations of malabsorption, CNS disease (ataxia, retinitis pigmentosa), and abnormal RBCs (acanthocytes).

Objective 2: To define and discuss diseases of the arterial system.

II. Overview
   A. Arteries can be **large elastic arteries** (e.g., aorta and its major branches, pulmonary arteries), **medium-sized muscular arteries** (e.g., distribution vessels; radial artery), and **arterioles** (peripheral resistance vessels).
   B. **Atherosclerosis** is the **most common disease afflicting the aorta**.
   C. **Diseases of the aorta** may result in aneurysm formation (e.g., abdominal aortic aneurysm), bleeding into the vessel wall with the potential for rupture (e.g., dissecting aortic aneurysm) or occlusion of the vessel lumen leading to absence of a pulse, visual disturbances, or stroke (e.g., Takayasu's arteritis).
   D. **Diseases involving muscular arteries** include atherosclerosis and immune disease, both of which predispose to vessel thrombosis leading to infarction.
   E. Immunocomplex disease (type III hypersensitivity) is the pathogenesis of disorders involving arterioles, capillaries, and venules and manifests itself as palpable purpura.
III. Arteriosclerosis
   A. **Arteriosclerosis** (hardening of the arteries) is subclassified as atherosclerosis (formation of atheromas), Mönckeberg's medial calcification, and arteriolosclerosis (hyaline and hyperplastic types).
   B. **Atherosclerosis** is primarily responsible for two of the top three leading causes of death in the United States, namely, AMI (first) and cerebral infarctions (stroke; third).
      1. It is **more common in males** than in females and is age related (more common but not invariably associated with increasing age).
      2. It primarily involves the **intima** of elastic and muscular arteries.
      3. **Two primary lesions** of atherosclerosis are the **fatty streak** (early lesion) and the **fibrous plaque** (advanced lesion).
      4. Proposed mechanisms of atherosclerosis are the **thrombogenic** (a mural thrombus is incorporated into an atheroma), **monoclonal** (monoclonal proliferation of smooth muscle cells), and **reaction to injury theory** (most popular).
         a. In the reaction to injury theory, endothelial cell injury (toxins in cigarette smoke, LDL, turbulence) is the initiating event in atherosclerosis.
         b. Circulating monocytes and lymphocytes (CD8 and CD4 T cells) adhere to the area of injury and emigrate into the vessel wall (monocytes become macrophages).
         c. The above cells release various cytokines (growth factors), some of which induce smooth muscle proliferation and directed chemotaxis of the smooth muscle cells to the intimal area of the vessel.
         d. Macrophages, lymphocytes, and smooth muscle cells imbibe LDL containing CH and become foam cells with subsequent development of fatty streaks (reversible lesions).
         e. Injured endothelial cells and macrophages also produce free radicals, which produce **oxidized LDL**, a potent enhancer of the atherosclerotic process.
         f. Fatty streaks continue to enlarge and eventually disrupt the endothelial surface.
         g. Platelets adhere to the damaged endothelium overlying the fatty streaks and release

platelet-derived growth factor, which further contributes to smooth muscle proliferation.

h. Over time, the proliferating smooth muscle cells located at the base of the fatty streak begin to synthesize collagen, elastin, and proteoglycans, which subsequently produce **fibrous plaques**.

i. Fibrous plaques undergo dystrophic calcification, hemorrhage, thrombosis, fissuring, and ulceration to form a **complicated atheromatous plaque**.

5. In descending order of frequency, atherosclerosis involves the abdominal aorta, coronary arteries, popliteal artery, descending thoracic aorta, internal carotid artery, and circle of Willis.

6. Atherosclerosis involving elastic and muscular arteries produces significant morbidity and mortality.

 a. **Thromboembolism** of plaque material to distant sites may result in infarction.

 b. It may weaken the wall of a vessel, resulting in an **aneurysm** (e.g., abdominal aortic aneurysm).

 c. It is the primary pathogenesis of **ischemic heart disease**.

 d. It is associated with **peripheral vascular disease**, which may lead to **claudication** (pain when walking) and **amputation** of an extremity.

 e. It may result in **CNS disease** (e.g., transient ischemic attacks, stroke, atrophy).

 f. It is the primary cause of **renovascular hypertension**.

 g. It may produce **gastrointestinal disease** (e.g., mesenteric angina, bowel infarction, ischemic strictures).

C. Mönckeberg's medial calcification is an age-related, clinically insignificant degenerative disease that commonly involves muscular arteries (e.g., femoral artery, uterine arteries).

D. **Arteriolosclerosis** is either hyperplastic (proliferative) or hyalinized.

1. The **hyperplastic type** is characterized by proliferation of smooth muscle cells in an "**onion-skin**" pattern with subsequent narrowing of the lumen (e.g., seen in renal vessels in malignant hypertension and progressive systemic sclerosis).

2. The **hyaline type** is associated with arterioles that have a glassy, pink appearance on H and E staining.

 a. It is the "**small-vessel disease**" of **diabetes mellitus** (DM) and **hypertension**.

 b. In DM, **nonenzymatic glycosylation** (glucose attached to amino acids) of the basement membrane of the vessels renders them permeable to proteins.

 c. In hypertension, the increased pressure imposed on the arteriolar walls drives protein into the vessel.

IV. Aneurysms

A. An aneurysm is a localized dilatation of an artery that results from weakening by atherosclerosis (most common), inflammation, a congenital abnormality (e.g., Ehlers-Danlos syndrome), trauma, or hypertension.

B. The natural history of an aneurysm is to **enlarge** and **rupture**.

C. **Aneurysms in the aorta** have different etiologies, depending on the location.

1. In the **ascending aorta**, they are most commonly secondary to a dissecting aortic aneurysm that has extended proximally (tertiary syphilis is no longer the most common cause).

2. In the **distal aorta** (thoracic [below the subclavian and above the diaphragm] and abdominal [below the renal arteries]) and in the extremities, they are most commonly secondary to atherosclerosis.

D. Aneurysms may be **fusiform** (spindle shaped), **saccular** (round), or **dissecting**.

E. **Abdominal aortic aneurysms** are the **most common overall aneurysm**.

1. They are most often seen in men over age 55.

2. They are due to weakening of the wall by **atherosclerosis** owing to lack of vasa vasorum below the renal artery orifices.

3. The majority are asymptomatic.

4. If symptomatic, they commonly present as a **pulsatile mass** with mid-abdominal to lower back pain and demonstrate an abdominal bruit (50%) on auscultation.

5. **Rupture** is the **most common complication** and is responsible for an abrupt onset of severe back pain (most rupture into the left retroperitoneum), hypotension, and a pulsatile mass in the abdomen.

6. **Abdominal ultrasound** is the gold standard test (sensitivity approaching 100%).

7. Size and risk for rupture influence the choice of treatment.

F. **Berry aneurysms** are most commonly located at bifurcations of the cerebral vessels (anterior communicating artery with anterior cerebral artery).

1. Most are **congenital** and are associated with vessels that lack an internal elastic membrane and muscle wall.

2. There is an association with **adult polycystic disease** (10–15%) and **coarctation of the aorta** (increased pressure in cerebral vessels).

G. **Mycotic aneurysms** are secondary to weakening of the vessel wall by an infectious process (e.g., septic embolism, infective endocarditis, fungal vasculitis (*Aspergillus, Mucor, Candida*).

H. A **syphilitic aneurysm** involving the arch of aorta is the **second most common manifestation of tertiary syphilis** (*Treponema pallidum*).

1. *T. pallidum* produces **endarteritis obliterans** (vasculitis; numerous plasma cells) of the vasa vasorum in the ascending and transverse portions of the arch of the aorta.

2. Ischemia in the outer adventitial and outer medial tissue of the aorta leads to weakening of the wall with subsequent aneurysm formation and aortic regurgitation from stretching of the aortic valve ring.

3. Aortic regurgitation is associated with a hyperdynamic circulation (e.g., water-hammer pulse, pulsating uvula).

4. Death usually occurs from rupture or heart failure.

I. **Dissecting aortic aneurysms** are the **most common catastrophic disorder** of the aorta.
   1. **Elastic tissue fragmentation** (95%) with or without **mucoid degeneration** (**cystic medial necrosis**) in the middle and outer part of the media weakens the wall of the vessel.
   2. Other **predisposing causes** are as follows:
      a. Marfan's syndrome (defect in fibrillin).
      b. Ehlers-Danlos syndrome (defect in collagen).
      c. Pregnancy (increased plasma volume).
      d. Copper deficiency (cofactor in lysyl oxidase).
      e. Coarctation of aorta (wall stress).
      f. Trauma.
   3. **Hypertension**, the single most important factor for initiating the dissection, applies a shearing force to the intimal surface, leading to an intimal tear usually within 10 cm of the aortic valve, followed by the entry of a column of blood that dissects through the weakened vessel.
      a. **Eventual sites of egress** include the **pericardial sac** (**most common cause of death**), mediastinum, or peritoneum or reentry through another tear to create a double-barreled aorta.
      b. **Type A aneurysms** (most common and worst type) involve the ascending aorta, while **type B aneurysms** begin below the subclavian artery.
   4. Dissections present with an acute onset of severe chest pain (described as tearing), which radiates to the back.
   5. There is an **increased aortic diameter** on chest x-ray in 80%, which is verified by a **retrograde arteriography** (gold standard test).

V. Arteriovenous fistulas
   A. Arteriovenous (AV) fistulas are abnormal communications between arteries and veins that are either congenital or acquired (most commonly due to penetrating knife injury).
   B. Large AV fistulas reduce systemic resistance and bypass the microcirculation, hence increasing venous return to the heart and producing high-output cardiac failure.

Objective 3: To define and review disorders involving the venous system.

VI. Overview
   A. Superficial veins (e.g., superficial saphenous veins) drain into the deep veins (e.g., deep saphenous veins) via communicating (penetrating) branches.
   B. Valves prevent blood flow from the deep into the superficial venous system except around the ankles, where blood flow is normally in that direction.
   C. Muscle contraction in the legs reduces hydrostatic pressure in the veins below the resting pressure, hence increasing the return of blood to the heart.

VII. Phlebothrombosis and thrombophlebitis
   A. **Phlebothrombosis** is thrombosis of a vein without inflammation.
      1. **Most venous clots develop in the legs** (90%), which in descending order of frequency are the deep saphenous vein in the calf, femoral vein, popliteal vein, and iliac vein.
      2. **Predisposing factors** for phlebothrombosis include damage to the vessel endothelium (e.g., inflammation, varicose veins), stasis of blood flow (e.g., bed rest), and hypercoagulability (e.g., oral contraceptive use).
         a. The clotting process begins in stasis areas such as the venous sinuses of the calf muscles and the valve cusps.
         b. Platelets form the initial clot in the valve cusps.
         c. The developing clot extends beyond the next branching point, at which juncture the clot becomes a venous clot (red thrombus) consisting of RBCs and fibrin.
         d. The venous clot propagates toward the heart in the direction of blood flow, hence the danger of embolization.
      3. **Clinical findings** in phlebothrombosis are swelling, pain, edema distal to the thrombosis, varicosities, and ulceration.
   B. **Deep venous thrombosis** (DVT) in the lower extremity produces **deep venous insufficiency,** or the **postphlebitic syndrome**.
      1. Thrombosis with subsequent obstruction of the deep saphenous vein lumen leads to an increased venous pressure and increased blood flow to the veins around the ankles that communicate with the superficial system.
      2. The veins in the ankles rupture, resulting in **stasis dermatitis** (swelling, hemorrhage, ulcers) and secondary varicosities in the superficial saphenous system owing to the increase in blood.
      3. **Complications** of venous thrombosis are as follows:
         a. Thromboembolism (with the potential for a pulmonary embolism with infarction [most commonly arising from the thigh vessels—iliac, femoral, popliteal, and pelvic veins]).
         b. Thrombophlebitis.
         c. Varicose veins.
      4. **Doppler (duplex) ultrasonography** (best test) or **impedance plethysmography** are the screening tests of choice, and **x-ray venography** is the gold standard test for confirmation.
   C. **Thrombophlebitis** is pain and tenderness along the course of a superficial vein.
      1. It usually occurs postoperatively in patients over 40 years of age.
      2. It is most commonly secondary to varicose veins but may be associated with phlebothrombosis (common), intravenous catheters, polycythemia, intravenous drug abuse, or a neighboring infection.
      3. The involved vein is a palpable cord with pain, induration, heat and erythema along the skin surface.
   D. **Migratory thrombophlebitis** is a subtype of thrombophlebitis in which venous thrombi disappear at one site and reappear at another (it may be a paraneoplastic sign of underlying pancreatic cancer [**Trousseau's sign**]).

VIII. Varicose veins
   A. Varicose veins are abnormally distended, length-

ened, and tortuous veins associated with the superficial saphenous veins, distal esophagus in portal hypertension, anorectal region (e.g., hemorrhoids), and left testicle (varicocele).

1. **Primary varicose veins** are due to valvular incompetence and weakened vessel walls and are frequently associated with a positive family history or certain occupations.
2. **Secondary varicose veins** are the result of valve damage from previous thrombophlebitis or deep vein thrombosis.

B. **Contributing factors** to varicosities include prolonged standing, obesity, and pregnancy.

C. **Complications** include phlebothrombosis, swelling of the extremity, stasis dermatitis (deep venous thrombosis), ulceration, and rupture.

IX. Syndromes

A. The **thoracic outlet syndrome** refers to abnormal compression of the neurovascular compartment in the neck owing to a cervical rib, spastic scalenus anterior muscle, or positional change in the neck and arms.

B. The **superior vena cava (SVC) syndrome** is secondary to extrinsic compression of the SVC from a primary lung cancer (90%; > 50% small-cell carcinoma) and less commonly to malignant lymphoma.

1. There is puffiness and blue to purple discoloration of the face, arms, and shoulders and CNS findings of dizziness, convulsions, and visual disturbances (congested retinal veins).
2. The jugular veins are visibly distended.

Objective 4: To review disorders involving the lymphatic system.

X. Lymphatic disorders

A. Lymphatic vessels have an incomplete basement membrane, hence predisposing them to infection and tumor invasion.

1. Drainage of infected material to regional lymph nodes results in reactive hyperplasia with enlarged, tender nodes.
2. Lymphatic drainage of tumor emboli first occurs in the subcapsular sinus.

B. **Acute lymphangitis** is inflammation of the lymphatics ("red streak") and is most commonly secondary to *Streptococcus pyogenes* (e.g., cellulitis) and *Staphylococcus aureus* to a lesser degree.

C. Lymphedema is an abnormal interstitial collection of lymphatic fluid due to congenital disease (e.g., Milroy's disease, Turner's syndrome) or blockage of the lymphatics (e.g., postmastectomy radiation therapy, peau d'orange of the breast in inflammatory carcinoma, filariasis). *elephantitis*

D. **Chylous effusions** are collections of lymphatic fluid (chylomicrons plus lymphocytes) in a body cavity secondary to a malignant lymphoma (the most common cause in the pleural cavity) or trauma.

Objective 5: To be familiar with the vasculitis syndromes and their pathogenesis.

XI. Benign and malignant tumors and tumor-like conditions

A. A **port wine stain** (PWS), or **nevus flammeus,** is a flat pink, red, or purple benign lesion located on the face that presents at birth.

B. The **Sturge-Weber syndrome** (SWS) is a benign port wine stain in the distribution of the ophthalmic branch of the trigeminal nerve that is also associated with leptomeningeal vascular abnormalities (they frequently calcify), mental retardation, and seizures.

C. **Pyogenic granulomas** are highly vascular benign lesions (they bleed easily) that result from trauma (most common) and have an increased incidence in pregnancy (located on the gingiva).

D. **Hereditary hemorrhagic telangiectasia (Osler-Weber-Rendu disease)** is a benign AD disease characterized by small aneurysmal telangiectasias on the skin and mucous membranes that commonly produce nosebleeds and gastrointestinal bleeds, often leading to iron deficiency.

E. **Spider telangiectasias** are small benign AV communications commonly located on the skin (face and upper thorax) in conditions associated with hyperestrinism (e.g., normal pregnancy, cirrhosis).

F. **Angiomyolipomas** are **hamartomatous tumors** composed of blood vessels, muscle, and mature adipose tissue that are most commonly found in the kidneys of patients with tuberous sclerosis.

G. **Bacillary angiomatosis** is an infectious disease caused by *Bartonella (Rochalimaea) henselae* and *Bartonella quintana* that is most commonly encountered in patients with AIDS.

1. Grossly, and to a lesser extent histologically, they simulate Kaposi's sarcomas due to herpesvirus 8.
2. Silver stains can identify the organisms in tissue.

H. **Capillary hemangiomas ("strawberry hemangiomas")** are benign tumors (possibly hamartomas) of mature capillary channels that are commonly seen on the skin in 10% of newborns and regress with age without treatment.

I. **Cavernous hemangiomas** are benign tumors located on skin, particularly the head and neck area, mucosal surfaces, and within viscera (liver, spleen, and placenta).

J. **Glomus tumors (glomangiomas)** are painful, elevated, red-blue nodular benign tumors derived from the glomus body that are most commonly located directly beneath the nail bed.

K. **Lymphangiomas** are benign tumors (possibly hamartomas) of lymphatic channels that develop during embryogenesis and present at birth as a **cystic mass (cystic hygroma)** in the neck and axilla.

L. **Angiosarcomas** (formerly designated lymphangiosarcomas) are malignant sarcomas derived from the vessel endothelium that may locate on the skin, within organs (breast, liver [association with vinyl chloride, arsenic, and Thorotrast exposure]), in soft tissue, or as a complication of chronic lymphedema.

M. **Kaposi's sarcoma** is a malignant tumor most likely arising from endothelial cells (controversial).

1. Variants include the **classic variant** in elderly men of Jewish/Mediterranean origin, an **African variant** noted in young adults and chil-

dren, an **immunodeficiency variant** (e.g., in people taking immunosuppressive drugs), and a variant associated with AIDS (most common cancer in AIDS; 35% of cases).

2. It is one of the criteria for defining AIDS in an HIV-positive patient.

3. The etiology is thought to be herpesvirus 8.

4. The lesions are solitary to multiple red-purple lesions that progress from a flat lesion (macule) to a plaque to a nodule that ulcerates.

5. They are commonly located on the skin, on mucocutaneous surfaces (oropharynx common location), and in visceral locations (75% of cases), most commonly the lung (common cause of death in this location) and gastrointestinal tract.

6. They are composed of spindle cells (neoplastic element) with increased mitotic activity surrounding slit-like spaces with protuberances into the lumen.

XII. Vasculitis

A. Vasculitis means inflammation of the blood vessel wall of elastic and muscular arteries, arterioles, capillaries, or venules.

B. **Immunologic mechanisms** (most commonly immunocomplexes) are responsible for most (not all) cases.

1. Soluble immunocomplexes (antigen excess complexes) deposit in areas of increased vessel permeability.

   a. Immunocomplexes activate the complement pathway with subsequent release of C5a, which is an anaphylatoxin (it further enhances increased vessel permeability) and a chemotactic agent for neutrophils.

   b. Neutrophils damage the vessel wall by releasing collagenases, elastases, and toxic free radicals.

   c. Endothelial damage predisposes to vessel thrombosis and ischemic changes in the tissue involved.

2. **Type IV hypersensitivity** has also been implicated in some types of vasculitis owing to the presence of granulomatous inflammation (e.g., temporal arteritis).

3. **Antineutrophil cytoplasmic antibodies (ANCAs)** are etiologic agents in some of the vasculitides (e.g., Wegener's granulomatosis), where they activate previously primed neutrophils (priming agents include interleukin-1 and other cytokines) with subsequent release of their degradative enzymes and free radicals.

C. Examples of **large-vessel vasculitis** (large to medium-sized muscular arteries) are giant cell arteritis (temporal arteritis) and Takayasu's arteritis.

1. **Giant cell (temporal) arteritis** is a granulomatous vasculitis that primarily involves the temporal artery and extracranial branches of the carotid artery in women > 50 years of age.

   a. **Signs** and **symptoms** include the following:
      (1) Fever.
      (2) Unilateral headache (most common symptom).
      (3) Temporary or permanent blindness.
      (4) Polymyalgia rheumatica (above findings plus pain and morning stiffness in the neck, shoulders, and hip).

   b. The **erythrocyte sedimentation rate** (ESR) is the screening test of choice and is subsequently followed by a temporal artery biopsy (positive in 60%).

   c. **Treatment** is immediate institution of corticosteroid therapy to prevent blindness.

2. **Takayasu's arteritis** (**pulseless disease**) is a granulomatous vasculitis involving the aortic arch vessels in young Asian women that is associated with visual disturbances and an absent pulse.

D. Examples of **medium-vessel vasculitis** (medium-sized muscular arteries to small arteries) are polyarteritis nodosa, Kawasaki's disease, thromboangiitis obliterans, and Churg-Strauss syndrome.

1. **Polyarteritis nodosa** (PAN) is a necrotizing immune vasculitis that is more common in men than women (3:1).

   a. The **pathogenesis** relates to immunocomplex deposition (type III hypersensitivity) and activation of neutrophils and monocytes by antineutrophil cytoplasmic antibodies.

   b. There is a strong association with **HBV antigenemia** (30–40%) and hypersensitivity to drugs (intravenous amphetamines).

   c. Organ systems involved in decreasing order of frequency are the kidneys (vasculitis, glomerulonephritis), coronary arteries, liver, and gastrointestinal tract.

   d. Vascular lesions are in **different stages of development** (acute or healing stage) and frequently involve only part of the vessel (nodosa = focal aneurysm formation).
      (1) Fibrinoid necrosis, neutrophilic/eosinophilic infiltrates, and nuclear debris are commonly found.
      (2) Multiple aneurysm formation is common.

   e. **Laboratory findings** include peripheral neutrophilic leukocytosis and eosinophilia, **positive antineutrophil cytoplasmic antibodies with perinuclear staining** (p-ANCA), and renal abnormalities (hematuria with RBC casts).

   f. Arteriography or biopsy of palpable nodulations in the skin or organ involved is confirmatory.

2. **Kawasaki's disease** is an acute febrile disease in children that is frequently associated a desquamating rash, mucosal inflammation, lymphadenopathy, and **coronary artery vasculitis,** often leading to aneurysm formation.

3. **Thromboangiitis obliterans** (**Buerger's disease**) is an inflammatory vasculitis involving the whole neurovascular compartment of tibial, popliteal, and radial arteries.

   a. It is seen in young to middle-aged **cigarette-smoking males.**

   b. The thrombus in vessels contains focal neutrophilic microabscesses and occasional multinucleated giant cells.

   c. Patients frequently have Raynaud's phenomenon (color changes in the digits) and distal gangrene often requiring amputation.

4. The **Churg-Strauss syndrome** involves granulomatous inflammation and necrotizing vasculitis of the upper and lower respiratory tract

associated with asthma and peripheral eosinophilia.

E. Examples of **small-vessel vasculitis** (arterioles, capillaries, and venules) are Henoch-Schönlein purpura, microscopic polyarteritis, cryoglobulinemic vasculitis, vasculitis associated with autoimmune disease, and vasculitis associated with serum sickness.

1. Small-vessel vasculitis is sometimes designated **hypersensitivity vasculitis** or **leukocytoclastic venulitis,** the latter referring to the presence of nuclear debris derived from neutrophils intermixed with fibrinoid necrosis.
   a. The vasculitis usually centers on the **postcapillary venules.**
   b. Inflammation is at the **same stage in all vessels.**
   c. **Immunocomplexes** are primarily involved in the pathogenesis.
   d. **Palpable purpura** is a common sign.

2. **Henoch-Schönlein purpura** (HSP) is an immune vasculitis mostly occurring in children following an upper respiratory infection.
   a. HSP is the **most common vasculitis in children.**
   b. IgA-C3 immunocomplexes deposit in the vessel wall.
   c. **IgA nephropathy** (**Berger's disease**) may be part of the syndrome complex.
   d. **Signs** and **symptoms** include the following:
      (1) Palpable purpura (often limited to the lower extremities and buttocks).
      (2) Polyarthritis.
      (3) Abdominal pain (sometimes with melena).
      (4) Renal disease presenting with hematuria.

3. **Microscopic polyarteritis** is a necrotizing vasculitis with few or no immune deposits that involves the pulmonary and glomerular capillaries in elderly patients.

4. **Cryoglobulinemic vasculitis** is a necrotizing vasculitis most commonly involving the skin and glomeruli in the elderly population.
   a. **Cryoglobulins** are immunoglobulins (most commonly IgM) that precipitate at 4°C and redissolve at 37°C.
   b. Cryoglobulins may be monoclonal, mixed monoclonal/polyclonal, or polyclonal.

5. **Vasculitis associated with autoimmune disease** most commonly involves the skin, kidneys, and brain in patients with SLE, progressive systemic sclerosis, and rheumatoid arthritis.   _—scleroderma_

6. **Vasculitis associated with serum sickness** involves the deposition of soluble immunocomplexes with antigen excess that develop in patients who are exposed to foreign antigens (e.g., rattlesnake antivenin).

F. Examples of **vasculitis involving vessels ranging from medium to small** (small arteries to venules to veins) are Wegener's granulomatosis and lymphomatoid granulomatosis.

1. **Wegener's granulomatosis** (WG) is a necrotizing granulomatous inflammation of the upper and lower respiratory tract (90–95% of cases) frequently accompanied by a necrotizing granulomatous vasculitis involving these same areas plus the kidneys (~75% of cases).
   a. **Antineutrophil cytoplasmic antibodies** (c-

ANCA type) have a pivotal role in the pathogenesis of WG.
   b. The **classic triad** of WG is acute necrotizing granulomatous inflammation involving the upper and lower respiratory tract (sinuses [90%], saddle nose deformity, nasopharynx [75%], lung [95%]), focal necrotizing vasculitis, and necrotizing glomerulonephritis (75%).
   c. **Cyclophosphamide** plus corticosteroids are useful treatment.

2. **Lymphomatoid granulomatosis** is similar to WG except for the absence of upper respiratory involvement and the potential for progression to malignant lymphoma (50% of cases).

G. **Raynaud's phenomenon** is arterial insufficiency of the digital vessels in response to cold or increased emotion.

1. Primary disease of the digital vessels is a rare cause.

2. Most cases are secondary to other diseases.
   a. It is a vasospastic disease that may be secondary to collagen vascular diseases (SLE, progressive systemic sclerosis [most common initial manifestation], CREST syndrome).
   b. Cold temperatures and stress are stimuli that may trigger color changes of the fingers from white to blue to red.
   c. The **CREST syndrome** is a limited variant of progressive systemic sclerosis that is associated with calcinosis of the finger tips, Raynaud's phenomenon, esophageal motility disorder, sclerodactyly, telangiectasia, and a positive anticentromere antibody.
   d. Other causes of Raynaud's phenomenon include thromboangiitis obliterans, Takayasu's arteritis, cryoglobulinemia, ergot poisoning, thoracic outlet syndrome, and cold agglutinin diseases (IgM).

H. **Infectious vasculitis** may involve a variety of microbial pathogens.

1. **Vessel-invading fungi** consist of *Candida, Aspergillus,* and *Mucor* species.

2. **Rocky Mountain spotted fever** is caused by *Rickettsia rickettsii,* which is transmitted by the bite of a tick.
   a. Organisms invade the vessel endothelium (arterioles and venules) and cause inflammation and rupture of weakened vessels leading to petechial lesions that begin on the soles and palms and spread to the trunk (centripetal spread).
   b. The **classic triad** of the disease is rash, fever, and history of a tick bite.

3. **Disseminated meningococcemia** (*Neisseria meningitidis*) is associated with capillary thrombosis and petechial hemorrhages, often progressing to the Waterhouse-Friderichsen syndrome.   _— adrenal insuff + vascular collapse due to hemorrhage/necrosis of adrenal cortex_

4. **Disseminated gonococcemia** (*Neisseria gonorrhoeae*) produces a small-vessel vasculitis that is commonly located on the hands, wrists, and feet.

5. **Viral vasculitis** is associated with hepatitis B and C (immunocomplex), rubella, and herpes zoster.

S₄ - diastolic filling

Objective 6: To understand the pathogenesis of essential hypertension and causes of secondary hypertension.

XIII. Hypertension
  A. Hypertension is defined as blood pressure ≥ 140/90 mm Hg in a person ≥ 18 years old.
    1. The prevalence is higher in industrialized countries and is more common in men than women and in African Americans than whites.
    2. The **control** of hypertension is the single most important factor that reduces mortality due to stroke (57% reduction) and mortality from coronary artery disease (CAD; 50% reduction).
    3. **Essential hypertension** accounts for 95% of cases with the remaining 5% representing secondary hypertension (most commonly renovascular hypertension).
    4. **Renal disease** (e.g., cystic disease, Wilms' tumor) is the most common cause of hypertension in **children**.
    5. **Oral contraceptive use** is the most common cause of hypertension in women of reproductive age.
  B. **Essential hypertension** is linked to sodium intake, obesity, sedentary life-style, stress, family history, and race.
    1. **Arterial blood pressure** (BP) is equal to the cardiac output (CO) times the total peripheral resistance (TPR), hence an increase in either or both of these components increases the BP.

    BP = CO × TPR

    2. Proposed mechanisms for producing hypertension either singly or in concert are the following:
       a. Salt retention leading to an increase in ECF volume, which increases the CO, which in turn increases TPR.
       b. An inherited defect that increases sodium concentration in the smooth muscle cells of the resistance arterioles (which increases TPR).
       c. Activation of the renin-angiotensin-aldosterone (RAA) system (which increases CO and TPR).
       d. Increased sympathetic nervous system activity (which increases TPR).
       e. Medications such as decongestants, appetite suppressants, NSAIDs (which block the vasodilator effect of prostaglandins), and estrogen (which increases angiotensinogen synthesis in the liver).
       f. Addicting agents such as cocaine (a potent vasoconstrictor and sympathetic nervous system stimulant), alcohol (which increases catecholamines), and smoking (which also increases catecholamines).
    3. Essential hypertension has a varied presentation.
       a. Most patients are asymptomatic.
       b. **Symptomatic patients** complain of morning headaches that subside before noon, dizziness, blurry vision, sweating, and chest pain.
       c. **Signs** of hypertension include the following:
          (1) Hypertensive retinopathy (e.g., silver and copper wiring, AV nicking, hemorrhages, exudate, microaneurysms).
          (2) Increased amplitude of the point of maximal impulse (PMI) from left ventricular hypertrophy (LVH) and an S₄ (fourth heart sound).
  4. **Primary consequences** of hypertension target many organ systems.
       a. It is a major risk factor for **CAD**, which in turn predisposes to AMI (most common cause of death in hypertension).
       b. It is the leading cause of **LVH** (concentric type).
       c. It is the major risk factor for initiating the intimal tear leading to a **dissecting aortic aneurysm**.
       d. It produces **hyaline arteriolosclerosis**.
       e. It predisposes to **intracerebral bleeds** (second most common cause of death due to hypertension).
       f. It produces **benign nephrosclerosis** (BNS), which may progress to malignant hypertension and renal failure.
  5. The laboratory workup for essential hypertension includes tests designed to exclude the following:
       a. Renal disease (e.g., urinalysis, serum BUN, and creatinine).
       b. Heart disease (e.g., ECG, chest x-ray).
       c. Mineralocorticoid excess states (e.g., serum electrolytes).
       d. Diabetes mellitus (e.g., serum glucose).
       e. Lipid abnormalities (e.g., lipid profiles).
  C. **Renovascular hypertension** is the most common secondary cause of hypertension in adults.
    1. Approximately two-thirds of cases are secondary to **proximal atherosclerotic plaque occlusion of the renal artery** in older men and one-third to **fibromuscular hyperplasia** (smooth muscle hyperplasia), which is more common in young to middle-aged women.
    2. In both conditions, the RAA system is activated (high renin hypertension).
    3. In either condition, the affected kidney is small and shrunken owing to persistent ischemia.
    4. **Clinical findings** include an abrupt onset of severe uncontrollable hypertension, the presence of an abdominal bruit (40% of patients), and resistance to standard medical therapy.
    5. **Screening tests** for renovascular hypertension consist of measurement of the plasma renin activity (PRA) and the captopril renogram (captopril plus a radionuclide scan of the kidneys), the latter representing the most popular screening test.
       a. A positive screen is followed up by a **renal arteriogram**, which is the gold standard confirmatory test, and catheterization of the inferior vena cava.
       b. The arteriogram reveals narrowing of the ostia due to atherosclerosis and a **"beading effect"** in fibromuscular hyperplasia owing to segmental hyperplasia of the smooth muscle.
       c. Also obtained are PRA samples from the inferior vena cava above and below the renal vein orifices and samples from both the left and right renal veins.
          (1) PRA activity in the renal vein draining the affected kidney should be increased.
          (2) PRA activity in the contralateral kidney should be suppressed, owing to suppression

of renin release by increased levels of angiotensin II.

Objective 7: To be familiar with the types of cardiac hypertrophy.

XIV. Cardiac hypertrophy
  A. **Hypertrophy** is a compensatory change that the heart (atria and ventricles) undergoes when subjected to an increased workload in response to increased pressure resistance (afterload) or volume overload (preload).
    1. Preload is the amount of blood in the heart during diastole, which is dependent on venous return to the right heart.
      a. It is equivalent to the left ventricular end-diastolic volume (LVEDV).
      b. It leads to stretching of the cardiac muscle, which invokes the Frank-Starling relationship, and subsequent increase in the force of contraction to increase the SV.
    2. Afterload is the resistance against which the ventricle must contract when ejecting blood during systole.
      a. The **Laplace relationship** involving wall stress is a better estimate of afterload.
      b. Tension in the left ventricle wall (T; wall stress, or force/cross-sectional area) during systole is equal to the product of the mean pressure in the wall of the ventricle (P) times the radius (r) of the lumen of the ventricle divided by 2 times the wall thickness (h): $T = P \times r/2\ (h)$.

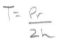
$$T = \frac{Pr}{2h}$$

      c. Sustained pressure in the cardiac chambers leads to changes in gene expression, resulting in an increase in protein synthesis.
        (1) The **stimulus for hypertrophy** is an increase in the wall stress (T) of the chamber.
        (2) Hypertrophy reduces wall stress by increasing wall thickness (h) and by reducing the radius (r) of the chamber.
        (3) Hypertrophy increases the force of contraction (more contractile elements in a hypertrophied muscle), hence increasing SV.
      d. **Physiologic hypertrophy** (reversible hypertrophy) is noted in well-trained athletes.
        (1) The increased force of contraction by hypertrophied muscle increases both the SV and the ejection fraction (EF), the latter representing SV divided by the left ventricular end-diastolic volume (LVEDV): **EF = SV/LVEDV**.
        (2) For example, if the normal SV is 80 mL and LVEDV is 120 mL, the EF is 0.66 (normal range, 0.55–0.80).
        (3) An athlete with physiologic hypertrophy who has an SV of 100 mL and an LVEDV of 120 mL has an EF of 0.83, which is increased.
  B. **Pathologic LVH** occurs as compensation for an increased afterload (e.g., essential hypertension, aortic stenosis) or as a response to an increase in preload (e.g., increased return of blood from the right heart [AV fistula], or valvular incompetence [aortic regurgitation]).
    1. **Concentric hypertrophy** of the chamber occurs with pressure resistance, while hypertrophy and dilatation occur with volume overload.
    2. **Dilatation of the left ventricle** increases wall

stress owing to an increase in the radius (r) and a decrease in wall thickness (h).
    3. In general, the heart responds better to volume than to pressure overload.
  C. **Pathologic right ventricular hypertrophy** (RVH) is similar in pathogenesis to LVH.
    1. Examples of **concentric RVH** secondary to increased afterload are pulmonary hypertension and pulmonic stenosis.
    2. **Volume overload** producing hypertrophy and dilatation are noted in pulmonic or tricuspid valve regurgitation or left-to-right shunting in congenital heart disease (e.g., ventricular septal defect).
    3. **Cor pulmonale** is RVH secondary to pulmonary hypertension (PH) that originates from primary lung disease (e.g., chronic obstructive pulmonary disease) or primary pulmonary vascular disease.
    4. **Biventricular hypertrophy** associated with a heart weighing in excess of 600–1000 g (normal weight, 300–350 g) is called **cor bovinum**.

Objective 8: To discuss the similarities and differences between left, right, and high-output cardiac failure.

XV. Congestive heart failure (CHF)
  A. **Symptoms** (what the patient complains about) predominate in left heart failure (dyspnea most commonly), while **signs** (what the physician detects on physical examination) are more prominent in right heart failure (neck vein distention and dependent edema most commonly).
  B. CHF is synonymous with a dysfunctional ventricular muscle that is unable to maintain a cardiac output sufficient to meet the demands of the body despite an adequate venous return to the right heart.
  C. **Forward failure** characterizes left heart failure due to a reduced cardiac output leading to tissue hypoxia, whereas **backward failure** highlights the systemic venous congestion associated with right heart failure.
    1. The **basic mechanisms** of heart failure are weakness or inefficiency of ventricular contraction (e.g., myocardial ischemia), restricted filling (noncompliance) of the chambers of the heart (e.g., restrictive cardiomyopathy), and increase in workload.
    2. An increase in workload can be an increase in afterload (e.g., essential hypertension) or in preload (e.g., valve incompetence).
    3. A reduction in cardiac output is common to both left and right heart failure, which ultimately causes the kidneys to reabsorb salt and water to restore volume.
  D. **Left heart failure** (LHF), the most common cause of CHF, is associated with a decrease in left ventricular cardiac output most commonly secondary to AMI or essential hypertension.
    1. The left ventricular SV is decreased, leading to incomplete emptying of the ventricle.
      a. The **LV end-diastolic pressure** (LVEDP) and **volume** (LVEDV) both increase (which increases preload), resulting in dilatation of the mitral valve (MV) ring to produce a **functional mitral valve regurgitation**.

ACE inhibitor

b. The increased LVEDP is reflected back into the left atrium with a subsequent increase in the hydrostatic pressure in the pulmonary veins that overrides the capillary oncotic pressure, resulting in **pulmonary edema** and **congestion**.

c. Vasoconstriction of the pulmonary artery (possibly an autoregulation mechanism) increases the afterload against which the right ventricle must contract, hence leading to right heart failure (RHF).

2. **Signs** and **symptoms** in LHF include the following:

   a. **Dyspnea** is the sensation of difficult or uncomfortable breathing (stimulation of J receptors).

   b. **Orthopnea** is dyspnea in the recumbent position (excess fluid returns to the failed left heart when the patient lies down).

   c. **Paroxysmal nocturnal dyspnea** (PND) is a choking sensation that awakens the patient (similar in pathogenesis to orthopnea).

   d. **"Cardiac asthma"** is due to peribronchiolar edema.

   e. S_3 is functional mitral regurgitation from stretching of the valve ring.

   f. **Bibasilar inspiratory rales** are associated with pulmonary edema.

3. **Laboratory abnormalities** consist of the following:

   a. **Prerenal azotemia** (a disproportionate increase in serum BUN over serum creatinine) is due to a reduction in the glomerular filtration rate and increased reabsorption of urea in the proximal tubules.

   b. **Perihilar congestion** ("bat wing configuration"), **Kerley's B lines** (septal edema at the costophrenic angle), and **patchy interstitial** and **alveolar infiltrates** are noted on chest x-ray.

E. **Right heart failure** (RHF) is most commonly due to LHF.

1. RHF is primarily characterized by **signs** and **symptoms** of the following:

   a. **Increased systemic venous pressure** (*sine qua non* of RHF) leading to jugular neck vein distention, liver congestion ("nutmeg liver"), splenomegaly, splanchnic congestion (anorexia, nausea, and vomiting), kidney congestion (oliguria), pitting edema of the lower extremities, and ascites in severe cases.

   b. A **functional tricuspid valve regurgitation** and S_3.

   c. **Neck vein distention** on compression of the liver (**hepatojugular reflux**).

2. **Laboratory abnormalities** associated with RHF consist of the following:

   a. **Hyponatremia** (hypotonic gain of more water than salt from the kidneys; see Chapter 5).

   b. **Prerenal azotemia** (related to a decreased cardiac output and reduction in the GFR).

F. **Treatment** of CHF consists of improving the performance of the failed ventricle by the following means:

1. Administering positive inotropic agents (e.g., digoxin, dopamine, dobutamine).

2. Reducing afterload (e.g., using vasodilators such as captopril, which reduce afterload by preventing the release of angiotensin II and also reduce preload by preventing the release of aldosterone).

3. Reducing preload by controlling salt and water retention (e.g., with thiazide diuretics or by limiting salt and water intake).

G. **High-output failure** (normal to increased cardiac output) may occur when one or more of the following are present:

1. **Increased blood volume** (e.g., excess infusion of isotonic saline), which increases the preload and increases the SV (by Frank-Starling mechanisms).

2. **Increased positive inotropism** (increases contractility; hyperthyroidism).

3. **Decreased blood viscosity** or **vasodilatation of arterioles**, which, according to Poiseuille's equation, reduces the total peripheral resistance (TPR) in arterioles, hence increasing venous return to the heart: $R = 8 n l / \pi r^4$, where R = resistance, n = viscosity of blood (decreased in anemia), l = length of the vessel, and r^4 = radius of the vessel to the fourth power (vasodilatation may be due to endotoxemia or thiamine deficiency).

4. **Increased venous return to the heart** due to an AV fistula, which decreases the TPR.

Objective 9: To outline the pathogenesis of the common acyanotic and cyanotic congenital heart diseases.

XVI. Congenital heart disease

A. Congenital heart disease (CHD) is the most common heart disease in children.

1. Most cases of CHD are not inherited and have no identifiable cause (~90%).

2. **Chromosomal abnormalities** (e.g., Down syndrome) and maternal factors (diabetes mellitus, alcohol, smoking, infection) account for a small number of cases.

3. Acyanotic and cyanotic variants are recognized.

B. **Acyanotic CHD** includes ventricular septal defects (VSD), atrial septal defects (ASD), patent ductus arteriosus (PDA), and coarctation of the aorta.

1. **VSDs** are the **most common** overall type of CHD (32%).

   a. The majority (75–80%) are associated with a defect in the membranous portion of the interventricular septum, which usually closes spontaneously.

   b. Associations with VSD include the **cri du chat syndrome** (partial deletion of chromosome 5) and **trisomy 18** (Edwards' syndrome).

   c. VSDs begin as a left-to-right shunt owing to the higher pressure in the left ventricle than that in the pulmonary vascular system.

      (1) Volume overload of the right ventricle produces RVH, which is further enhanced by the development of pulmonary hypertension (PH).

(2) Excess volume of blood returning to the left ventricle is a stimulus for LVH and dilatation.

(3) When right ventricular pressure overrides left ventricular pressure, blood flow moves from right to left (**Eisenmenger's syndrome**).

(4) Mixing of unoxygenated blood from the right ventricle with oxygenated blood in the left ventricle lowers the arterial oxygen saturation (SaO_2), leading to the **late onset of cyanosis (cyanosis tardive)**.

2. **ASDs** are primarily associated with patency of the foramen ovale (ostium secundum type) and account for 8% of CHD.

   a. There is an increased incidence in newborns with the **fetal alcohol syndrome**.

   b. The **ostium primum type** often involves the whole endocardial cushion (combined ASD and VSD), and these defects are commonly present in Down syndrome (Chapter 7).

   c. In the **ostium secundum type**, blood initially flows from the left into the right atrium.

      (1) Volume overflow of the right and left heart results in hypertrophy and dilatation, PH, and Eisenmenger's syndrome.

      (2) Volume overload of the right heart produces **fixed splitting of the second heart sound** (delayed closure of the pulmonic valve keeps the split in the second heart sound on expiration as well as inspiration).

3. **PDA** is most frequently secondary to hypoxemia, acidosis, or prematurity, all of which delay normal ductus closure in the newborn.

   a. It is most commonly an isolated defect but may accompany other defects (e.g., VSDs, ASDs, transposition of the great vessels, and coarctation of the aorta).

   b. There is an association with **congenital rubella**.

   c. It begins as a left-to-right shunt with blood moving from the high-pressure aorta into the low-pressure pulmonary artery through the ductus.

      (1) Blood refluxing to and fro in the ductus during systole and diastole produces a **machinery murmur**.

      (2) Overload of the pulmonary artery results in the same sequence of events described for both VSD and ASD, namely, Eisenmenger's syndrome as well as RVH and LVH with dilatation.

      (3) With reversal of the shunt, unoxygenated blood is delivered distal to the subclavian artery, hence the upper body appears pink (well oxygenated), while the lower part of the body is cyanotic (**differential cyanosis**).

      (4) Medical closure of a PDA is enhanced by giving **indomethacin**, which blocks cyclooxygenase and the synthesis of prostaglandins.

4. A **coarctation** is a localized constriction of the aorta either before the ductus (**preductal**) or after the ductus (**postductal**).

   a. It is subdivided into **infantile** (70% of cases; preductal type) and **adult** types (30% of cases; postductal type), the former having an association with Turner's syndrome and both having an increased incidence of bicuspid aortic valves.

   b. **Preductal types** are symptomatic at birth, whereas the **postductal type** becomes clinically apparent in adolescents or adults.

   c. In the **adult type**, there is proximal dilatation of the aorta and the aortic valve leading to aortic regurgitation, a potential for dissecting aortic aneurysm, and an increased incidence of berry aneurysms in the cerebral vessels (increased pressure in the intracranial vessels).

   d. The following are **additional findings** in the adult type:

      (1) **Increase in upper body musculature** over that of the lower body.

      (2) **Inequality of the blood pressure** (> 10 mm Hg) and pulse between the upper and lower extremities.

      (3) Development of **collateral circulations** through the internal mammary (which connects with the superficial epigastric artery) and intercostal arterial systems (producing **rib notching**).

      (4) **Diastolic hypertension** due to activation of the renin-angiotensin-aldosterone system from reduced blood flow distally.

C. **Cyanotic CHD** includes *t*etralogy of Fallot, *t*ransposition of the great vessels, *t*runcus arteriosus, *t*otal anomalous pulmonary venous return, and *t*ricuspid atresia (mnemonic: 5 T's).

   1. **Right-to-left intracardiac shunts** are responsible for cyanotic CHD.

      a. Hypoxemia stimulates the release of erythropoietin, leading to **secondary polycythemia**.

      b. Right-to-left shunts bypass the normal filtering action of the lungs, hence predisposing patients to **septicemia** and **metastatic abscess** formation (most commonly in the brain).

   2. **Tetralogy of Fallot**, accounting for ~8% of CHD, is the most common cause of cyanotic CHD.

      a. It has four components:

         (1) A **dextrorotated aorta** (overriding the interventricular septum).

         (2) **Subpulmonary pulmonic valve stenosis** (stenosis below the valve).

         (3) RVH.

         (4) VSD (membranous type).

      b. The magnitude of the right-to-left shunt and the potential for cyanosis is dependent on the **degree of subpulmonic valve stenosis**.

         (1) **Less stenosis** permits more blood to enter the pulmonary artery for oxygenation (newborns are not cyanotic).

         (2) **Severe stenosis** directs more unoxygenated blood through the VSD into the left ventricle (newborns are cyanotic).

   3. **Transposition of the great vessels** accounts for ~5% of CHD.

      a. There is an increased incidence of **maternal diabetes mellitus**.

      b. In the **most common type** of transposition, the right ventricle is emptied by the aorta and the left ventricle is emptied by the pulmonary artery.

         (1) The left atrium receives oxygenated blood from the pulmonary veins, and the right atrium receives unoxygenated venous blood from the venae cavae.

         (2) **Survival** depends on the presence of shunts, which allow blood to pass in both directions (i.e., left-to-right [ASD and PDA] and right-to-left [VSD]).

(3) Oxygenated blood from the left atrium flows into the right atrium, where it mixes with venous blood (steps up the SaO_2).

(4) Blood passes into the right ventricle, where a portion is pumped into the aorta to the rest of the body.

(5) If a PDA is present, some of the blood enters the pulmonary artery for oxygenation (left-to-right shunt).

(6) The remainder of the blood passes from the right ventricle to the left ventricle (right-to-left shunt) through the VSD owing to the greater systemic resistance on the right side of the heart.

(7) The left ventricle is emptied by the pulmonary artery, which delivers the blood to the lungs for oxygenation.

Objective 10: To review the pathogenesis of ischemic heart disease.

XVII. Ischemic heart disease (IHD)

A. IHD is the **most common cause of death** in the United States (25% of all deaths) despite an approximate 40% decline in death rate over the last few years.

B. The **clinical manifestations** of IHD consist of **angina pectoris** (most common), **AMI, sudden cardiac death syndrome**, **chronic ischemic heart disease**, and **cardiac arrhythmias**.

C. IHD, whether asymptomatic or symptomatic, is associated with myocardial ischemia secondary to occlusive atherosclerosis of the coronary arteries.

1. The **left anterior descending** (LAD) coronary artery supplies the anterior wall of the left ventricle and the anterior two-thirds of the interventricular septum, respectively.

2. The **right coronary artery** (RCA) nourishes the entire right ventricle, posteroinferior wall of the left ventricle (including the posteromedial papillary muscle), and posterior third of the interventricular septum and supplies 90% of the blood to the atrioventricular node.

3. The **left circumflex coronary artery** (LCA) has marginal branches that supply the lateral free wall of the LV.

D. **Sudden cardiac death** (SCD) **syndrome** is death within 1 hour of chest pain.

1. Ischemia provokes a fatal ventricular arrhythmia, usually ventricular fibrillation.

2. SCD accounts for ~50% of all deaths associated with IHD and almost 25% of deaths in the United States.

3. At autopsy, most patients have severe, fixed atherosclerotic CAD involving one or more coronary arteries; however, a grossly obvious coronary thrombosis or acute changes in the myocardium (coagulation necrosis) are not usually present.

E. **Angina pectoris**, the most common manifestation of occlusive atherosclerotic CAD, is recurrent episodes of precordial chest pain associated with myocardial ischemia.

$T = \frac{P r}{2 h}$

1. **Myocardial oxygen consumption** (MVO_2) of the left ventricle is primarily dependent on heart rate, contractility, and ventricular wall tension (wall stress).

2. **Three clinical variants** of angina are exertional, Prinzmetal's, and unstable (crescendo, preinfarction) angina.

a. **Exertional (classical) angina** is the most common variant.

(1) There is a sudden onset of exercise-induced substernal chest pain lasting 1–15 minutes that is relieved by resting or by nitroglycerin.

(2) Severe, fixed CAD atherosclerosis is present on coronary arteriography.

b. **Prinzmetal's angina** is characterized by chest pain at rest and is secondary to vasospasm of the coronary arteries possibly owing to the vasoconstrictive effects of thromboxane A_2 released from small platelet thrombi.

c. **Unstable (crescendo) angina** is frequent bouts of chest pain at rest and is associated with eccentric stenosis of vessels with disrupted plaques and nonocclusive thrombus formation.

3. The **stress electrocardiogram** (ECG) is the screening test of choice for determining the type of angina present.

a. A **positive test** is the presence of either ST depression (subendocardial ischemia; exertional angina) or ST elevation (transmural ischemia; Prinzmetal's angina).

b. **Coronary arteriography** is the gold standard confirmatory test after a positive stress ECG.

F. **Acute myocardial infarction** (AMI) incidence increases with age, particularly in men over 45 years of age.

1. Approximately 25% of patients either succumb to a terminal ventricular arrhythmia prior to reaching the hospital (sudden cardiac death) or suffer a similar event while in the critical care unit.

2. The majority (> 90%) demonstrate occlusion of a coronary artery by a fresh thrombus (composed of platelets and fibrin) overlying a ruptured atheromatous plaque.

3. The **coronary vessels most commonly involved** in decreasing order of frequency are the LAD, RCA, and LCA.

4. Most AMIs are located in the left ventricle and the interventricular septum.

a. A **Q wave infarction** is the presence of a Q wave (area of necrosis on an ECG) either with or without transmural (all layers involved) disease.

b. A **non–Q wave infarction** is more likely to be subendocardial and less likely to show occlusive thrombi in the coronary artery.

5. AMIs follow a progressive series of gross, microscopic, and enzyme alterations (Table 10–1).

6. **Signs** and **symptoms** that have a high predictive value for diagnosing an AMI follow:

a. Substernal chest pain with radiation into the left arm, left shoulder, or jaw.

b. Pain described as pressure that lasts longer than 30–45 minutes and is not relieved by nitroglycerin.

c. Pain associated with a diaphoresis (e.g., perspiration, nausea).

7. **Complications** plague the majority (> 80%) of AMIs.

TABLE 10–1. Gross, Microscopic, and Laboratory Changes in the Natural History of Acute Myocardial Infarction (AMI)

Time Post-AMI	Gross Abnormalities	Microscopic Abnormalities	Laboratory Abnormalities
0–24 hours	0–4 hours: no change. 4–12 hours: no change. 12–24 hours: early pallor of coagulation necrosis (18–24 hours).	0–4 hours: no change. 4–12 hours: coagulation necrosis beginning after 6 hours. 12–24 hours: coagulation necrosis with nuclear pyknosis, loss of striations, eosinophilia, interstitial neutrophil infiltrate.	0–4 hours: no change. 4–12 hours: ↑ total CK (4–6 hours); slight ↑ CK-MB (begins in 4–8 hours); ↑ total LDH and LDH ½ flip (begins to appear in 10 hours); AST ↑ (begins in 6–12 hours). 12–24 hours: same as 4–12 hours; CK-MB peaks in 24 hours.
1–3 days	Definite pallor. Some hyperemia around areas of pallor.	Advanced coagulation necrosis. Marked neutrophilic infiltrate.	↑ Total CK (disappears in 3–4 days); CK-MB disappears in 3 days; LDH ½ flip peaks in 2–3 days; AST ↑ (peaks 1–2 days).
3–7 days	Central yellow area with well demarcated hyperemic border. Period of maximal softness (time for ruptures).	Dissolution of myocardial fibers. Macrophages from hyperemic area migrate into necrotic tissue.	Total CK absent by 3–4 days. LDH ½ flip decreasing (gone in 7 days). Total LDH decreasing. AST disappears in 5–9 days.
7–10 days	Same as 3–7 days.	More advanced repair with macrophages, fibroblasts, and neovascularization. Collagen deposition beginning.	Total LDH normal after 10–14 days. No LDH ½ flip.
>10 days	Central softening and yellow discoloration maximal by 20 days. Patchy areas of fibrosis (scar).	Continuation of repair. Collagen deposition continues over subsequent 1–3 weeks, and inflammatory infiltrate recedes. Dense fibrous tissue after 4 weeks.	No enzyme abnormalities after 2 weeks.

a. **Ventricular extrasystoles** often serve as warning signals for impending ventricular fibrillation (the most common cause of death) and cardiac standstill.
b. **CHF** and **cardiogenic shock** commonly occur in the first 24 hours.
c. **Mural thrombi** overlying the damaged subendocardium usually develop in the first week and have the potential for embolization.
d. The soft, necrotic myocardial tissue during the third through tenth day predisposes to **rupture of the left ventricle** (most commonly the anterior free wall; LAD thrombosis), **posteromedial papillary muscle** (RCA thrombosis), or **interventricular septum**.
e. **Reinfarction** is characterized by the reappearance of CK-MB after 3 days.
f. **Acute fibrinous pericarditis** occurs with a transmural infarction usually within 2–3 days.
g. **Ventricular aneurysms** may occur as an early complication developing in the first 2 weeks or they may occur after several months (10–15%).
   (1) **Complications** associated with aneurysms include CHF (the most common cause of aneurysm-related death) and thromboembolization.
   (2) Rupture is uncommon owing to the presence of scar tissue.
h. **Dressler's syndrome** is an autoimmune pericarditis that occurs weeks to months after an AMI.
i. **Right ventricular infarcts** occur in one-third of patients with inferior myocardial infarctions.

8. The **electrocardiogram** (ECG), **cardiac enzymes**, and **cardiac-specific troponin-I assays** are the mainstays in confirming an AMI.
   a. The **classic electrocardiographic evolution** of an AMI is as follows:
      (1) Peaked (hyperacute) T waves (area of ischemia).
      (2) ST segment elevation (area of injury, loss of normal myocardial cell membrane ion pumps).
      (3) Symmetric T wave inversion (area of ischemia).
      (4) Q wave (area of infarction with cell death).
   b. **Anterior AMIs** have Q waves in leads V1 through V4.
   c. **Lateral wall AMIs** have Q waves in leads I and aVL.
   d. **Inferior AMIs** have Q waves in leads II, III, and aVF.
   e. **Posterior wall AMIs** have a large R wave and ST depression in V1, V2, and/or V3.
   f. The **cardiac enzymes** consist of serum creatine kinase (CK) and its isoenzyme CK-MB, lactate dehydrogenase (LDH) and its LDH isoenzyme fractions 1 and 2, and aspartate aminotransferase (AST).
      (1) **Total CK** first increases in 4–6 hours, peaks in 12–24 hours, and subsides in 3–4 days.
      (2) **CK-MB** first appears in 4–8 hours, peaks in 24 hours, and returns to normal in 1.5–3 days.
      (3) **Total LDH** and the **LDH ½ flip** begin to increase in 10 hours after an AMI, peak in 48–72 hours, and return to normal in 7–10 days.

(a) LDH 2 isoenzyme is normally > LDH 1.
(b) LDH 1 in cardiac muscle is released with infarction and becomes > LDH 2 (flip).
(4) Aspartate aminotransferase (AST) first appears in 6–12 hours, peaks in 1–2 days, and returns to normal in 5–9 days.

  g. Cardiac-specific troponin-I assays are replacing CK-MB; they first increase in 2–6 hours, peak in 15–24 hours, and return to normal in 7 days.

  h. The **prognosis** depends on the degree of left ventricular dysfunction.

G. Chronic IHD is the result of myocardial ischemia leading to progressive, focal replacement of cardiac muscle by scar tissue.

Objective 11: To understand the pathogenesis of congenital and acquired valvular disorders.

XVIII. Valvular disorders

A. **Rheumatic fever** (RF) is a multisystem immunologic disorder generally involving children from ages 5 to 15.

  1. RF is preceded by infections with certain serotypes of **group A β-hemolytic streptococci** that most commonly produce an exudative pharyngitis.

  2. Shortly after the infection, problems occur in the heart (carditis), joints (polyarthritis; most common), skin (erythema marginatum), basal ganglia (chorea), and soft tissues (subcutaneous nodules).

  3. Cytotoxic antibodies develop against the M protein (virulence factor) of the streptococcus, which has antigens similar (antigen mimicry) to those in the heart and other tissues, resulting in damage to these structures.

  4. The **Aschoff body** is the **pathognomonic lesion** of RF and consists of a collection of **Anichkov's myocytes** (reactive histiocytes) and **Aschoff multinucleated giant cells** within an area of fibrinoid necrosis located in the myocardium, endocardium, or both.

    a. **Valvular disease** in order of decreasing frequency affects the **mitral** (most common), **mitral and aortic**, and tricuspid and pulmonic valves (rare).

    b. Sterile, nonembolic, warty (verrucous) **vegetations** occur along the **lines of closure** (edge) of the involved valve, often leading to regurgitation murmurs.

    c. With **recurrent attacks** of RF, the valve leaflets undergo repair by fibrous tissue and dystrophic calcification, resulting in interadherence of the valve leaflets leading to stenosis (**mitral stenosis** most common) and less commonly regurgitation murmurs (aortic regurgitation).

  5. The **diagnosis** of acute RF must comply with the **Jones major** and **minor criteria**.

    a. The Jones major criteria are the following:
      (1) Migratory asymmetric polyarthritis (~75%).
      (2) Carditis (~35%).
      (3) Chorea (~10%).
      (4) Subcutaneous nodules (~10%).
      (5) Erythema marginatum (~10%).

    b. The Jones minor criteria include fever and prolonged PR interval.

  6. The **prognosis** in acute RF depends on the severity of the initial attack, number of recurrences, and degree of valvular involvement.

  7. **Heart failure** from chronic valvular disease (usually mitral stenosis) is the most common cause of death.

B. **Mitral stenosis** is most commonly caused by **chronic rheumatic heart disease**.

  1. There is an abnormality in mitral valve opening (diastole), leading to volume overload in the left atrium and lungs.

  2. **Signs** and **symptoms** include the following:

    a. **Accentuated** S_1.

    b. **Opening snap** (OS) followed by a **mid-diastolic rumbling murmur** heard best at apex.

    c. **Dyspnea** and **hemoptysis** secondary to pulmonary congestion.

    d. **Atrial fibrillation** secondary to left atrial dilatation and hypertrophy.

    e. **Systemic embolization** from clots in the left atrium dislodged by atrial fibrillation.

    f. **Dysphagia** for solids owing to left atrial enlargement.

C. **Mitral valve prolapse** (MVP) is the most common valvular disease.

  1. The valve leaflets (anterior and/or posterior [most common]) undergo **myxomatous degeneration**, resulting in redundant (voluminous) valve leaflets that prolapse into the left atrium during systole.

  2. An **AD** inheritance pattern is seen in some cases.

  3. There is an association with **Marfan's** and **Ehlers-Danlos** syndromes.

  4. **Signs** and **symptoms** include the following:

    a. There is a **mid-systolic click** when the valve prolapses into the left atrium and suddenly stops.

    b. The click is followed by a **mid- or late systolic murmur** (element of mitral regurgitation).

    c. Anxiety, with an increase in heart rate, and decreasing venous return to the heart (by standing or the Valsalva maneuver) cause the click and murmur to occur earlier in systole (closer to S_1).

    d. Lying down, squatting, sustained hand grip exercise, and passive leg lifting in the supine position increase venous return and cause the click and murmur to occur later in systole.

    e. Symptomatic cases (most are asymptomatic) present with palpitations, chest pain, and fatigue.

    f. Most patients are women who are tall and thin.

    g. Rupture of the chordae produces acute mitral insufficiency.

  5. The **diagnosis** is best made by **echocardiography**.

  6. **Calcium channel blockers** or **β-blockers** are used as treatment in symptomatic cases.

D. **Mitral regurgitation** (insufficiency) is most commonly due to MVP.

  1. It is an abnormality in mitral valve closing in systole, leading to reflux of blood into the left

Valsalva maneuver — ↑ in intraabdominal P by expiring vs. closed glottis

atrium and volume overload in the left ventricle.

2. **Signs** and **symptoms** include the following:
   a. Pansystolic murmur with radiation into the axilla heard best at the apex.
   b. Pulmonary symptoms (dyspnea, cough) late in the disease.

E. **Aortic stenosis** is most frequently secondary to a calcified **congenital bicuspid valve** (>50% of cases).
   1. It is caused by a reduction in the valve orifice area, which offers increased resistance to the ejection of blood during systole, leading to pressure overload in the left ventricle and concentric LVH.
   2. **Signs** and **symptoms** include the following:
      a. Narrow pulse pressure.
      b. Ejection type murmur during systole that radiates into the carotids.
      c. Angina and/or syncope with exertion (most common valvular lesion producing these findings).

F. **Aortic regurgitation** is most frequently secondary to chronic rheumatic heart disease.
   1. Less common causes consist of infective endocarditis, syphilitic aortic aneurysms, dissecting aortic aneurysms, ankylosing spondylitis, Marfan's syndrome, and coarctation of the aorta.
   2. It is a problem with volume overload in the left ventricle from an incompetent valve that leaks blood back into the ventricle during diastole.
      a. It produces LVH with dilatation.
      b. The stroke volume increases (often > 100 mL) owing to Frank-Starling mechanisms.
      c. The **pulse pressure widens**, resulting in a hyperdynamic circulation (e.g., water-hammer pulse).

G. **Tricuspid stenosis** is usually associated with mitral stenosis post–chronic rheumatic heart disease.

H. **Tricuspid regurgitation** is most commonly due to stretching of the tricuspid valve ring in right heart failure.

I. **Carcinoid heart disease** is associated with the carcinoid syndrome consisting of the triad of cutaneous flushing, diarrhea, and valvular disease (tricuspid regurgitation and pulmonic stenosis).

J. **Endocarditis** is usually accompanied by vegetations, which represent depositions of platelets held together by fibrin on the endothelial surface of the heart, most commonly the valve leaflets.
   1. Vegetations may become infected by microbial pathogens (e.g., acute and subacute infective endocarditis), remain sterile (e.g., marantic vegetations), or be a manifestation of an autoimmune disease (e.g., rheumatic fever, SLE).
   2. **Infective endocarditis** (IE) is most commonly secondary to bacterial pathogens.
      a. **Predisposing factors** include bacteremia (e.g., due to intravenous drug abuse, indwelling venous catheter, dental manipulation), previous valvular disease (e.g., mitral stenosis), or the presence of prosthetic heart valves.
      b. Organisms associated with **acute IE** are generally more virulent (most commonly *S.*

aureus) and may infect previously normal or abnormal valves.
      c. Pathogens associated with **subacute IE** are usually less virulent (most commonly *Streptococcus viridans*) and infect previously damaged valves.
      d. In patients with **prosthetic heart valves**, coagulase-negative staphylococci are the most common pathogens.
      e. In **intravenous drug abusers**, *S. aureus* is the most common pathogen.
      f. The **mitral valve** is most frequently involved; however, in intravenous drug abuse, the tricuspid or aortic valves are equally affected.
      g. The **valve vegetations** are usually multiple, bulky, and extremely friable, hence predisposing to systemic embolization (embolic strokes, splenic infarcts).
      h. Immunocomplex disease (type III hypersensitivity) due to antibodies against bacterial antigens assumes a prominent role in the pathogenesis of organ damage in IE (e.g., Osler's nodes).
      i. The following are **signs** (immunocomplex-mediated) and **symptoms** of IE:
         (1) Roth's retinal hemorrhages, splinter hemorrhages under the nails, Osler's nodes (painful nodules on the hands and feet), Janeway's lesions (painless nodules on the hands and feet), and glomerulonephritis with hematuria (all immunocomplex mediated).
         (2) Fever (most consistent sign).
      j. Blood cultures are positive in 95% of cases.
   3. **Libman-Sacks endocarditis** is an uncommon, usually uneventful immune endocarditis associated with SLE (10–20%).
      a. Nonembolic, verrucous vegetations are randomly scattered over the valves, chordae, and endocardial surfaces.
      b. It is more often a postmortem finding than a serious complication during the course of the disease.
   4. **Nonbacterial thrombotic endocarditis** (**marantic vegetations**) demonstrates bulky, sterile vegetations.
      a. The vegetations are most commonly located on the **mitral valve**.
      b. They may develop as part of a **paraneoplastic syndrome** in malignancies associated with a hypercoagulable state, such as mucinous carcinomas of the colon, pancreas, or lungs.
   5. **Prosthetic heart valves** are associated with the following complications:
      a. Thromboembolism (most common).
      b. Infective endocarditis.
      c. Microangiopathic hemolytic anemia.
      d. Mechanical dysfunction with heart failure.

Objective 12: To outline the pathogenesis of diseases involving the myocardium.

XIX. Disorders involving the myocardium
   A. **Myocarditis** is secondary to invasive microbial pathogens, bacterial toxins, hypersensitivity reactions, or drugs.

1. Consequences of myocarditis include progression to congestive cardiomyopathy, heart failure, arrhythmias, and sudden cardiac death.
2. **Infectious myocarditis** is most commonly due to viruses (usually coxsackie B).
3. **Autoimmune myocarditis** is sometimes associated with rheumatoid arthritis, SLE, progressive systemic sclerosis, or rheumatic fever.
4. **Toxic myocarditis** is frequently secondary to drugs such as doxorubicin and tricyclic antidepressants.
5. Sarcoidosis may produce a granulomatous myocarditis.
6. **Hypersensitivity reactions** may be associated with penicillin, methyldopa, sulfonamides, and anticonvulsants.

B. **Cardiomyopathies** (primary and secondary types) commonly present with signs and symptoms related to myocardial dysfunction (e.g., heart failure, arrhythmias).
1. **Congestive cardiomyopathy** (the most common type) primarily occurs in young adults and is most frequently idiopathic.
   a. It presents with signs of both left and right heart failure manifested by a massively dilated heart on chest x-ray.
   b. Acquired forms are associated with previous viral myocarditis, the postpartum state, alcoholism (due to direct toxicity or thiamine deficiency [globoid heart]), hypothyroidism (myxedema heart), and drug toxicities (e.g., doxorubicin).
2. **Hypertrophic cardiomyopathy** (idiopathic hypertrophic subaortic stenosis, or IHSS) is a disorder afflicting young adults.
   a. It demonstrates disproportionate hypertrophy of the interventricular septum and hypertrophy of the free wall of the left ventricle resulting in diminution of the left ventricle chamber.
   b. **Myofiber disarray** and **abnormalities in the conduction system** (causing increased sudden death syndrome) are frequently noted in autopsy tissue.
   c. The **pathophysiology** of outflow obstruction relates to a combination of asymmetric hypertrophy of the septum plus apposition of the anterior leaflet of the mitral valve drawn against the septum during systole.
   d. **Increasing preload** in the ventricle by **decreasing inotropism** (e.g., with β-blockers or calcium channel blockers) and/or **increasing venous return of blood to the right heart** (e.g., by squatting or lying down) results in clinical improvement. *[handwritten: Inotropism = Contractility]*
   e. **Reducing preload** in the ventricle (e.g., with the Valsalva maneuver, venodilators, positive inotropic agents) worsens clinical signs and symptoms.
   f. The diagnosis is confirmed by **echocardiography**.
3. **Restrictive cardiomyopathy** is characterized by decreased compliance (distensibility) of the myocardium with subsequent decrease in diastolic filling and cardiac output.
   a. **Primary diseases** include **Loeffler's endomyocarditis** (association with eosinophil

infiltrates and eosinophilia) and **endocardial fibroelastosis**.
   (1) Fibroelastosis is present in 10% of patients with CHD, most commonly aortic stenosis or the infantile type of coarctation.
   (2) Endocardial biopsies reveal increased deposition of collagen and elastic tissue.
   b. **Acquired causes** consist of **infiltrative diseases** such as Pompe's disease (glycogenosis), hemochromatosis or hemosiderosis, sarcoidosis (granulomatous myocarditis), mucopolysaccharidoses (e.g., Hurler's syndrome), and amyloidosis.

C. **Primary tumors** of the heart are rare.
1. A **cardiac myxoma** is the most common (35–50%) primary benign tumor of the heart.
   a. Myxomas are derived from mesenchyme and are almost exclusively located in the left atrium (~75%).
   b. They restrict blood flow into the left ventricle, embolize (often to the brain), and demonstrate constitutional signs of fever, weight loss, and anemia.
2. **Rhabdomyomas** are the second most common benign tumor of heart muscle in adults and are associated with tuberous sclerosis. *[handwritten: 1st most common in kids]*
3. **Metastatic disease** (lung cancer most frequently) is more common than primary cancer of the heart.

Objective 13: To be familiar with disorders involving the pericardium.

XX. Disorders involving the pericardium
A. **Acute pericarditis** is most commonly secondary to viruses, usually coxsackie B (also the most common cause of myocarditis).
1. **Pyogenic pericarditis** is most frequently a consequence of direct spread from a subjacent lung infection caused by *S. aureus* or *Streptococcus pneumoniae*.
2. **Fibrinous pericarditis** ("bread and butter pericarditis") is associated with uremia, acute myocardial infarction, rheumatic fever, SLE (very common), radiation, or metastasis.
3. **Signs** and **symptoms** include the following:
   a. Precordial chest pain.
   b. A friction rub (often has three components).

B. **Constrictive pericarditis** occurs when the visceral or parietal pericardium becomes noncompliant.
1. **Tuberculosis** is the most common cause worldwide, while open heart surgery, purulent infections, and trauma are more frequent causes in the United States.
2. Stiffness of the pericardium is often enhanced by dystrophic calcification.
   a. Ventricular filling is normal in early diastole but is abruptly reduced later in diastole when the dilated ventricle reaches the confines of the thickened pericardial shell (cause of a pericardial knock).
   b. The mean pressures in the chambers of the heart, the pulmonic veins, and systemic veins are all equally elevated (~20 mm Hg; LVEDP is normally ≥ 12 mm Hg).
   c. The return of venous blood to the right

heart is also compromised, resulting in pulsus paradoxus and Kussmaul's sign.

C. **Pericardial effusions** are collections of fluid in the pericardial sac beyond the 30–50 mL normally present.

1. They are often due to an alteration of Starling's forces related to an increase in hydrostatic pressure or a decrease in oncotic pressure.

2. When an effusion compromises the normal filling of the heart, the condition is referred to as **cardiac tamponade.**

   a. In tamponade, the increased intrapericardial pressure impedes diastolic filling of both atria and both ventricles by restricting expansion of the cardiac chambers (most evident in the ventricles).

   b. As the intrapericardial pressure increases, the end-diastolic pressures in all the cardiac chambers also increase in order to prevent chamber collapse.

3. Three classic physical diagnostic signs of cardiac tamponade (**Beck's triad**) are hypotension, elevated jugular venous pulse, and muffled heart sounds.

4. An **echocardiogram** is the best test to document a pericardial effusion.

5. A chest x-ray exhibits a "**water bottle**" configuration of the heart.

QUESTIONS

DIRECTIONS. (Items 1–26): Each of the numbered items or incomplete statements in this section is followed by answers or by completions of the statement. Select the ONE lettered answer or completion that is BEST in each case. Correct answers and explanations are given at the end of the chapter.

1. The left atrium of the heart in this photograph is opened and the arrows point to the mitral valve orifice of a 52-year-old woman with a long history of heart disease. Which of the following would least likely have been present in the heart or lungs at some time during the course of her disease?

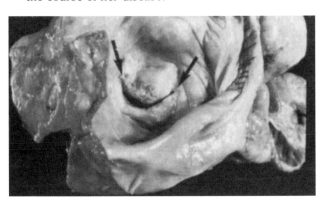

(A) Aschoff bodies
(B) Atrial fibrillation
(C) Pulmonary congestion
(D) Left ventricular hypertrophy
(E) Opening snap

2. The lesion in the left side of the heart was an incidental finding at autopsy in a 71-year-old man who was killed in an automobile accident. Which of the following physical diagnostic findings would most likely have been present in this man?

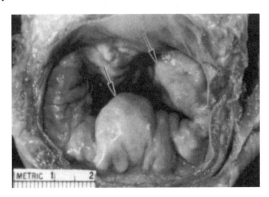

(A) Opening snap
(B) Mid-systolic ejection click
(C) Pulsus paradoxus
(D) Accentuated A2
(E) Mid-diastolic rumble

3. The pathology of this lesion in the aorta is most closely related to

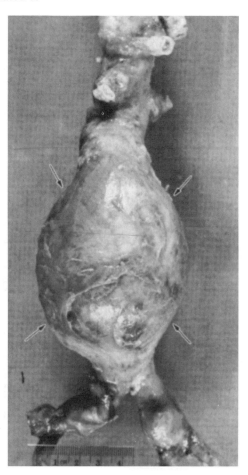

(A) elastic tissue fragmentation
(B) a primary defect in collagen synthesis
(C) endarteritis obliterans of the vasa vasorum
(D) severe atherosclerosis
(E) previous bacterial septicemia

4. The pathogenesis of the lesion depicted in this heart with attached aorta would most likely have come from a patient with

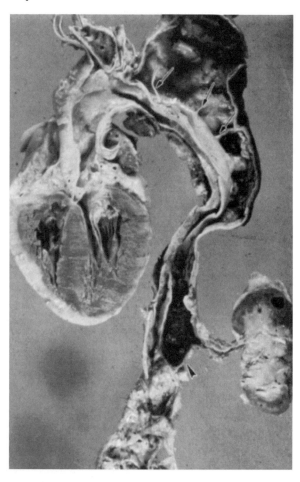

(A) a positive syphilis serology
(B) mitral valve prolapse
(C) a history of essential hypertension
(D) a previous history of intravenous drug abuse
(E) ischemic heart disease

5. The gross specimen represents the left side of the heart removed at autopsy from a 56-year-old man who presented with chest pain 4 days prior to his death. A microscopic slide illustrates the primary event responsible for his death. The patient most likely died of complications secondary to

(A) thrombosis of the left anterior descending coronary artery
(B) thrombosis of the right coronary artery
(C) acute rheumatic fever involving the mitral valve
(D) infective endocarditis involving the mitral valve
(E) mitral valve prolapse with rupture of the papillary muscle

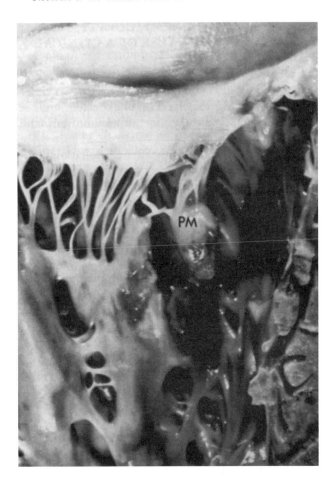

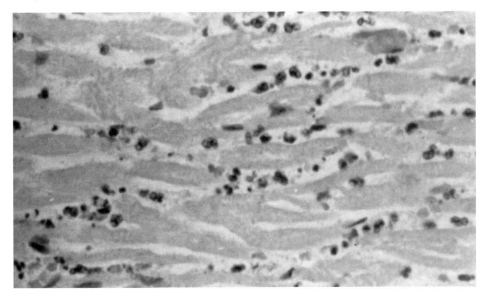

6. The autopsy finding depicted in this heart most likely came from a patient who had a positive

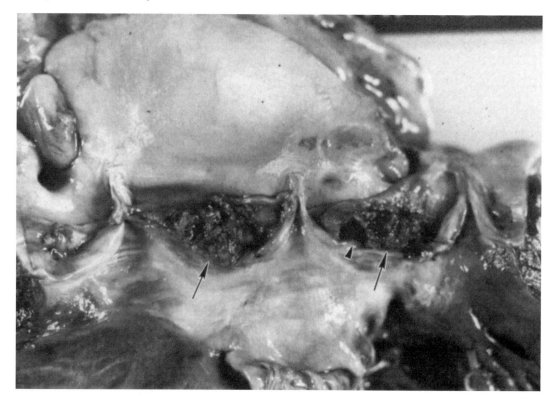

(A) blood culture that isolated *Staphylococcus aureus*
(B) blood culture that isolated *Streptococcus viridans*
(C) blood culture that isolated group A streptococci
(D) anti–streptolysin O (ASO) antibody titer
(E) antinuclear antibody test

7. The heart depicted in this photograph most likely came from a patient who had

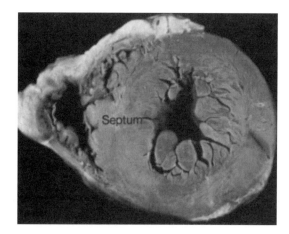

(A) syncopal episodes with exercise
(B) a long history of essential hypertension
(C) an aortic aneurysm with aortic valve regurgitation
(D) long-standing mitral stenosis
(E) thrombosis of the left anterior descending coronary artery

8. You would expect the patient with this finding in the aortic valve to have had

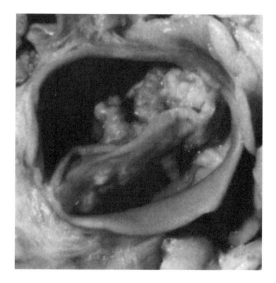

(A) a positive blood culture
(B) Aschoff bodies in the myocardium
(C) a systolic ejection murmur
(D) a wide pulse pressure
(E) a diastolic blowing murmur after S_2

9. Which of the following groupings of vascular disease have the same etiology (e.g., neoplastic, infectious, immune, congenital, malformation)?

   (A) Mycotic aneurysm and berry aneurysm
   (B) Polyarteritis nodosa and Henoch-Schönlein purpura
   (C) Kaposi's sarcoma and bacillary angiomatosis
   (D) Kawasaki's disease and cavernous hemangioma
   (E) Pyogenic granuloma and capillary hemangioma

10. Stasis dermatitis is best described as a/an

    (A) atopic dermatitis
    (B) complication of deep venous thrombosis
    (C) manifestation of arterial insufficiency
    (D) complication of superficial thrombophlebitis
    (E) immunocomplex vasculitis

11. A 68-year-old man has a long history of exertional angina and chronic obstructive pulmonary disease due to smoking. His father died of an acute myocardial infarction at 40 years of age. Recently, a diagnosis of type II diabetes was made for which he is presently on a low-fat, high-fiber diet to lose weight. His blood pressure has averaged 160/98 mm Hg on three separate office visits. A recent lipid profile revealed a serum cholesterol of 320 mg/dL, a serum triglyceride of 400 mg/dL, and an HDL of 20 mg/dL. How many major risk factors for coronary artery disease does the patient have at the present time?

    (A) 5
    (B) 6
    (C) 7
    (D) 8
    (E) 9

12. A 29-year-old man with substernal chest pain has an abnormal stress electrocardiogram with ST depression > 2 mm. His father died of an acute myocardial infarction at 30 years of age, and his 30-year-old brother just had an angioplasty performed for three-vessel coronary artery disease. On physical examination, the man has a nodular lesion on his Achilles tendon. You suspect the patient would have which of the following laboratory abnormalities?

    (A) LDL > 160 mg/dL
    (B) Turbid supranate on a standing chylomicron test
    (C) Turbid infranate on a standing chylomicron test
    (D) HDL > 60 mg/dL
    (E) Serum cholesterol < 200 mg/dL

13. Which of the following is least likely operative in the formation of a fibrous plaque in atherosclerosis?

    (A) Smooth muscle cells
    (B) Platelets
    (C) Macrophages
    (D) T cells
    (E) Natural killer cells

14. Which of the following signs or symptoms is common to both left and right heart failure?

    (A) Wet inspiratory rales
    (B) Exercise intolerance
    (C) Dependent pitting edema
    (D) Orthopnea
    (E) Jugular neck vein distention

15. High-output cardiac failure would most likely be associated with

    (A) hypertrophic cardiomyopathy
    (B) renovascular hypertension
    (C) severe anemia
    (D) hypothyroidism
    (E) drugs producing venodilation

16. A 29-year-old woman with hypertension most likely

    (A) has primary renal disease
    (B) has fibromuscular hyperplasia of the renal artery
    (C) has essential hypertension
    (D) has occlusive atherosclerosis of the proximal renal artery
    (E) is taking oral contraceptives

17. Study the following oxygen saturation values from a patient with congenital heart disease.

	Normal Value	Patient
Right atrium	75%	75%
Right ventricle	75%	75%
Pulmonary artery	75%	90%
Pulmonary vein	95%	95%
Left atrium	95%	95%
Left ventricle	95%	95%

    The patient most likely has
    (A) tetralogy of Fallot
    (B) a patent ductus arteriosus
    (C) a ventricular septal defect
    (D) an atrial septal defect
    (E) complete transposition of the great vessels

18. Study the following oxygen saturation values from a patient with congenital heart disease.

	Normal Value	Patient
Right atrium	75%	85%
Right ventricle	75%	85%
Pulmonary artery	75%	85%
Pulmonary vein	95%	95%
Left atrium	95%	95%
Left ventricle	95%	95%

    The patient most likely has
    (A) tetralogy of Fallot
    (B) a patent ductus arteriosus
    (C) a ventricular septal defect
    (D) an atrial septal defect
    (E) complete transposition of the great vessels

19. Diastolic hypertension, leg claudication, and rib notching on a chest x-ray is most likely associated with which one of the additional abnormalities listed below?

    (A) Congenital rubella
    (B) Down syndrome
    (C) Fetal alcohol syndrome
    (D) Bicuspid aortic valve
    (E) Maternal diabetes mellitus

20. A 62-year-old man with an acute myocardial infarction involving the anterior wall of the left ventricle experiences chest pain on day 4 in the coronary care unit. Bibasilar rales, neck vein distention, and a positive hepatojugular reflux are identified on examination. No murmurs are present. An S_3 is present. A CK-MB is elevated, and there is an LDH $\frac{1}{2}$ flip. Which of the following diagnostic groups best describes the events that have occurred in this patient?

    (A) Reinfarction with progression to both left and right heart failure
    (B) Reinfarction associated with rupture of the posteromedial papillary muscle leading to both left and right heart failure
    (C) Reinfarction associated with rupture of the free wall of the left ventricle
    (D) Right ventricular infarction with right heart failure
    (E) Right ventricular infarction with left and right heart failure

21. An elevated serum CK-MB and a normal LDH isoenzyme study would be expected in a patient with

    (A) an acute myocardial infarction with rupture of the left ventricle
    (B) an acute myocardial infarction and development of a ventricular aneurysm
    (C) an acute myocardial infarction associated with Dressler's syndrome
    (D) an acute myocardial infarction that is 8 hours old
    (E) unstable angina and substernal chest pain less than 24 hours old

22. Severe coronary artery atherosclerosis is most likely responsible for substernal chest pain in a patient with

    (A) Prinzmetal's angina
    (B) dissecting aortic aneurysm
    (C) aortic stenosis
    (D) mitral valve prolapse
    (E) exertional angina

23. Granulomatous inflammation often associated with necrotizing vasculitis involving the upper airways, lungs, and glomeruli is also likely to be associated with a positive

    (A) serum antinuclear antibody test
    (B) serum antineutrophil cytoplasmic antibody test (c-ANCA)
    (C) serum antineutrophil cytoplasmic antibody test (p-ANCA)
    (D) hepatitis B surface antigen
    (E) anticentromere antibody

24. The most common cause of both myocarditis and pericarditis is most likely a/an

    (A) neoplastic process
    (B) viral infection
    (C) metabolic abnormality
    (D) immunologic disease
    (E) drug

25. Pulsus paradoxus, Kussmaul's sign, and a pericardial knock in a patient recently transferred to the United States from a developing country most likely are due to

    (A) acute pericarditis
    (B) a pericardial effusion
    (C) constrictive pericarditis
    (D) metastatic disease to the pericardium
    (E) cor pulmonale

26. Which one of the following would improve the cardiac output in a patient with hypertrophic cardiomyopathy?

    (A) Calcium channel blockers
    (B) Digoxin
    (C) Valsalva's maneuver
    (D) Venodilator drugs
    (E) Standing up

Directions. (Items 27–30): Each set of matching questions in this section consists of a list of lettered options followed by several numbered items. For each numbered item, select the ONE option that is most closely associated with it. Each lettered option may be selected once, more than once, or not at all.

    (A) Cardiac myxoma
    (B) Libman-Sacks endocarditis
    (C) Cardiac amyloidosis
    (D) Congestive cardiomyopathy
    (E) Endocardial fibroelastosis
    (F) Nonbacterial thrombotic endocarditis
    (G) Rhabdomyoma
    (H) Carcinoid heart disease

27. Generalized cardiomegaly and heart failure in a 23-year-old woman who is 6 weeks post partum.

28. Constitutional signs and symptoms, embolization, and syncope.

29. Part of a paraneoplastic syndrome.

30. Right-sided valvular disease.

ANSWERS AND EXPLANATIONS

1. The answer is D: left ventricular hypertrophy. The left atrium is dilated and the mitral valve orifice has a fish-mouth appearance consistent with mitral stenosis. Chronic rheumatic heart disease is the most common cause of mitral stenosis. Stenosis is a problem with opening the valve, hence an increase in left atrial pres-

sure is required to open the nonpliable valve in diastole. Sudden opening of the valve under pressure produces an opening snap followed by a mid-diastolic rumble. Since less blood enters the left ventricle, there is no stimulus for left ventricular hypertrophy. The back pressure of blood into the left atrium leads to hypertrophy and dilatation of that chamber, which predisposes to thrombus formation and atrial fibrillation. Pulmonary venous pressures also increase, leading to pulmonary edema and congestion. Eventually, pulmonary hypertension develops with subsequent hypertrophy of the right ventricle. Aschoff bodies are pathognomonic lesions in the myocardium in rheumatic fever. They contain reactive histiocytes (Anichkov's myocytes) surrounded by fibrinoid necrosis. (Photograph reproduced, with permission, from F.J. Schoen and M. St. John Sutton. Contemporary issues in the pathology of valvular disease. Hum Pathol 18:568, 1987.)

2. The answer is B: mid-systolic ejection click. The posterior leaflets of the mitral valve are voluminous and balloon into the left atrium. These gross findings are consistent with mitral valve prolapse (MVP). MVP is usually asymptomatic. It is due to myxomatous degeneration of the valve leaflets, leading to redundancy of the tissue. During systole, the affected valves are ballooned into the left atrium by blood (like air catching beneath a parachute), resulting in a systolic ejection click. Usually this is followed by a systolic murmur. In some cases, there is an AD inheritance pattern. There is an increased incidence in Marfan's syndrome and Ehlers-Danlos syndrome. Symptomatic patients (e.g., with palpitations or chest pain) are usually given a calcium channel blocker. An opening snap and mid-diastolic rumble are heard in mitral stenosis. Pulsus paradoxus is a drop in pulse and blood pressure secondary to restricted filling of the right heart during inspiration (e.g., pericardial effusion). An accentuated A2 is noted in essential hypertension. (Photograph reproduced, with permission, from R. Virmani, J.B. Atkinson, and J.J. Fenoglio. *Cardiovascular Pathology.* Philadelphia, W.B. Saunders Co., 1991, p. 428.)

3. The answer is D: severe atherosclerosis. The photograph depicts an abdominal aortic aneurysm located below the renal arteries and above the bifurcation. These are most commonly due to atherosclerosis, which weakens the wall, thereby predisposing it to aneurysmal enlargement and the potential for rupture. There are no vasa vasorum below the renal arteries, hence the aorta lacks its own blood supply, which may explain why the abdominal aorta is the most common location for these aneurysms. Elastic tissue fragmentation is a feature of a dissecting aortic aneurysm. A primary defect in collagen synthesis is noted in Ehlers-Danlos syndrome, which also predisposes to dissecting aortic aneurysms. Endarteritis obliterans of the vasa vasorum is the pathogenesis of syphilitic aortic aneurysms involving the arch of the aorta. Previous bacterial septicemia may predispose to mycotic aneurysms. (Photograph reproduced, with permission, from R. Virmani, J.B. Atkinson, and J.J. Fenoglio. *Cardiovascular Pathology.* Philadelphia, W.B. Saunders Co., 1991, p. 13.)

4. The answer is C: a history of essential hypertension. The photograph exhibits a dissecting aortic aneurysm. The intimal tear is located at the arrow, which is just distal to the subclavian artery. The false lumen extends distally and ends just below the renal artery (type B dissection). The lumen is filled with thrombus and fibrous strands. Hypertension applies the shearing force necessary to tear the intima. Elastic tissue fragmentation and cystic medial necrosis in the media of the aorta weaken the wall, hence allowing a column of blood under increased pressure to dissect through the areas of weakness. Most dissections extend proximally (type A) and egress into the pericardial sac, producing

cardiac tamponade. Other associations include Marfan's syndrome, Ehlers-Danlos syndrome, pregnancy, trauma, and copper deficiency. Mitral valve prolapse, intravenous drug abuse, and ischemic heart disease are not associated with dissections. Syphilitic aortic aneurysms are localized to the arch of the aorta. (Photograph reproduced, with permission, from R. Virmani, J.B. Atkinson, and J.J. Fenoglio. *Cardiovascular Pathology.* Philadelphia, W.B. Saunders Co., 1991, p. 14.)

5. The answer is B: thrombosis of the right coronary artery. The gross specimen reveals a ruptured posteromedial (PM) papillary muscle and the microscopic slide exhibits classic coagulation necrosis with dissolution of the myocardial fibers. Vague outlines of cardiac muscle remain. Neutrophils infiltrate the necrotic tissue. The RCA supplies the posterior part of the heart and the papillary muscle. The heart is softest during the third to tenth day, hence the danger of rupture is greatest during this time frame. The LAD supplies the anterior portion of the left ventricle and the anterior two-thirds of the interventricular septum. No vegetations are noted on the mitral valve to implicate acute rheumatic fever or infective endocarditis. The valve leaflets are normal, hence excluding mitral valve prolapse. (Photographs reproduced, with permission, from R. Virmani, J.B. Atkinson, and J.J. Fenoglio. *Cardiovascular Pathology.* Philadelphia, W.B. Saunders Co., 1991, pp. 24 and 95.)

6. The answer is A: blood culture that isolated *Staphylococcus aureus*. Two of the three aortic valve cusps have bulky vegetations. The cusp with the arrowhead has a perforation. Since the valves are otherwise unremarkable, the organism must be virulent enough to colonize a previously undamaged valve, so *Staphylococcus aureus* is the best answer. *Streptococcus viridans* is not a virulent organism and requires a previously damaged valve for colonization. Although group A streptococci are virulent, they are not the most common cause of acute infective endocarditis. The vegetations are too bulky to represent the sterile vegetations of acute rheumatic fever, which is caused by group A streptococci (positive ASO titer). In rheumatic fever, immunologic damage to the valve provides a site for platelet thrombi, which represent the verrucal vegetations that develop along the lines of closure of the valve. In addition, valve perforation does not occur in rheumatic fever. Libman-Sacks endocarditis, which is associated with SLE (positive ANA), produces vegetations similar to those of rheumatic fever except that they are randomly scattered over the valve surfaces. (Photograph reproduced, with permission, from J.B. Atkinson and R. Virmani. Infective endocarditis: Changing trends and general approach for examination. Hum Pathol 18:603, 1987.)

7. The answer is B: a long history of essential hypertension. The heart exhibits concentric left ventricular hypertrophy (LVH), the most common cause of which is essential hypertension. Owing to an increase in peripheral resistance, the ventricle must contract against an increased afterload, leading to concentric LVH. Volume overload secondary to increased venous return to the right heart or valvular incompetence (e.g., aortic or mitral regurgitation) would produce hypertrophy and dilatation of the left ventricle. Syncopal episodes with exercise are noted with aortic stenosis, which does produce concentric LVH but it is not the most common cause of this type of hypertrophy. Mitral stenosis demonstrates reduced filling of the left ventricle, hence LVH is not a feature of the disease. There is no evidence of a pale infarction to implicate a thrombosis of the LAD.

(Photograph reproduced, with permission, from W.D. Edwards. Cardiomyopathies. Hum Pathol 18:625, 1987.)

8. The answer is C: a systolic ejection murmur. The aortic valve is bicuspid and stenotic secondary to dystrophic calcification of the cusps. Most cases of aortic stenosis are secondary to a congenital bicuspid valve. Since the aortic valve opens in systole, the murmur of aortic stenosis is in systole and of the ejection type (crescendo/decrescendo) with radiation into the carotids. The pulse pressure (difference between the systolic and diastolic pressure) is diminished, since the systolic pressure is reduced owing to the stenotic valve. Concentric LVH is present as well. Aschoff bodies are pathognomonic of rheumatic fever, which most commonly affects the mitral valve. A diastolic blowing murmur after S_2 characterizes aortic valve regurgitation, since regurgitation murmurs are valve closure abnormalities (the aortic valve closes in diastole). (Photograph reproduced, with permission, from F.J. Schoen and M. St. John Sutton. Contemporary issues in the pathology of valvular disease. Hum Pathol 18:568, 1987.)

9. The answer is B: polyarteritis nodosa and Henoch-Schönlein purpura. Both PAN and HSP have an immune etiology. In PAN, antinuclear cytoplasmic antibodies attack neutrophils and monocytes in muscular arteries, causing the release of free radicals and enzymes that damage the vessel wall, leading to focal aneurysmal dilatations ("nodosa"). Immunocomplex formation associated with hepatitis B surface antigenemia has been implicated as well. HSP produces a small-vessel vasculitis (leukocytoclastic venulitis) with IgA-C3 immunocomplexes producing vessel damage, rupture, and clinical findings of palpable purpura limited to the buttocks and lower extremities. Mycotic aneurysms are secondary to septicemia, whereas berry aneurysms are most commonly congenital. Kaposi's sarcoma is a malignancy of endothelial cells (the most common cancer in AIDS), while bacillary angiomatosis is an infectious disease caused by *Bartonella (Rochalimaea) henselae* that produces gross vascular lesions resembling those seen in Kaposi's sarcoma. Kawasaki's disease is an acute febrile disease in childhood that is associated with a coronary artery vasculitis (probably immune-mediated), whereas a cavernous hemangioma is a neoplasm of vessels (the most common benign tumor in the liver, placenta, and spleen). A capillary hemangioma is a neoplasm (possible hamartoma) of capillary channels that is raised and regresses over time ("strawberry hemangioma" in a newborn). Pyogenic granulomas are reactive tumor-like growths that develop after trauma. They bleed very easily and are sometimes noted on the gingiva in pregnancy ("pregnancy tumor").

10. The answer is B: complication of deep venous thrombosis. Thrombosis of the deep saphenous vein in the lower extremity causes a backup of venous blood into the veins around the ankle, leading to swelling, hemorrhage with hemosiderin deposition in the skin, ulceration, and varicosities in the superficial saphenous vein. The skin lesion just described is referred to as stasis dermatitis. Atopic dermatitis is a manifestation of a type I IgE-mediated hypersensitivity reaction. Arterial insufficiency in the peripheral vessels produces gangrene of the digits. Superficial thrombophlebitis develops in areas of thrombosis of the superficial saphenous veins or in varicosities. It is not associated with stasis dermatitis. Stasis dermatitis is not an immunocomplex vasculitis, although the lower extremity is a common site for small-vessel vasculitis (e.g., rheumatoid vasculitis).

11. The answer is C: 7. The patient is a male over 45 years of age (1 risk factor) who is a smoker (1 risk factor) and has diabetes mellitus (1 risk factor) and essential hypertension (1 risk factor). His father died of an AMI before 55 years of age (1 risk factor). His lipid profile reveals a calculated LDL of 220 mg/dL (calculated LDL = cholesterol [320 mg/dL] − HDL [20 mg/dL] − triglyceride [400 mg/dL/5] = 220 mg/dL; ≥ 160 mg/dL is a major risk factor). The HDL is < 35 mg/dL (1 risk factor).

12. The answer is A: LDL > 160 mg/dL. The young man has familial hypercholesterolemia (type II hyperlipoproteinemia), which has an AD inheritance pattern. The Achilles tendon xanthoma is pathognomonic for the disease. The family history of premature coronary artery disease is also suggestive of a genetic disorder. Owing to a defect in the LDL receptor, the LDL fraction is elevated in these patients. The HDL would likely be < 35 mg/dL, the serum cholesterol would likely be > 240 mg/dL, and the standing chylomicron test would likely be normal, since an increase in cholesterol does not produce turbidity in plasma. Presence of a supranate is secondary to chylomicrons (diet-derived triglyceride), whereas a turbid infranate indicates an increase in VLDL (liver derived triglyceride).

13. The answer is E: natural killer cells. Natural killer cells, or large granular lymphocytes, are neither B nor T cells. They are important in antibody-dependent cytotoxicity reactions (type II hypersensitivity), graft-versus-host reactions, and the elimination of virally infected and neoplastic cells. They serve no function in the formation of fibrous plaques (late manifestation of atherosclerosis). Macrophages and smooth muscle cells imbibe LDL and become the foam cells of a fatty streak, the early lesion of atherosclerosis. Platelets contribute growth factors that increase smooth muscle cell proliferation in the vessel. T cells release various cytokines that contribute to atherosclerosis.

14. The answer is B: exercise intolerance. Left heart failure (LHF) is characterized by symptoms (what the patient complains about), while right heart failure (RHF) is associated with signs (what the physician discovers on physical examination). LHF is associated with dyspnea (pulmonary congestion), pillow orthopnea (dyspnea when reclining owing to increased return of blood to the heart), paroxysmal nocturnal dyspnea (similar to orthopnea except the patient gasps for breath), and nocturia (increased venous return at night "normalizes" the glomerular filtration rate, hence a greater urine flow). RHF is characterized by signs of systemic venous congestion consisting of neck vein distention, hepatomegaly ("nutmeg" liver), splenomegaly, and dependent pitting edema. Both LHF and RHF demonstrate a reduced cardiac output, hence both are associated with exercise intolerance due to tissue hypoxia.

15. The answer is C: severe anemia. High-output failure (normal to increased cardiac output) may occur when there is an increase in blood volume (e.g., excess infusion of isotonic saline), an increase in positive inotropism (e.g., hyperthyroidism), decreased blood viscosity (e.g., anemia), or vasodilatation of arterioles, which increases venous return to the heart. According to Poiseuille's equation, the total peripheral resistance in arterioles (R) = 8 n l / π r^4, where R = resistance, n = viscosity of blood (decreased in anemia), l = the length of the vessel, and r^4 = the radius of the vessel

to the fourth power. Hence, a decrease in viscosity (anemia) and vasodilatation (e.g., endotoxemia, thiamine deficiency) reduces resistance, increasing venous return to the heart. Increased venous return to the heart also occurs with an AV fistula, which shunts blood directly from arterioles to venules. Hypertrophic cardiomyopathy reduces the cardiac output, renovascular hypertension (renal artery stenosis secondary to atherosclerosis or fibromuscular hyperplasia) increases peripheral resistance, hypothyroidism increases peripheral resistance, and venodilation reduces venous return to the heart.

16. The answer is E: is currently taking oral contraceptives. Estrogen in oral contraceptives increases liver synthesis of angiotensinogen, hence increasing levels of aldosterone (which increases plasma volume) and angiotensin II (a peripheral arteriole vasoconstrictor), both of which contribute to hypertension. Primary renal disease is the most common cause of hypertension in children. Fibromuscular hyperplasia of the renal artery is a cause of renovascular hypertension in young women, but it is not more common than oral contraceptive use as a cause of hypertension. Essential hypertension would be unusual in a young woman. Occlusive atherosclerosis of the proximal renal artery is the overall most common cause of secondary hypertension. It produces renovascular hypertension by activation of the renin-angiotensin-aldosterone system. It is more likely to occur in elderly men than in young women.

17. The answer is B: a patent ductus arteriosus. Note that there is a step-up in oxygen saturation (SaO_2) in the pulmonary artery owing to a left-to-right shunt from the aorta through the patent ductus into the pulmonary artery. In tetralogy of Fallot, there would be a drop in SaO_2 in the left ventricle and aorta owing to subpulmonic pulmonary stenosis, leading to RVH and shunting of unoxygenated blood from the right ventricle to the left ventricle through a VSD. In a VSD, there would be a step-up of SaO_2 in the right ventricle and pulmonary artery owing to a left-to-right shunt. In an ASD, there would be a step-up of SaO_2 in the right atrium, right ventricle, and pulmonary artery owing to a left-to-right shunt through a patent foramen ovale. In complete transposition of the great vessels, there is a step-up of SaO_2 in the right atrium and right ventricle from a left-to-right shunt through an ASD (the pulmonary vein empties oxygenated blood into the left atrium). In the left ventricle, there is a slight step-down in SaO_2 owing to a right-to-left shunt through a VSD. The pulmonary artery has a slight step-up in SaO_2, since it normally contains venous blood but now contains mixed venous and arterial blood from the left ventricle. The aorta has a step-down in SaO_2, since it is draining the right ventricle and does not have the usual full complement of oxygenated blood returning from the lungs.

18. The answer is D: an atrial septal defect. Note the step-up in the SaO_2 in the right atrium, right ventricle, and pulmonary artery owing to the left-to-right shunt through a patent foramen ovale. Refer to the discussion in question 17 for explanations of the other congenital heart disease findings.

19. The answer is D: bicuspid aortic valve. The presence of diastolic hypertension, leg claudication, and rib notching on a chest x-ray is consistent with an adult type of coarctation of the aorta, which has an increased incidence of bicuspid aortic valves. Congenital rubella is associated with a patent ductus arteriosus, Down syndrome with combined atrial and ventricular septal defects (endocardial cushion defect), fetal alcohol syndrome with atrial septal defects, and maternal diabetes mellitus with transposition of the great vessels.

20. The answer is A: reinfarction with progression into both left and right heart failure. By definition, the patient has reinfarction because of the presence of CK-MB after 3 days, when it normally disappears. Since no murmurs are present and the anterior wall is infarcted, indicating a thrombosis of the LAD coronary artery, a rupture of the posteromedial papillary muscle is unlikely (thrombosis of the RCA and mitral regurgitation would be present). Since heart sounds are audible, a rupture of the free wall of the left ventricle is unlikely, because cardiac tamponade would muffle heart sounds. A right ventricular infarct is excluded, since the RCA supplies the right ventricle and the patient has evidence of left heart failure (bibasilar rales and an S_3), which should not be present in a right ventricular infarct. Neck vein distention and a positive hepatojugular reflux (pressing the congested liver refluxes blood back to the jugular veins) indicate right heart failure. An LDH $\frac{1}{2}$ flip would be expected on day 4 and does not contribute to the diagnosis.

21. The answer is D: an acute myocardial infarction that is 8 hours old. Since serum CK-MB first appears in 4–8 hours, peaks in 24 hours, and returns to normal in 1.5–3 days and the LDH $\frac{1}{2}$ flip begins to increase in 10 hours, peaks in 48–72 hours, and returns to normal in 7–10 days, the most likely explanation is a patient with an AMI of 8 hours' duration. Ruptures in the heart after an AMI usually occur between days 3 and 10, when CK-MB has disappeared and an LDH $\frac{1}{2}$ flip is present. Ventricular aneurysms begin to develop later in the week and would not be expected during the time when CK-MB is present. Dressler's syndrome, or autoimmune pericarditis, first manifests a few weeks after an AMI. Unstable angina is not usually associated with elevation of CK-MB.

22. The answer is E: exertional angina. This variant of angina is most commonly related to severe occlusive atherosclerosis of the coronary arteries. Prinzmetal's angina is due to vasospasm of the coronary arteries secondary to the release of thromboxane A_2 from small platelet thrombi. Dissecting aortic aneurysms produce substernal chest pain owing to the dissection of blood through the weakened vessel wall. Aortic stenosis produces chest pain on exertion as a result of an inadequate supply of oxygen to the hypertrophied myocardium. Mitral valve prolapse produces chest pain owing to arrhythmias and/or mitral valve regurgitation.

23. The answer is B: serum antineutrophil cytoplasmic antibody test (c-ANCA). Granulomatous inflammation often associated with necrotizing vasculitis involving the upper airways, lungs, and glomeruli is characteristic of Wegener's granulomatosis (WG). The serum antineutrophil cytoplasmic antibody test (c-ANCA) is positive in most cases and an excellent index of disease severity. The serum antinuclear antibody test in WG is negative, since it is not an autoimmune disease. The serum antineutrophil cytoplasmic antibody test (p-ANCA) is positive in polyarteritis nodosa (PAN) and microscopic polyarteritis. PAN also has a high incidence of hepatitis B surface antigenemia. The anticentromere antibody is diagnostic of the CREST syndrome, which is a limited variant of progressive systemic sclerosis. (CREST = *c*alcinosis of the digits, *R*aynaud's phenomenon, *e*soph-

ageal motility disorder, *s*clerodactyly, and *t*elangiectasia.)

24. The answer is B: viral infection. Coxsackie B viruses are the most common cause of myocarditis and pericarditis. Metastasis to the pericardium commonly produces a hemorrhagic pericardial effusion. Uremia is associated with a fibrinous pericarditis. SLE and Dressler's syndrome are associated with fibrinous pericarditis. Drugs are more likely to produce myocarditis.

25. The answer is C: constrictive pericarditis. The patient most likely has constrictive pericarditis secondary to tuberculosis. Constrictive pericarditis occurs when the visceral or parietal pericardium becomes noncompliant owing to fibrosis and calcification. Ventricular filling is normal in early diastole but is abruptly reduced later in diastole when the dilated ventricle reaches the confines of the thickened pericardial shell (the cause of a pericardial knock). The mean pressures in the chambers of the heart, pulmonic veins, and systemic veins are all equally elevated. The return of venous blood to the right heart is also compromised, resulting in pulsus paradoxus and Kussmaul's sign. Acute pericarditis without an effusion would not restrict blood entering the right heart and produce Kussmaul's sign (neck vein distention on inspiration) and pulsus paradoxus (drop in pulse amplitude and blood pressure on inspiration). A pericardial effusion would not be associated with a knock, since fluid is between the heart and the thickened pericardium. Metastatic disease to the pericardium could produce a constrictive pericarditis, but the latter disease is most commonly caused by TB, particularly in developing countries. Cor pulmonale refers to pulmonary hypertension associated with right ventricular hypertrophy.

26. The answer is A: calcium channel blockers. The pathophysiology of outflow obstruction in hypertrophic cardiomyopathy (idiopathic hypertrophic subaortic stenosis) relates to a combination of asymmetric hypertrophy of the septum plus apposition of the anterior leaflet of the mitral valve drawn against the septum during systole. Increasing preload in the ventricle by decreasing inotropism (e.g., with β-blockers or calcium channel blockers) and/or increasing venous return of blood to the right heart (e.g., by squatting or lying down) results in clinical improvement. Reducing preload in the ventricle (e.g., by Valsalva's maneuver, venodilators, positive inotropic agents) worsens the clinical signs and symptoms.

27. The answer is D: congestive cardiomyopathy. Generalized cardiomegaly and heart failure in a 23-year-old woman who is 6 weeks post partum is characteristic of congestive cardiomyopathy. Both the left and right heart are usually dilated, hence both left and right heart failure are commonly present. Other causes include previous myocarditis, alcoholism, and drug use (e.g., doxorubicin).

28. The answer is A: cardiac myxoma. Constitutional signs and symptoms (fever, weight loss), embolization, and syncope characterize cardiac myxomas, which are the most common primary tumor of the heart. They are derived from mesenchyme and are almost exclusively located in the left atrium (~75%). They restrict blood flow into the left ventricle by dropping on top of the valve orifice. They frequently embolize to the brain.

29. The answer is F: nonbacterial thrombotic endocarditis. Nonbacterial thrombotic endocarditis (marantic vegetations) demonstrate bulky vegetations on the mitral valve that are sterile. They may develop as part of a paraneoplastic syndrome in malignancies associated with a hypercoagulable state, such as mucinous carcinoma of the colon, pancreas, or lungs. Embolization is commonly encountered.

30. The answer is H: carcinoid heart disease. Carcinoid heart disease is associated with the carcinoid syndrome, which consists of a triad of cutaneous flushing, diarrhea, and valvular disease (tricuspid regurgitation and pulmonic stenosis).

CHAPTER ELEVEN

DISORDERS OF THE LUNG, MEDIASTINUM, AND PLEURA

SYNOPSIS

OBJECTIVES

1. To be familiar with the calculation of the alveolar-arterial (A-a) gradient and its use in the workup of respiratory failure.
2. To discuss common upper respiratory disorders.
3. To review disorders associated with atelectasis.
4. To be familiar with common locations in the lung associated with the aspiration of particulate matter.
5. To review diseases produced by common respiratory microbial pathogens.
6. To discuss vascular diseases in the lungs.
7. To understand the interstitial (restrictive) lung disorders.
8. To be familiar with obstructive lung disorders.
9. To discuss the natural history of lung cancer.
10. To review the mediastinal compartments and the most common diseases in each compartment.
11. To understand the pathogenesis of pleural effusions and pleural diseases.

Objective 1: To be familiar with the calculation of the alveolar-arterial (A-a) gradient and its use in the workup of respiratory failure.

I. Calculation of the alveolar-arterial (A-a) gradient
   A. **Hypoxemia** is a low partial pressure of oxygen dissolved in arterial blood (PaO_2).
   B. The partial pressure of *al*veolar oxygen (PAO_2) rarely matches the partial pressure of *ar*terial oxygen (PaO_2) owing to small ventilation/perfusion (V/Q) mismatches throughout the lungs.
   C. The difference between the PAO_2 and PaO_2 is called the **alveolar-arterial gradient** (A-a gradient, which normally is 5–15 mm Hg).
      1. A medically significant A-a gradient is $\geq$ 30 mm Hg.
      2. The PAO_2 is the difference between the amount of oxygen inspired, or PiO_2 (% O_2 × 713 mm Hg), and the amount exchanged in the lungs with CO_2 ($PaCO_2/0.8$); thus, $PAO_2 = PiO_2 - PaCO_2/0.8$.
      3. For example, a person breathing room air (21%

oxygen) who has a normal $PaCO_2$ (40 mm Hg) and a PaO_2 of 90 has an A-a gradient of 10 mm Hg: $PAO_2 = 0.21 (713) - 40/0.8 = 100$ mm Hg $- 90$ mm Hg $= 10$ mm Hg.
   D. An **abnormal A-a gradient** is always associated with hypoxemia and indicates an abnormality in the lungs or heart.
      1. In the lungs, the abnormality may involve one of the following disorders or combinations of these disorders:
         a. Ventilation (no ventilation [e.g., atelectasis] but perfusion produces an intrapulmonary shunt).
         b. Perfusion (ventilation but no perfusion produces an increase in dead space) as in a pulmonary embolus.
         c. Diffusion of gas at the alveolocapillary interface (e.g., interstitial fibrosis, pulmonary edema).
      2. In the heart, the abnormality is produced by right-to-left shunts (e.g., tetralogy of Fallot).

II. Respiratory failure
   A. Respiratory failure is any PaO_2 < 60 mm Hg (normal, 75–100 mm Hg).
   B. It may be due to respiratory acidosis or to any of the lung factors listed in ¶I.D.1 that prolong the A-a gradient.
   C. **Respiratory acidosis** may result from depression of the respiratory center (e.g., by barbiturates), chest bellows dysfunction (thoracic cage plus the muscles of respiration; e.g., paralysis of the diaphragm), or obstructive lung disease (e.g., COPD).
   D. In respiratory failure, the A-a gradient is normal if the hypoxemia relates to respiratory center depression or chest bellows dysfunction and prolonged if it is secondary to a ventilation, perfusion, or diffusion abnormalities.

Objective 2: To discuss common upper respiratory disorders.

III. Upper respiratory disorders
   A. **Choanal atresia** is a neonatal disease characterized by incomplete development of the nasal passages.

B. **Nasal polyps** are associated with allergic disease (most common), infection (inflammatory polyps), cystic fibrosis (15%), and triad asthma (aspirin ingestion, asthma, and nasal polyps).

C. **Sinusitis** is secondary to an accumulation of mucus in one or more of the paranasal sinuses (maxillary most often) owing to obstruction of drainage in the nasal cavity, most commonly by inflammation (e.g., allergic rhinitis).
   1. In **acute sinusitis**, there is facial pain, headache, fever, and postnasal discharge, often leading to a chronic cough.
   2. The most common organisms are *Streptococcus pneumoniae* and *Haemophilus influenzae*.

D. **Wegener's granulomatosis** is a necrotizing granulomatous vasculitis that involves the nasal cavity, sinuses, or both, in 90% of cases.

E. The most common **malignancy** of the **nasal cavities** and **paranasal sinuses** is **squamous cell carcinoma**.

F. **Adenocarcinoma** of the nasal cavity is associated with exposure to wood dust.

G. **Nasopharyngeal carcinoma** accounts for 85% of cancers arising in the nasopharynx.
   1. It is associated with Epstein-Barr virus and is commonly found in parts of Africa and southern China.
   2. It commonly metastasizes to cervical lymph nodes and may go undiagnosed without a biopsy of the nasopharynx.

H. **Acute epiglottitis**, most commonly due to *H. influenzae* type B, presents with high fever, drooling, inspiratory stridor, and severe dyspnea in children from 2 to 7 years of age.

I. **Laryngotracheobronchitis** (**croup**), due to the parainfluenza virus, most commonly occurs in children from 3 months to 5 years of age and presents with low-grade fever and inspiratory stridor.

J. **Diphtheria** is due to *Corynebacterium diphtheriae*, a gram-positive bacillus.
   1. The bacterium produces a toxin that inhibits ribosomal synthesis and impairs fatty acid oxidation in host cells; toxin damage to the heart is the leading cause of death.
   2. In the oropharynx and larynx, it produces an inflammatory gray-white pseudomembrane (toxin induced) that may obstruct breathing and produce dysphonia (speaking difficulties).
   3. Susceptibility to diphtheria can be determined by the Schick test.
   4. Erythromycin is the treatment of choice, and vaccination is the most important means of prevention.

K. **Squamous papillomas** of the vocal cord, secondary to human papillomavirus (HPV) types 6 and 11, may remit during puberty or, in some cases, progress to squamous cell carcinoma.

L. **Squamous cell carcinoma** of the **larynx** is associated with smoking, heavy alcohol consumption (additive effect with smoking), and asbestos exposure.
   1. Approximately 50% of tumors are supraglottic (epiglottis, false vocal cords, ventricle) and 35% are glottic (true vocal cords, ventricles) in their location.
   2. Hoarseness is the most common initial symptom, and death is usually due to direct extension.

Objective 3: To review disorders associated with atelectasis.

IV. Disorders associated with atelectasis
   A. Atelectasis is imperfect expansion of the lung or parts of the lung secondary to obstruction (most common), compression of lung tissue (e.g., tension pneumothorax), or loss of surfactant (respiratory distress syndrome).
      1. Grossly, the lung surface is depressed and has a bluish-gray appearance.
      2. Fever occurring within 24 to 48 hours of surgery is almost always due to atelectasis.
      3. Consequences of atelectasis include intrapulmonary shunting (no ventilation, only perfusion), hypoxemia, and a predisposition to bronchopneumonia.

   B. **Respiratory distress syndrome** (RDS) along with congenital defects is the most common cause of neonatal death.
      1. It is secondary to a decrease in pulmonary surfactant (lecithin, or phosphatidylcholine), which normally is synthesized by type II pneumocytes.
         a. Surfactant is measured in amniotic fluid and reported as a **lecithin/sphingomyelin ratio** (L/S ratio > 2 indicates adequate surfactant).
         b. Synthesis is enhanced by cortisol and thyroxine and inhibited by insulin.
         c. It reduces the alveolar surface tension during expiration, hence preventing alveolar collapse.
         d. Deficiency may be due to prematurity (reduced synthesis), delivery by cesarean section (lack of cortisol-induced stress associated with vaginal delivery), or maternal diabetes (inhibitory effect of fetal insulin on surfactant production in response to maternal hyperglycemia).
      2. Atelectasis results in massive intrapulmonary shunting as well as hypotension, respiratory acidosis, and hypoxemia, leading to reduced perfusion (acidosis- and hypoxemia-induced vasoconstriction).
      3. The lungs have a solid, red appearance, and histologic sections reveal diffuse atelectasis and protein-rich fluid lining the alveoli (hyaline membranes).
      4. Respiratory difficulties (tachypnea, grunting, cyanosis) begin at birth or within a few hours after birth.
      5. A chest x-ray reveals a "ground glass" appearance.
      6. Oxygen-related injury (free radical injury) may result in **retrolental fibroplasia** (now called the retinopathy of prematurity) and **bronchopulmonary dysplasia**.
      7. Other complications include intraventricular hemorrhage (due to CNS hypoxia), necrotizing enterocolitis (ischemic necrosis, bowel invasion by microbial pathogens), and patent ductus (due to persistent hypoxemia).
      8. Overall mortality is 20–30% in newborns of > 28 weeks' gestation.

   C. **Adult respiratory distress syndrome** (ARDs) is associated with diffuse alveolar damage (DAD) characterized by leaky pulmonary capillaries, hyaline membranes, atelectasis, and massive intrapulmonary shunts (most important defect).

1. Precipitating factors include gram-negative sepsis (most common), pulmonary infection, severe trauma, aspiration of gastric contents, burns, and DIC.
2. Neutrophils damage the pulmonary endothelium, resulting in release of inflammatory agents that produce pulmonary vasoconstriction, increased vessel permeability ("**leaky capillary syndrome**"), and hyaline membranes in the alveoli.
3. Damage to type II pneumocytes produces surfactant deficiency with subsequent widespread atelectasis and intrapulmonary shunting.
4. Lung compliance is decreased (stiff lungs on inspiration), and defects occur in ventilation, perfusion, and diffusion.
5. Patients present with rapid onset of dyspnea and respiratory failure.
6. ABGs exhibit severe hypoxemia, respiratory acidosis, and a markedly prolonged A-a gradient that does not improve with 100% oxygen (indicating an intrapulmonary shunt).
7. The chest x-ray reveals diffuse or patchy bilateral infiltrates with both an interstitial and an alveolar pattern.
8. Mortality exceeds 50%.
D. Pneumothorax is air in the pleural cavity that results in a rise in intrapleural pressure and subsequent collapse of the lung.
1. It may occur spontaneously (from idiopathic or underlying lung disease) or as a result of chest trauma (knife wound, subclavian line insertion).
2. The **idiopathic type** is due to rupture of localized subpleural bullae (> 1 cm) at the apex of the lung.
3. Patients present with sudden onset of a localized pleuritic chest pain (sharp stabbing pain), dyspnea, and ipsilateral hyperresonance (tympanitic percussion note), absent breath sounds, absent fremitus (no chest vibration when talking), and deviation of the trachea to the ipsilateral side.
4. In a **tension pneumothorax**, air continues to enter the pleural space from a tear in the pleura, which causes a contralateral shift in the mediastinal structures and trachea and compression atelectasis of the lung.

Objective 4: To be familiar with common locations in the lung associated with the aspiration of particulate matter.

V. Aspiration disorders
A. Aspiration of particles and their location in the lung depend on the position of the patient:
1. **Standing or sitting**, posterobasal segment of the right lower lobe.
2. **Lying down**, superior segment of the right lower lobe.
3. **Lying on the right side**, right middle lobe or the posterior segment of the right upper lobe.
4. **Lying on the left side**, lingula of the left lung.
B. **Aspiration of gastric contents**, a common cause of ARDs, produces damage to the lungs that is most dependent on the pH of the gastric acid (the lower the pH, the more severe the disease).
C. **Aspiration of lipids** (**exogenous lipid pneumonia**)

occurs primarily in the elderly with impaired swallowing (due to stroke) and evokes a granulomatous reaction, leading to fibrosis.

Objective 5: To review diseases produced by common respiratory microbial pathogens.

VI. Respiratory infections
A. **Community-acquired pneumonias** are subdivided into typical and atypical types (*Mycoplasma pneumoniae* [most common], *Chlamydia pneumoniae*, viruses).
1. **Typical pneumonias** present with sudden onset of fever, productive cough, and signs of consolidation in the lungs on physical examination (dull percussion note, increased tactile fremitus, crackles).
a. *Streptococcus pneumoniae* (gram-positive diplococcus) is the most common bacterial cause of community-acquired pneumonia.
b. *Klebsiella pneumoniae* (gram-negative rod with mucus) is commonly associated with alcoholism.
c. *Pseudomonas aeruginosa* and *Legionella pneumophila* are water-loving (spread via respirator or water cooler, respectively) gram-negative rods that produce pneumonia.
2. **Atypical pneumonias** present with an insidious onset, lowgrade fever, nonproductive cough, flu-like symptoms, and a chest x-ray with interstitial, patchy infiltrates.
a. **Respiratory syncytial virus** is the most common cause of pneumonia and bronchiolitis in infants and children.
b. **Influenzavirus** increases morbidity and mortality in the elderly owing to superimposed bacterial pneumonias (*S. aureus* most commonly).
B. **Nosocomial** (**hospital-acquired**) **pneumonias** are most commonly due to enteric gram-negative bacteria (e.g., *E. coli* and *P. aeruginosa*).
C. **Bacterial pneumonias** have lobar and bronchopneumonic types.
1. **Bronchopneumonia** first involves the bronchus and then spreads to the alveoli, where it produces raised areas of reddish-gray consolidation in the lung parenchyma.
2. **Lobar pneumonia** involves the entire lobe of a lung without bronchial involvement and, if left untreated, passes through the following stages:
a. **Congestion** (12–36 hours) correlates with the onset of the illness described for typical pneumonias.
b. **Red hepatization** (2–4 days) is marked by brick red lungs (vascular congestion) and a neutrophilic infiltrate (liquefactive necrosis).
c. **Gray hepatization** (4–8 days) is associated with numerous neutrophils.
d. **Resolution** (8–10 days) is characterized by macrophages and contracted clumps of digested debris called **Masson bodies**.
e. Lobar pneumonia resolves with less scar tissue than bronchopneumonia, which often heals with scar tissue formation.
3. **Laboratory abnormalities** in both types include an absolute neutrophilic leukocytosis with left

shift and a positive sputum Gram's stain (most important step in the initial workup).

4. **Complications** include lung abscess, empyema (pus in the pleural space), suppurative pericarditis, and septicemia.

D. **Tuberculosis** (TB), the most common cause of death due to infectious disease in the world, is contracted by droplet infection.

1. It has primary (which usually develops in children) and secondary (reactivation) types.

2. **Primary TB** initially locates in a subpleural location (**Ghon's focus** with caseation necrosis) in the upper part of the lower lobes or the lower part of the upper lobes and subsequently spreads to the hilar nodes (**Ghon's complex**).

   a. Organisms initially phagocytosed by alveolar macrophages are disseminated throughout the body (**preallergic lymphohematogenous spread**) without producing systemic disease.

   b. Most cases resolve once the immune system becomes activated and the organisms are destroyed by the macrophages in concert with CD4 T helper cells.

   c. Less commonly, primary disease may result in severe pneumonia or miliary spread limited to the lungs or throughout the body (CNS disease in particular).

3. Secondary, or reactivation, TB is usually reactivation of TB organisms from a previous primary infection in the lung or in one or more preallergic lymphohematogenous sites.

   a. Corticosteroids or immunosuppressants are often responsible for reactivation.

   b. Reactivation occurs in the oxygen-rich apex of the lungs, where it produces extensive destruction and cavity formation.

   c. Scar formation, calcification, bronchiectasis, aspergilloma (fungus ball), and scar cancer are potential complications.

   d. Possible outcomes of reactivation TB include miliary spread only in the lungs (bronchus invasion, invasion of the pulmonary artery or lymphatics) or miliary spread throughout the body (via entry into a pulmonary vein tributary).

E. **Systemic fungi** may involve the lungs.

1. *Candida albicans* (budding yeast and pseudohyphae) invades pulmonary vessels, leading to hemorrhagic infarcts.

2. *Coccidioides immitis* (spherules with endospores) is acquired by inhaling arthrospores in dust in the Southwest or San Joaquin Valley in California ("valley fever").

   a. It presents with flu-like symptoms and erythema nodosum (painful nodules on the lower legs).

   b. It most commonly produces a solitary granuloma (eggshell cavity) in the lower lobes.

3. *Cryptococcus neoformans* (budding yeast with narrow-based buds) is the most common fungal opportunistic infection in immunocompromised hosts.

   a. It may be contracted from living or working near pigeon excreta.

   b. It produces a granulomatous reaction if immunity is intact but no inflammatory reaction if the host is immunocompromised.

4. *Histoplasma capsulatum* (yeast in macrophages) is the most common systemic fungal infection and is most common in the Midwest.

   a. It is associated with exposure to bats (e.g., in caves) and birds (not pigeons).

   b. It simulates TB (primary and reactivation disease) and characteristically produces extensive dystrophic calcification in the granulomas.

5. *Blastomyces dermatitidis* (yeast with broad-based buds) is a male-dominant disease that primarily occurs in the Southeast and Midwest and involves the skin and/or lungs.

6. *Aspergillus fumigatus* (fruiting body, narrow-angled, branching septate hyphae) may be associated with an aspergilloma (fungus ball that develops in a preexisting cavity in the lung), allergic bronchopulmonary disease (asthma), and a necrotizing bronchopneumonia with infarction (vessel invader).

7. *Absidia, Mucor, Rhizopus* species (wide-angled hyphae without septae) are vessel invaders (causing hemorrhagic infarction in the lungs) that produce lung disease in patients who have diabetes or are immunosuppressed.

8. *Pneumocystis carinii* (reclassified as a fungus) is the most common initial infection in AIDS.

   a. Cysts attach to type I pneumocytes and are well visualized with silver and Giemsa's stains but not with Gram's stain.

   b. It produces a foamy alveolar infiltrate.

   c. It occurs when the CD4 T helper count is < 200 cells/μL.

   d. It produces diffuse alveolar and interstitial infiltrates on a chest x-ray.

   e. Trimethoprim/sulfamethoxazole is the treatment of choice.

F. A pulmonary abscess is a local suppurative process that most commonly originates from aspiration of infected oropharyngeal material.

1. It may also occur as a complication of bronchopneumonia or lobar pneumonia, septic embolization, or infection behind a neoplastic process obstructing a bronchus.

2. The most commonly isolated organisms are aerobic and anaerobic bacteria (gram-positive and -negative organisms), *S. aureus*, and *K. pneumoniae*.

Objective 6: To discuss vascular diseases in the lungs.

VII. Vascular disorders

A. **Pulmonary emboli** (PE) most commonly originate (90%) from thromboemboli in the proximal deep saphenous veins of the thighs (iliac, femoral, popliteal) and pelvis.

1. **Predisposing factors** include the postpartum period, postsurgery period, trauma, immobilization (congestive heart failure), and hypercoagulability (e.g., from malignancy or oral contraceptive use).

2. **Saddle emboli** can block the main pulmonary artery or the bifurcation.

3. **Massive pulmonary embolization** (50–75% occlusion of the large pulmonary vessels) results in the sequence of acute right heart strain, right

heart failure, acute cor pulmonale, and sudden death.

4. **Medium-sized emboli** occlude peripheral vessels and initially produce perfusion defects followed in 48 hours by intrapulmonary shunting (atelectasis from a loss of surfactant).

5. **Infarction** (coagulation necrosis) occurs in only 10–15% of cases and mainly in the presence of preexisting lung disease.
   a. Infarctions are hemorrhagic and triangular shaped with the base located along the pleura (and commonly produce a hemorrhagic pleural effusion).
   b. Dyspnea is the most common symptom and tachypnea ($\geq$ 20/min) the most common sign.

6. **Laboratory test abnormalities** include hypoxemia ($PaO_2 < 80$ mm Hg), prolonged A-a gradient, respiratory alkalosis ($PaCO_2 < 33$ mm Hg), and an abnormal ECG with a right ventricular strain pattern ($S_1Q_3T_3$).

7. **Perfusion radionuclide scans** are the first step in the workup of a suspected PE, while pulmonary angiography is the gold standard test in equivocal cases.

B. **Pulmonary hypertension** (PH) arises from intimal fibrosis and medial smooth muscle hypertrophy as a primary or secondary process.
1. The pathophysiology involves the following:
   a. Reduction in cross-sectional area of the PA bed (e.g., COPD, recurrent embolization).
   b. Increased pulmonary venous pressure (e.g., mitral stenosis).
   c. Increased PA flow (e.g., left-to-right shunt [VSD]).
   d. Increased blood viscosity (e.g., polycythemia).
2. **Primary PH** is most frequently noted in young to middle-aged women, who present with progressive dyspnea, fatigue, and chest pain.
3. The pulmonary arteries often exhibit atherosclerosis (increased PA pressure).
4. Patients present with right heart failure, right ventricular hypertrophy (RVH), and accentuation of P_2.
5. **Cor pulmonale** is RVH originating from PH that has developed from either primary pulmonary vascular disease or primary lung disease (it does not include PH secondary to cardiovascular disease).

C. **Wegener's granulomatosis** is a necrotizing granulomatous vasculitis involving the upper respiratory tract (nose, paranasal sinuses, and nasopharynx), lungs, and kidneys.

Objective 7: To understand the interstitial (restrictive) lung disorders.

VIII. Interstitial (restrictive) lung disorders
A. Interstitial lung diseases (ILDs) produce diffuse interstitial fibrosis leading to reduced lung compliance (decreased expansion of the lungs on inspiration), increased elasticity (increased lung recoil on expiration), and diffusion defects.
B. There is widespread disruption of the alveolar walls, leading to a functional loss in alveolar capillary units and an increase in interstitial fibrosis as a reaction to injury.

C. The arterial blood gases (ABGs) exhibit hypoxemia with exercise, respiratory alkalosis ($PaCO_2 < 33$ mm Hg), and an increase in the A-a gradient.
D. The pulmonary function tests (PFTs) reveal the following:
1. Generalized diminution of all the lung volumes and capacities (e.g., total lung capacity [TLC], tidal volume [TV]).
2. Decreased forced expiratory volume 1 second (FEV_{1sec}), i.e., how much air is expelled from the lungs in 1 second after a maximal inspiration (normal, 4 L).
3. Decreased forced vital capacity (FVC), i.e., total amount of air expelled after a maximal inspiration (normal, 5 L).
4. Increased FEV_{1sec}/FVC ratio (normal, 0.80; in ILDs, it is often 1.0), since the increased elasticity expels all available air in 1 second, hence the FEV_{1sec} and FVC are frequently equal.
5. Decreased diffusion capacity with carbon monoxide (DL_{CO}) owing to increased fibrosis at the alveolar-arterial interface.

E. **Pneumoconiosis**, the most common cause of ILD, refers to a group of occupational diseases characterized by inhalation of dust particles that may predispose to pulmonary damage.
1. **Coal workers' pneumoconiosis** (CWP), or **black lung disease**, varies in severity from deposition of coal dust (anthracotic pigment) in the parenchyma (**simple CWP**) to a crippling lung disease called **progressive massive fibrosis** (PMF).
   a. Alveolar macrophages that have phagocytosed coal dust release interleukin-1 (IL-1), which stimulates fibrogenesis.
   b. Nodular masses in the lungs are composed of collagen intermixed with anthracotic pigment.
   c. CWP plus rheumatoid lung disease is called **Caplan's syndrome**.
   d. There is an increased incidence of TB but not of cancer.
2. **Silicosis** is due to inhalation of crystalline silicon dioxide (found in quartz).
   a. Nodules in the lungs are composed of concentric areas of fibrosis entrapping polarizable silica particles.
   b. There is an increased incidence of TB but not of cancer.
3. **Asbestosis** is due to inhalation of asbestos fibers, leading to fibrosis of the pulmonary parenchyma.
   a. Asbestos used to be found in pipe fittings, brake linings in vehicles, cement pipes, and insulation material (still a risk during demolition of old buildings).
   b. It is a crystalline silicate with two subfamilies: serpentines (chrysotile, a curly fiber) and amphiboles (crocidolite, thin and needle-like).
   c. **Asbestos bodies** are composed of iron (**ferruginous bodies**) and protein surrounding a core of asbestos.
   d. Asbestos exposure plus smoking predisposes to primary lung cancer (most common cancer in asbestosis), while asbestos without smoking increases the risk for mesothelioma.
4. Exposure to **beryllium** may produce acute exu-

dative pneumonitis, chronic noncaseating granulomatous disease, and an increased incidence
of lung cancer.
F. The **hypersensitivity pneumonitides** produce an
exudative lung reaction (immunocomplex disease
initially and granulomatous disease later) upon re-
petitive exposure to a specific external antigen.
1. **Farmer's lung** is associated with exposure to
moldy hay containing thermophilic actinomycetes (external antigen).
2. **Silo filler's disease** may occur after inhalation
of nitrous oxide fumes originating from fer-
menting corn.
3. **Bagassosis** is lung disease that develops after
repeated exposure to moldy sugar cane.
4. **Byssinosis** is associated with exposure to cotton, hemp, or linen.
G. **Noninfectious interstitial pneumonias** (e.g., usual,
desquamative, or lymphoid interstitial pneumonitis
types) start out as an alveolitis and progress to a
fibrosing alveolitis, resulting in a honeycomb pattern in lung tissue (**Hamman-Rich lung**).
H. **Sarcoidosis** (second most common ILD) is a
multisystem granulomatous (noncaseating) disease
of unknown etiology that frequents adults (usually
African Americans) from 20 to 40 years of age.
1. It primarily targets the lungs (reticulonodular
densities and hilar adenopathy) and face (uveal
tract [uveitis], salivary glands).
2. Laboratory abnormalities include an increase in
angiotensin-converting enzyme, hypercalcemia,
polyclonal gammopathy, and anergy to skin testing (low CD4 T helper cell count).
I. **Drugs** that commonly produce ILD include nitrofu-
rantoin, amiodarone, bleomycin, busulfan, and cyclophosphamide.
J. Most **collagen vascular diseases** (RA, SLE, PSS,
Sjögren's syndrome) produce lung disease.
K. **Goodpasture's syndrome** is a male-predominant
disease initially presenting with hemoptysis and
then acute glomerulonephritis owing to the presence of anti–basement membrane antibodies directed against pulmonary and glomerular capillaries.

Objective 8: To be familiar with obstructive lung disorders.

IX. Obstructive lung disorders
A. **Chronic obstructive lung disease** (COPD) is progressive airway obstruction due to destruction of
the respiratory unit (respiratory bronchioles, alveolar ducts, alveoli) or damage to the conducting
pathways.
B. Cigarette smoking is the main cause of COPD,
which is usually either chronic bronchitis (CB) or
emphysema.
C. Other obstructive diseases include bronchial
asthma, bronchiectasis, and cystic fibrosis.
D. COPD is characterized by an increase in lung compliance and a decrease in lung elasticity.
1. PFTs exhibit an increase in TLC and residual
volume (air left in the lung after maximal expiration) and a decrease in vital capacity and tidal
volume.
2. FEV_{1sec}, FVC, and FEV_{1sec}/FVC ratio are all decreased.

3. Hypoxemia and a prolonged A-a gradient are
invariably present.
4. Chest x-ray reveals an increased anteroposterior
diameter and flattening of the diaphragms.
E. **CB** is a clinical diagnosis defined as excessive sputum production for at least 3 months for 2 consecu-
tive years.
1. There is increased mucous gland hyperplasia,
goblet cell hyperplasia, and inflammation in the
terminal (nonrespiratory) bronchioles (most
significant obstructive component).
2. It is associated with marked ventilation/perfu-
sion defects, retention of CO_2 (respiratory acidosis), hypoxemia, and cyanosis ("blue bloater").
F. **Emphysema** is a histologic diagnosis defined as
permanent enlargement of air spaces of the respiratory unit with irreversible damage to their elastic
tissue support due to neutrophil-derived elastase
and inactivation of α_1-antitrypsin (AAT) by chemicals in smoke.
1. In **centrilobular emphysema** (seen in smokers
and CWP), the structural support in the respiratory bronchiole is primarily destroyed (upper
lobe disease).
2. **Panacinar emphysema** (seen in smokers and in
AAT deficiency) characteristically is associated
with the entire respiratory unit (lower lobe disease).
3. Ventilation/perfusion defects are equally
matched (both respiratory unit and capillaries
are destroyed), hypoxemia is not as severe as
in CB, and the PCO_2 is either normal or low
(respiratory alkalosis ensues and patients are
termed "pink puffers").
G. **Bronchial asthma** is an episodic respiratory disease characterized by reversible small airway obstruction (in terminal bronchioles) manifested by
inspiratory and expiratory wheezing.
1. Inflammation secondary to the release of chemical mediators (e.g., histamine; leukotrienes C_4,
D_4, and E_4) is the primary cause of bronchocon-
striction.
2. Most cases are secondary to type I IgE-mediated
hypersensitivity disease.
H. **Bronchiectasis** is a congenital (e.g., immotile cilia
syndrome) or acquired (e.g., cystic fibrosis, TB)
lung disease associated with irreversible dilatation
of the bronchi owing to weakening of the support-
ive structures by obstruction and inflammation.
1. It is characterized by coughing up copious foul-
smelling sputum in the morning.
2. Dilated bronchi extend to the periphery of the
lung.
3. CF is the most common cause in the United
States and TB worldwide.
I. The pulmonary system is most affected in **cystic
fibrosis**, and progressive respiratory failure is the
most common cause of death.

Objective 9: To discuss the natural history of lung cancer.

X. Lung cancer
A. In both men and women, lung cancer is the most
common cause of cancer death and the second
most common cancer.
B. **Predisposing factors** for primary lung cancer in-

clude cigarette smoking (~90% of cases), asbestosis (enhanced risk with smoking), chromates, arsenic, radon gas (from uranium), and beryllium.

C. Cough is the most common presenting symptom.

D. There are **small-cell** and **non–small-cell types**, the latter including adenocarcinoma (most common overall lung cancer), squamous cell carcinoma, and large-cell undifferentiated carcinoma.

1. **Squamous cell carcinoma** (SCC) and **small-cell carcinoma** are centrally located tumors that are strongly associated with smoking; SCC may secrete a parathormone-like peptide (causing hypercalcemia).

2. **Adenocarcinomas** are more peripherally located and are the most common cancer in nonsmokers.

3. **Bronchioloalveolar carcinomas** derive from Clara cells (nonciliated epithelium) and characteristically spread along the walls of the terminal and respiratory bronchioles, alveolar ducts, and alveoli in a hobnail (picket fence) fashion.

4. **Small-cell**, or **oat cell**, **carcinomas** are of neural crest origin (they contain dense-core neurosecretory granules) and can ectopically produce ACTH (causing Cushing's syndrome) and ADH (causing inappropriate ADH syndrome).

E. Common sites of distant metastasis of lung cancers are the adrenals (50%), liver (30%), brain (20%), and bone.

F. **Pancoast's syndrome** is invasion of the brachial plexus (usually T1–T2) and the cervical sympathetic chain (**Horner's syndrome**) by a primary lung cancer.

G. **Bronchial carcinoid tumors** are low-grade malignant neuroendocrine tumors with no relationship to smoking.

H. **Metastatic disease** to the lung is the most common lung cancer (breast cancer is the leading cause).

I. Greater than 75% of **solitary coin lesions** are benign (usually granulomas), while < 25% are malignant (primary SCC or adenocarcinoma).

Objective 10: To review the mediastinal compartments and the most common diseases in each compartment.

XI. Mediastinum disorders

A. The most common mediastinal mass in older patients is metastatic disease originating in the lung.

B. In younger patients, most mediastinal masses are primary diseases originating in the mediastinum.

C. Most mediastinal masses are located in the anterior compartment, followed by the posterior and middle mediastinum.

D. The most common primary mediastinal masses, in descending order, are neurogenic tumors (posterior), thymomas (anterior), primary cysts (middle), and malignant lymphomas (anterior).

E. **Thymomas** may be associated with myasthenia gravis and pure RBC aplasia.

Objective 11: To understand the pathogenesis of pleural effusions and pleural diseases.

XII. Pleural disorders

A. A **pleural exudate** is defined by any one of the following criteria: pleural fluid (PF) protein/serum protein ratio > 0.5, PF LDH/serum LDH ratio > 0.6, or a PF LDH greater than two-thirds of the upper limit of serum LDH.

1. Causes of **PF exudates** include pneumonia, infarction, and lymphatic obstruction by tumor (primary lung cancer most commonly).

2. TB causes a lymphocyte-predominant type of exudate.

3. Rheumatoid arthritis is associated with a pseudochylous effusion (increased cholesterol and neutrophils) and low PF glucose values.

B. **PF transudates** have smaller values than those given above and represent an alteration in Starling's forces (increased hydrostatic pressure or decreased oncotic pressure).

C. **Mesotheliomas** are primary malignant tumors of the pleura that, in the majority of cases, are associated with asbestos exposure (usually crocidolite fibers).

QUESTIONS

DIRECTIONS. (Items 1–17): Each of the numbered items or incomplete statements in this section is followed by answers or by completions of the statement. Select the ONE lettered answer or completion that is BEST in each case. Correct answers and explanations are given at the end of the chapter.

1. The photograph is of an H and E–stained bronchoscopy biopsy specimen taken from the right main stem bronchus of a 62-year-old man with chronic cough, weight loss, and a 40-year history of cigarette smoking. Which of the following best characterizes this patient's lung disease?

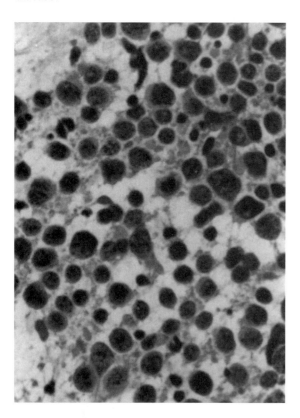

(A) Tumor derived from Clara cells
(B) Neurosecretory tumor
(C) Hamartoma
(D) Metastatic disease
(E) Tumor associated with keratin production

2. The photograph exhibits silver stain–positive structures that are located within a foamy intraalveolar exudate. The biopsy was performed on a 32-year-old male who presented with fever, weight loss, dyspnea, generalized lymphadenopathy, and a diffuse, bilateral infiltrate in the lungs on chest x-ray. Which of the following tests would be most useful in confirming the pathogenesis of this patient's disease?

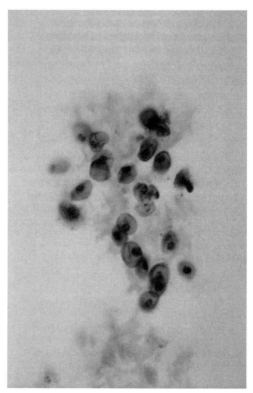

(A) Serologic tests for histoplasmosis
(B) Culture to rule out *Cryptococcus neoformans*
(C) PPD skin test
(D) HIV antibody test
(E) Lymph node biopsy

3. This is a Papanicolaou-stained slide ($\times 650$) of sediment from a bronchoalveolar lavage performed on a 60-year-old retired enlisted man in the Navy. He spent most of his naval career either at sea or in a shipyard. He has a 50-year history of cigarette smoking and is currently being evaluated for the etiology of a centrally located left lung mass. Which of the following best applies to the findings in this patient?

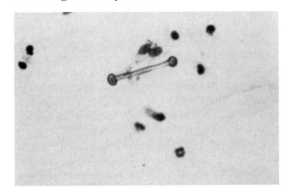

(A) The sediment finding has no direct relationship to his lung mass
(B) Smoking has no direct relationship to his lung mass
(C) A culture will likely grow out *Aspergillus fumigatus*
(D) The structure represents crystalline material from eosinophils
(E) The structure represents material that he inhaled while working in a shipyard

4. Which of the following is present in both interstitial (restrictive) and obstructive lung disease?

(A) Decreased diffusion capacity (DL_{CO})
(B) Increased total lung capacity (TLC)
(C) Decreased FEV_{1sec}/FVC ratio
(D) Normal vital capacity (VC)
(E) Increased residual volume (RV)

5. You would expect a normal alveolar-arterial (A-a) gradient in a patient with

(A) coal workers' pneumoconiosis (CWP)
(B) adult respiratory distress syndrome (ARDS)
(C) paralysis of the diaphragms
(D) cystic fibrosis
(E) farmer's lung

6. Decreased tactile fremitus and dullness to percussion at the right lung base would most likely indicate

(A) spontaneous pneumothorax
(B) right lower lobe bacterial pneumonia
(C) right lower lobe viral pneumonia
(D) pleural effusion
(E) lung abscess

7. A PaO_2 of 40 mm Hg (normal, 75–100 mm Hg), a $PaCO_2$ of 80 mm Hg (normal, 33–44 mm Hg), an arterial pH of 7.20 (normal, 7.35–7.45), and an A-a gradient of 70 mm Hg (normal, 5–15 mm Hg) in a patient receiving oxygen would be most consistent with

(A) sarcoidosis
(B) a Hamman-Rich lung
(C) progressive massive fibrosis

(D) depression of the CNS respiratory center
(E) chronic bronchitis with an acute exacerbation

8. Which of the following disease/location relationships is correct?

(A) Laryngeal cancer: subglottis
(B) Neurogenic tumor: posterior mediastinum
(C) Reactivation tuberculosis: lower lobe
(D) Lung abscess in a person with alcoholism and poor dentition: left upper lobe
(E) Foreign body aspiration while lying down: postero-basal segment of right lower lobe

9. A 14-year-old boy with cystic fibrosis has cough productive of cupfuls of foul-smelling fluid. The pathogenesis of this finding is most closely related to

(A) patchy atelectasis
(B) cor pulmonale
(C) bronchiectasis
(D) a lung abscess
(E) lobar pneumonia

10. Atelectasis is least likely operative in a patient with

(A) fever on the fourth postoperative day
(B) respiratory distress syndrome (RDS)
(C) a tension pneumothorax
(D) mucous plugs in the small airways
(E) adult respiratory distress syndrome (ARDS)

11. Obstruction has an insignificant role in the pathogenesis of

(A) bronchiectasis
(B) endogenous lipoid pneumonia
(C) bronchial asthma
(D) aspiration pneumonia
(E) sarcoidosis

12. Both chronic bronchitis (CB) and emphysema are associated with

(A) respiratory acidosis
(B) excessive sputum production
(C) severe ventilation/perfusion (V/Q) mismatches
(D) irreversible destruction of the respiratory unit
(E) a low PaO_2

13. Cough, weight loss, a smoking history, and hypercalcemia would be most consistent with a diagnosis of

(A) scar carcinoma
(B) metastatic lung disease
(C) primary adenocarcinoma of the lung
(D) primary squamous cell carcinoma of the lung
(E) primary small-cell carcinoma of the lung

14. Which of the following infectious disease relationships is correct?

(A) Rhinovirus: antigen drifts and shifts
(B) Respiratory syncytial virus: laryngotracheobronchitis
(C) Parainfluenza: most common cause of pneumonia in children
(D) *Chlamydia pneumoniae*: pneumonia in a bird fancier
(E) *Mycoplasma pneumoniae*: bullous myringitis

15. Which of the following infectious disease relationships is correct?

 (A) Histoplasmosis: increased incidence in pigeon breeders
 (B) Coccidioidomycosis: increased incidence in earthquakes
 (C) Cryptococcosis: increased incidence in cave explorers
 (D) Blastomycosis: increased incidence in the Midwest and Southwest
 (E) Aspergillosis: increased incidence in workers in the textile industry

16. On the second postoperative day, an obese 24-year-old woman presents with a sudden onset of fever, tachypnea, dyspnea, and pain on inspiration. The pathogenesis of her condition is most closely related to

 (A) a defect in ventilation
 (B) a defect in perfusion
 (C) a defect in diffusion
 (D) intrapulmonary shunting
 (E) a nosocomial infection

17. Cigarette smoking is most likely to assume a pivotal role in the pathogenesis of

 (A) progressive massive fibrosis (PMF)
 (B) cor pulmonale
 (C) mesothelioma
 (D) triad asthma
 (E) bagassosis

ANSWERS AND EXPLANATIONS

1. The answer is B: neurosecretory tumor. The slide reveals small cells with hyperchromatic nuclei and increased mitotic activity. These cells along with a smoking history and a central location are most consistent with a small (oat) cell carcinoma of the lungs. This tumor is derived from the neural crest (they contain neurosecretory granules on ultrastructural examination). They are not usually amenable to surgical removal and commonly secrete ACTH and ADH. A tumor derived from Clara cells is the bronchioloalveolar adenocarcinoma. A bronchial hamartoma is nonneoplastic and contains mature cartilage. Although metastatic disease is the most common lung cancer, the history, morphology of the tumor, and its location argue against metastasis. A squamous cell carcinoma is associated with keratin production. (Photomicrograph reproduced, with permission, from T.V. Colby, C. Lombard, S.A. Yousem, and M. Kitaichi. *Atlas of Pulmonary Surgical Pathology*. Philadelphia, W.B. Saunders Co., 1991, p. 101.)

2. The answer is D: HIV antibody test. The photograph reveals the cyst walls of *Pneumocystis carinii*. This infection usually occurs in the setting of AIDS and other immunocompromised conditions. An HIV antibody test would be most useful in arriving at the pathogenesis of his disease. Pneumocystis is the most common initial presentation in AIDS and is best treated with trimethoprim/sulfamethoxazole. A PPD skin test and bacterial, acid-fast, and fungal cultures should also be performed on the lung material to rule out other microbial pathogens. A lymph node biopsy would not be useful in the initial workup of this patient. (Photomicrograph reproduced, with permission, from T.V. Colby, C. Lombard, S.A. Yousem, and M. Kitaichi. *Atlas of Pulmonary Surgical Pathology*. Philadelphia, W.B. Saunders Co., 1991, p. 198.)

3. The answer is E: the structure represents material that he inhaled while working in a shipyard. The structure is a dumbbell-shaped asbestos (ferruginous) body, which is an asbestos fiber (chrysotile or crocidolite) coated by iron. The patient most likely inhaled asbestos fibers while working around pipes insulated with asbestos. It requires at least 15–20 years from first exposure before cancer presents. The combination of smoking and asbestos, both of which are carcinogens, markedly increases the chances that the lung mass is a primary lung cancer. The structure is not a hypha from *Aspergillus* (which would be septate) and is not a Charcot-Leyden crystal (degenerated crystalline material from eosinophils), commonly noted in the sputum of people with asthma. (Photomicrograph reproduced, with permission, from J.B. Henry. *Clinical Diagnosis and Management by Laboratory Methods*, 18th ed. Philadelphia, W.B. Saunders Co., 1991, p. 516.)

4. The answer is A: decreased diffusion capacity (DL_{CO}). In restrictive disease, all lung volumes and capacities are decreased owing to decreased compliance (decreased expansion of the lungs on inspiration) from an increase in interstitial fibrosis. Elasticity (recoil of the lungs on expiration) is increased. Because of the increased elasticity, the FEV_{1sec} (amount of available air forced out of the lungs in 1 second after a maximal inspiration; normally 4 L) and FVC (total amount of available air forced out of the lungs after maximal inspiration; normally 5 L), though decreased, are often the same (e.g., 3 L). Therefore, the FEV_{1sec}/FVC ratio is either normal (0.80) or increased over normal (3/3 = 1.0). In obstructive lung disease, there is an increase in lung compliance (easy expansion of the lungs on inspiration) and a decrease in lung elasticity (elastic tissue is destroyed by neutrophil-derived elastases). The PFTs exhibit an increase in the TLC owing to an increase in the residual volume (RV; air left in the lung after maximal expiration) related to air trapped in the lungs on expiration behind collapsed airways. The expanding RV eventually decreases all the other volumes and capacities. The FEV_{1sec}, FVC, and FEV_{1sec}/FVC ratio are all decreased. The diffusing capacity (DL_{CO}) evaluates the movement of CO through the alveolocapillary interface to Hb in RBCs in the pulmonary capillaries. It is dependent on the amount of CO that (1) reaches the alveoli, (2) crosses the alveolocapillary interface (which depends on the thickness of the interface and its total cross-sectional area), and (3) binds to Hb in RBCs (which depends on the pulmonary capillary blood volume). It is decreased in both restrictive and obstructive lung disease, the former from thickening of the alveolo-

capillary interface from fibrosis and the latter from destruction of the capillary bed.

5. The answer is C: paralysis of the diaphragms. The difference between the PAO_2 and PaO_2 is called the A-a gradient (normally, 5–15 mm Hg). It is due to the normal mismatch between ventilation and perfusion in the lungs. An abnormal A-a gradient is associated with hypoxemia and indicates a primary problem in the lungs (ventilation, perfusion, diffusion problem) or heart (right-to-left shunt; e.g., tetralogy of Fallot). CWP, ARDS, cystic fibrosis, and farmer's lung (hypersensitivity pneumonitis due to inhalation of thermophilic actinomycetes) all produce lung disease involving one or more of the above abnormalities that increase the A-a gradient. Paralysis of the diaphragm reduces the ventilation to the lung, hence decreasing the PAO_2; however, there is nothing wrong with gas exchange (perfusion, diffusion). Hence, the PaO_2 is also decreased without alteration of the normal gradient of 5–15 mm Hg (e.g., PAO_2 = 60 mm Hg, PaO_2 = 50 mm Hg, A-a gradient = 10 mm Hg).

6. The answer is D: pleural effusion. Tactile fremitus represents the vibrations on the chest that are normally felt when a patient speaks. When increased, it indicates a lung consolidation (e.g., bacterial pneumonia) and when decreased, it may represent a pleural effusion or pneumothorax (collapsed lung). It is not affected by viral pneumonia, which usually produces interstitial inflammation. Decreased percussion may indicate a lung consolidation or fluid in the pleural cavity. A tympanitic percussion note indicates only air in the chest cavity (pneumothorax) or an increase in the AP diameter (COPD, asthma). Hence, a reduction in both tactile fremitus and percussion note is most consistent with a pleural effusion.

7. The answer is E: chronic bronchitis with an acute exacerbation. The ABGs indicate a respiratory acidosis (acid pH, $PaCO_2$ >44 mm Hg) with severe hypoxemia and a medically significant A-a gradient even while the patient is on oxygen. The only lung disease resulting in retention of CO_2 that could produce the above findings among the choices listed is chronic bronchitis, which is the most common cause of COPD. A superimposed infection exacerbates the degree of obstruction in CB, hence increasing the severity of respiratory acidosis. Sarcoidosis is a restrictive lung disease, which produces either normal ABGs or mild respiratory alkalosis. Depression of the CNS respiratory center produces all the ABG findings in this patient; however, the A-a gradient is normal, since there is no alteration in perfusion or diffusion in the lungs (see the discussion of question 5). A Hamman-Rich lung (honeycomb lung) is an end-stage lung associated with noninfectious interstitial pneumonias (e.g., usual, desquamative, or lymphoid interstitial pneumonitis), which starts out as an alveolitis and progresses to a fibrosing alveolitis. The ABG findings are those of restrictive lung disease. Progressive massive fibrosis is the crippling lung disease associated with coal workers' pneumoconiosis and silicosis, both of which produce restrictive lung disease findings.

8. The answer is B: neurogenic tumor: posterior mediastinum. Neurogenic tumors are the most common mediastinal tumors, and most are located in the posterior compartment. There is a greater chance that they are malignant in children (neuroblastoma) than in adults (usually a benign ganglioneuroma). Laryngeal cancer (squamous cell carcinoma) is most commonly due to smoking and is most commonly supraglottic (false vo-

cal cords, ventricle) rather than subglottic (below the true vocal cords). Reactivation tuberculosis (a strict aerobe) is most commonly in the apex of the lungs. A person with alcoholism and poor dentition would most likely aspirate infected oropharyngeal material into the posterobasal segment of the right lower lobe if sitting or standing, superior segment of the right lower lobe if lying down (explanation for choice E), right middle lobe or posterior segment of the right upper lobe if lying down on the right side, or lingula of the left lung if lying down on the left side. Aspiration is uncommon in the left upper lobe.

9. The answer is C: bronchiectasis. Cystic fibrosis (CF) is the most common cause of bronchiectasis (dilated bronchi filled with pus) in the United States. The copious foul-smelling sputum is characteristic owing to pooling of pus in dilated bronchial segments that have been destroyed by obstruction of the airways by inspissated mucous plugs and repeated infections. All the other choices listed may occur in the lungs of patients with CF; however, the amount of sputum produced by this patient is not characteristic of any of those disorders.

10. The answer is A: fever on the fourth postoperative day. Fever that develops within 24–48 hours of surgery is most commonly due to atelectasis. After that time, fever is most commonly due to pneumonia. Both RDS and ARDS demonstrate surfactant deficiencies with collapse of the alveoli (atelectasis). Resorption atelectasis occurs behind points of obstruction in the small airways. A tension pneumothorax allows air to accumulate in the pleural cavity through a tear in the pleura, hence shifting the lungs to the contralateral side and producing compression atelectasis of the lung.

11. The answer is E: sarcoidosis. Sarcoidosis is a multisystem granulomatous (noncaseating) disease of unknown etiology that frequents adults between 20 and 40 years of age. It is a restrictive and not an obstructive type of lung disease. Obstruction and infection are operative in the pathogenesis of bronchiectasis (question 9). Endogenous lipoid pneumonia (golden pneumonia), characterized by an accumulation of cholesterol-laden macrophages in the lungs, invariably develops behind obstructive lesions in the airways (e.g., cancer). Bronchial asthma is a reversible, obstructive type of small airway disease. Aspiration pneumonia involves the introduction of foreign material (e.g., gastric juice) into the airways with subsequent inflammation.

12. The answer is E: a low PaO_2. Both CB and emphysema interfere with gas exchange in the lungs, resulting in a low PaO_2 (hypoxemia). CB is more likely to demonstrate respiratory acidosis, while emphysema is likely to either have a normal or low $PaCO_2$ (respiratory alkalosis). Excessive sputum production is primarily seen in CB (mucous gland hyperplasia). Severe V/Q mismatches are more likely in CB owing to obstruction in the terminal (nonrespiratory bronchioles), hence affecting a greater cross-sectional area of lung. The V/Q losses in emphysema are evenly matched (airway and capillary destruction). Emphysema is characterized by irreversible destruction of the respiratory unit (respiratory bronchioles, alveolar ducts, alveoli).

13. The answer is D: primary squamous cell carcinoma of the lung. Primary squamous cancers of the lung can ectopically secrete a parathormone-like peptide, resulting in hypercalcemia. Along with small-cell carcinoma, it has a strong association with smoking; however, that cancer does not secrete a PTH-like peptide.

Adenocarcinomas do not ectopically secrete hormones and are not as strongly associated with smoking. Metastatic disease to the lungs does not fit the case scenario and relationship to smoking. Scar cancers are most commonly adenocarcinomas.

14. The answer is E: *Mycoplasma pneumoniae*: bullous myringitis. *M. pneumoniae*, in addition to producing bullous myringitis, is the most common cause of atypical pneumonia. Rhinovirus is the most common cause of the common cold. Influenzavirus is associated with mutations in hemagglutinins resulting in antigen drifts (minor mutation) and shifts (major mutation). Respiratory syncytial virus is the most common cause of pneumonia and bronchiolitis in children. Parainfluenza virus is the most common cause of laryngotracheobronchitis (croup) in children. *Chlamydia pneumoniae* is a common cause of atypical pneumonia and should not be confused with *Chlamydia psittaci*, which may be associated with handling of psittacine birds (parakeets, parrots).

15. The answer is B: coccidioidomycosis: increased incidence in earthquakes. The arthrospores of *C. immitis* are present in dust, hence the increase in lung disease in earthquakes in the Southwestern states (particularly southern California). Histoplasmosis is increased in cave explorers owing to exposure to bird and bat dung (cryptococcosis is associated with pigeons). Blastomycosis is increased in the Midwest and Southeastern states. Byssinosis is a hypersensitivity pneumonitis associated with exposure to cotton, hemp, or linen in the textile industry and has no relationship with aspergillosis.

16. The answer is B: a defect in perfusion. The patient has a classic history for a pulmonary embolus (PE) with infarction and pleuritic chest pain. A PE is commonly seen in the postoperative state owing to lack of movement and stasis in the leg veins. A PE initially produces a perfusion defect, while ventilation defects with intrapulmonary shunting occur after 48 hours. Diffusion defects are not prominent in a PE. A nosocomial (hospital-acquired) infection does not fit this case scenario.

17. The answer is B: cor pulmonale. Smoking produces COPD (CB and emphysema), which in turn can produce cor pulmonale (pulmonary hypertension and right ventricular hypertrophy). Smoking is not associated with PMF (coal workers' pneumoconiosis, silicosis), mesothelioma, triad asthma (aspirin, asthma, nasal polyps), or bagassosis (hypersensitivity pneumonitis associated with exposure to moldy sugar cane).

CHAPTER TWELVE

DISORDERS OF THE RED AND

WHITE BLOOD CELLS AND

BONE MARROW

SYNOPSIS

OBJECTIVES

1. To understand normal and abnormal hematopoiesis in the bone marrow.
2. To be familiar with the components of a complete blood cell count (CBC) and their significance in the workup of anemia.
3. To describe the normal components of the bone marrow examination.
4. To review microcytic, normocytic, and macrocytic anemias with reference to pathogenesis, clinical features, and laboratory abnormalities.
5. To understand benign quantitative and qualitative white blood cell disorders.
6. To describe the myeloproliferative disorders and the differential diagnosis of polycythemia.
7. To review the myelodysplastic syndrome and acute and chronic leukemias.
8. To discuss sepsis and selected disorders that commonly involve blood.

Objective 1: To understand normal and abnormal hematopoiesis in the bone marrow.

I. Hematopoiesis
   A. Hematopoiesis (blood cell formation) in the bone marrow is promulgated by a self-perpetuating pool of multipotential stem cells consisting of pluripotential stem cells, lymphoid stem cells (which subsequently develop into B and T cells in the bone marrow and thymus, respectively), and trilineage myeloid stem cells that further subdivide into committed stem cells that produce red blood cells (RBCs), white blood cells (WBCs), and platelets.
   B. Severe anemias (e.g., sickle cell disease) that impose a severe stress on the bone marrow to produce RBCs expand the marrow cavity, producing such physical findings as a "chipmunk" face, frontal bossing of the skull, and "hair-on-end" appearance on skull x-rays.

   C. Extramedullary (outside the marrow) hematopoiesis may occur in organs such as the spleen and liver in severe anemias or when there is intrinsic disease in the marrow (e.g., myelofibrosis).
   D. **Erythropoiesis** is the production of RBCs in the bone marrow.
      1. It is dependent on the hormone erythropoietin, which is synthesized in the kidneys.
      2. Pathologic stimuli prompting enhanced release of erythropoietin leading to accelerated erythropoiesis (RBC hyperplasia) include a low PaO_2 (hypoxemia), moderately severe anemia (< 7 g/dL) and a left-shifted oxygen dissociation curve (ODC; a high affinity for oxygen produces less release of oxygen to tissue and tissue hypoxia).
      3. Peripheral blood manifestations of accelerated erythropoiesis include the presence of shift cells (see Figure 12–1N), or marrow reticulocytes (which require 2–3 days to become mature RBCs), and an increase in peripheral blood reticulocytes (which require 24 hours to become mature RBCs; Figure 12–1M).
         a. Both types of reticulocytes contain RNA filaments, which can only be identified with supravital stains when performing a reticulocyte count.
         b. A reticulocyte count is the most cost-effective method of determining whether the marrow is responding appropriately to anemia (effective erythropoiesis), since peripheral blood reticulocytes alone or in concert with marrow reticulocytes are released prematurely from the marrow.
            (1) A reticulocyte count is normally reported as a percentage (normal, 0.5–1.5%).
            (2) By convention, the count is based on the number of peripheral blood (24-hour-old) reticulocytes rather than marrow reticulocytes (which are 2–3 days old); an increase in the latter falsely elevates the count.
            (3) The count is first corrected for the degree of anemia (if present) with the following formula:

**Corrected reticulocyte count =
(patient Hct/45) × reticulocyte count,** where 45 represents the normal Hct.

Example: Patient Hct = 15%, reticulocyte count = 9%, corrected count = 3% (15/45 × 9% = 3%).

(4) The presence of marrow reticulocytes (shift cells) requires an additional correction, which is made by dividing the corrected count by 2 (the result is called the reticulocyte index; in the above example, 3/2 = 1.5%).

(5) After the above is applied to the raw reticulocyte count, a count > 3% is considered a good response to anemia, whereas a count < 2% is considered a poor response (something is wrong in the bone marrow).

4. Mature RBCs are biconcave disks with a central area of depression.
   a. They are anucleate cells that are devoid of mitochondria, hence they lack the following biochemical systems: citric acid cycle, β-oxidation of fatty acids, and oxidative phosphorylation.
   b. They metabolize glucose by anaerobic glycolysis (lactate is the end product), generate glutathione (GSH) via a pentose phosphate shunt, reduce heme iron from +3 (methemoglobin) to the ferrous (+2) state (which binds oxygen) utilizing a methemoglobin reductase system, synthesize 2,3-bisphosphoglycerate (which right-shifts the oxygen dissociation curve) via the Rapoport-Luebering shunt, and have ABO and Rh antigens on their membranes.
   c. Senescent RBCs are removed mainly by extravascular hemolysis (macrophage removal in the spleen), the end product of which is lipid-soluble unconjugated bilirubin.
   d. To a lesser extent, senescent RBCs are destroyed intravascularly with the release of free Hb, which is immediately bound to haptoglobin (a protein synthesized in the liver) to form a complex that is subsequently removed by macrophages in the spleen, liver, and bone marrow.
   e. In pathologic extravascular hemolysis (e.g., congenital spherocytosis), the increase in unconjugated bilirubin may produce jaundice.
   f. In pathologic intravascular hemolysis (e.g., microangiopathic hemolytic anemia), serum haptoglobin is reduced and Hb may be excreted in the urine as free Hb (hemoglobinuria) or as hemosiderin (a breakdown product of Hb absorbed into renal tubular cells).

E. **Granulopoiesis** is the formation of granulocytes (neutrophils, eosinophils, and basophils) in the marrow.
   1. Myeloblasts, progranulocytes (which contain nonspecific or azurophilic granules), and myelocytes (the last cell capable of dividing and the first cell to produce specific granules) are able to divide, and so they represent the mitotic granulocyte pool.
   2. Metamyelocytes, band neutrophils, and segmented neutrophils are unable to divide (they represent the postmitotic granulocyte pool)

and are released from the marrow into the peripheral blood in inflammatory conditions (via interleukin-1 and tumor necrosis factor stimulation) to produce an absolute neutrophilic leukocytosis and shift to the left (>10% band neutrophils in a 100–leukocyte cell count).

3. Neutrophils in the peripheral circulation are equally divided between the circulating pool (population of cells reported in an automated WBC count) and the marginating pool (neutrophils adhering to the endothelium because of adhesion molecules).

Objective 2: To be familiar with the components of a complete blood cell count (CBC) and their significance in the workup of anemia.

II. Complete blood cell count (CBC)
   A. The "rule of 3" states that the Hb times 3 should approximate the Hct (e.g., Hb of 9 g/dL × 3 = Hct of 27%).
   B. The Hct is the ratio of RBC mass to that of whole blood expressed as a percent.
   C. Variables that affect the reference intervals for Hb and Hct are age (newborns have a greater concentration than infants and children), sex (men have a greater concentration than women), place of residence (high-altitude residents have a greater concentration than those living at sea level), tobacco use (smokers have a greater concentration than nonsmokers), and pregnancy (pregnant women have a lower concentration than nonpregnant women).
   D. Newborns have ~70–90% HbF (2 α- and 2 γ-globin chains), 10–30% HbA (2 α- and 2 β-globin chains), and < 1% HbA$_2$ (2 α- and 2 δ-globin chains).
      1. During the 3 months following birth, the Hb drops from a mean of 18.5 g/dL at birth to 11 g/dL as fetal RBCs are destroyed (physiologic anemia), hence replenishing low iron stores and offsetting the possibility of nutritional iron deficiency from iron-poor breast milk.
      2. In the newborn, fetal RBCs are replaced by RBCs containing HbA (> 97%), HbA$_2$ (< 2.5%), and HbF (< 1%), the latter over a period of 6–9 months.
   E. Hb electrophoresis is the gold standard test for evaluating patients with a suspected hemoglobinopathy (abnormalities in globin chain structure [e.g., sickle cell disease] or globin chain synthesis [e.g., thalassemias]).
   F. As a rule, the **RBC count** parallels the Hb and Hct concentration; however, in the thalassemias, the RBC count is frequently normal to increased in the presence of a low Hb and Hct.
   G. The **RBC indices** include the mean corpuscular volume (MCV), mean corpuscular Hb (MCH), and mean corpuscular Hb concentration (MCHC).
      1. MCV is the average volume of millions of RBCs passing through a preset aperture in an automated cell counter.
         a. It lends itself to a classification scheme for anemias based on size, hence the designations microcytic (< 80 fL), normocytic (80–100 fL), and macrocytic (> 100 fL) anemias.
         b. Variables affecting the MCV include the age

of the patient (e.g., newborns have an increased MCV) and pregnancy (increased if women are not on folate supplements).

2. The MCHC correlates with the Hb concentration in RBCs.

   a. When Hb production is decreased, as it is in the microcytic anemias, the MCHC is decreased (hypochromasia) and the RBCs have a greater central area of pallor in the peripheral smear.

   b. Spherical RBCs (spherocytes; Figure 12–1B) have an increased MCHC and no central area of pallor.

H. Unlike the MCV, which reports average RBC cell size (which could be reported as normal if RBCs are a mixture of microcytic and macrocytic cells), the **red blood cell distribution width** (RDW) detects whether RBCs are a mixture of microcytic and macrocytic cells or whether there is significant variation in size of RBCs that are predominantly microcytic, normocytic, or macrocytic cells.

I. The **white blood cell** (WBC) **count** on an automated instrument includes neutrophils, eosinophils, basophils, lymphocytes, and monocytes.

   1. A 100-cell differential leukocyte count subdivides the cell types according to percentage and further classifies neutrophils as segmented or band neutrophils.

   2. In adults, the total leukocyte count ranges between 4500 and 11,000 cells/µL, with the following normal differential in percentage: segmented neutrophils, 54–62%; band neutrophils, 3–5%; eosinophils, 1–3%; basophils, 0–1%; lymphocytes, 23–33%; and monocytes, 3–7%.

   3. The leukocyte percentage multiplied by the total WBC count equals the absolute number of cells (e.g., 50% segmented neutrophils × 10,000 cells/µL = 5000 cells/µL).

      a. An increase in the absolute number of leukocytes is called absolute leukocytosis, which can be subdivided according to individual cell types (e.g., absolute neutrophilic leukocytosis, eosinophilia).

      b. A decrease in the absolute number of leukocytes is called absolute leukopenia (e.g., absolute neutropenia, absolute lymphopenia).

      c. A relative increase in leukocytes refers to an increase in the percentage of cells without a corresponding increase in the absolute number.

   4. Variables affecting the total leukocyte count include age (children have a greater number of lymphocytes than adults), ethnicity (African Americans have lower total leukocyte counts than whites), tobacco use (smokers have higher neutrophil counts than nonsmokers), and drugs (phenytoin increases the lymphocyte count; corticosteroids increase the neutrophil count).

J. A **smear of peripheral blood** should be evaluated for **RBC morphology** (Figure 12–1) including shape (poikilocytosis) and size (anisocytosis; correlates with RDW), Hb concentration in individual RBCs (i.e., the degree of hypochromasia or hyperchromasia), WBC morphology and number (Figure 12–2), and platelet morphology and number.

Objective 3. To describe the normal components of the bone marrow examination.

III. Normal components of the bone marrow examination

A. Normal components include an assessment of cellularity (normally a 30% fat to 70% cell ratio), a calculation of the M/E ratio (usually 3/1), an evaluation of hematopoietic cell morphology, an appraisal of the adequacy of megakaryocytes, and an estimate of the status of iron stores using the Prussian blue stain (absent in iron deficiency, increased in anemia of chronic inflammation and the sideroblastic anemias).

B. Regarding the M/E ratio, only cells in the myeloid (granulocytic series) and erythroid cells are counted.

   1. An increase in total erythropoiesis (RBC hyperplasia) produces a decreased ratio (e.g., 1/1), while a decrease in total erythropoiesis increases the ratio (e.g., 6/1).

   2. A major limitation of the M/E ratio is that it provides only a static picture of marrow events without indicating how many of the RBCs are finding their way into the peripheral circulation (effective erythropoiesis) in response to an anemia (this is provided by a reticulocyte count).

Objective 4: To review microcytic, normocytic, and macrocytic anemias with reference to pathogenesis, clinical features, and laboratory abnormalities.

IV. Anemia

A. Anemia signifies a decrease in Hb or Hct concentration and represents a sign of an underlying disease rather than a specific diagnosis.

   1. The following are accepted definitions for anemia: Hb < 13.5 g/dL in a male, < 12.5 g/dL in an adult woman, < 11 g/dL in pregnancy, < 14 g/dL in a preterm infant, ≤ 13.5 g/dL in a full-term newborn, and < 11 g/dL in children between 6 months and 8 years of age.

   2. In anemia, the SaO_2 (percentage of heme groups occupied by oxygen) and PaO_2 (amount of oxygen dissolved in plasma) are normal, since oxygen exchange in the lungs is normal; however, the oxygen content (total amount of oxygen available to tissue) is decreased owing to the reduction in Hb concentration.

B. Classification of anemia based on the MCV (morphologic classification) is used here and is summarized in Table 12–1.

C. Symptoms associated with anemia are primarily those of tissue hypoxia and consist of dyspnea with exertion (uncomfortable awareness of breathing), weakness, fatigue, anorexia (intestinal hypoxia), insomnia, inability to concentrate, and dizziness (CNS hypoxia).

D. A thorough history and physical examination are critical to arriving at the cause of a patient's anemia.

E. Table 12–2 summarizes the key abnormalities associated with the **microcytic anemias**.

   1. A defect in Hb synthesis underlies the pathogenesis of all microcytic anemias.

   2. Reduced Hb concentration in developing nor-

Iron def
Thalassemia

A. Target cell

Too much membrane

Alcoholism
Hemoglobinopathy
Liver disease
Splenectomy

B. Spherocyte

Too little membrane

Congenital
 spherocytosis
ABO incompatibility
Autoimmune hemolytic
 anemia
Burns

C. Schistocytes

Prosthetic heart valve
DIC
Thrombotic thrombo-
 cytopenic purpura/
 hemolytic uremic
 syndrome

D. Basophillic stippling

Ribosomes

Iron deficiency (fine
 granules)
Thalassemias (fine
 granules)
Anemia of chronic
 inflammation (fine
 granules)
Lead poisoning
 (coarse granules)

E. Howell-Jolly body

Nuclear
 remnant

Splenectomy
Autosplenectomy in
 HbSS disease

F. Tear drop

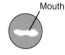

Myelofibrosis
Thalassemia

G. Stomatocyte

Mouth

Alcoholism

H. Bite cell

Glucose-6-phosphate
 dehydrogenase
 deficiency

I. Dimorphic RBCs

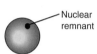

Macrocyte

Microcyte

Microcytic/macrocytic
 anemia
Myelodysplastic
 syndrome

J. Macroovalocyte

Egg-shaped

Pernicious anemia
Folate deficiency

**K. Pappenheimer
bodies***

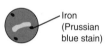

Iron
 (Prussian
 blue stain)

Sideroblastic anemias
Iron overload conditions

L. Heinz bodies*

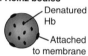

Denatured
 Hb

Attached
 to membrane

Glucose-6-phosphate
 dehydrogenase
 deficiency

FIGURE 12–1. Red blood cell morphology.

M. Reticulocyte*

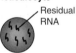

Residual
 RNA

Hemolytic anemias
Posttreatment for iron
 deficiency/B$_{12}$ defici-
 ency/folate deficiency
Myelophthisic anemia

N. Shift cell

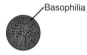

Basophilia

Severe hemolytic anemias

O. Sickle cell

HbSS disease
HbS/thalassemia

P. Elliptocyte/ovalocyte

Hereditary disease
Iron deficiency

Q. Ringed sideroblast*

Iron in
 mitochondria

Sideroblastic anemias
Myelodysplasia

R. Acanthocytes

Fulminant liver failure
Abetalipoproteinemia

S. Rouleaux

Increased γ-globulins
 or fibrinogen

T. Agglutination

Increased IgM

U. Burr cells

Uremia

*Special stain needed.

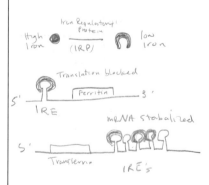

TABLE 12–1.   Classification of Anemia on the Basis of Mean Corpuscular Volume (MCV)

Microcytic Anemias (MCV < 80 fL)

Iron deficiency (most common) [handwritten: → defective heme synthesis]
Anemia of chronic disease
Thalassemia [handwritten: -defective globin synthesis]
Sideroblastic anemia (least common)

Macrocytic Anemias (MCV > 100 fL)

B_{12} deficiency
Folate deficiency (most common)
Alcoholic liver disease

Normocytic Anemias (MCV 80–100 fL)

*Reticulocyte Count (<2%)	↑ Reticulocyte Count > 3% Intrinsic RBC Defect (MAD)	↑ Reticulocyte Count > 3% Extrinsic RBC Defect

*Acute blood loss (<7 days)
Early iron deficiency
Aplastic anemia
Anemia of chronic disease
Renal disease
	*Membrane defects
	  Congenital spherocytosis/elliptocytosis
	  Paroxysmal nocturnal hemoglobinuria (PNH)
	*Abnormal hemoglobins
	  Sickle cell disease/variants (HbS-C, HbC)
	*Deficient enzymes
	  Glucose-6-phosphate dehydrogenase deficiency
	    (most common)
	  Pyruvate kinase deficiency
		Autoimmune hemolytic anemias (warm and cold)
		Paroxysmal cold hemoglobinuria (PCH)
		Microangiopathic hemolytic anemia

* Acute bleed > 7 days: reticulocyte count > 3%.
Reticulocyte count: the count after all corrections are made for anemia and for shift cells, if they are present.
Intrinsic defect: something is wrong with the RBC that causes a hemolytic anemia (membrane, Hb, enzyme defect).
Extrinsic defect: nothing is wrong with the RBC; however, something outside the RBC is causing hemolytic anemia (antibody, prosthetic valve, fibrin strands in DIC).
Mechanisms of hemolytic anemia: intravascular (hemolysis within the vascular system) or extravascular (macrophages remove RBCs and destroy them, usually in the spleen [MC], liver, or bone marrow).

moblasts increases the number of mitoses, resulting in the formation of microcytic cells.

3. When iron stores are reduced or absent, transferrin synthesis is increased (e.g., iron deficiency anemia), whereas increased iron stores reduce transferrin synthesis (e.g., sideroblastic anemias, ACD).

4. Hb synthesis involves the formation of heme (iron + protoporphyrin), which primarily occurs in the mitochondria and the synthesis of globin chains (α, β, δ, and γ) on the ribosomes.

5. Iron deficiency, ACD, and sideroblastic anemia all have abnormalities in heme synthesis, whereas the thalassemias have defective globin chain synthesis.

6. Approximately 10% of dietary iron is normally reabsorbed (1–2 mg/d) in the duodenum.

   a. The percentage increases in pregnancy and lactation as well as in any anemia regardless of type.

   b. Most iron in the adult male and female is attached to Hb, while the remainder is stored in macrophages in the marrow (1000 mg in men and 400 mg in women).

   c. Ascorbic acid is the most important factor for reducing ferric (+3) iron in nonheme foods (plants) to the absorbable ferrous (+2) form (heme in meat is already in the ferrous state).

   d. Iron homeostasis is maintained by regulating the amount of iron reabsorbed (mucosal block theory), which appears to be a function of the amount of ferritin in the mucosal cell.

7. Serum iron, total iron-binding capacity (TIBC; represents transferrin), percent saturation ([serum iron/TIBC] × 100), and serum ferritin (circulating fraction of storage iron; single best test) are important in the diagnosis of iron deficiency, ACD, and sideroblastic anemia.

8. Hb electrophoresis is the gold standard for diagnosing mild β-thalassemia (there is an increase in HbA_2 and HbF), while mild α-thalassemia is a diagnosis of exclusion (HB electrophoresis is normal).

9. Table 12–3 provides a summary of the main differential points between the microcytic anemias.

F. Table 12–4 provides a summary of the main causes of the **macrocytic anemias**, namely, folate deficiency (most common), B_{12} deficiency, and alcohol-related liver disease.

   1. The primary mechanisms for producing a macrocytic anemia include defective DNA synthesis (B_{12}/folate deficiency) and increased RBC membrane (from lipid alterations associated with alcohol use).

   a. Vitamin B_{12} (cobalamin, Cbl) retrieves a methyl group from N^5-methyltetrahydrofolate (N^5-methyl-FH_4; circulating form of folate) to produce tetrahydrofolate (FH_4), which is converted to $N^{5,10}$-methylene-FH_4, which converts deoxyuridine monophosphate (dUMP) to deoxythymidine monophosphate (dTMP; integrated into DNA), resulting in the formation of oxidized dihydrofolate, which is reduced back to FH_4 by dihydrofolate reductase (inhibited by methotrexate and trimethoprim).

TIBC = total iron binding Capacity ≈ transferrin

TABLE 12–2. Microcytic Anemias

Anemia Characteristics	Pathogenesis	Causes	Clinical Findings	Treatment	Laboratory Tests
Iron deficiency (most common overall anemia). **MCV:** microcytic (begins normocytic). **Reticulocyte count:** <2%. **Key findings:** hypochromic cells (hypochromasia), thrombocytosis in chronic disease.	**Decreased Hb synthesis:** reduced heme synthesis. **Hypoproliferative:** iron lack. _BM_	**Bleeding:** most common overall cause, usually gastrointestinal (GI). **Prematurity:** loss of iron each day fetus is not in utero; blood loss from phlebotomy. **6 months–2 years of age:** nutritional (milk baby). **Child:** GI bleed (Meckel's diverticulum). **Pregnancy:** net loss of 500 mg if iron supplements are not taken. Lactation depletes iron. **Female <50 years:** menorrhagia (>80 mL loss/period). **Male <50 years:** peptic ulcer disease (duodenal most common). **Male/female >50 years:** GI bleed (rule out colon cancer).	Iron is a cofactor for many enzymes in the GI tract and is responsible for spoon nails (koilonychia), Plummer-Vinson syndrome (esophageal web, achlorhydria, glossitis, and intestinal malabsorption. **Stages of development in succession:** **No anemia:** decreased iron stores → decreased ferritin → decreased iron, increased TIBC, decreased % saturation. **Anemia:** normocytic → microcytic.	Ferrous sulfate/gluconate (see an increase in Hct after a 1-week lag period of 0.5–1 Hct point/day). Stools turn black.	**Serum iron:** decreased. **TIBC:** increased. **% Saturation:** decreased. **Serum ferritin:** decreased. **RDW:** increased. —_hypochromic_ **MCHC:** decreased. —_hypochromic_ **Free RBC protoporphyrin (FEP):** increased. _Protoporphyrin + Iron = heme_
Anemia of chronic inflammation (ACD). **MCV:** microcytic or normocytic (most common). **Reticulocyte count:** <2%. **Key findings:** similar to iron deficiency.	**Decreased Hb synthesis.** **Hypoproliferative:** iron blockade in macrophages (lactoferrin from neutrophils delivers iron to macrophages). Also decreased synthesis of transferrin by the liver in inflammation (related to interleukin-1 and tumor necrosis factor). **Mild hemolytic component** (extravascular hemolysis; not enough to increase reticulocytes).	**Chronic inflammation:** microbial, rheumatoid arthritis. **Malignancy:** ACD is the most common anemia.	Hb is rarely <9 gm/dL. It may be combined with iron deficiency (e.g., GI blood loss + rheumatoid arthritis).	Treat the underlying disease. Iron therapy is not indicated. Erythropoietin is useful in some cases.	**Serum iron:** decreased. **TIBC:** decreased. **% Saturation:** decreased. **Serum ferritin:** increased. **RDW:** normal. **MCHC:** decreased. **Free RBC FEP:** increased.

Thalassemia (α and β). MCV: microcytic. Reticulocyte count: <2% in mild thalassemia; >3% in severe types. Key findings: *basophilic stippling* (Figure 12–1D; persistence of ribosomes; indicates a problem with Hb synthesis), *target cells* (Figure 12–1A; excess RBC membrane bulges in the center of the RBC; an excellent marker of an Hb disorder), *tear drop cells* (Figure 12–1F; possibly due to the removal of excess globin chains by macrophages), *α-globin chain inclusions* in severe β-thalassemia (Cooley's anemia; inclusions are toxic to RBCs, leading to hemolysis).	**Decreased Hb synthesis. Maturation disorder:** cytoplasmic maturation defect. **α-Thalassemia:** decreased α-globin chain synthesis (gene deletions on chromosome 16), but β-, δ-, and γ-globin chain syntheses are normal, hence HbA $(2\alpha/2\beta)$, HbA$_2$ $(2\alpha/2\delta)$, and HbF $(2\alpha/2\gamma)$ are all reduced. **β-Thalassemia:** decreased β-globin chain synthesis on chromosome 11 (**point mutation producing splicing defect most common**). α-, and γ-globin chains are synthesized: **increased synthesis of HbA$_2$ and F.** No β-globin chain synthesis is β^0. Some β-globin chain synthesis is β$^+$. **β-Thalassemia minor** (β/β$^+$): common among Asians, Blacks, Greeks, Italians. Mild protective effect against falciparum malaria. **β-Thalassemia major (Cooley's anemia;** β^0/β$^-$): hemolytic component.	**Autosomal recessive. One-gene deletion:** silent carrier. **Two-gene deletion:** α-thalassemia trait (African American and Asian types are slightly different). **African Americans** $(\alpha-/\alpha-)$: one-gene deletion on each chromosome. **Asian** $(\alpha\alpha/--)$: both deletions on the same chromosome (danger for Hb Bart's disease, since fetus could have no α-globin genes). **Three-gene deletion:** HbH disease (HbH = 4 β-globin chains). Hemolytic anemia. **Four-gene deletion:** Hb Bart's disease (Hb Bart's = four γ-globin chains). Incompatible with life. Spontaneous abortion (hydrops fetalis). Increased risk of molar disease (hydatidiform mole and choriocarcinoma).	**α-Thalassemia:** Asians, African Americans. **β-Thalassemia:** African Americans, Italians, Greeks. **Terms:** minor, intermedia, and major connote degree of severity. Severe thalassemia does not manifest at birth (γ-globin chains, not β-globin chains predominate). First manifestation occurs at 6–9 months of age. Both α- and β-thalassemia decrease severity of sickle disease (α-chains prefer normal β-chains; decreased β-chain synthesis reduces the total amount of HbS).	**Iron studies:** normal in the mild varieties. **RBC count:** normal to increased. **MCV/RBC ratio:** <13. **RDW:** normal. **Hb electrophoresis: α-thalassemia minor (one- and two-gene deletions):** normal. **α-Thalassemia (three-gene deletions) or HbH disease:** HbH increased. **α-Thalassemia (four-gene deletions) or Hb Bart's disease:** Hb Bart's increased. **β-Thalassemia minor:** increase in HbA$_2$ (best parameter) and HbF.	α- and β-thalassemia minor require no treatment. Severe thalassemia requires transfusions. There is a danger of iron overload and transmission of infectious diseases.
Sideroblastic anemia: Lead (Pb) poisoning. MCV: microcytic. Reticulocyte count: often >3% owing to a mild hemolytic component. Key findings: *coarse basophilic stippling* (Figure 12–1D; prominent ribosomes).	**Decreased Hb synthesis. Sideroblastic anemia. Maturation disorder:** cytoplasmic maturation defect. **Pb denatures enzymes:** ferrochelatase (binds iron to protoporphyrin), ALA dehydrase (converts δ-aminolevulinic acid [ALA] to porphobilinogen), and ribonuclease (cannot degrade ribosomes; coarse basophilic stippling).	**Child:** eating old Pb-based paint. **Adult:** working in or living near a battery factory, drinking moonshine (Pb in old radiators), using Pb-glazed pottery, sniffing gasoline, eating foods fertilized with sewage.	**Abnormal craving (pica) for paint and plaster. Lead colic:** severe abdominal pain. **Peripheral neuropathy:** wristdrop (radial nerve), claw hand (ulnar nerve). **Encephalopathy:** cerebral edema, convulsions. **Learning disability. Bone:** Pb is the only heavy metal that deposits in the epiphysis (visible on radiographs). **Proximal renal tubular acidosis:** Pb denatures proximal tubule cells (nephrotoxic; type of coagulation necrosis).	**Blood Pb levels:** increased (best screen and confirmatory test). **Urine δ-ALA:** increased. **RBC protoporphyrin:** increased. **Serum iron:** increased. **TIBC:** decreased. **% Saturation:** increased. **Serum ferritin:** increased. **Bone radiographs:** deposits in the epiphyses.	Combination of dimercaprol (BAL), EDTA, and penicillamine.

Handwritten annotations: "MCV ↑", "hypochromic cells", "→ Use chelating agents ex Desferal", "Hb H = β$_4$", "Hb barts = γ$_4$", "– due to toxic or inclusions"

Table continued on following page

TABLE 12–2. Microcytic Anemias *Continued*

Anemia Characteristics	Pathogenesis	Causes	Clinical Findings	Treatment	Laboratory Tests
Sideroblastic anemias. MCV: microcytic (most cases; some macrocytic). Reticulocyte count: <2%. Key findings: *siderocytes* (Figure 12–1K; called Pappenheimer bodies; common in iron overload diseases such as hemosiderosis), *ringed sideroblasts in the bone marrow* (Figure 12–1Q; present in all sideroblastic anemias; iron enters mitochondria located around the nucleus but cannot exit; iron stains blue with Prussian blue stain).	**Decreased Hb synthesis (defect in heme synthesis). Maturation disorder:** cytoplasmic maturation defect.	**Alcoholism:** most common cause owing to alcohol being a mitochondrial poison. **Pyridoxine (B₆) deficiency:** association with isoniazid therapy in tuberculosis. **Drugs:** alkylating agents. **Pb poisoning. Myelodysplastic (MDS) syndromes.**	Depend on the cause of the anemia.	Depends on the cause of the anemia.	**Serum iron:** increased. **TIBC:** decreased. % **Saturation:** increased. **Serum ferritin:** increased. **Bone marrow:** ringed sideroblasts. Bone marrow examination is mandatory, since ringed sideroblasts are required to make the diagnosis. Pb poisoning does not require a bone marrow test, since blood Pb levels are sufficient.

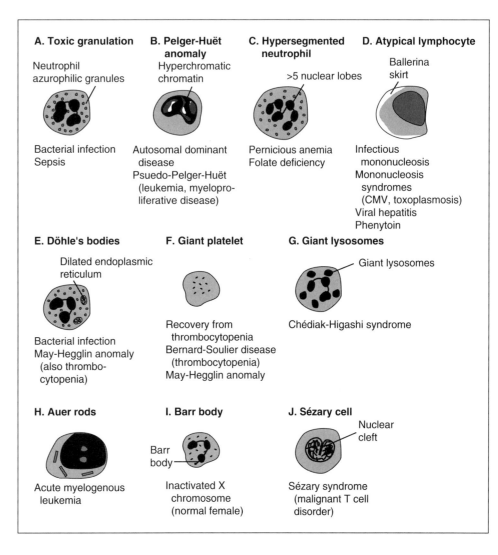

FIGURE 12–2. White blood cell and platelet morphology.

b. Deficiency of either B₁₂ or folate results in defective DNA maturation, while cytoplasmic maturation is unaffected, hence the formation of large hematopoietic cells (megaloblastic anemia) within the marrow and the peripheral blood.

c. Vitamin B₁₂ is found only in animal products and requires intrinsic factor (IF), synthesized in the parietal cells of the stomach, for reabsorption as an IF-B₁₂ complex in the terminal ileum (the liver stores a 6- to 9-year supply).

Text continued on page 162

TABLE 12–3. Differential Features of the Microcytic Anemias

Laboratory Test	Iron Deficiency	ACD	α, β-Thalassemia Minor	Sideroblastic
MCV	Low	Low	Low	Low
Serum iron	Low	Low	Normal	High
TIBC	High	Low	Normal	Low
% Saturation	Low	Low	Normal	High
Serum ferritin	Low	High	Normal	High
RDW	High	Normal	Normal	Normal
RBC count	Low	Low	High	Low
RBC FEP*	High	High	Normal	High (Pb poison)
Hb electrophoresis	Normal	Normal	α-Thalassemia: normal β-Thalassemia: ↑ Hb A₂ and F	Normal
Marrow iron	Absent	High	Normal	High
Miscellaneous	Ferritin best test	Most commonly normocytic	Hb electrophoresis gold standard test	Coarse basophilic stippling in Pb poisoning

* FEP, free erythrocyte protoporphyrin.

TABLE 12–4. Macrocytic Anemias

Anemia Characteristics	Pathogenesis	Causes	Clinical Findings	Treatment	Laboratory Tests
Folate deficiency (most common macrocytic anemia). **MCV:** macrocytic. **Reticulocyte count:** <2%. **Key findings:** *macroovalocytes* (egg-shaped RBCs; Figure 12–1J), megaloblastic bone marrow (immature nuclei due to defective DNA synthesis), *hypersegmented neutrophils* (Figure 12–2C; >5 nuclear lobes; first marker of the disease and last cell to disappear with treatment), *pancytopenia* (destruction of cells by macrophages in the bone marrow), giant bands.	**Defect in DNA synthesis. Maturation defect:** nuclear maturation defect (cytoplasm matures normally). Unlike in B$_{12}$ deficiency, there is no defect in propionate metabolism, hence no CNS disease.	**Alcoholism:** most common cause. **Poor diet:** missing in goat's milk, diet poor in vegetables. **Pregnancy/lactation:** increased utilization of folate owing to only 3 to 4 month supply in the liver (therefore it is a prenatal vitamin supplement). **Drugs:** block dihydrofolate reductase (methotrexate, trimethoprim), block intestinal conjugase and conversion of polyglutamates to monoglutamates (phenytoin), block intestinal reabsorption of monoglutamate (birth control pills). **Malabsorption:** celiac disease. **Increased turnover of cells:** high-grade malignancy (leukemia).	**Glossitis** (not present in beer-drinking alcoholics; beer is rich in folates).	Folic acid in pharmacologic doses. Will correct hematologic findings in B$_{12}$ deficiency as well but not the neurologic disease.	**Serum folate:** low. **RBC folate:** low (best test of overall supply of folate). **Serum homocysteine:** increased (also increased in B$_{12}$ deficiency; associated with vessel damage and thrombosis). **Urine FIGlu** (formiminoglutamic acid): increased owing to the role of FIGlu in transferring carbon units to tetrahydrofolate). **Serum LDH:** increased owing to increased marrow destruction of RBCs.

154

B₁₂ deficiency.
MCV: macrocytic.
Reticulocyte count: <2%.
Key findings: same as for folate deficiency.

Defect in DNA synthesis.
Maturation defect: nuclear maturation defect (cytoplasm matures normally). B₁₂ deficiency produces a defect in propionate (odd-chain fatty acid). Deficiency increases propionate, which produces demyelination in the CNS (posterior column and lateral corticospinal tract).

Pernicious anemia: most common cause (autoimmune destruction of parietal cells).
Pure vegan diet: B₁₂ found only in animal products.
Terminal ileal disease (site of intrinsic factor–B₁₂ complex reabsorption): Crohn's disease.
Fish tapeworm.
Chronic pancreatitis: cannot cleave R factor from B₁₂.
Bacterial overgrowth: diverticular disease, decreased peristalsis from autonomic neuropathy, replacement of muscle with collagen (progressive systemic sclerosis).

Patient: sallow, waxy complexion. Elderly women of Scandinavian origin (not always). Blue eyes. Premature graying. Blood group A.
Glossitis: smooth, sore tongue. Atrophy of papillae.
Autoimmune disease: pernicious anemia (PA) most common cause of B₁₂ deficiency. Increased incidence of other autoimmune diseases (Hashimoto's thyroiditis, vitiligo [autoimmune destruction of melanocytes producing hypopigmentation], and Addison's disease). **Atrophic gastritis of body and fundus** owing to autoimmune destruction of parietal cells. Predisposition for achlorhydria and adenocarcinoma (10%).
Neurologic disease: see above. Decreased vibratory sensation first neurologic sign (posterior column disease). Upper motor neuron signs (lateral corticospinal tracts). Dementia, impaired memory, depression, and psychosis.

Serum B₁₂: decreased.
Serum homocysteine: increased (no methylcobalamin to transfer to homocysteine; associated with vessel damage and thrombosis). Also increased in folate deficiency.
Urine methylmalonic acid: increased (see propionate reaction). Only B₁₂ deficiency. Serum homocysteine and methylmalonic acid most sensitive tests. Use only when B₁₂ testing is equivocal.
Schilling test: abnormal.
Correction with intrinsic factor: pernicious anemia.
Correction following antibiotics: bacterial overgrowth.
Correction following pancreatic extracts: chronic pancreatitis.
No correction with any of the above: probable terminal ileal disease.

Treatment: B₁₂ injections.

TABLE 12–5. Normocytic Anemias: Nonhemolytic with Corrected Reticulocyte Count <2%

Anemia Characteristics	Pathogenesis	Causes	Clinical Findings	Treatment	Laboratory Tests
Acute/chronic blood loss. **MCV:** normocytic. **Reticulocyte count:** <2% (>3% if the bleed is over 5–7 days). **Key findings:** normal peripheral blood until there is a reticulocyte response (Figure 12–1M) with shift cells (Figure 12–1N) indicating a bone marrow response to the blood loss.	**Hemorrhage.** **Chronic blood loss (hypoproliferative):** iron lack from chronic bleeding. Initially no anemia owing to an equal loss of plasma and RBC mass.	**Gastrointestinal bleed: upper GI:** peptic ulcer disease (duodenal > gastric) most commonly. **Lower GI:** diverticulosis, angiodysplasia, colon cancer (>50 years). **Miscellaneous:** splenic rupture (abdominal trauma), ruptured aortic aneurysm, Meckel's diverticulum (particularly in a child).	Positive tilt test (blood pressure drops and pulse increases when patient moves from supine to upright position). **Lower left rib tenderness:** consider ruptured spleen. **Fractures:** pelvic fractures followed by femoral fractures can be associated with significant internal bleeding. **Exacerbation of angina.** **Increased pulse pressure with a potential for high-output cardiac failure:** anemia reduces blood viscosity, which decreases the total peripheral resistance.	Packed cell transfusion if the patient is symptomatic.	No specific laboratory tests. **General:** do a stool guaiac, dipstick test of urine for blood.
Aplastic anemia. **MCV:** normocytic (sometimes slightly macrocytic). **Reticulocyte count:** <2%. **Key findings:** pancytopenia due to a hypocellular bone marrow.	**Stem cell disease:** suppression of the trilineage stem cell in the bone marrow.	**Idiopathic:** most common cause. **Genetic:** Fanconi's syndrome. **Chemical:** benzene (increased risk for acute leukemia). **Drugs:** chloramphenicol, phenylbutazone. **Infection:** NANB hepatitis most commonly. **Irradiation.** **Anemia:** aplastic crisis in HbSS disease, congenital spherocytosis; "spent marrow" (self-limited). May be associated with parvovirus infection. **Pure RBC aplasia** (no bone marrow RBC precursors): parvovirus infection (infection of the erythroid stem cell), thymoma (anterior mediastinal mass), Blackfan-Diamond syndrome (genetic disease).	Bleeding (thrombocytopenia), fever (infection associated with neutropenia), fatigue (anemia).	Patient <50 years old: consider a bone marrow transplantation with an HLA-identical sibling (60–70% survival). **Other treatment:** antithymocyte globulin, antilymphocyte globulin, cyclosporine. Avoid transfusions if the patient is a transplant candidate.	**CBC:** pancytopenia. **Bone marrow:** hypocellular (lymphoid cells still present).

Renal disease. MCV: normocytic. **Reticulocyte count:** <2%. **Key findings:** *burr cells* (Figure 12–1U).	**Hypoproliferative:** decreased erythropoietin.	**Diabetes mellitus** (most common cause of chronic renal disease). **Chronic glomerulonephritis.** **Adult polycystic kidney disease.** **Chronic pyelonephritis.** **Other anemias in renal disease:** iron and folate deficiency from dialysis.	Degree of anemia correlates with the degree of renal failure (not present until the creatinine clearance is <40 mL/min).	Recombinant erythropoietin.	**Serum BUN/creatinine:** increased.
Malignancy. MCV: normocytic. **Reticulocyte count:** <2%. **Key findings:** immature neutrophil precursors and nucleated RBCs if marrow metastasis has occurred (called a **leukoerythroblastic smear**).	**Hypoproliferative:** iron lack from ACD (most common cause).	**Lung cancer:** most common cause of death due to cancer in men and women. **Breast cancer:** most common cancer in women. **Prostate cancer:** most common cancer in men. **Colon cancer:** second most common cancer in both men and women. **Other anemias in malignancy:** metastasis to the marrow with replacement of hematopoietic elements (**myelophthisic anemia**), marrow suppression from chemotherapy, blood loss (colon cancer), autoimmune hemolytic anemia (chronic lymphocytic leukemia), folate deficiency (increased utilization, poor diet).	Anemia is multifactorial and may be due to more than one cause.	Packed RBC transfusions if symptomatic.	**Bone marrow biopsy:** if metastasis is suspected.

TABLE 12–6. Normocytic Anemias: Hemolytic with Corrected Reticulocyte Count >3%

Anemia Characteristics	Pathogenesis	Causes	Clinical Findings	Treatment	Laboratory Tests
Congenital spherocytosis. MCV: normocytic. **Reticulocyte count:** >3%. **Key findings:** *spherocytes* (Figure 12–1B; no central pallor since the RBC is a sphere rather than a biconcave disk), *shift cells.*	**Hemolytic anemia:** macrophage phagocytosis. **Intrinsic hemolytic anemia with extravascular hemolysis.** Defect in spectrin in the cell membrane resulting in a low surface-to-volume ratio and loss of the biconcave disk. Spherocytes are trapped and phagocytosed in the splenic cords.	**Autosomal dominant disease** (highest prevalence in people of Northern European extraction) **Acquired causes** include ABO hemolytic disease of newborns, burns, autoimmune hemolytic anemia.	Triad of anemia, splenomegaly, and jaundice (unconjugated hyperbilirubinemia). Splenectomy should be considered when there is a history of splenectomy in the family or increased incidence of gallstones (jet black calcium bilirubinate stones) at an early age.	Splenectomy (spherocytes remain in the peripheral blood after splenectomy). Must give vaccines to protect against sepsis from *Streptococcus pneumoniae* and *Haemophilus influenzae.*	**Osmotic fragility:** increased. Spherocytes begin hemolysis at 0.65% (increased fragility), whereas normal cells begin to hemolyze at 0.50%. Incubation increases test sensitivity. **Total bilirubin:** increased (primarily unconjugated bilirubin from extravascular hemolysis).
Paroxysmal nocturnal hemoglobinuria (PNH). MCV: normocytic. **Reticulocyte count:** >3%. **Key findings:** pancytopenia, iron deficiency in chronic stages.	**Hemolytic anemia: intravascular hemolysis. Intrinsic hemolytic anemia with intravascular hemolysis.** Acquired deficiency of decay accelerating factor (DAF) on trilineage myeloid stem membrane. Affects RBCs, WBCs, and platelets.	**Abdominal pain.** Signs of iron deficiency in chronic cases due to loss of iron in the urine from hemoglobinuria.	**Episodic hemoglobinuria** noted in the first morning void. Platelet destruction predisposes to vessel **thrombosis** (by releasing thromboxane A$_2$), leading to **hepatic vein thrombosis** (Budd-Chiari syndrome). Possible acute leukemia as a terminal event.	Blood transfusions. Prednisone is useful in some cases when hemolysis is active. Androgens may correct the anemia.	**Sugar-water test:** initial screen for PNH. Sugar water enhances complement attachment to RBCs, leading to RBC hemolysis. **Acidified serum test (Ham's test):** confirmatory test for PNH. **Urine hemosiderin:** usually positive owing to the chronic hemolytic state.
Sickle cell trait and disease. MCV: normocytic. **Reticulocyte count:** >3%. **Key findings:** *sickle cells* (Figure 12–1O), *Howell-Jolly bodies* (Figure 12–1E; remnants of nucleus) when spleen becomes nonfunctional, *target cells* (marker of hemoglobinopathies). Trait has no abnormalities in the peripheral blood.	**Hemolytic anemia: macrophage removal of RBCs. Intrinsic hemolytic anemia with extravascular hemolysis. Mutation:** point mutation with substitution of valine for glutamic acid in the sixth position of the β-globin chain. **Factors that induce sickling:** concentration of HbS in RBC >60% (most important factor), reduced oxygen tension, high altitude, low oxygen tension in renal medulla, presence of other Hbs combined with HbS (e.g., HbC), dehydration (↑MCHC → ↑HbS concentration), acidosis (right-shifts ODC → ↑oxygen released to tissue → ↑amount deoxygenated Hb → sickling). HbF inhibits sickling (high oxygen affinity prevents deoxygenation).	**Prevalence:** HbSS afflicts 1:600 African Americans (most common Hb disorder). 8% of African Americans have HbAS (trait). **Autosomal recessive:** A S A AA AS S AS **SS** 25% disease (SS) 25% normal (AA) 50% trait (AS)	**Two main problems:** chronic hemolytic anemia and vaso-occlusive disease. **Newborns with HbSS do not sickle** until HbF concentration is decreased (takes 6 months to as long as a year before HbF <1%). **Vaso-occlusive disease:** combination of sickled cells blocking the microvasculature and nonsickled cells sticking to the endothelium. **Vaso-occlusive crises** with organ damage are the most common clinical manifestation. **Crises may occur in the following sites:** **hands and feet (dactylitis):** first occurs in a 6- to 9-month old. Bone infarcts produce painful swelling of the hands and feet. **brain:** leads to strokes at an early age. **lungs:** infarction, acute chest syndrome (fever, infiltrate, chest pain), hypoxemia. **liver:** liver cell necrosis. **RBC aplastic crisis:** triggered by a parvovirus infection. Anemia present *without reticulocytosis* (no RBCs produced) or RBC precursors in the bone marrow.	**Painful crises:** managed by hydration (not blood transfusions), analgesics, and oxygen if hypoxemia is present. **Crises requiring blood transfusion:** acute chest syndrome, strokes, aplastic and sequestration crises. **Other treatment:** hydroxyurea increases synthesis of HbF and reduces the number of crises per year. Immunize with Pneumovax and *Haemophilus influenzae* b vaccine. Give prophylactic penicillin.	**Sickle cell screen:** positive. *Solubility test* (Sickledex; uses dithionite) has high specificity for HbS (fewer false positives), but poor sensitivity (more false negatives). *Sodium metabisulfite* reduces oxygen tension and induces sickling (visible sickle cells; both sensitive and specific; better of the two tests). Positive screen always confirmed with a Hb electrophoresis. **Hb electrophoresis** (gold standard test): must document amount of HbS, HbF, or other Hbs that may ameliorate the disease (e.g., HbS/thalassemia). Amount of Hb is quantitated and expressed as a percentage. In **sickle disease:** HbS 90–95%, no HbA, 5–10% HbF. In **sickle trait:** HbS 40–45%, HbA 55–60%. **Sickle cells present peripherally** only in HbSS or HbS/thalassemia but not trait (HbAS). **Low (often zero) erythrocyte sedimentation rate:** sickled cells cannot aggregate to increase their overall density.

Splenic sequestration crisis: marked splenomegaly from sickle cells jammed up in the cords, anemia, and *reticulocytosis* (RBCs are still produced in the marrow).

Complications:

aseptic necrosis of femoral head: infarction of bone with new, reactive bone formation. X-rays reveal increased density. MRI most sensitive test.

pigmented gallstones: due to increased extravascular hemolysis.

functional asplenia: by 2–3 years of age, spleen is nonfunctional. Splenomegaly is present. Howell-Jolly bodies appear in the blood, indicating splenic dysfunction.

autosplenectomy: spleen eventually becomes small and fibrosed due to repeated infarctions.

osteomyelitis: predisposition for *Salmonella* osteomyelitis (*Staphylococcus aureus* still most common osteomyelitis).

increased susceptibility to infections: most commonly *Streptococcus pneumoniae* (most common cause of death in children) and *H. influenzae.* Trait offers some protection against falciparum malaria.

priapism: continual painful erection.

leg ulcers: usually occur around the ankles.

microhematuria: may occur in both sickle trait and disease. Low oxygen tension in renal medulla induces sickling → microinfarctions → hematuria, dilution and concentration defects, and potential for renal papillary necrosis. All African Americans with microhematuria should have a sickle cell screen.

Generalized growth impairment.

Retinal vascular lesions: potential for detachment.

Prenatal diagnosis: in normal genes, **MSTII endonuclease** cleaves the gene on the β-globin chain at the same point mutation site involved in sickle cell trait/disease, hence converting a segment 1.35 kb long into two fragments: one that is 1.15 kb long and one that is 0.2 kb long. MSTII endonuclease cannot cleave this site if the point mutation is present. In HbAS, one chromosome is involved and the other is normal, hence the abnormal chromosome has no cleavage of the 1.35 kb segment, but the normal chromosome splits into one 1.15 kb fragment and one 0.2 kb fragment. In HbSS, both chromosomes are affected, hence there are two 1.35 kb long segments and no smaller fragments.

Table continued on following page

TABLE 12–6. Normocytic Anemias: Hemolytic with Corrected Reticulocyte Count >3% *Continued*

Anemia Characteristics	Pathogenesis	Causes	Clinical Findings	Treatment	Laboratory Tests
Glucose-6-phosphate dehydrogenase (G6PD) deficiency (most common hemolytic anemia due to an enzyme deficiency). **MCV:** normocytic. **Reticulocyte count:** >3%. **Key findings:** *Heinz bodies* (denatured Hb) present in acute hemolytic episodes (Figure 12–1L; need a supravital stain), *bite cells* (Figure 12–1H; macrophage removal of portion of the membrane).	**Hemolytic anemia:** macrophage removal of RBCs. **Intrinsic hemolytic anemia with intravascular** (predominant) **and extravascular hemolysis** (lesser extent). Lack of G6PD leads to a reduction in glutathione (GSH), which is necessary to neutralize peroxide. Peroxide derived from oxidant injury (drugs) and infections (most commonly) denatures Hb, forming **Heinz bodies,** and damages RBC membrane. Heinz bodies attached to RBC membrane are removed by splenic macrophages, resulting in permanent injury to the membrane **(bite cells),** or the total RBC is destroyed extravascularly. Patients are prone to infection owing to the small amount of NADPH available to neutrophils and monocytes that require NADPH as a cofactor for NADPH oxidase in the oxygen-dependent myeloperoxidase system of killing bacteria (for this reason, infection is most common precipitating factor of hemolysis).	**Sex-linked recessive disease** (see Chapter 7). A weak variant occurs in **African Americans** (10%). Defective enzyme (decreased half-life) only present in older RBCs (less severe hemolysis). **Mediterranean variant** has decreased synthesis and defective enzyme present in **all RBCs,** young and old (more severe hemolysis). **Oxidant drugs (mnemonic: AAA) precipitate hemolytic episodes (lag phase of 2–3 days);** *antibiotics* (sulfa drugs), *antimalarials* (primaquine, not chloroquine), *antipyretics* (acetanilid, not aspirin or acetaminophen). **Fava beans** precipitate hemolysis in the Mediterranean variant.	Hemoglobinuria, back pain, dizziness, and palpitations are common in acute hemolytic episodes. G6PD deficiency offers protection against falciparum malaria. G6PD deficiency should always be considered when hemolysis is associated with a drug. Also consider drug-induced autoimmune hemolytic anemia (see below). Coombs' test is the best discriminator of the two anemias.	Avoidance of drugs known to precipitate hemolysis. Splenectomy is of no benefit.	**Active hemolysis:** a Heinz body preparation is used. Enzyme assay may be normal owing to hemolysis of RBCs lacking the enzyme while remaining RBCs have the enzyme. **Asymptomatic state:** an enzyme assay is used.

Disease	Pathophysiology	Etiology	Signs/Symptoms	Treatment	Diagnosis
Autoimmune hemolytic anemia (AIHA). MCV: normocytic. Reticulocyte count: >3%. Key findings: *spherocytes, shift cells, erythrophagocytosis* in the bone marrow.	**Hemolytic anemia:** macrophage removal of RBCs. **Extrinsic hemolytic anemia with extravascular or intravascular hemolysis.** Warm (IgG) type: usually extravascular. Cold (IgM) type: could be intravascular (most common) or extravascular.	**Warm (IgG) type:** systemic lupus erythematosus (most common cause), drugs (penicillin and methyldopa; both are type II hypersensitivity reactions). **Cold (IgM) type:** infection (*Mycoplasma pneumoniae* with anti-I antibodies), infectious mononucleosis with anti-I antibodies, chronic lymphocytic leukemia, drugs (quinidine, isoniazid; immunocomplex or type III hypersensitivity reaction).	Fever, jaundice (unconjugated type when extravascular hemolysis is present), hepatosplenomegaly in both cold and warm types, and generalized lymphadenopathy.	**Avoidance of transfusions if possible.** In most cases, the transfused cells are destroyed. **Warm AIHA:** corticosteroids, if unsuccessful → splenectomy, if unsuccessful → immunosuppressive therapy. May have to use intravenous γ-globulins to block macrophage Fc receptors for IgG to prevent RBC phagocytosis. **Cold AIHA:** alkylating agents. **Drug induced AIHA:** discontinue the offending drug and instruct the patient to never use the drug again.	**Direct Coombs' test:** positive in the majority of cases. **Indirect Coombs' test:** often positive. **Direct Coombs':** RBCs coated by IgG, IgM, or C3 do not agglutinate. Rabbit antibodies against IgG, IgM, or C3 (Coombs' reagent) cross-link subjacent RBCs, causing visible agglutination. Direct Coombs' detects IgG, IgM, or C3 on the RBC membrane. **Indirect Coombs'** (antibody screen): detects antibodies in patient serum (IgM or IgG). First, antibodies must bind to antigens on test blood group O cells (e.g., anti-D against D antigen). Then Coombs' reagent is added, and RBCs with antibodies visibly agglutinate. Specificity of the antibody (anti-D, anti-Kell) requires further testing using antibody panels.
Microangiopathic hemolytic anemia. MCV: normocytic. Reticulocyte count: >3%. Key findings: *schistocytes* (Figure 12–1C; fragmented RBCs).	**Hemolytic anemia:** intravascular. **Extrinsic hemolytic anemia with intravascular hemolysis.**	Prosthetic heart valves. Disseminated intravascular coagulation (DIC). Thrombotic thrombocytopenic purpura. Hemolytic uremic syndrome. Runner's anemia in long-distance runners. HELLP syndrome (preeclampsia + hemolytic anemia).	Varies with the underlying disease state.		**Serum haptoglobin:** decreased. **Urine hemosiderin:** increased. **Iron studies:** iron deficiency may be present owing to the loss of Hb in the urine.

d. Folate is present in both animal and plant products and is primarily reabsorbed in the jejunum and stored in the liver (only a 3- to 4-month supply).

2. Alcohol-related macrocytosis differs from the macrocytosis of B_{12} and folate deficiency in that the macrocytes are round (not egg-shaped), target cells (see Figure 12–1A) are commonly present, and hypersegmented neutrophils and megaloblastic changes in the marrow are not present.

G. Table 12–5 summarizes the **normocytic anemias with a corrected reticulocyte count < 2%**.

H. Table 12–6 summarizes the important differential points of the **hemolytic normocytic anemias with a corrected reticulocyte count > 3%**.

1. Hemolytic anemias are intrinsic, in which something is wrong with the RBC (membrane defect, abnormal Hb, deficient enzyme), or extrinsic, in which something outside the RBC is responsible for hemolysis.

2. The mechanism of hemolysis may be intravascular (within the circulation; reduced serum haptoglobin, hemoglobinuria, hemosiderinuria) or extravascular (RBCs removed by macrophages; increased unconjugated bilirubin).

3. Complications associated with hemolytic anemia include a self-limited aplastic crisis (often associated with a parvovirus infection in sickle cell disease), folate and iron deficiency (rapid turnover of RBCs), extramedullary hematopoiesis, calcium bilirubinate gallstones (chronic extravascular hemolysis—congenital spherocytosis, HbSS), and kernicterus in newborns (e.g., Rh hemolytic disease).

[handwritten margin note: Intravascular ↓ haptoglobin Extravascular ↑ bilirubin]

Objective 5: To understand benign quantitative and qualitative white blood cell disorders.

V. Benign quantitative and qualitative WBC disorders

A. Benign quantitative WBC disorders are summarized in Table 12–7.

B. Qualitative defects may involve structure (e.g., microtubules) or leukocyte function (e.g., problems with adherence, chemotaxis, phagocytosis, or killing).

1. Clues suggesting a qualitative disorder include the presence of unusual pathogens, such as coagulase-negative *Staphylococcus*, frequent infections complicated by growth failure in children, and lack of an inflammatory response to an infection (so-called cold abscess).

2. Laboratory tests frequently used to detect qualitative defects include the nitroblue tetrazolium (NBT) dye test (in which a colorless dye phagocytosed by neutrophils is converted to a colored dye if superoxide is produced in the oxygen-dependent MPO system) and specialized tests for adhesion, chemotaxis, and phagocytosis.

3. Acquired MPO deficiencies are commonly seen in newborns, in pregnancy, and in the neoplastic leukocytes of chronic myelogenous leukemia.

4. The **Chédiak-Higashi** syndrome is an autosomal recessive disease with a primary defect in the polymerization of microtubules in leukocytes leading to abnormalities in chemotaxis,

phagocytosis, phagolysosome formation, and bacterial killing (see Figure 12–2G).

5. **Chronic granulomatous disease** (CGD) of childhood is a sex-linked recessive disease characterized by the absence of NADPH oxidase, leading to an absent respiratory burst mechanism (abnormal NBT dye test).

6. Acquired chemotactic problems are noted in newborns, in leukemic neutrophils, and in people with diabetes, particularly in the setting of ketoacidosis, where hyperosmolarity inhibits chemotaxis.

7. Adhesion defects most often present at birth with failure to separate the umbilical cord, since neutrophils are unable to emigrate from the vasculature to produce an inflammatory response.

Objective 6: To describe the myeloproliferative disorders and the differential diagnosis of polycythemia.

VI. Myeloproliferative disorders (MPDs)

A. MPDs are acquired, neoplastic stem cell disorders characterized by autonomous (unregulated) proliferation or accumulation of one or more hematopoietic elements (RBCs, WBCs, platelets) in the bone marrow, splenomegaly, and a propensity for reactive bone marrow fibrosis during the course of the disease.

B. **Polycythemia vera** (PV) is an MPD associated with an increase in RBCs, WBCs, and platelets.

1. In the workup of PV, other causes of polycythemia (increased RBC count) must be excluded.

2. Polycythemia may be absolute (true increase in RBC mass reported as mL/kg) or relative (normal RBC mass but decreased plasma volume, hence increasing the RBC count in cells/μL).

3. An arterial blood gas measurement determines whether polycythemia is appropriate (e.g., hypoxemia/hypoxia stimulation of erythropoietin) or inappropriate (e.g., no hypoxemia/hypoxia stimulus for erythropoietin).

4. The classification of the polycythemia states is summarized Table 12–8, and their differential features are further summarized in Table 12–9.

C. **Chronic myelogenous (granulocytic) leukemia** (CML) is an MPD having primarily an increase in WBCs and platelets to a lesser extent.

D. **Agnogenic myeloid metaplasia** (AMM) is an MPD characterized by massive hepatosplenomegaly owing to extramedullary hematopoiesis secondary to reactive myelofibrosis in the bone marrow.

E. **Essential thrombocythemia** (ET) is an MPD with a primary increase in platelets (>600,000 cells/μL) and WBCs to a lesser extent.

F. MPDs may evolve into each other or terminate as acute leukemia, the latter invariably occurring in CML.

G. Table 12–10 summarizes the MPDs.

Objective 7: To review the myelodysplastic syndrome and acute and chronic leukemias.

VII. Myelodysplastic syndrome (MDS) and acute and chronic leukemias

TABLE 12–7. Benign Quantitative White Blood Cell Disorders

Leukocyte Disorder Characteristics	Pathogenesis	Causes	Clinical Findings	Laboratory Findings
Absolute neutrophilic leukocytosis. **Definition:** absolute count >7000 cells/μL. **Key findings:** *left shift* (presence of immature neutrophils in the peripheral blood [>10% band neutrophils] or any neutrophil younger than a band), *toxic granulation* (Figure 12–2A; increase in azurophilic granules), *cytoplasmic vacuoles* (phagolysosomes, indicating the presence of phagocytosis), and *Döhle's bodies* (Figure 12–2D; dull gray inclusions representing parallel strands of rough endoplasmic reticulum).	**Increased production:** infection. **Decreased margination (decreased adhesion):** corticosteroids, epinephrine. **Increased release from marrow postmitotic pool:** infection.	**Infections:** acute appendicitis. **Sterile inflammation:** myocardial infarction, blood in body cavities. **Physiologic:** stress. **Myeloproliferative disease:** polycythemia rubra vera, chronic myelogenous leukemia. **Metabolic disease:** uremia, ketoacidosis. **Hematologic disease:** acute hemolytic disease. **Drugs (decrease adhesion molecule synthesis):** corticosteroids, lithium, epinephrine. **Endocrine:** pheochromocytoma, Cushing's syndrome. **Miscellaneous:** smoking, tumor necrosis.	Varies with the clinical condition.	**Complete blood cell count (CBC) with a 100 WBC differential count.** **Bone marrow examination:** usually not necessary. **Blood cultures:** if infection is suspected.
Leukemoid reaction. **Definition:** >30,000 (often >50,000) leukocytes/μL. May involve any leukocyte (neutrophil, eosinophil, lymphocyte). **Key findings:** absence of myeloblasts or lymphoblasts in the peripheral blood or bone marrow.	Exaggerated benign leukocyte response to infection (common in children) or malignancy (especially those with increased necrosis) with a superimposed infection.	**Infections:** tuberculosis, whooping cough, infectious lymphocytosis, perforated acute appendicitis.	Frequently confused with leukemia (especially chronic myelogenous leukemia). **Factors favoring a leukemoid reaction** include fever, resolution with treatment of infection, increased leukocyte alkaline phosphatase score (see laboratory findings), absence of splenomegaly or abnormal chromosomes (e.g., Philadelphia chromosome), bone marrow examination with reactive leukocytosis.	**Leukocyte alkaline phosphatase (LAP) score:** LAP is present in specific granules and is a marker of a mature neutrophil. Neutrophils are stained for alkaline phosphatase and scored (0 to 4) for the intensity of uptake of the stain in a 100 cell count. Leukemoid reactions have an increased LAP score, since this is a benign reactive process. Chronic myelogenous leukemia has a low score, since the cells are neoplastic.
Leukoerythroblastic reaction. **Definition:** *immature WBCs* (myeloblasts, progranulocytes) and *nucleated RBCs* in the peripheral blood.	Peripheralization of bone marrow elements secondary to metastasis, severe bone fractures, or replacement of the bone marrow by fibrosis, an overgrowth of bone, or abnormal cells.	**Metastasis:** breast cancer (most common cause), lung cancer. **Fibrosis:** agnogenic myeloid metaplasia, metastasis with reactive fibrosis, leukemia (chronic myelogenous leukemia), polycythemia vera. **Abnormal cells:** leukemia. **Fracture:** pelvic fracture, multiple comminuted fractures. **Excess bone:** osteopetrosis (Chapter 20).	Extramedullary hematopoiesis with massive hepatosplenomegaly often accompanies marrow replacement by fibrosis.	**Bone marrow examination:** identifies the source of the reaction.
Absolute neutropenia. **Definition:** absolute count 1000–1500 cells/μL (mild), 500–1000 cells/μL (moderate), <500 cells/μL (severe).	**Decreased production.** **Increased destruction.** **Increased margination (increased adhesion molecule synthesis).** **Maturation defect** (failure of neutrophils to mature in the marrow; "arrested development" at a stage of development).	**Hematologic disorders:** production problem (aplastic anemia), destruction problems (B$_{12}$/folate deficiency, paroxysmal nocturnal hemoglobinuria). **Drugs (production problem):** chloramphenicol, alkylating agents (busulfan the worst), phenylbutazone (NSAID), propylthiouracil (antithyroid medication), methotrexate. **Chemicals (production problems):** benzene (also danger of acute leukemia), insecticides. **Infectious diseases:** typhoid (characteristic finding), NANB hepatitis (aplastic anemia). **Increased destruction:** autoimmune neutropenia (SLE), Felty's syndrome (autoimmune neutropenia + rheumatoid arthritis). **Increased margination:** endotoxins in gram-negative sepsis, a normal finding in African Americans.	**Counts <500 cells/μL impose a serious risk for infection** (neutropenia + fever = infection). **Bacteria:** gram negatives. **Fungi:** *Candida.* **Viruses:** Herpes simplex. **Cyclic neutropenia:** occurs about every 21 days and is associated with fever, aphthous ulcers, and furuncles. Probable stem cell defect.	CBC. **Bone marrow examination:** rule out aplastic anemia versus maturation defect versus increased margination.

Table continued on following page

163

TABLE 12–7. Benign Quantitative White Blood Cell Disorders *Continued*

Leukocyte Disorder Characteristics	Pathogenesis	Causes	Clinical Findings	Laboratory Findings
Absolute lymphocytosis. **Definition:** **Adults:** >4000 cells/μL. **Children:** >8000 cells/μL. **Infants:** 11,000–17,000 cells/μL. **Atypical lymphocytes:** antigen stimulated lymphocytes (Figure 12–2D), with prominent nucleoli and bluish discoloration of the cytoplasm (RNA synthesis).	**Increased production of lymphocytes** (antigen driven): viral infections. **Increased release from lymph nodes** (decreased adhesion in efferent lymphatics): whooping cough.	**Infections:** **viral:** infectious mononucleosis (IM), cytomegalovirus (CMV), infectious lymphocytosis, mumps, measles, roseola, varicella, hepatitis, mononucleosis-like syndrome in the initial seroconversion in HIV. **bacterial:** whooping cough (lymphocytosis promoting factor), tuberculosis, brucellosis, *Mycoplasma*. **parasitic:** toxoplasmosis. **Autoimmune disease:** SLE. **Endocrine:** Graves' disease. **Drugs:** phenytoin. **Malignancy:** acute and chronic lymphocytic leukemia.	**Conditions with atypical lymphocytes:** IM (most common cause), CMV, toxoplasmosis, phenytoin, viral hepatitis, roseola, mumps, measles, varicella. **Conditions with mature** (nonreactive) **lymphocytes:** whooping cough, infectious lymphocytosis (probably viral; self-limited). Children commonly respond to infections with a pronounced lymphocytosis, often in leukemoid ranges.	**CBC:** atypical lymphocytosis is >10% atypical lymphocytes in a 100 cell differential count. **Viral cultures:** CMV (urine best to culture). **Serologic tests:** hepatitis, toxoplasmosis, HIV. **Bone marrow examination:** to rule out acute/chronic lymphocytic leukemia versus leukemoid reaction.
Infectious mononucleosis (IM): atypical lymphocytosis. **Definition:** infection by Epstein-Barr virus (EBV). **Key findings:** atypical lymphocytes designated *Downey cells*.	Transmitted by saliva, blood transfusion. Virus initially replicates in the oropharynx and salivary glands. EBV infects B cells (all B cells have EBV receptors; CD21) and remains in B cells indefinitely. Atypical lymphocytes (Figure 12–2D) are T cells reacting against infected B cells.	**Epstein-Barr virus.** **Other EBV associations:** hairy leukoplakia on the tongue (often precedes onset of AIDS), sex-linked lymphoproliferative syndrome, nasopharyngeal carcinoma, polyclonal malignant lymphoma, primary CNS malignant lymphoma (in association with HIV). **Mononucleosis-like syndromes:** CMV (most common), toxoplasmosis, seroconversion stage in HIV. Less severe pharyngitis and lymphadenopathy in CMV and toxoplasmosis than in IM.	**Common findings:** exudative tonsillitis (due to the virus or group A streptococcus), petechiae on the palate, sudden onset of a rash when ampicillin is given, posterior cervical adenopathy, tender hepatosplenomegaly (jaundice is uncommon), generalized painful lymphadenopathy.	**CBC:** atypical lymphocytosis >20%. **Serologic tests:** positive heterophile antibody test (e.g., Monospot) in >96% of cases (false negatives more common in children <2 years old and the elderly). Heterophile antibody is an IgM antibody against sheep RBCs and horse RBCs (basis of the Monospot test). **EBV serologies:** anti-VCA (viral capsid antigen) IgM best test (sensitivity of 100%). Anti-EA (early antigen) has 70% sensitivity in acute IM. Anti-EBNA (Epstein-Barr nuclear antigen) antibodies occur late in the disease.
Absolute lymphopenia. **Definition:** **adults:** <1500 cells/μL. **children:** <3000 cells/μL.	**Decreased production.** **Increased destruction.** **Decreased release from lymph nodes** (increased adhesion in the efferent lymphatics). **Loss of lymphocytes.**	**Drugs:** corticosteroids (increased adhesion), alkylating agents (cyclophosphamide), antilymphocyte serum. **Autoimmune destruction:** SLE. **Immunodeficiency syndromes:** DiGeorge syndrome (T-cell deficiency), AIDS, severe combined immunodeficiency. **Direct loss:** protein-losing enteropathies associated with lymphatic blockage (intestinal lymphangiectasia, increased lymphatic pressure from chronic heart failure). **Endocrine:** Cushing's syndrome (effect of cortisol).	Clinical findings in B- and T-cell deficiencies are discussed in Chapter 4. **Corticosteroids have multiple effects on leukocytes:** absolute neutrophilic leukocytosis (decreased adhesion molecule synthesis), absolute lymphopenia (increased lymphocyte adhesion in lymph nodes and lymphocytotoxicity effect), and eosinopenia (toxic effect on eosinophils).	**CBC.**

Eosinophilia/Eosinopenia. **Definition:** Eosinophilia: >700 cells/μL. Eosinopenia: notable absence of eosinophils on a peripheral smear.	**Eosinophilia:** release of eosinophil chemotactic factor from mast cells/basophils in type I IgE-mediated hypersensitivity reactions. **Eosinopenia:** toxic effect on eosinophils.	**Eosinophilia:** **Type I hypersensitivity reactions:** asthma, hay fever, drug reactions (penicillin, iodides). **Parasitic diseases:** invasive helminthic (not protozoal, pinworm, or adult ascariasis) diseases such as the larval (not adult) phase of ascariasis, strongyloidiasis, ancylostomiasis, trichinosis. **Neoplasia:** chronic myelogenous leukemia, Hodgkin's disease. **Myeloproliferative diseases:** polycythemia vera, chronic myelogenous leukemia. **Endocrine:** Addison's disease. **Autoimmune disease:** polyarteritis nodosa. **Pulmonary disease:** Loeffler syndrome, allergic bronchopulmonary aspergillosis, hypereosinophilic syndrome. **Eosinopenia:** acute stress, corticosteroid use, Cushing's syndrome.	Eosinophils have crystalline material in their granules, which form **Charcot-Leyden crystals** in the sputum of asthmatics. Eosinophil count is not a good indicator of type I hypersensitivity reactions.	**CBC.** **Nasal smear for eosinophils:** allergic rhinitis. **Urine stain for eosinophils:** rule out drug-induced acute interstitial disease as a cause of oliguria, skin rash, and azotemia. **Total eosinophil count:** No longer a practical test.
Basophilia. Definition: >110 cells/μL.	Unknown.	**Myeloproliferative diseases:** excellent marker for polycythemia rubra vera, chronic myelogenous leukemia. Greater than 5% basophils in a WBC differential is highly suggestive of a myeloproliferative disorder. **Miscellaneous:** hypersensitivity reactions, myxedema, varicella, ulcerative colitis.	Mast cells and basophils in the skin may degranulate after a warm bath or shower, with subsequent release of histamine and the onset of severe pruritus.	CBC.
Monocytosis. Definition: >800 cells/μL.	Usually associated with chronic inflammation.	**Chronic infection:** tuberculosis, subacute bacterial endocarditis, syphilis, brucellosis. **Chronic inflammation:** autoimmune disease (SLE, rheumatoid arthritis), ulcerative colitis, Crohn's disease. **Malignancy:** malignant lymphoma, carcinoma, acute and chronic monocytic leukemia. **Miscellaneous:** recovery phase in the marrow after acute infections or neutrophil suppression, myelodysplasia syndrome.	Marker of chronic inflammation.	**CBC.** **Bone marrow examination:** if monocytic leukemia or myelodysplasia is suspected.

TABLE 12–8. Differential Diagnosis of the Polycythemia Disorders

Condition	RBC Mass	Plasma Volume	SaO₂*	Erythropoietin
Polycythemia vera	Increased	Increased	Normal	Decreased
Chronic obstructive pulmonary disease	Increased	Normal	Decreased	Increased
Cyanotic congenital heart disease	Increased	Normal	Decreased	Increased
Renal adenocarcinoma	Increased	Normal	Normal	Increased
Smoker's polycythemia	Increased	Decreased	Variable	Variable
Stress polycythemia	Normal	Decreased	Normal	Normal
Dehydration	Normal	Decreased	Normal	Normal

* SaO_2 = arterial oxygen saturation.

A. MDS is a malignant stem cell disorder characterized by cytopenias in the peripheral blood, megaloblastic change in the marrow, ringed sideroblasts, and a propensity for progressing to acute leukemia (Table 12–11).

B. Leukemia is a malignancy of hematopoietic stem cells within the bone marrow that may involve all cell lines including neutrophils, lymphocytes, monocytes, megakaryocytes, and erythroid cells.

1. Leukemic cells ultimately replace the bone marrow, enter the peripheral blood, and infiltrate tissues throughout the body.

2. They are subdivided into acute and chronic types, the former characterized by an abrupt onset and > 30% blasts (e.g., myeloblasts, lymphoblasts, etc.) in the bone marrow, while the latter has an insidious onset, some evidence of maturation of cells in both the peripheral blood and bone marrow, and < 30% blasts in the bone marrow (see Table 12–11).

3. Leukemia may be lymphocytic or myelogenous (nonlymphocytic), the latter referring to leukocytes derived from the trilineage myeloid stem cell (neutrophils, monocytes, eosinophils, basophils, megakaryocytes, and erythroid cells).

4. The frequency of these leukemias by age bracket is as follows: newborn to 14 years, acute lymphoblastic leukemia; 15–39 years, acute myelogenous leukemia; 40–60 years, acute myelogenous leukemia (~60%) and chronic myelogenous leukemia (~40%); and > 60 years, chronic lymphocytic leukemia.

5. Leukemic cells crowd out other hematopoietic elements, hence producing anemia, thrombocytopenia, and peripheralization of blasts and other marrow elements (leukoerythroblastic reaction).

6. Cytogenetic abnormalities are common and often have diagnostic and prognostic significance (e.g., Philadelphia chromosome).

7. Predisposing causes of leukemia include chromosomal abnormalities (e.g., trisomy 21 in Down syndrome), ionizing radiation (atomic bomb), chemicals (e.g., benzene), alkylating agents (particularly busulfan), and immunodeficiency syndromes (e.g., Wiskott-Aldrich syndrome).

8. Clinical features include fever (usually related to infection), fatigue (anemia), bleeding (thrombocytopenia), organomegaly (e.g., hepatosplenomegaly), generalized lymphadenopathy, bone pain (leukemic expansion of the marrow space and invasion of the periosteum), and disseminated intravascular coagulation (particularly acute progranulocytic leukemia).

9. Laboratory abnormalities consist of a normocytic anemia, leukoerythroblastic reaction (immature leukocytes plus nucleated RBCs in the peripheral blood), leukocytosis with circulating blasts, thrombocytopenia, and a hypercellular bone marrow packed with blasts.

10. Important special stains include peroxidase, Sudan black B, and specific esterases (naphthol ASD chloroacetate) for the granulocytic leukemias; nonspecific esterase for the monocytic leukemias; periodic acid–Schiff (PAS) for lymphoblasts and the bizarre erythroblasts of Di Guglielmo's erythroleukemia; tartrate-resistant acid phosphatases (TRAPs) for the neoplastic B cells of hairy cell leukemia; platelet peroxidases for acute megakaryocytic leukemia; and immunophenotyping of leukocytes in identifying B and T cell leukemias.

Objective 8: To discuss sepsis and selected disorders that commonly involve blood.

VIII. Sepsis

A. Sepsis is the systemic response of the host to severe infection.

1. Microbial infections in the blood include bacteremia (bacteria), fungemia (fungi), parasitemia (parasitic organisms), and viremia (viruses).

2. The systemic response includes fever > 38°C or < 36°C, heart rate > 90 beats/min, increased respiratory rate (> 20 breaths/min), and WBC count > 12,000 cells/μL or < 4000 cells/μL with > 10% of the neutrophils representing bands (left-shifted smear).

3. Sepsis may be associated with gram-positive or -negative bacteria, fungi, certain viruses, and rickettsial organisms and often progresses to septic shock and multisystem organ failure.

4. Patient risk factors include immunosuppression (e.g., treatment of cancer), previous splenectomy, diabetes mellitus (e.g., glucose is an excellent culture medium), therapeutic procedures (e.g., indwelling urinary catheters [the

main source of gram-negative sepsis in the hospital] and ventilators [which transmit *Pseudomonas aeruginosa*, a water-loving bacterium]).

5. Hospital risk factors consist of venipuncture and any intravenous or indwelling line in place for over 48 hours (*Staphylococcus aureus* is the most common pathogen).

6. Some diseases predisposing to sepsis are pyelonephritis (*Escherichia coli*), burns (*P. aeruginosa*), pneumonia (*Streptococcus pneumoniae*), biliary tract infections, and AIDS.

B. Blood cultures are important in the workup of sepsis.

1. Volume of blood collected for blood culture (aerobic and anaerobic) is more important than the timing of collection.

2. Indications for blood cultures include fever of unknown origin (FUO), localized infections (e.g., typhoid fever), suspected infective endocarditis, and unexpected rapid deterioration in any patient.

3. The two most common pathogens isolated in blood are *S. aureus* and *E. coli*.

4. The most common contaminants are *Bacillus* species, *Corynebacterium* species, and coagulase-negative *Staphylococcus*.

IX. Selected disorders

A. **Relapsing fever** is caused by *Borrelia recurrentis*, a gram-negative spirochete.

1. Ticks and the human body louse are potential vectors for the disease.

2. The relapses of high fever are secondary to the emergence of new antigen types.

3. The organisms are commonly visualized in peripheral smears during relapses (70% of cases).

B. **Leptospirosis**, or **Weil's syndrome**, is most commonly caused by the spirochete *Leptospira interrogans*.

1. *Leptospira* is a tightly wound spirochete with a crook at the end that resembles a shepherd's staff (best visualized by darkfield microscopy in urine).

2. Important reservoirs for the spirochetes are rodents and domesticated animals (most commonly dogs), which shed the organisms in their urine.

3. Leptospirosis is biphasic, having a septicemic and an immune phase.

4. Severe disease (Weil's) is associated with jaundice, an extensive hemorrhagic diathesis, and renal failure (tubulointerstitial disease).

5. Urine is the best body fluid in which to identify the organism.

C. Hemoflagellates are protozoans that produce disease via organisms that may be intracellular (within macrophages), in which case they are called leishmania (amastigotes), or extracellular (in blood), in which case they are called trypanosomes (trypomastigotes).

1. In **leishmaniasis**, only the leishmanial forms are present in humans; in **African trypanosomiasis**, only the extracellular, or trypanosomal form, is present; and in **American trypanosomiasis**, or **Chagas' disease**, both the intracellular and extracellular forms are present.

2. **African trypanosomiasis**, or **sleeping sick-**

ness, is caused by *Trypanosoma brucei gambiense* or *Trypanosoma brucei rhodesiense*, which is introduced into humans by the bite of an infected tsetse fly *(Glossina)*.

a. Trypanosomes invade the blood and lymphatics (lymphadenopathy; Winterbottom's sign in the posterior cervical nodes) early in the disease.

b. Later in the disease, trypanosomes enter the CNS, where in addition to fever, they produce headache and diffuse encephalitis characterized by somnolence (due to sleep mediators produced by the organism).

c. Starvation is the most common cause of death.

d. Trypanosomes are capable of antigen variation (thus, the persistent elevation of IgM early in the disease).

e. Suramin or pentamidine is used for treatment in non-CNS disease, while melarsoprol is preferred for CNS infection.

3. **American trypanosomiasis** is caused by *Trypanosoma cruzi*, which is a flagellated protozoan that is transmitted to humans by the bite of the reduviid bug (*Triatoma*, or kissing bug).

a. The bite usually occurs during the night (often around the eye) and is introduced into the skin after the bug defecates on the wound site and the material is rubbed into the wound by the patient (Romaña's sign).

b. In South America, it is the major cause of progressive heart failure leading to death.

c. Trypanosomes circulate in the blood, and leishmanial forms invade macrophages in the liver and spleen (hepatosplenomegaly), heart muscle (myocarditis, arrhythmias), CNS (meningoencephalitis), and gastrointestinal tract (motility disturbances in the distal esophagus [acquired achalasia] and distal colon [acquired Hirschsprung's disease]).

d. The laboratory diagnosis is secured by finding trypanosomes in the blood or leishmanial forms in tissue.

e. Xenodiagnosis refers to the use of sterile reduviid bugs in confirming the diagnosis (they feed on the patient and then are sacrificed for organism identification).

f. Nifurtimox is the drug of choice.

4. **Leishmaniasis** is a complex of three different diseases: visceral leishmaniasis due to *Leishmania donovani* complex; cutaneous leishmaniasis due to *Leishmania tropica* complex; and mucocutaneous leishmaniasis due to *Leishmania viannia* (formerly *braziliensis*), *mexicana*, or *tropica*; or mucocutaneous leishmaniasis secondary to *Leishmania viannia braziliensis*.

a. Organisms are introduced into humans by the bite of an infected sandfly (*Phlebotomus, Lutzomyia, Psychodopygus*).

b. **Visceral leishmaniasis**, or **kala-azar**, is characterized by intracellular invasion of macrophages by leishmanial forms, leading to massive hepatosplenomegaly and anemia.

c. The laboratory diagnosis of visceral leishmaniasis is secured by performing a bone marrow aspirate and identifying the leish-

TABLE 12–9. Myeloproliferative Disorders (MPDs)

Definition	Pathogenesis	Clinical Findings	Treatment	Laboratory Findings
Polycythemia vera (PV). **Definition:** Hct >52% in an adult male, Hct >48% in an adult female, Hct >65% in a newborn.	**Adult:** clonal expansion of the trilineage myeloid stem cell associated with a primary increase in RBC mass, plasma volume, and granulocytes and platelets to a lesser extent. Only MPD with an increase in RBC mass (RBC mass is not equivalent with RBC count). **Newborn:** placental insufficiency with hypoxemia-induced polycythemia, a twin-to-twin bleed in a monochorionic placenta, or a patient with Down syndrome who is subject to developing myeloproliferative disease.	Slightly more common in men than women. Median age of 60 years. **Hypervolemia:** increase in plasma volume. Unique to PV and no other causes of polycythemia. **Hyperviscosity:** increased RBC mass. Predisposes to thrombotic episodes (most common cause of death) including myocardial infarction, stroke, bowel infarction, hepatic vein thrombosis (Budd-Chiari syndrome), retinal vein thrombosis. **Hyperuricemia (70%):** increased breakdown of nucleated cells and increase in purine metabolism. **Histaminemia:** increased release of histamine from basophils and mast cells. Associated with vasodilation (plethoric-appearing face) and pruritus (release reaction of mast cells after warm baths), and peptic ulcer disease from histamine stimulation of gastric acid. **Miscellaneous findings:** splenomegaly (70%), GI bleeding (qualitative platelet abnormalities; iron deficiency), acute myelogenous leukemia (rare terminal event), enhanced atherosclerosis (possible relationship with thrombocytosis). **Differential diagnosis from other polycythemias:** see text.	**Phlebotomy:** phlebotomy alone is the treatment of choice. Purpose is to reduce RBC mass and to render the patient iron deficient, so there is less RBC production in the bone marrow. **Phlebotomy plus chemotherapy (hydroxyurea).** **Phlebotomy plus radioactive ^{32}P** (danger of acute leukemia). **Average survival:** 10–16 years.	**Category A criteria:** A1: increased RBC mass. A2: oxygen saturation >92%. A3: splenomegaly. **Category B criteria:** B1: thrombocytosis with a platelet count >400,000 cells/μL. B2: leukocytosis with a WBC count >12,000 cells/μL in the absence of fever. B3: elevated leukocyte alkaline phosphatase score (>100). B4: serum B$_{12}$ >900 pg/mL (due to increase in neutrophils, which carry B$_{12}$ bound to transcobalamin I). **Scoring system:** A1 + A2 + A3 present = PV. A1 + A2 and two parameters from category B = PV. **Note:** RBC mass (^{51}chromium study) is not the same as an increase in RBC count or an increase in Hct, although they sometimes parallel each other. RBC mass is expressed in RBC mL/kg of body weight, while RBC count is cells/μL. Hence, a decrease in plasma volume (dehydration) increases the RBC count, but the RBC mass is normal. **Plasma volume (radioisotope test):** increased (only MPD with an increase in plasma volume). **Bone marrow examination:** always indicated in any MPD. Marrow is hypercellular, and all hematopoietic elements are increased (except lymphocytes). Iron deficiency is frequently present (low MCV) if the patient has been phlebotomized or has persistent GI bleeding. Marrow fibrosis is common. **Plasma erythropoietin:** low, since RBC mass and total oxygen content are increased (useful test in distinguishing PV from the other causes of polycythemia). **Peripheral blood:** packed RBCs, increased platelets, neutrophils (mature, not a left-shifted smear), possible pseudo-Pelger-Huët cells (Figure 12–2B; condensed, hyperchromatic nuclei), basophilia/eosinophilia (excellent markers for MPD), giant platelets. **Note:** if iron deficiency is present, microcytic cells and hypochromasia are present. The Hb concentration may be in the normal range, the MCV low, and the RBC count elevated, the latter two findings similar to those seen in thalassemia.

Chronic myelogenous (granulocytic) leukemia (CML).

Definition: neoplastic clonal expansion of the pluripotential stem cell, so virtually any cell lineage may be involved including RBCs, granulocytes, megakaryocytes, B and T cells.

Predisposing factors: radiation (1945 atomic bomb), benzene.
Chromosome abnormality: t9;22 translocation of **abl** oncogene from chromosome 9 to chromosome 22 with fusion at the **break cluster region (bcr)** to form a fusion gene → continual tyrosine kinase activity → increased mitotic activity. Presence of **bcr-c-abl fusion gene** (present in 100%; sensitivity of 100% and 100% specific for CML). **Chromosome 22 is Philadelphia chromosome** (high sensitivity for CML but not 100% specific).

Second most common leukemia between age 40 and 60 years. Slightly male dominant.
Signs of anemia: malaise, fatigue.
Hypermetabolic state: due to the increased turnover of large numbers of cells. Associated with hyperuricemia, fever, weight loss, and sweating.
Hepatosplenomegaly and generalized lymphadenopathy: splenic infarcts are common.
Soft tissue collections of leukemic cells: called **chloromas** (granulocytic sarcoma). In children, they commonly locate in the orbit.
Accelerated phase/blast crisis: After ~3 years progresses to accelerated phase (new cytogenetic abnormalities) or a blast crisis with 70% of blasts representing myeloblasts and 30% lymphoblasts. **Lymphoid blast crises** (25-30% of cases).

Busulfan or hydroxyurea is the mainstay of therapy. Bone marrow transplantation is the only curative treatment. α-Interferon therapy is also used. Philadelphia chromosome is not lost in treatment. About 85% of patients die when in the blast crisis. Prognosis is poorer if Philadelphia chromosome is absent.

CBC:
Normocytic normochromic anemia.
WBC findings: mature and immature WBCs (myelocyte most abundant cell) with counts between 50,000-200,000 cells/μL. Pseudo-Pelger-Huët cells (Figure 12-2B). Increased basophils/eosinophils. Myeloblasts <10% of total cells. Leukoerythroblastic smear with immature granulocyte elements and nucleated RBCs.
Platelets: Thrombocytosis (40-50% of cases) or thrombocytopenia. Only leukemia with potential for thrombocytosis.
Bone marrow examination: hypercellular bone marrow. Marrow fibrosis common. Increased M/E ratio and <10% myeloblasts.
Chromosome studies: Philadelphia chromosome positive in 95%. Positive bcr fusion gene study in 100%.
LAP score: low (very useful in distinguishing it from other disorders having an increased neutrophil count).

Agnogenic myeloid metaplasia (AMM).

Definition: proliferation of neoplastic stem cells that begins in the bone marrow (replaced by fibrosis) and later relocates in the spleen, where the primary process continues as a trilineage production of RBCs, granulocytes, and platelets (extramedullary hematopoiesis).

Bone marrow fibrosis is benign reactive fibroblast proliferation. Megakaryocytes secrete transforming growth factor-β and platelet-derived growth factor, which stimulate marrow fibrosis. Residual RBCs are deformed by fibrous tissue when entering the sinusoids, hence producing the classic **teardrop** (Figure 12-1F) appearance.

Uncommon in patients <60 years of age.
Massive splenomegaly: secondary to extramedullary hematopoiesis. Splenic infarcts are common (friction rub over the infarction site + left-sided pleural effusion as a reaction to injury).
Portal hypertension: backup of blood into the portal vein from the splenic vein (portal vein = splenic vein + superior mesenteric vein). Myelofibrosis in the marrow must be differentiated from metastatic disease to the marrow (reactive myelofibrosis). Crowding out of hematopoietic elements produces anemia (called **myelophthisic anemia**).
Blast crisis: occurs in 10% of cases.

No specific treatment. Splenectomy does not improve survival. Median survival is 1-5 years from the initial diagnosis.

CBC:
Normocytic normochromic anemia with teardrop cells.
WBC findings: WBC count between 10,000 and 50,000 cells/μL. Leukoerythroblastic smear. Basophilia/eosinophilia present.
Platelets: thrombocytosis in 50%.
Bone marrow examination: bone marrow fibrosis (dry tap is common).
LAP score: normal to high LAP score (helps distinguish it from CML).
Chromosome studies: absent Philadelphia chromosome.

Essential thrombocythemia (EP).

Definition: stem cell disease with a platelet count >600,000 cells/μL (often >1,000,000) and abnormal-appearing megakaryocytes in the bone marrow.

Clonal stem cell disorder with a preference for proliferation of megakaryocytes.

Patients generally >50 years old. Least common MPD.
Bleeding abnormalities: common finding owing to qualitative platelet defects. Bleeding is usually gastrointestinal and produces iron deficiency. Distinction between chronic iron deficiency with reactive thrombocytosis and essential thrombocythemia is important.
Neurologic findings: transient ischemic attacks are common.
Splenomegaly (80%).

Alkylating agents and platelet pheresis. Compatible with a long life (best prognosis of the MPDs).

CBC:
Normocytic to microcytic anemia (if bleeding present).
WBC findings: neutrophilic leukocytosis between 10,000 and 40,000 cells/μL. Basophilia/eosinophilia present.
Platelets: count >600,000 cells/μL and often in the millions. Platelets have abnormal morphology (see Figure 12-2F) and abnormal function (prolonged bleeding time).
Bone marrow examination: increased numbers of dysplastic (abnormal) megakaryocytes.

TABLE 12–10. Classification of Polycythemia*

Subtype of Polycythemia	Causes/Discussion
Absolute polycythemia: appropriate ($\downarrow PaO_2/SaO_2$)	**Chronic obstructive pulmonary disease:** most common cause in this category. **High altitude residents:** percentage of oxygen is 21% but the atmospheric pressure is decreased, leading to low PaO_2. **Cyanotic congenital heart disease:** right to left shunt. **Hypoventilation syndromes (sleep apnea, pickwickian syndrome):** retention of CO_2 leads to automatic reduction in PaO_2. **Left-shifted oxygen dissociation curve:** decreased release of oxygen to tissue leads to tissue hypoxia; e.g., CO poisoning (low SaO_2, normal PaO_2), methemoglobinemia (low SaO_2, normal PaO_2), increased Hb F (newborn).
Absolute polycythemia: inappropriate (normal PaO_2/SaO_2); low and high erythropoietin types	**Polycythemia vera:** normal PaO_2/SaO_2 and low erythropoietin (total oxygen content of blood is increased owing to increased Hb concentration). **Renal disorders:** increased erythropoietin. Renal adenocarcinoma, Wilms' tumor, renal cysts, hydronephrosis. **Endocrine disorders:** Cushing's syndrome (cortisol and 17-ketosteroids stimulate erythropoiesis). **Miscellaneous:** Uterine leiomyomas (compression of ureters). Cerebellar hemangioblastoma (part of Lindau–von Hippel disease: increased incidence of renal adenocarcinoma). Hepatocellular carcinoma (ectopic erythropoietin production).
Relative polycythemia: $\downarrow$ plasma volume, normal RBC mass	**Smoker's polycythemia:** unexplained effects of CO in smoke on increased RBC mass and tobacco smoke lower plasma volume. **Stress polycythemia (Gaisböck's syndrome):** individuals under constant stress. Typically males with hypertension and obesity. **Dehydration:** volume contraction.

* PaO_2, partial pressure of arterial oxygen; SaO_2, arterial oxygen saturation.

manial forms in macrophages (similar in appearance to *Histoplasma*).

d. **Cutaneous** and **mucocutaneous leishmaniasis** limit themselves to the skin alone (ulcers) in the former disease and skin plus mucous membranes in the latter variant.

e. The diagnosis of cutaneous or mucocutaneous leishmaniasis is made by biopsy, culture, skin testing, or serologic tests.

f. Stibogluconate is the treatment of choice (pentamidine may be added for antimony resistance).

D. *Babesia microti* is the sporozoan responsible for **babesiosis**.

1. The organism parasitizes RBCs after it is introduced into the patient by the bite of an infected ixodid tick (the same tick that transmits *Borrelia burgdorferi* to produce Lyme disease).

2. Babesiosis is endemic in the United States along the Eastern seaboard, particularly in Massachusetts (Martha's Vineyard) and New York (Long Island).

3. Clinically, patients present with chills, fever, headache, and a mild hemolytic anemia.

4. The laboratory diagnosis is secured by examining the peripheral blood for intraerythrocytic organisms (similar in morphology to malaria and *Bartonella*) or by using serologic tests or hamster inoculation.

5. Clindamycin plus quinine is used for treatment.

E. **Malaria** is a sporozoan disease consisting of four *Plasmodium* species that are pathogenic to humans: *P. vivax* (the most common), *P. falciparum* (the most deadly), *P. malariae*, and *P. ovale*.

1. Similarly to *Babesia*, malarial organisms infect RBCs.

2. Table 12–12 summarizes these species with regard to their frequency, peripheral blood findings, fever patterns, and existence of relapses (reinfection of the liver).

3. The female *Anopheles* mosquito is the vector for malaria and is where the sexual cycle (schizogony) develops.

4. The asexual cycle (sporogony) develops in humans.

5. Reinfection of hepatocytes by merozoites as in *P. vivax* and *P. ovale* infestations is responsible for relapses with these variants of disease.

6. People with sickle cell trait/disease, glucose-6-phosphate dehydrogenase deficiency, or β-thalassemia (all frequently encountered among African Americans) are resistant to *P. falciparum* infections.

7. African Americans are usually Duffy blood group (Fy) antigen negative, which renders them resistant to *P. vivax* infections, since the organism requires the antigen as a receptor before it parasitizes the RBC.

8. The pathogenesis of anemia in malaria relates to both intravascular and extravascular hemolysis of RBCs, the latter by removal of infected cells by macrophages.

9. The clinical presentation for the "benign" forms of malaria encompasses periodic paroxysms of shaking chills (correlating with intravascular rupture of RBCs) followed by high fever (having a specific pattern in some types) and pronounced diaphoresis as the temperature falls.

   a. Splenomegaly is a consistent feature of all malarias, and the spleen may even spontaneously rupture.

   b. *P. falciparum* is the most severe form of malaria owing to its greater degree of parasitemia.

      (1) It causes RBCs to agglutinate and stick to blood vessels, resulting in CNS hemorrhage (classic "ring hemorrhages" in the brain) and disseminated intravascular coagulation.

      (2) Massive intravascular hemolysis results in hemoglobinuria, which turns a black color in the presence of an acid pH, hence the term "blackwater fever."

      (3) *P. malariae* is associated with the formation of immunocomplexes leading to membranous glomerulonephritis and the nephrotic syndrome.

   c. The laboratory diagnosis of malaria is facili-

TABLE 12–11. Myelodysplasia/Acute and Chronic Leukemias

Definition	Pathogenesis	Clinical Findings	Treatment	Laboratory Findings
Myelodysplastic syndrome (MDS). **Definition:** stem cell disease that frequently progresses to acute leukemia, hence the term preleukemia. **FAB* classification:** Refractory anemia (24%). Refractory anemia with ringed sideroblasts (24%). Refractory anemia with excess blasts (23%). Refractory anemia with excess blasts in transformation (9%). Chronic myelomonocytic leukemia (16%).	Clonal stem cell disorder characterized by maturation defects resulting in ineffective erythropoiesis (anemia), granulopoiesis (neutropenia), and thrombopoiesis (thrombocytopenia) and a megaloblastic-appearing bone marrow similar to that seen in B_{12}/folate deficiency. Pancytopenia is the rule. **Chromosome abnormalities are common** (50%), particularly 5q− and trisomy 8. May be acquired from previous chemotherapy or irradiation, usually given within the previous 5 years.	Primarily a disease of the elderly (60–75 years old) and of men more than women. **Profile:** elderly person with severe cytopenias, severe anemia and a constant transfusion requirement. Half of patients are asymptomatic, and 10–40% progress to acute myelogenous leukemia. **MDS must be differentiated from other causes of pancytopenia** including B_{12}/folate deficiency, chemotherapy effect on the bone marrow, and acute leukemia (those types with cytopenias in the peripheral blood rather than a leukocytosis). **Key features that distinguish FAB subgroups** include the percentage of blasts in the peripheral blood or marrow, percentage of ringed sideroblasts in the marrow, frequency of cytogenetic abnormalities, frequency of transformation into an acute myelogenous leukemia (refractory anemia with excess blasts in transformation has the highest rate, and refractory anemia with ringed sideroblasts has the lowest incidence).	Transfusions (danger of iron overload), erythropoietin, pyridoxine (B_6), colony-stimulating factors, low-dose chemotherapy, in some cases. **Median survival is 9–29 months.**	CBC: **Normocytic to macrocytic anemia with a dimorphic RBC population** (microcytic and macrocytic RBCs). **Pancytopenia.** **Leukoerythroblastic reaction** is common. **Peripheral blood myeloblasts** are usually <5% and may have Auer rods (Figure 12–2H). **Bone marrow examination:** ringed sideroblasts, increased myeloblasts (<30%; otherwise it is called acute leukemia). Megaloblastic change is common. **Abnormal marrow chromosome studies are common,** and chromosome studies should be ordered, since they have some prognostic significance.
Acute lymphoblastic leukemia (ALL). **Definition:** stem cell disorder arising from the lymphoid stem cell. **FAB classification:** L1 subgroup: 85% of childhood ALL. L2 subgroup: 65% of adult ALL. L3 subgroup: frequently have t8;14 translocation (Burkitt type; worst prognosis). **Immunophenotype classification** of ALL is based on marker studies. **Early pre-B: CALLA† antigen positive** (most common overall; 55–60%). **CALLA† antigen negative.** **Pre-B** (20%). **Mature B** (1–2%). **Immature T** (15%).	Clonal stem cell disease associated in some cases with Down syndrome, immunodeficiency disorders, chromosome instability syndromes, viruses, drugs. About 90% of patients have cytogenetic abnormalities, which include translocations (poor prognosis) and hyperdiploidy (good prognosis).	Most common leukemia and overall type of cancer in children. Most children are <15 years old with a mean age of onset of 4 years. Slightly more frequent in boys and in whites than in African Americans. Accounts for 15% of adult leukemia. **Fever** and **bone pain** (leukemic infiltration in the marrow) are common presentations. **Generalized lymphadenopathy.** **Epistaxis and ecchymoses from thrombocytopenia.** **Hepatosplenomegaly** is common. **Testicular and CNS involvement** are common.	**Remission/induction therapy** (usually prednisone, vincristine, and asparaginase) is followed by **consolidation therapy** (short doses of the same drugs) and then **maintenance therapy** (6-mercaptopurine + methotrexate). Since the CNS is a common site for residual blasts, neuraxis irradiation and intrathecal methotrexate are used to eradicate disease in this area. **Bone marrow transplantation** has improved overall survival. Overall, there is a 60% 5-year survival. Immunophenotyping and determining the type of ALL is most important prognostic factor. Early pre-B, CALLA† antigen positive has best prognosis.	CBC: **Normocytic anemia in all patients often with nucleated RBCs in the peripheral blood.** **WBC findings:** WBC counts most commonly between 10,000 and 100,000 cells/μL. WBC counts most commonly between 10,000 and 100,000 cells/μL with lymphoblasts present. Absolute neutropenia in 80%. **Platelets:** thrombocytopenia (90%). **Bone marrow examination:** bone marrow packed with lymphoblasts.

Table continued on following page

TABLE 12–11. Myelodysplasia/Acute and Chronic Leukemias *Continued*

Definition	Pathogenesis	Clinical Findings	Treatment	Laboratory Findings
Chronic lymphocytic leukemia (CLL). **Definition:** B cell (most common) leukemia arising from lymphoid stem cells.	Neoplastic disorder of virgin B cells, which are long-lived but cannot differentiate into plasma cells (reason for hypogammaglobulinemia). About 50% have chromosomal abnormalities (trisomy 12 most common).	Most common overall leukemia. Most common leukemia in patients over age 60 and cause of generalized lymphadenopathy in an elderly patient. More common in men than in women. Median age of 60 years. Never seen in the Asian population. **About 25% are asymptomatic at presentation** (good prognostic sign). **Generalized, nonpainful lymphadenopathy. Hepatosplenomegaly. Increased Incidence of autoimmune hemolytic anemia** (warm and cold types), autoimmune **thrombocytopenia, hypogammaglobulinemia, and second malignancies.**	Treatment depends on degree of anemia and thrombocytopenia. Prednisone and chlorambucil are commonly used. Transformation to acute leukemia is rare, thus differing from CML. About 50% die of infection related to hypogammaglobulinemia. Median survival is 4–6 years.	**CBC:** **Normocytic anemia** (50%). **WBC findings:** absolute lymphocytosis (15,000–200,000 cells/ μL) with smudge cells (fragile lymphocytes; very characteristic). Absolute neutropenia. **Platelets:** thrombocytopenia (40%). **Bone marrow examination:** usually diffuse infiltration of the marrow. **Miscellaneous:** monoclonal IgM spike is common. Hypogammaglobulinemia is common.
Adult T cell leukemia. **Definition:** malignant T cell leukemia associated with the HTLV-1 retrovirus.	Stem cell disease.	Most common in Japan and sporadic in USA. Majority of patients are men. Presents at a median age of 34 years. **Generalized lymphadenopathy. Hepatosplenomegaly.** **Skin infiltration** (common with any T cell neoplasms in general). **Lytic lesions in bone (lymphoblasts secrete osteoclast activating factor)** often associated with hypercalcemia (90%).	Majority die in 1 year despite chemotherapy.	**CBC:** **Normocytic anemia.** **WBC findings:** WBC counts of 10,000–50,000 cells/μL. Lymphoblasts with T cell markers. **Platelets:** thrombocytopenia. **Bone marrow examination:** lymphoblasts. **Miscellaneous:** hypercalcemia.
Hairy cell leukemia (HCL). **Definition:** stem cell disease associated with malignant B cells with cytoplasmic projections.	Stem cell disease.	Most common in middle-aged men. **Splenomegaly is the most common physical finding** (90%): leukemic cells specifically infiltrate the red rather than the white pulp, which is unusual in leukemia and characteristic of HCL. The spleen is an important site for proliferation of the neoplastic cells, which is the reason for splenectomy. **Hepatomegaly** (20%). **Lymphadenopathy** is conspicuously absent (unusual in leukemia). **Increased incidence of autoimmune syndromes:** vasculitis, arthritis. **Lytic bone lesions. Increased incidence of *Mycobacterium avium-intracellulare.***	Splenectomy followed by human leukocyte interferon and α-interferon therapy and pentostatin, which blocks adenine deaminase (adenine is toxic to lymphocytes). About 50% 5-year survival.	**CBC:** **Normocytic anemia.** **Pancytopenia** is characteristic. **WBC findings:** malignant B cells with hairy projections. **Positive tartrate resistant acid phosphatase** (TRAP) **stain.** Electron microscopy of cells reveals characteristic complex lamellae. **Platelets:** thrombocytopenia. **Bone marrow examination:** the bone marrow is always packed. Malignant cells resemble fried eggs, with ample cytoplasm and a small nucleus (yolk).

Acute nonlymphocytic leukemias.
Definition: stem cell disorders that may involve the granulocytic, monocytic, erythrocytic, and megakaryocytic series.

FAB classification:

M0: minimally differentiated acute myelogenous leukemia (2–3%).

M1: acute myelogenous leukemia without differentiation (20%).

M2: acute myelogenous leukemia with maturation (30–40%).

M3: acute progranulocytic leukemia (5–10%).

M4: acute myelomonocytic leukemia (15–20%).

M5: acute monocytic leukemia (10%).

M6: acute erythroleukemia (Di Guglielmo's disease; 5%).

M7: acute megakaryocytic leukemia (1%).

Clonal stem cell disease that may be associated with irradiation, alkylating agents, benzene, immunodeficiency states, Down syndrome.

Most common type of leukemia between 15 and 39 years of age and slightly more common than CML in the 40–59 age bracket. Majority present with bleeding (thrombocytopenia), fever (infection), fatigue, and bone pain.

M0: no Auer rods (Figure 12–2H) in the myeloblasts.

M1: rare Auer rods present in myeloblasts.

M2: most common AML. Auer rods easily found in myeloblasts. Association with a t(8;21) translocation is favorable.

M3: numerous Auer rods. Blasts have a granular cytoplasm. Most common leukemia associated with DIC. A t(15;17) translocation is characteristic. Relationship with abnormal retinoic acid metabolism and high doses of vitamin A may induce remission.

M4: Auer rods are uncommon. Chromosome 6 abnormalities (inversion) associated with increased eosinophils indicate a better prognosis.

M5: no Auer rods. Gum infiltration is characteristic. High association with organ infiltration (liver, spleen, nodes).

M6: bizarre, multinucleated and often megaloblastoid-appearing erythroblasts that are PAS positive. More common in advanced age. Increased numbers of myeloblasts.

M7: myelofibrosis in the marrow. Platelet peroxidase stain is positive and is identified by electron microscopy.

Remission-induction (daunorubicin plus cytarabine), consolidation with repeated intensive chemotherapy, high-dose chemotherapy plus bone marrow transplant (autologous or donor). Overall long-term survival is 10–15%. Majority die of infection, hemorrhage, or combinations of the two.

CBC:
Normocytic anemia.
WBC findings: blasts are commonly present. Counts range from <10,000 cells/μL to >200,000 cells/μL.
Platelets: thrombocytopenia.
Bone marrow examination: hypercellular and packed with blasts. Blast count >30%.

---

* FAB, French-American-British.
† CALLA, common acute lymphoblastic leukemia antigen.

TABLE 12–12. Differential Features of the *Plasmodium* Species

Plasmodium Species	Frequency	Peripheral Blood Findings	Fever Pattern/Relapses
Plasmodium vivax	55%	Macrocytic RBCs. Schüffner's dots present. All forms present in peripheral blood.	**Tertian:** temperature spike every 48 hours. **Relapses:** yes
Plasmodium falciparum	40%	Normocytic. Schüffner's dots not present. Only ring forms (multiple infestation) and gametocytes (banana shaped) present in peripheral blood.	**Quotidian:** intermittent fever spikes. **Relapses:** no
Plasmodium malariae	5%	Normocytic. Schüffner's dots present. All forms present in peripheral blood.	**Quartan:** temperature spike every 72 hours. **Relapses:** no
Plasmodium ovale	<1%	Macrocytic. Schüffner's dots not present. All forms present in peripheral blood. Probably evolved from *P. vivax*.	**Tertian:** temperature spike every 48 hours. **Relapses:** yes

tated by noting the parasites in thin and thick smears of the peripheral blood.

(1) *P. falciparum* has only ring forms (which frequently multiply infect an RBC) with or without gametocytes (banana-shaped organisms) in the peripheral blood, whereas the other types have ring forms, merozoites, schizonts, and gametocytes.

(2) Schüffner's dots are a golden pigment in the RBCs that are present in *P. vivax* and *P. malariae*.

d. In general, chloroquine is used for prevention in all types of malaria, while primaquine is primarily used to eradicate *P. vivax* and *P. ovale*.

(1) Chloroquine kills blood schizonts and is gametocidal to all malaria species except falciparum, while primaquine is a tissue schizonticide (e.g., liver) and is gametocidal to *P. falciparum*.

(2) Mefloquine and doxycycline are the drugs of choice in treating chloroquine-resistant *P. falciparum*.

QUESTIONS

DIRECTIONS. (Items 1–17): Each of the numbered items or incomplete statements in this section is followed by answers or by completions of the statement. Select the ONE lettered answer or completion that is BEST in each case. Correct answers and explanations are given at the end of the chapter.

1. The peripheral smear is representative of the findings of a 26-year-old African American woman who presents for a routine physical examination. The examination is normal except for conjunctival pallor. The CBC reveals a low MCV, low Hb and Hct, low RBC count, and normal WBC count and differential. You expect further studies would reveal

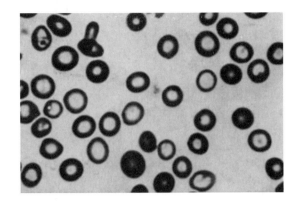

(A) a positive sickle cell screen
(B) an increase in HbA₂ and F
(C) a low serum ferritin level
(D) increased blood lead levels
(E) increased RBC osmotic fragility

2. This peripheral smear is from a 22-year-old man with right upper quadrant pain 30 minutes after eating fatty foods. Physical examination reveals point tenderness on deep palpation in the right upper quadrant and moderate, nontender splenomegaly. His CBC exhibits a mild normocytic anemia with an uncorrected reticulocyte count of 15% and Hb of 10 g/dL (13.5–17.5 g/dL). His mother had her spleen removed as a teenager for a "problem with her blood." Which of the following tests would be most useful in arriving at the diagnosis in this patient?

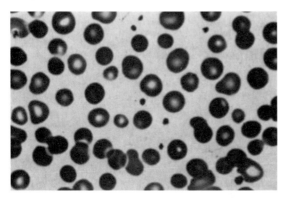

(A) Osmotic fragility test
(B) Sugar water test
(C) Direct Coombs' test
(D) Serum ferritin
(E) Heinz body preparation

3. This peripheral smear comes from a 65-year-old white woman with fatigue and a sore tongue. She has a past history of Hashimoto's thyroiditis for which she has had a thyroidectomy. Physical examination reveals pallor of the conjunctiva and palmar creases. Her tongue is beefy red and smooth. Vibratory sensation is absent in the lower extremities. You would expect additional studies to reveal

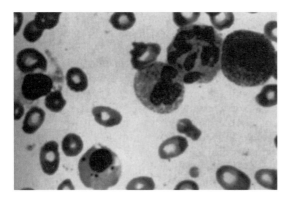

(A) low serum and RBC folate levels
(B) a normal MCV
(C) a normal Schilling's test
(D) a hypocellular bone marrow aspirate
(E) an increase in urine methylmalonic acid

4. The patient with this peripheral smear is a 21-year-old college student who presents with fever and a sore throat. He states that for the last 3 days he has not been able to move out of bed owing to extreme fatigue. Physical examination shows a febrile patient with an exudative tonsillitis, tender anterior and posterior cervical lymph nodes, and tender hepatosplenomegaly. The peripheral smear is representative of the type of cells that accounted for 25% of the cells in the differential count. There is no anemia or thrombocytopenia. Which of the following tests would most likely be abnormal in this patient?

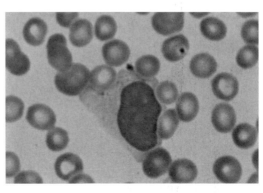

(A) Acidified serum test (Ham's test)
(B) Direct and indirect Coombs' tests
(C) Leukocyte alkaline phosphatase score
(D) Specific esterase stain of the cells
(E) Heterophil antibody test

5. Which of the following is present in iron deficiency, lead poisoning, and β-thalassemia minor?

(A) Abnormality in serum ferritin concentration
(B) Microcytic RBC indices
(C) Abnormal Hb electrophoresis
(D) Abnormal total iron-binding capacity (TIBC)
(E) Abnormal concentration of free erythrocyte protoporphyrin (FEP)

6. Which of the following differentiates pernicious anemia from other causes of B_{12} or folate deficiency?

(A) Abnormal proprioception
(B) Megaloblastic bone marrow
(C) Hypersegmented neutrophils
(D) Pancytopenia
(E) Achlorhydria

7. In which of the following patient descriptions would you expect the patient to have a normocytic anemia with a corrected reticulocyte count < 2%?

(A) Patient with episodic hemoglobinuria in the first morning void
(B) Patient with chronic renal failure secondary to type I diabetes mellitus
(C) Patient with untreated long-standing peptic ulcer disease
(D) Patient with a positive sickle cell screen and a normal peripheral smear
(E) Patient with a family history of hemolytic anemia after eating fava beans

8. A 42-year-old African American missionary returning from Africa presented to his physician with shaking chills and fever. A diagnosis of malaria due to *Plasmodium vivax* was made after examination of his peripheral smear. He was treated and 3 days later presented with dyspnea, dizziness, back pain, and a history of sudden onset of reddish-brown urine. His Hb was 7 g/dL, MCV normal, and WBC count slightly elevated with an absolute neutrophilic leukocytosis, and the reticulocyte count corrected for anemia and the presence of shift cells was 18%. The peripheral blood also had bite cells present. The urine dipstick for blood was positive. Which of the following tests would be most useful in arriving at a preliminary diagnosis?

(A) Enzyme assay of RBCs
(B) Direct Coombs' test
(C) Heinz body preparation
(D) Hb electrophoresis
(E) Osmotic fragility test

9. A patient with systemic lupus erythematosus (SLE) presents with fever and fatigue. She is presently taking corticosteroids to control her disease. Physical examination reveals a moon face consistent with Cushing's syndrome, generalized lymphadenopathy, conjunctival pallor, and hepatosplenomegaly. The CBC exhibits a normocytic anemia with an Hb of 6 g/dL, an increased MCHC, neutrophilic leukocytosis, absolute lymphopenia, borderline thrombocytopenia, eosinopenia, and a corrected reticulocyte count of 20%. Shift cells and spherocytes are reported to be present in the smear. Which of the following tests would best confirm the cause of the patient's anemia?

(A) Heinz body preparation
(B) Enzyme assay of RBCs
(C) Bone marrow aspirate
(D) Direct Coombs' test
(E) Osmotic fragility test

10. Which of the following anemia/confirmatory test relationships is correct?

(A) α-Thalassemia minor: Hb electrophoresis
(B) Sideroblastic anemia secondary to alcoholism: bone marrow aspirate
(C) Microangiopathic hemolytic anemia: Coombs' test
(D) Paroxysmal cold hemoglobinuria: Ham's test
(E) Lead poisoning: free erythrocyte protoporphyrin assay

11. Which of the following disorders will most likely show a normal percentage of eosinophils in the peripheral blood?

(A) Strongyloidiasis
(B) Hookworm infestation
(C) Drug allergy
(D) Contact dermatitis
(E) Addison's disease

12. A 49-year-old woman with a history of a modified radical mastectomy for infiltrating ductal carcinoma 2 years ago presents with fatigue, right upper quadrant pain, and pain in the lower lumbar area. Physical examination reveals mild hepatomegaly and point tenderness over the lower lumbar vertebra. A CBC exhibits microcytic RBC indices, thrombocytosis, and the presence of progranulocytes, myelocytes, and nucleated RBCs scattered throughout the smear. Liver function studies reveal slight elevation of alkaline phosphatase, γ-glutamyltransferase, and lactate dehydrogenase, but the total bilirubin and transaminases are in normal range. The stool guaiac is negative. You would least expect which of the following in this patient?

(A) Low serum ferritin
(B) Metastatic disease to bone
(C) Low serum iron
(D) Metastatic disease to liver
(E) Low total iron-binding capacity (TIBC)

13. Absolute lymphocytosis without atypical lymphocytosis would be expected in

(A) whooping cough
(B) a cytomegalovirus infection
(C) an Epstein-Barr virus infection
(D) a patient taking phenytoin
(E) toxoplasmosis

14. In a patient with significant blood loss within the last 24 hours, you would expect a/an

(A) low Hb and Hct
(B) low RBC count
(C) increase in the reticulocyte count
(D) positive tilt test
(E) low MCV

15. In a patient with pancytopenia, a normal MCV, and a corrected reticulocyte count < 2%, you would expect the mechanism of disease to be

(A) renal failure with reduction in erythropoietin
(B) suppression or destruction of the trilineage myeloid stem cell
(C) a DNA maturation defect
(D) chronic blood loss
(E) increased susceptibility of hematopoietic cells to complement destruction

16. In a febrile 4-year-old child with sickle cell disease and a CBC exhibiting a normocytic anemia, increased corrected reticulocyte count, absolute leukocytosis, > 10% band neutrophils, toxic granulation, sickle cells, target cells, and Howell-Jolly bodies, you would strongly suspect

(A) a viral infection
(B) salmonella osteomyelitis
(C) *Streptococcus pneumoniae* sepsis
(D) tuberculosis
(E) a systemic fungal infection

17. A 5-year-old African American foster child presents with abdominal pain, growth retardation, a severe microcytic anemia, and bone x-rays exhibiting increased densities in the epiphyseal plates of the bones in both hands. Additional findings would likely include

(A) coarse basophilic stippling of RBCs
(B) normal iron studies
(C) an abnormal Hb electrophoresis
(D) a positive sickle cell screen
(E) a "hair-on-end" appearance in a skull x-ray

Items 18–19

	RBC Mass	Plasma Volume	SaO$_2$*	Erythropoietin Concentration
(A)	Increased	Normal	Normal	Increased
(B)	Normal	Decreased	Normal	Normal
(C)	Increased	Increased	Normal	Low
(D)	Increased	Normal	Low	Increased
(E)	Increased	Decreased	Variable	Variable

* SaO$_2$ = oxygen saturation.

18. A 65-year-old man with a long history of chronic bronchitis, who presents with clinical evidence of cyanosis of the mucous membranes.

19. A 55-year-old man with a ruddy complexion, dizziness, splenomegaly, basophilia in the peripheral blood, and a hypercellular bone marrow.

Items 20–23

(A) Acute lymphoblastic leukemia
(B) Acute myelogenous leukemia
(C) Hairy cell leukemia
(D) HTLV-1 T cell leukemia
(E) Chronic myelogenous leukemia
(F) Acute progranulocytic leukemia
(G) Acute monocytic leukemia
(H) Chronic lymphocytic leukemia

20. A 45-year-old man with hepatosplenomegaly, a leukocyte count $> 150,000$ cells/μL with $< 1\%$ blasts, normocytic anemia, thrombocytopenia, a low leukocyte alkaline phosphatase (LAP) score, and an abnormal chromosome study.

21. A 70-year-old man with generalized, nontender lymphadenopathy, hepatosplenomegaly, a leukocyte count of ~80,000 cells/μL with "smudge cells" present in the peripheral smear, normocytic anemia, and thrombocytopenia.

22. A 65-year-old man with pancytopenia, hepatosplenomegaly, and abnormal-appearing cells in the peripheral blood that stain positive for tartrate-resistant acid phosphatase.

23. A 23-year-old man with disseminated intravascular coagulation who has leukemic cells that are hypergranular and contain numerous Auer rods.

ANSWERS AND EXPLANATIONS

1. The answer is C: a low serum ferritin level. The patient most likely has iron deficiency, the most common overall microcytic anemia. The smear reveals microcytic cells with hypochromasia (increased pallor). Serum ferritin is low in iron deficiency. Sickle cell disease is a normocytic anemia. An increase in HbA$_2$ and F is β-thalassemia minor, which is microcytic, but the RBC count is normal to elevated. An increased blood lead level is noted in lead poisoning (microcytic anemia). She would most likely be symptomatic, and coarse basophilic stippling would have been noted in the smear. Increased RBC osmotic fragility is seen in congenital spherocytosis (spherocytes are not present in this smear), which is a normocytic hemolytic anemia with an increased reticulocyte count. (Photomicrograph reproduced, with permission, from J.B. Henry. *Clinical Diagnosis and Management by Laboratory Methods,* 19th ed. Philadelphia, W.B. Saunders Co., 1996, p. 577.)

2. The answer is A: osmotic fragility test. The patient has congenital spherocytosis (normocytic anemia with a corrected reticulocyte count $> 3\%$) as evidenced by the spherical cells (defect in spectrin) with no central area of pallor, splenomegaly, and a family history of anemia requiring splenectomy. Congenital spherocytosis is an extravascular hemolytic anemia with an autosomal dominant (AD) inheritance pattern. There is an increased amount of unconjugated bilirubin generated from macrophage removal of RBCs, hence more bilirubin is cleared by the liver, which predisposes the patient to calcium bilirubinate gallstones. The corrected reticulocyte count in this case is 10%: Hb of 10 g/dL = Hct of 30%; (30/45) $\times$ 15% = 10%. An osmotic fragility test is the confirmatory test. The sugar water test is a screening test for paroxysmal nocturnal hemoglobinuria (PNH). The direct Coombs' test detects IgG, IgM, or C3 on the surface of RBCs in autoimmune hemolytic anemias. Serum ferritin is the screening test of choice for iron deficiency and ACD. A Heinz body preparation uncovers glucose-6-phosphate dehydrogenase deficiency in the active hemolytic stage. (Photomicrograph reproduced, with permission, from J.B. Henry. *Clinical Diagnosis and Management by Laboratory Methods,* 19th ed. Philadelphia, W.B. Saunders Co., 1996, p. 578.)

3. The answer is E: an increase in urine methylmalonic acid. The patient has B$_{12}$ deficiency, most likely pernicious anemia because of the history of another autoimmune disease. B$_{12}$ deficiency is associated with severe anemia, glossitis, macroovalocytes and hypersegmented neutrophils (> 5 lobes) in the peripheral smear, and absent vibratory sensation in the lower extremities (posterior column disease). The urine methylmalonic acid levels are invariably elevated in B$_{12}$ deficiency, since the vitamin is involved in propionate metabolism and the conversion of methylmalonyl-CoA to succinyl-CoA. B$_{12}$ deficiency, unlike folate deficiency, is associated with neurologic disease, since deficiency increases

propionates, leading to demyelination in the CNS (dementia and spinal cord disease involving the posterior columns and lateral corticospinal tracts). A low serum and RBC folate is expected in folate deficiency, which would not be associated with neurologic disease. MCV would be increased, since the anemia is macrocytic (defect in DNA maturation). Schilling's test would be abnormal owing to malabsorption of B_{12} related to a deficiency of intrinsic factor (pernicious anemia), chronic pancreatitis (the R factor cannot be cleaved off), or terminal ileal disease (the IF-B_{12} complex cannot be reabsorbed). A bone marrow aspirate would be hypercellular and megaloblastic (large immature nucleus). (Photomicrograph reproduced, with permission, from J.B. Henry. *Clinical Diagnosis and Management by Laboratory Methods,* 19th ed. Philadelphia, W.B. Saunders Co., 1996, p. 621.)

4. The answer is E: heterophil antibody test. The patient has infectious mononucleosis owing to the history of fatigue, the presence of atypical lymphocytes (large cells with abundant cytoplasm) in the peripheral smear, hepatosplenomegaly, exudative tonsillitis (usually related to the Epstein-Barr virus), and cervical adenopathy. The Monospot test identifies the heterophil antibody that is specific for infectious mononucleosis. The acidified serum test (Ham's test) is the confirmatory test for PNH. The direct and indirect Coombs' tests are used in the diagnosis of autoimmune hemolytic anemias. A leukocyte alkaline phosphatase (LAP) score differentiates neoplastic granulocytes (chronic myelogenous leukemia; low score) from a benign neutrophilic leukocytosis (high score). Specific esterase stains identify cells of granulocytic origin. (Photomicrograph reproduced, with permission, from J.B. Henry. *Clinical Diagnosis and Management by Laboratory Methods,* 19th ed. Philadelphia, W.B. Saunders Co., 1996.)

5. The answer is B: microcytic RBC indices. Iron deficiency, lead poisoning, and β-thalassemia minor are all microcytic anemias. Only iron deficiency and lead poisoning have an abnormality in the serum ferritin concentration (low in the former, high in the latter), TIBC (high in the former, low in the latter), and FEP (high in both). Only β-thalassemia minor has an abnormal Hb electrophoresis ($\uparrow$ HbA$_2$ and F). Since there is a defect in globin chain synthesis, heme synthesis is not affected and iron metabolism is normal in mild forms of the disease.

6. The answer is E: achlorhydria. Pernicious anemia is an autoimmune disease with destruction of the parietal cells in the body and fundus of the stomach, hence producing a deficiency of intrinsic factor (necessary for B_{12} absorption in the terminal ileum) and a deficiency in acid production (achlorhydria). All causes of B_{12} deficiency have the potential for abnormal proprioception (posterior column disease). Furthermore, all causes of B_{12} and folate deficiency have a megaloblastic bone marrow (DNA maturation defect), hypersegmented neutrophils, and pancytopenia (massive destruction of megaloblastic cells in the bone marrow; ineffective erythropoiesis).

7. The answer is B: patient with chronic renal failure secondary to type I diabetes mellitus. Chronic renal failure results in a normocytic anemia with a corrected reticulocyte count < 2% owing to a decrease in erythropoietin production by the kidneys. The remaining choices, except (D), have an elevated reticulocyte count. A patient with episodic hemoglobinuria in the first morning void most likely has PNH with absence of decay-acceler-

ating factor on the membranes, leading to complement destruction and intravascular hemolysis. A patient with untreated long-standing peptic ulcer disease probably has a microcytic anemia related to iron deficiency. A patient with a positive sickle cell screen and a normal peripheral smear would most likely have sickle cell trait, which would not include anemia. A patient with a family history of hemolytic anemia after eating fava beans most likely has glucose-6-phosphate dehydrogenase (G6PD) deficiency of the Mediterranean type, since fava beans precipitate intravascular hemolysis.

8. The answer is C: Heinz body preparation. The patient most likely has the African American variant of G6PD deficiency precipitated by the use of primaquine to treat malaria secondary to *Plasmodium vivax*. Deficiency of G6PD leads to decreased glutathione, which is necessary to detoxify the hydrogen peroxide generated by oxidizing drugs and infection. Increased peroxide damages Hb (producing Heinz bodies), leading to combined intravascular (primary event; reason for hemoglobinuria in this patient) and extravascular hemolysis (lesser event). Bite cells (which have a defect in the RBC membrane from macrophage removal of Heinz bodies) and a positive Heinz body preparation are important findings in active hemolysis. Enzyme assay of RBCs is reserved for confirmation after the hemolytic episode has subsided and RBCs without the enzyme are present in the peripheral blood. A direct Coombs' test is used in the diagnosis of autoimmune hemolytic anemia. Hb electrophoresis is the confirmatory test of β-thalassemia and hemoglobinopathies such as sickle cell trait/disease. The osmotic fragility test is the confirmatory test for congenital spherocytosis (increased fragility in hypotonic salt solutions).

9. The answer is D: direct Coombs' test. Any patient with an autoimmune disease, in this case SLE, who has an anemia is strongly suspect for having another autoimmune disease (autoimmune hemolytic anemia, thrombocytopenia, neutropenia, or lymphopenia). The normocytic anemia, increased corrected reticulocyte count, and presence of spherocytes (macrophages remove IgG and C3 from the RBC membrane) in the peripheral blood in this patient all suggest autoimmune hemolytic anemia. A direct Coombs' test is the confirmatory test. The patient also exhibits the effect of corticosteroids on hematopoietic cells, i.e., absolute neutrophilic leukocytosis (decreased adhesion molecule synthesis, hence releasing the marginating pool), lymphopenia (lymphocytotoxicity of steroids), and eosinopenia (destruction of eosinophils). A Heinz body preparation is used in the diagnosis of G6PD deficiency in the active hemolytic stage, while the enzyme assay of RBCs is the confirmatory test that is positive in the quiescent stage of the disease. A bone marrow aspirate is generally not indicated in autoimmune hemolytic anemia (it would show RBC hyperplasia and erythrophagocytosis by macrophages). An osmotic fragility test is reserved for confirming congenital spherocytosis, not acquired spherocytosis.

10. The answer is B: sideroblastic anemia secondary to alcoholism: bone marrow aspirate. Alcohol is a mitochondrial poison and hence interferes with heme synthesis (iron + protoporphyrin). The result is a sideroblastic anemia, since iron enters the damaged mitochondria but cannot exit. This leads to the formation of ringed sideroblasts (mitochondria laden with iron encircling a normoblast nucleus). These cells must be identified with a bone marrow aspirate and Prussian

blue staining to confirm the diagnosis. α-Thalassemia minor is associated with a normal Hb electrophoresis, since α-globin chains are reduced, leading to an equal reduction in HbA (2α/2β), A_2 (2α/2δ), and F (2α/2γ). Microangiopathic hemolytic anemias are intravascular hemolytic anemias, hence low serum haptoglobin levels, hemoglobinuria, and hemosiderinuria would be expected, *not* a positive Coombs' test. Paroxysmal *cold* hemoglobinuria is an intravascular hemolytic anemia associated with the formation of a bithermal antibody called the Donath-Landsteiner antibody. Ham's test is the confirmatory test for paroxysmal *nocturnal* hemoglobinuria. Lead poisoning is best diagnosed by blood lead levels rather than free erythrocyte protoporphyrin assays (increased), as formerly. When this test was positive, a blood lead level was used to confirm the diagnosis.

11. The answer is D: contact dermatitis. Contact dermatitis is a type IV hypersensitivity reaction, which should not be confused with a type I hypersensitivity reaction producing dermatitis (eczema), the latter often associated with eosinophilia. Invasive helminthic infections such strongyloidiasis and hookworm infestation (not pinworms) are associated with eosinophilia. Drug allergy is one of the most common causes of eosinophilia. Hypocortisolism associated with Addison's disease leads to eosinophilia, the opposite of Cushing's syndrome, in which hypercortisolism destroys eosinophils.

12. The answer is A: low serum ferritin. The patient most likely has metastatic breast cancer to the vertebral column (reason for bone pain) and liver (reason for hepatomegaly and elevated liver enzymes). The peripheral blood findings are those of both ACD and a leukoerythroblastic reaction, whereby malignant cells have pushed immature WBCs and nucleated RBCs into the peripheral blood. ACD is the most common anemia in malignancy and would be expected to have an elevated serum ferritin, low serum iron, low TIBC, and low percent saturation.

13. The answer is A: whooping cough. Whooping cough, due to *Bordetella pertussis*, produces an absolute lymphocytosis frequently in leukemoid range (> 50,000 cell/μL). The lymphocytes have a normal appearance rather than an antigenically stimulated appearance (atypical lymphocyte). Infectious lymphocytosis is another childhood disease with similar findings. Cytomegalovirus and *Toxoplasma* often produce a mononucleosis-like syndrome similar to Epstein-Barr virus infections in that atypical lymphocytosis is a prominent feature. Phenytoin also produces an atypical lymphocytosis.

14. The answer is D: positive tilt test. A patient with a significant blood loss within the last 24 hours would not be expected to have a low Hb and Hct, a low RBC count, a low MCV, or an increase in the reticulocyte count. The reasons are that acute blood loss results in an equal loss of RBCs and plasma, the bone marrow requires at least 5–7 days to generate RBCs and release reticulocytes into the peripheral blood, and a low MCV from iron deficiency would require weeks to months to develop. A positive tilt test (increase in heart rate and decrease in blood pressure when moving from sitting to standing) would be expected owing to the presence of hypovolemia. Over the ensuing days, plasma is replaced before RBCs, thereby uncovering the deficit in RBCs and leading to low Hb, Hct, and RBC counts.

15. The answer is B: suppression or destruction of the trilineage myeloid stem cell. A patient with pancytopenia, a normal MCV and a corrected reticulocyte count < 2% would most likely have aplastic anemia, which is a stem cell disease secondary to immune suppression or destruction of the trilineage myeloid stem cell. Drugs (e.g., chloramphenicol), chemicals (e.g., benzene), and infection (e.g., NANB hepatitis) are potential causes of aplastic anemia, characterized by hypocellularity of the bone marrow. Renal failure with reduction in erythropoietin does not produce pancytopenia. A DNA maturation defect is associated with B_{12}/folate deficiency. Chronic blood loss would result in a microcytic anemia secondary to iron deficiency. Increased susceptibility of hematopoietic cells to complement destruction is a feature of PNH, which does produce pancytopenia; however, the reticulocyte count is > 3% in the early stages of the disease.

16. The answer is C: *Streptococcus pneumoniae* sepsis. A febrile 4-year-old child with sickle cell disease, the presence of a left-shifted smear (> 10% band neutrophils and toxic granulation), and Howell-Jolly bodies (indicating splenic hypofunction) most likely has sepsis secondary to *S. pneumoniae*. This is the most common cause of death in children with sickle cell disease. A viral infection, tuberculosis, salmonella osteomyelitis, and a systemic fungal infection would not be associated with this constellation of findings.

17. The answer is A: coarse basophilic stippling of RBCs. A 5-year-old child with abdominal pain, growth retardation, severe microcytic anemia, and bone x-rays with densities in the epiphyseal plates has lead poisoning most likely contracted from eating old lead-based paint. Coarse basophilic stippling of RBCs is virtually pathognomonic for the disease owing to the denaturation of ribonuclease by lead, leaving ribosomes intact. Since lead poisoning is an example of sideroblastic anemia (a defect in heme synthesis with production of ringed sideroblasts), iron studies are those of iron overload, mainly an elevated serum iron, low TIBC, increased percent saturation, and increased serum ferritin. Abnormal Hb electrophoresis is noted in β-thalassemia and other hemoglobinopathies, a positive sickle cell screen is present in sickle cell trait/disease, and a "hair-on-end" appearance in a skull x-ray is seen in severe anemias where the marrow cannot keep pace with RBC destruction (e.g., sickle cell disease).

18. The answer is D: RBC mass, increased; plasma volume, normal; SaO_2, low; erythropoietin concentration, increased. A 65-year-old man with a long history of chronic bronchitis and clinical evidence of cyanosis has an appropriate secondary polycythemia owing to the hypoxemic stimulus of a low PaO_2 and the release of erythropoietin. The plasma volume is normal in all of the absolute polycythemias with the exception of polycythemia vera (PV), where it is increased.

19. The answer is C: RBC mass, increased; plasma volume, increased; SaO_2, normal; erythropoietin concentration, low. A 55-year-old man with a ruddy complexion, dizziness, splenomegaly, basophilia in the peripheral blood, and a hypercellular bone marrow has PV. PV is a myeloproliferative disease involving the trilineage myeloid stem cell in the bone marrow. It is an absolute polycythemia in that the RBC mass is increased, but it is inappropriate, since the SaO_2 is normal. Erythropoietin is low because the oxygen content of blood is high, hence suppressing erythropoietin release. It is the only absolute polycythemia in which the increase in RBC mass is matched by an increase in plasma volume. Choice A represents an absolute polycythemia that is

inappropriate, since the SaO_2 is normal. However, the erythropoietin level is high and the plasma volume normal, hence excluding PV and ruling in ectopic production of erythropoietin as the primary disorder (e.g., renal adenocarcinoma, etc.). Choice B represents a relative polycythemia with a reduction in plasma volume hemoconcentrating the blood, leading to an increase in the RBC count without affecting the RBC mass. This occurs in dehydration and stress polycythemia. Choice E represents smoker's polycythemia, in which there is a combination of hemoconcentration from the loss of plasma volume and the effect of carbon monoxide on increasing RBC mass.

20. The answer is E: chronic myelogenous leukemia. A 45-year-old man with hepatosplenomegaly, a leukocyte count > 150,000 cells/μL with < 1% blasts, normocytic anemia, thrombocytopenia, a low LAP score, and an abnormal chromosome (Philadelphia chromosome) has CML. This is the second most common leukemia in the age bracket of 40–60 years (acute myelogenous is more common). It is a myeloproliferative disorder that qualifies as a chronic leukemia owing to < 30% blasts in the marrow (usually < 10%) and evidence of maturation in the peripheral blood and marrow. A low LAP score (alkaline phosphatase is a marker of mature granulocytes) and the Philadelphia chromosome (t9;22), which is chromosome 22 with the *abl* oncogene fused to the break cluster region (bcr) of the chromosome, clinch the diagnosis of CML. Most patients have a blast crisis within a few years and die.

21. The answer is H: chronic lymphocytic leukemia. A 70-year-old man with generalized, nontender lymphadenopathy, hepatosplenomegaly, a leukocyte count of ~80,000 cells/μL (mostly mature-looking lymphocytes) with "smudge cells" (fragile neoplastic lymphocytes) present in the peripheral smear, normocytic anemia, and thrombocytopenia has CLL, a B-cell leukemia. This is the most common cause of generalized lymphadenopathy in patients over 60 years of age. Hypogammaglobulinemia, autoimmune cytopenias and second malignancies are commonly associated with CLL.

22. The answer is C: hairy cell leukemia. A 65-year-old man with pancytopenia, hepatosplenomegaly, and abnormal appearing cells in the peripheral blood that stain positive for tartrate-resistant acid phosphatase has a B-cell leukemia called hairy cell leukemia. Splenomegaly is the most consistent feature of the disease. The spleen is the favored site for neoplastic cell proliferation limited to the red pulp (unusual in leukemia).

23. The answer is F: acute progranulocytic leukemia. A 23-year-old man with disseminated intravascular coagulation who has leukemic cells that are hypergranular and contain numerous Auer rods has acute progranulocytic leukemia. Although all leukemias predispose to DIC, this type often presents with DIC. Regarding the other choices, acute lymphoblastic leukemia is the most common leukemia in children, acute myelogenous leukemia is the most common leukemia from 15 to 59 years of age, acute monocytic leukemia characteristically infiltrates the gums, and HTLV-1 T-cell leukemia is commonly associated with hypercalcemia.

CHAPTER THIRTEEN

DISORDERS OF THE LYMPH NODES AND SPLEEN

SYNOPSIS

OBJECTIVES

1. To understand how lymph node architecture relates to diseases involving the lymph nodes.
2. To be apprised of the causes and clinical significance of lymphadenopathy.
3. To gain an improved understanding of diseases that produce reactive hyperplasia in lymph nodes.
4. To understand non-Hodgkin's lymphomas with regard to their classification and clinical significance.
5. To have an improved understanding of Hodgkin's disease.
6. To be familiar with the plasma cell disorders that produce monoclonal gammopathies.
7. To be apprised of the role that mast cells play in disease.
8. To appreciate the functional aspects of the spleen and disorders that have an impact on the spleen.

Objective 1: To understand how lymph node architecture relates to diseases involving the lymph nodes.

I. Lymph node architecture and function
   A. **B cells** are located in the germinal follicles, **T cells** in the paracortex (interfollicular area), and **histiocytes** in the sinuses.
   B. Presentation of antigen to B cells in the follicles by dendritic reticular cells with the aid of interleukins secreted by helper T cells leads to the following sequential morphologic changes in the lymphocytes: small cleaved → large cleaved → small noncleaved → large noncleaved → immunoblasts → plasma cells (which produce antibodies specific for the antigen) or memory B cells.
      1. The **primary response** by immunoglobulins to first exposure to antigen is **IgM**, which first increases in 3–5 days and peaks in ~10 days.
      2. Reexposure to the same antigenic stimulus produces an accelerated **secondary response**, whereby **IgG** is produced earlier (within 2–3 days) and reaches higher concentrations than in the primary response.
      3. Lymphomas arising from follicular B cells assume the morphology of the types of cells previously described (e.g., small cleaved lymphocytic lymphoma).
   C. The **T-cell antigenic response** in the paracortical tissue results in the production of T-cell immunoblasts or memory T cells.
   D. The **histiocytic response** to antigen stimulation is called sinus histiocytosis.

Objective 2: To be apprised of the causes and clinical significance of lymphadenopathy.

II. Lymphadenopathy
   A. Lymphadenopathy (enlargement of lymph nodes) may be secondary to reactive hyperplasia involving B and or T cells (e.g., infection, autoimmune disease), phagocytic hyperplasia (e.g., sinus histiocytosis), and infiltrative disease (e.g., metastasis, malignant lymphoma).
   B. Drainage patterns leading to localized lymphadenopathy include the following:
      1. **Submental nodes:** metastatic squamous carcinoma in the oral pharynx.
      2. **Anterior cervical nodes:** tonsillitis due to group A streptococci.
      3. **Cervical nodes in general:** metastasis from tumors of the head and neck (e.g., laryngeal cancer, papillary thyroid cancer).
      4. **Left-sided supraclavicular nodes (Virchow's nodes):** abdominal tumors (e.g., adenocarcinoma of the stomach).
      5. **Right supraclavicular nodes:** metastatic lung and esophageal cancers.
      6. **Axillary nodes:** metastatic breast cancer.
      7. **Hilar nodes:** metastatic primary lung cancers and infectious disease (e.g., tuberculosis, sarcoidosis, and systemic fungal infection).
      8. **Abdominal and retroperitoneal nodes:** malignant lymphomas and metastatic germ cell tumors of the testes.

Objective 3. To gain an improved understanding of diseases that produce reactive hyperplasia in lymph nodes.

III. Reactive lymph node hyperplasia
   A. Painful lymphadenopathy that occurs in response to an immunologic reaction is called **reactive hyperplasia**.
   B. It often simulates a neoplastic process, resulting in

a false-positive diagnosis of malignant lymphoma or Hodgkin's disease.

C. **Patterns of reactive hyperplasia** are associated with different diseases.

1. The **follicular pattern** (B-cell response) is associated with rheumatoid arthritis (increased plasma cells), primary and secondary syphilis (increased plasma cells; abundant spirochetes), Castleman disease (mediastinal location; hyalinized vessel in the center of an atrophic follicle), and HIV-related lymphadenopathy.

2. The **interfollicular** or **paracortical pattern** (T-cell response) is noted in patients with eczematous lesions (dermatopathic lymphadenitis with pigmented macrophages simulating malignant melanoma).

3. A **mixed follicular** (B- and T-cell response) is represented by cat-scratch disease (granulomatous microabscesses associated with *Bartonella [Rochalimaea] henselae*) and toxoplasmosis (clusters of epithelioid cells).

4. A **sinus pattern** (histiocyte response) is present in nodes draining tumor (sinus histiocytosis in breast cancer).

5. A **diffuse pattern** (effacement of the node) is present in nodes draining a vaccination site, in EBV infection (infectious mononucleosis) and in patients taking phenytoin.

Objective 4. To understand non-Hodgkin's lymphomas with regard to their classification and clinical significance.

IV. Non-Hodgkin's lymphoma

A. Approximately 60% of malignant lymphomas are non-Hodgkin's lymphoma (NHL), while the remaining 40% represent Hodgkin's disease (HD).

B. They are primary malignancies most commonly arising in lymph nodes (the stomach is the most common primary extranodal site).

C. Low-grade lymphomas often metastasize to the bone marrow and peripheral blood (leukemic phase), hence simulating leukemia.

D. Metastasis is the most common malignancy in lymph nodes, and carcinomas are the most common primary cancer.

1. The subcapsular sinus is the first area involved in metastasis.

2. Immunohistochemical stains (e.g., CD45-positive in 90% of NHLs), identification of translocations (e.g., t[8;14] in Burkitt's lymphoma), and detection of immunoglobulin gene arrangements (e.g., identifying monoclonality of a lymphocyte proliferation) are useful in the workup of NHL.

E. Approximately 60% of patients with NHL are men over 50 years of age.

F. NHL accounts for 60% of cases of lymphomas in children, with Burkitt's lymphoma (B-cell malignancy) and lymphoblastic lymphoma (T-cell malignancy) representing the most common types (HD accounts for the remainder).

G. **Predisposing factors** for NHL include the following:

1. Disease related to HIV positivity (primary CNS lymphomas, EBV-related lymphomas).

2. Autoimmune disease (e.g., Sjögren's syndrome).

3. Congenital immunodeficiency syndromes (e.g., ataxia telangiectasia, Wiskott-Aldrich syndrome,

common variable immunodeficiency, [EBV-related] X-linked immunoproliferative disease).

4. Immunosuppressive therapy (e.g., in recipients of organ or bone marrow transplants, patients taking alkylating agents).

5. High-dose radiation.

6. History of EBV infection.

H. Geographical patterns noted among types of NHL include the following:

1. **Burkitt's lymphoma** in equatorial Africa (strong relationship with EBV).

2. **HTLV-1 leukemia/lymphoma** in Japan.

3. **Small intestine lymphoma** in the Middle East (relationship with IgA heavy chain disease).

I. **Classification of NHL** is confusing owing to emphasis on different aspects of lymph node pathology (e.g., pattern, morphology, function).

1. The **Rappaport classification** is based on pattern (nodular or diffuse) and morphology (lymphocytic or histiocytic).

2. The **Lukes-Collins classification** is based on function (marker studies) and morphology.

3. The **Kiel classification** uses terms such as centrocytic (low-grade) and centroblastic (high-grade) lymphomas.

4. The **Working Formulation** translates the various systems into low-, intermediate-, and high-grade categories of lymphomas.

5. Nodular lymphomas have a better prognosis than diffuse lymphomas, diffuse lymphomas often arise from previous nodular lymphomas, and lymphocytic lymphomas have a better prognosis than histiocytic lymphomas.

J. **B-cell lymphomas** originate from follicular B cells (follicular lymphomas, Burkitt's lymphoma), medullary B cells (small-cell lymphomas), and immunoblastic B cells (diffuse immunoblastic lymphoma).

1. **FCC lymphoma of the small cleaved type** is a low-grade lymphoma.

   a. It is the most common overall NHL (~23% of cases).

   b. Most cases have a leukemic phase, and ~50% involve the marrow (stage IV).

   c. There is a t(14;18) translocation involving the *bcl*-2 gene, which normally inhibits apoptosis (programmed cell death).

2. **Small lymphocyte lymphocytic lymphoma** is a low-grade lymphoma that may be confused with chronic lymphocytic leukemia (CLL), since it metastasizes to the marrow and has a leukemic phase in the peripheral blood.

3. **Small noncleaved lymphocytic lymphoma (Burkitt's lymphoma)** is a high-grade lymphoma that is more common in children (34% of cases of NHL) than in adults.

   a. The **African variant** most commonly locates in the jaw and has a greater relationship with EBV (100%) than does the **American variant**, which most commonly presents in the abdominal cavity (boys, small intestine; girls, pelvic organs; adults, stomach and colon) and has an EBV relationship in only 5–15% of cases.

   b. There is a characteristic t(8;14) translocation with the c-*myc* oncogene translocated to chromosome 14.

c. Marrow involvement and a leukemic phase are common.

d. Lymph nodes have a characteristic diffuse pattern with a "starry sky" appearance.

4. **Diffuse large-cell immunoblastic lymphoma** is a high-grade lymphoma having an association with angioimmunoblastic lymphadenopathy (fever, weight loss, Coombs'-positive hemolytic anemia; relationship with viral infections and drugs), CLL, Sjögren's syndrome, and immunosuppression (from renal transplant).

K. **T-cell lymphomas** derive from thymic T cells (lymphoblastic lymphoma), mature T cells (peripheral T-cell lymphomas such as mycosis fungoides), or immunoblastic T cells (diffuse immunoblastic lymphoma).

1. **Mycosis fungoides** (MF) is a malignancy of CD4 T helper cells that occurs in patients between 40 and 60 years of age.

a. It begins in the skin and progresses to lymph nodes, lung, liver, and spleen.

b. **Pautrier's microabscesses** (collections of neoplastic T cells) are located in the epidermis, and a band-like infiltrate of neoplastic cells is noted in the dermis.

c. The presence of neoplastic T cells in the peripheral blood (a characteristic nuclear cleft is present; see Figure 12-2J) is called **Sézary syndrome**.

2. **Lymphoblastic lymphomas** are high-grade lymphomas that most commonly occur in children (29% of cases of NHL in children).

a. They primarily involve the mediastinum and less commonly the bone marrow, CNS, and peripheral blood.

b. They are the tissue equivalent of acute lymphoblastic leukemia.

L. Neoplastic disorders associated with histiocytes are uncommon.

1. Most patients with a **histiocytic lymphoma (malignant histiocytosis)** are adult males who typically have fever, diffuse lymphadenopathy, and hepatosplenomegaly.

a. Malignant histiocytes are noted in the sinusoids of the lymph nodes and liver and in the red pulp of the spleen.

b. The cells are large and frequently multinucleated and commonly phagocytose RBCs and other hematopoietic elements.

2. **Histiocytosis X** is predominantly a childhood disease.

a. It encompasses three diseases: **eosinophilic granuloma, Hand-Schüller-Christian disease**, and **Letterer-Siwe disease**.

b. Its true histiocytic origin (**Langerhans' cells; CD1 positive**) is documented on electron microscopy by the presence of **Birbeck granules**, which have a tennis racket appearance.

c. Histiocytes on H and E staining have a characteristic grooved nucleus, giving the nucleus a coffee bean appearance.

d. **Eosinophilic granuloma** is a benign variant of histiocytosis X associated with unifocal lytic lesions in bones (skull, ribs, and femur) that commonly produce pain and present with pathologic fractures.

e. **Hand-Schüller-Christian disease** is a disabling variant of histiocytosis X that is charac-

terized by a triad of multifocal cystic defects in the skull, diabetes insipidus due to neoplastic involvement of the hypothalamus, and exophthalmos from infiltration of the orbit by histiocytes.

f. **Letterer-Siwe diseas**e, the most aggressive variant of histiocytosis X, is characterized by a diffuse eczematous rash, organ involvement, and multifocal cystic defects in the skull, pelvis, and long bones.

M. Median **survival** is 6.5 years for low-grade lymphomas, 2.5 years for intermediate-grade lymphomas, and 1.5 years for high-grade lymphomas.

Objective 5: To have an improved understanding of Hodgkin's disease.

V. Hodgkin's disease

A. Hodgkin's disease (HD) is slightly more common in men than women (except for nodular sclerosing HD), adults than children, and whites than African Americans.

1. It has a **bimodal age distribution** with the first large peak in the third decade and the second, smaller peak in individuals over 45–50 years of age.

2. It is frequently associated with a past history of **Epstein-Barr virus infection** (> 50% demonstrate the EBV genome in tissue biopsy specimens).

B. Lymph nodes on cut surface have a "fish flesh" appearance.

C. In comparison with NHL, HD involves younger people; is more commonly associated with fever (Pel-Ebstein fever); rarely involves Waldeyer's ring (tonsils, adenoids), skin, or the gastrointestinal tract; and is more likely to present with unilateral adenopathy.

D. The **Reed-Sternberg** (RS) **cell** is the neoplastic cell in HD.

1. It is of B-cell origin in some variants and T-cell origin in others and is essential for making the initial diagnosis of HD in lymph nodes.

2. It has an "owl's eye" appearance as a single large cell with two or more nuclei or nuclear lobes with a large inclusion body–like eosinophilic nucleolus surrounded by a halo of clear nucleoplasm.

3. **RS variants** (mononuclear rather than binucleate) occur in different subtypes (see below) of HD: L and H cells with lymphocyte-predominant HD, lacunar cells with nodular sclerosing HD, and mononuclear variants with mixed-cellularity HD.

E. The four subtypes of HD are lymphocyte predominance (LP; 5% of cases), nodular sclerosis (NS; 60% of cases), mixed cellularity (MC; 30% of cases), and lymphocyte depletion (LD; 5% of cases).

1. Using the following sequence of the HD subtypes—LP → NS → MC → LD—the age of the patient progresses from youngest to oldest (LP youngest, LD oldest), the number of RS cells from least to greatest (LP the least, LD the most), and the prognosis from best to worst (LP the best, LD the worst).

2. **LP** most commonly presents in a young male with isolated lymphadenopathy involving the

cervical or supraclavicular nodes (90% 5-year survival; increased incidence of second malignancy [NHL]).

3. **NS**, the most common type of HD, most commonly presents as a mediastinal mass with additional involvement of cervical or supraclavicular nodes (stage IIA; ~70% 5-year survival).
   a. RS cells are difficult to identify; however, RS variants called **lacunar cells** are commonly noted in artifactually created spaces (formalin-fixed tissue).
   b. Broad bands of birefringent collagen separate nodular areas.
4. **MC**, the second most common type of HD, is associated with numerous RS cells interspersed among plasma cells and eosinophils (~50% 5-year survival).
5. **LD**, the most aggressive variant of HD, occurs in men > 40–50 years old and is frequently associated with anaplastic-appearing RS cells (~20% 5-year survival).

F. The two main factors that determine **prognosis in HD** are clinical stage (most important) and type of HD (LP the best, LD the worst).
1. More than 80% of patients present with lymphadenopathy above the diaphragm often involving the supraclavicular nodes and the anterior mediastinum.
2. In addition to location of involved lymph nodes and extranodal sites above and below the diaphragm, patients who are asymptomatic are designated A, whereas those who are symptomatic (having fever > 38°C, drenching night sweats, 10% weight loss during the past 6 months) are designated B.
3. Advances in radiation therapy and chemotherapy have resulted in cure of HD in > 75% of patients.
4. A complication of radiation therapy and chemotherapy is an increased risk for second malignancies, usually NHL.

Objective 6: To be familiar with the plasma cell disorders that produce monoclonal gammopathies.

VI. Plasma cell disorders associated with monoclonal gammopathies
   A. Plasma cell disorders are a group of neoplastic or potentially neoplastic disorders characterized by the proliferation of an uncontrolled clone of plasma cells.
   1. The neoplastic plasma cells frequently secrete immunoglobulin and/or light chains that produce a **monoclonal spike** (**M spike**) on serum protein electrophoresis (SPE; Chapter 3).
   2. Owing to their small molecular weight, κ or λ light chains are excreted in the urine, where they are designated **Bence Jones** (BJ) **protein** (best detected by urine electrophoresis).
   B. The **classification** of the monoclonal gammopathies (MGs) includes the following types:
   1. **Monoclonal gammopathy of undetermined significance** (MGUS), the most common MG, frequents patients > 70 years of age and pursues a stable course in some and a progressive course into multiple myeloma or a related disorder in others (~24% of cases).

2. **Multiple myeloma** (MM), the second most common MG, is also the most common primary malignancy of bone.
   a. It occurs more frequently in males than females (3:2 ratio), in African Americans than whites (2:1), and in patients over 40 years of age (median age, 61).
   b. There is an increased risk with radiation exposure and antigenic stimulation (e.g., allergy injections).
   c. M spikes occur in 80–90% of cases (IgG followed by IgA, followed by light chains only) and urine BJ protein in 60–80% of cases.
   d. Sheets of malignant plasma cells > 10% of cells are invariably present in the marrow.
   e. Anemia, bone pain (lytic bone lesions), pathologic fracture, recurrent infection (most common cause of death), unexplained hypercalcemia, and renal failure without hypertension are commonly observed.
   f. Median survival without treatment is 6 months.
3. **Solitary plasmacytomas of bone** (vertebra, ribs, and pelvis) often progress to MM (75%) within 10 years.
4. **Extramedullary plasmacytomas** are most commonly located in the upper respiratory tract (nasopharynx, sinuses, larynx) and rarely progress to MM.
5. **Waldenström's macroglobulinemia** is associated with neoplastic lymphoplasmacytoid cells that secrete IgM, often resulting in a **hyperviscosity syndrome** (e.g., retinal hemorrhages).
6. **Heavy-chain diseases** (α [most common], γ, and μ types) are extremely rare, do not have BJ protein in the urine, and frequently involve lymph nodes (γ and μ types) or the small bowel (α type), the latter associated with malabsorption and an increased risk for small bowel lymphoma.
7. **Amyloidosis** is associated with interstitial tissue deposition of amyloid, leading to organ dysfunction.
   a. It has the following properties: twisted β-pleated sheet by crystallography; eosinophilic staining in H and E–stained tissue; Congo red positivity; apple-green birefringence under polarized light; and a non-branching fiber with a hollow core on electron microscopy.
   b. It is derived from different proteins including light chains (called the primary type; associated with MM), serum-associated amyloid (called the secondary type; associated with chronic inflammation in rheumatoid arthritis, tuberculosis, and leprosy), prealbumin (associated with senile amyloidosis), β-proteins (coded for by chromosome 21; associated with Down syndrome; toxic to neurons, hence predisposing to Alzheimer's disease), and peptide hormones such as calcitonin (associated with medullary carcinoma of the thyroid).
   c. Common sites of involvement include the heart (restrictive cardiomyopathy), spleen (splenomegaly), tongue (macroglossia), adrenals (Addison's disease), liver (hepatomegaly), and kidneys (nephrotic syndrome).

d. The diagnosis is secured by a biopsy of rectal mucosa, gingiva, omental fat pad, or the organ involved.

e. The median survival in the primary (light chain) type is 13 months.

Objective 7: To be apprised of the role that mast cells play in disease.

VII. Mast cell diseases (mastocytosis)

A. Toluidine blue and Giemsa's are two metachromatic stains commonly used to identify mast cells in tissue.

B. **Urticaria pigmentosa** is primarily limited to the skin, where it is associated with small, reddish-brown macules (flat) or papules (raised) that when scratched produce swelling, erythema, and pruritus (owing to release of histamine from mast cells).

C. **Systemic mastocytosis** may be diagnosed by bone marrow aspiration or biopsy of lesions in the target organ sites.

Objective 8: To appreciate the functional aspects of the spleen and disorders that have an impact on the spleen.

VIII. Disorders of the spleen

A. Spleen disorders can involve the red pulp, which contains the sinusoids and the cords of Billroth; the white pulp, which contains the T cells surrounding the artery (periarteriolar lymphocyte sheath, or PALS) and B cells peripheral to the mantle of T cells; or combinations of the two areas.

B. The spleen has the following functions:

1. It filters the blood (e.g., removes senescent RBCs and encapsulated bacteria).

2. It traps and processes antigens in macrophages.

3. It is a reservoir for platelets.

C. Splenomegaly may be secondary to one of the following:

1. Reactive hyperplasia of the white pulp (infection, inflammation).

a. **Infectious mononucleosis** is associated with infiltration of the capsule by immunoblasts, which renders the spleen subject to rupture, most commonly during contact sports (e.g., football, wrestling).

b. **Kala-azar**, or visceral leishmaniasis, produces massive splenomegaly (*Leishmania* is present in macrophages).

c. **Malaria** is a frequent cause of splenomegaly in developing countries.

d. Splenomegaly is common with bacteria associated with macrophage involvement (e.g., typhoid fever).

e. Splenomegaly commonly occurs in SLE and rheumatoid arthritis owing to lymphoid hyperplasia (SLE is also associated with hyperplastic arteriolosclerosis, in which the penicilliary arteriole becomes like onionskin).

2. Infiltrative disease.

a. **Gaucher's disease**, an autosomal recessive lysosomal storage disease, produces massive splenomegaly owing to an accumulation of glucocerebroside in macrophages (the cytoplasm has a fibrillary appearance).

b. **Niemann-Pick disease**, an autosomal recessive lysosomal storage disease, produces massive splenomegaly owing to an accumulation of sphingomyelin in macrophages (the cytoplasm is foamy).

c. **Myeloproliferative diseases** (e.g., polycythemia rubra vera, agnogenic myeloid metaplasia) are associated with splenomegaly secondary to **extramedullary hematopoiesis** (hematopoiesis occurs in the sinusoids).

d. **Leukemia** (acute and chronic) is invariably associated with splenomegaly owing to leukemic infiltration of the red and white pulp (the exception is hairy cell leukemia, which involves only the red pulp).

e. **Malignant lymphoma** (e.g., NHL and HD) is the most common metastasis and malignancy of the spleen.

f. **Primary tumors** are most commonly due to a benign hemangioma.

3. Vascular congestion.

a. Portal hypertension (PH) is generally secondary to cirrhosis and produces **congestive splenomegaly**, leading to perisplenitis ("sugar-coated" spleen) and precipitation of calcium and iron in fibrous tissue, forming **Gamna-Gandy bodies**.

b. **Hypersplenism** is an exaggeration of normal splenic function that leads to sequestration and destruction of RBCs, WBCs, and platelets, either singly or in combination.

4. Phagocytic (macrophage) proliferation.

a. **Congenital spherocytosis** is associated with macrophage destruction of spherocytes (cords of Billroth are congested but sinuses are empty owing to macrophage destruction of spherocytes).

b. **Sickle cell disease** begins with splenomegaly owing to entrapment of RBCs in the cords and sinuses (eventually the spleen undergoes autosplenectomy).

c. **Autoimmune hemolytic anemia and thrombocytopenia** produce splenomegaly owing to the removal of IgG- or C3-coated cells by macrophages.

D. **Felty's syndrome** consists of the combination of rheumatoid arthritis, splenomegaly, and neutropenia (autoimmune neutropenia).

E. **Splenic rupture** is usually secondary to trauma and surgery.

F. **Splenic infarctions** are most commonly pale owing to arterial embolization of material (e.g., thrombus, vegetations) originating from the left side of the heart.

G. **Congenital asplenia** is associated in > 80% of cases with malformations in the heart.

H. **Splenectomy** (or functional asplenia [sickle cell disease]) predisposes to infections (septicemia, peritonitis) by *Streptococcus pneumoniae* (most common) followed by *Haemophilus influenzae*.

I. **Hematologic abnormalities accompanying splenectomy** include the presence of nucleated RBCs, Howell-Jolly bodies (nuclear remnants in the cytoplasm), increased reticulocytes (the RBC membrane is not removed by macrophages), target cells (excess membrane cannot be removed), Heinz bodies (denatured Hb), and an increase in platelets (thrombocytosis).

QUESTIONS

DIRECTIONS. (Items 1–10): Each of the numbered items or incomplete statements in this section is followed by answers or by completions of the statement. Select the ONE lettered answer or completion that is BEST in each case. Correct answers and explanations are given at the end of the chapter.

1. The photomicrograph is a high-power magnification of an abnormal cell identified in a right supraclavicular lymph node removed from a 32-year-old asymptomatic woman. The node was firm, moveable, nontender, and nodular on cut section. A chest x-ray revealed a mass in the anterior mediastinum. The remainder of her physical examination was unremarkable. Based on these findings you would expect

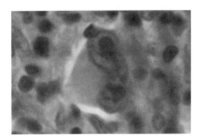

   (A) the lymph node to contain broad bands of birefringent collagen and lacunar cells
   (B) the lymph node to have a nodular infiltrate of small cleaved neoplastic lymphocytes
   (C) the patient to have a high-grade malignant lymphoma and stage IV disease
   (D) the lymph node to have a "starry sky" appearance on low-power examination
   (E) the patient to have a positive heterophil antibody test and atypical lymphocytes in the peripheral blood

2. The skull x-ray and the bone marrow aspirate are from a 58-year-old man who presented to his physician with a pathologic fracture of a rib after coughing. Physical examination revealed generalized bone tenderness. A CBC exhibited a normocytic anemia, extensive rouleaux, and mild thrombocytopenia. An x-ray of the ribs revealed lesions similar to those noted in the skull x-ray. You would least expect the patient to have

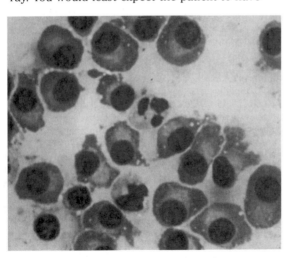

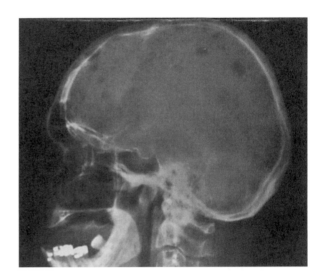

   (A) hypercalcemia related to the lesions noted in the skull and ribs
   (B) an abnormal serum protein electrophoresis
   (C) an abnormal urine electrophoresis
   (D) sheets of malignant cells in the bone marrow
   (E) a clonal proliferation of lymphoplasmacytoid cells secreting IgM

3. Which of the following clinical pictures is more consistent with reactive hyperplasia than with a neoplastic process involving the lymph nodes?

   (A) Submental lymphadenopathy in a 65-year-old man with alcoholism who smokes
   (B) Isolated inguinal lymphadenopathy in a 22-year-old man who presents with an indirect inguinal hernia
   (C) Left supraclavicular lymph node enlargement in a 49-year-old Japanese man who has weight loss and epigastric distress
   (D) Right axillary adenopathy in a 48-year-old woman with low back pain and a dragging sensation in her right upper quadrant
   (E) CT scan evidence of enlarged para-aortic lymph nodes in a 28-year-old man with a history of cryptorchidism as a child

4. Hodgkin's disease differs from non-Hodgkin's lymphoma in that it is more likely to

   (A) be generalized in its initial presentation
   (B) have a diffuse infiltrate of neoplastic B cells
   (C) involve the bone marrow
   (D) be associated with fever, night sweats, and weight loss
   (E) occur in children than in adults

5. Which of the following reactive lymph node relationships is correct?

   (A) Syphilis: spirochetes rarely identified in primary and secondary types
   (B) Rheumatoid arthritis: sinus histiocytosis is a marker of increased disease activity
   (C) Cat-scratch disease: granulomatous microabscesses are similar to lymphogranuloma venereum
   (D) Dermatopathic lymphadenitis: is commonly associated with vaccinations
   (E) HIV-related lymphadenopathy: onset occurs with the development of opportunistic infections

6. Massive splenomegaly in the United States is most commonly secondary to which of the following groups of diseases?

   (A) Malaria and infectious mononucleosis
   (B) Kala-azar and polycythemia rubra vera
   (C) Lysosomal storage disease and acute myelogenous leukemia
   (D) Myeloproliferative disease and chronic lymphocytic leukemia
   (E) Congenital spherocytosis and sickle cell disease

7. Which of the following relationships in the spleen is correct?

   (A) Systemic lupus erythematosus: hyaline arteriolosclerosis of the penicilliary arteriole
   (B) Portal hypertension: splenomegaly secondary to proliferation of the white pulp
   (C) Hypersplenism: splenomegaly associated with hyperfunction most commonly secondary to infiltrative disease
   (D) Splenectomy: thrombocytosis, target cells, Howell-Jolly bodies in the peripheral blood
   (E) Congenital asplenia: high incidence of Felty's syndrome

8. Which of the following diseases or physical diagnostic findings is least likely an association with amyloidosis?

   (A) Congestive cardiomyopathy
   (B) Peripheral neuropathy
   (C) Nephrotic syndrome
   (D) Alzheimer's disease
   (E) Hepatosplenomegaly

9. The most common cause of a monoclonal spike on serum protein electrophoresis would most likely be present in a

   (A) 75-year-old man who initially presented with a condition seemingly unrelated to the monoclonal gammopathy
   (B) 65-year-old man with anemia, renal failure, and Bence Jones proteinuria
   (C) 60-year-old man with retinal hemorrhages secondary to a hyperviscosity syndrome
   (D) 4-year-old child with exophthalmos, cystic lesions in the skull, and diabetes insipidus
   (E) 40-year-old man with reddish-brown lesions that when stroked become swollen, erythematous, and pruritic

10. Which of the following proteins is involved in the pathogenesis of dementia in a 40-year-old man with Down syndrome?

    (A) Prealbumin
    (B) β-Protein
    (C) Calcitonin
    (D) Light chains
    (E) Serum-associated amyloid protein

ANSWERS AND EXPLANATIONS

1. The answer is A: the lymph node to contain broad bands of birefringent collagen and lacunar cells. The patient most likely has nodular sclerosing HD with supraclavicular and mediastinal lymph node involvement. The photograph depicts a binucleate RS cell with nucleoli surrounded by a clear halo. This is the most common variant of HD and, unlike the other types, is female dominant. Lacunar cells are an RS variant located in spaces created by artifactual distortion secondary to previous formalin fixation of the node. Regarding the other choices, infiltrates of small cleaved neoplastic lymphocytes (FCC lymphoma) or a "starry sky" appearance of a lymph node (Burkitt's lymphoma) would not be associated with RS cells. The patient is most likely to be stage IIA, since there are no symptoms (A) and the disease is limited to two lymph node groups above the diaphragm. A positive heterophil antibody test and atypical lymphocytes in the peripheral blood indicates infectious mononucleosis, which produces generalized, tender adenopathy. There is a relationship between HD and previous EBV-related infectious mononucleosis. (Photomicrograph reproduced, with permission, from J.B. Henry. *Clinical Diagnosis and Management by Laboratory Methods,* 19th ed. Philadelphia, W.B. Saunders Co., 1996.)

2. The answer is E: a clonal proliferation of lymphoplasmacytoid cells secreting IgM. The patient has multiple myeloma (MM). Lytic lesions are noted in the skull x-ray, and the marrow contains sheets of malignant plasma cells with eccentric nuclei and perinuclear clearing. MM is the second most common type of monoclonal gammopathy, which produces an M protein spike on serum protein electrophoresis and Bence Jones (light chains) proteinuria on urine electrophoresis. Serum and urine immunoelectrophoresis identify the immunoglobulin (usually IgG) and light chain involved (usually kappa). Other uninvolved immunoglobulins are suppressed. Hypercalcemia is secondary to the release of osteoclast-activating factor from the malignant plasma cells. Osteoclast-activating factor is also responsible for the lytic areas in the bone, bone pain, and the tendency for pathologic fractures. A clonal proliferation

of lymphoplasmacytoid cells secreting IgM is seen in Waldenström's macroglobulinemia. Lytic lesions in bone are not present in this disorder, which behaves more like a malignant lymphoma. (Photomicrograph reproduced, with permission, from J.C. Bennett and F. Plum. *Cecil Textbook of Medicine*, 20th ed. Philadelphia, W.B. Saunders Co., 1996, p. 963.)

3. The answer is B: isolated inguinal lymphadenopathy in a 22-year-old man who presents with an indirect inguinal hernia. Inguinal lymph nodes and anterior cervical nodes draining the neck are common sites for drainage of infected material. A 22-year-old man with isolated inguinal lymphadenopathy with or without a hernia would most likely have benign disease (> 80% in patients < 30 years old). Submental lymphadenopathy in a 65-year-old man with alcoholism who smokes is most likely secondary to metastatic squamous cell carcinoma from a primary cancer in the oral cavity. Left supraclavicular lymph node enlargement (Virchow's node) in a 49-year-old Japanese man who has weight loss and epigastric distress is most consistent with metastatic adenocarcinoma of the stomach, which is the most common primary malignancy in Japan. Right axillary adenopathy in a 48-year-old woman with low back pain and a dragging sensation in her right upper quadrant is most likely the result of metastatic disease (vertebral column, liver, and axillary nodes) secondary to breast cancer. CT scan evidence of enlarged para-aortic lymph nodes in a 28-year-old man with a history of cryptorchidism is most likely the result of metastatic disease from a seminoma in a testicle. Seminomas are the most common germ cell tumor of the testicle that are associated with maldescent of the testicles.

4. The answer is D: be associated with fever, night sweats, and weight loss. HD is more likely than NHL to present with signs and symptoms of an infectious disease. It is more likely to be localized in its initial presentation rather than generalized as NHL is. The neoplastic cell in HD is the RS cell, which is derived from either a B or a T cell, depending on the subtype of HD. Diffuse infiltrates of RS cells are limited to the uncommon lymphocyte depletion type of HD, whereas NHL commonly is associated with a diffuse infiltrate of neoplastic B cells. HD is unlikely to present with stage IV disease (bone marrow involvement). NHLs commonly involve the marrow, particularly the low-grade B-cell lymphomas such as FCC of the small cleaved type and the small lymphocyte type. HD accounts for 40% of malignant lymphomas in children, while NHL accounts for 60% of cases in children (Burkitt's lymphoma, followed closely by lymphoblastic lymphoma).

5. The answer is C: cat-scratch disease: granulomatous microabscesses are similar to lymphogranuloma venereum. Cat-scratch disease is due to a gram-negative organism (*Bartonella [Rochalimaea] henselae*) identifiable only by a Warthin-Starry silver stain. The granulomatous microabscesses are similar to those found in lymph nodes in lymphogranuloma venereum, which is due to *Chlamydia trachomatis*. Spirochetes are easily identified in lymph nodes with the Warthin-Starry silver stain in both primary and secondary types of syphilis. Rheumatoid arthritis is associated with a follicular pattern and a heavy infiltrate of plasma cells. Sinus histiocytosis is a marker of increased histiocyte stimulation, as in nodes draining tumor or infection, and is not a feature of rheumatoid arthritis. Dermatopathic lymphadenitis is associated with eczematous diseases (e.g., psoriasis) with drainage of melanin pigment to the

lymph nodes and subsequent uptake by macrophages. It is often confused with metastatic malignant melanoma. Postvaccinal lymphadenitis is not associated with melanin pigmentation in lymph nodes. HIV-related lymphadenopathy is noted at the onset of HIV-positivity and in AIDS-related complex during the interval between the onset of disease and overt AIDS.

6. The answer is D: myeloproliferative disease and chronic lymphocytic leukemia. Myeloproliferative diseases (e.g., polycythemia rubra vera, agnogenic myeloid metaplasia, chronic myelogenous leukemia, essential thrombocythemia) are always associated with splenomegaly. Splenomegaly is often related to the presence of extramedullary hematopoiesis. CLL is the most common leukemia after 60 years of age and is associated with massive splenomegaly. Acute myelogenous leukemias are also associated with splenomegaly, but not to the same degree as the chronic leukemias. Congenital spherocytosis is associated with mild splenomegaly owing to extravascular removal of spherocytes. Sickle cell anemia is associated with splenomegaly in the first decade of life, following which autosplenectomy occurs from repeated infarctions. Malaria and kala-azar (visceral leishmaniasis) produce massive splenomegaly, but they are more common in developing countries than in the United States. Infectious mononucleosis commonly presents with mild splenomegaly. Lysosomal storage diseases, such as Gaucher's disease and Niemann-Pick disease, produce massive splenomegaly, but they are uncommon.

7. The answer is D: splenectomy: thrombocytosis, target cells, Howell-Jolly bodies in the peripheral blood. Splenectomy is associated with numerous hematologic abnormalities owing to its normal role as a filtering organ. In addition to the above findings, Heinz bodies (denatured Hb) and an increase in reticulocytes and nucleated RBCs may be seen in the peripheral blood. Systemic lupus erythematosus is associated with hyperplastic (onionskin) arteriolosclerosis of the penicillary arteriole rather than with hyaline arteriolosclerosis, which is a feature of diabetes mellitus and hypertension. Portal hypertension produces vascular congestion in the red pulp as a result of an increase in hydrostatic pressure in the portal vein (most commonly the result of cirrhosis). Hypersplenism is associated with splenomegaly and overactivity, leading to isolated or multiple cytopenias of hematopoietic elements. It is most commonly secondary to vascular congestion in patients with portal hypertension. Congenital asplenia has a high incidence of cardiac abnormalities. Felty's syndrome is the combination of rheumatoid arthritis, splenomegaly, and autoimmune neutropenia.

8. The answer is A: congestive cardiomyopathy. Restrictive rather than congestive cardiomyopathy (dilated heart) is more likely to be seen in amyloidosis. Amyloid is a protein that infiltrates interstitial tissue, resulting in progressive dysfunction in the organ or tissue involved. Peripheral neuropathy (e.g., carpal tunnel syndrome due to involvement of the median nerve), the nephrotic syndrome (seen in primary amyloidosis involving light chains), Alzheimer's disease (β-protein encoded by chromosome 21 is converted to amyloid that is toxic to neurons), and hepatosplenomegaly are commonly encountered in the spectrum of disease associated with amyloidosis.

9. The answer is A: 75-year-old man who initially presented with a condition seemingly unrelated to the monoclonal gammopathy. Monoclonal gammopathy of

undetermined significance (MGUS) is the most common type of monoclonal gammopathy. In three-fourths of patients, M spikes are uncovered as an unexpected finding in the workup of a seemingly non–plasma cell–related condition. A 65-year-old man with anemia, renal failure, and Bence Jones proteinuria most likely has multiple myeloma. A 60-year-old man with retinal hemorrhages secondary to a hyperviscosity syndrome probably has Waldenström's macroglobulinemia. A 4-year-old child with exophthalmos, cystic lesions in the skull, and diabetes insipidus most likely has histiocytosis X (Hand-Schüller-Christian variant of the disease). A 40-year-old man with reddish-brown lesions that when stroked become swollen, erythematous, and pruritic has urticaria pigmentosa, a benign, localized form of mastocytosis (in which the mast cells release histamine).

10. The answer is B: β-protein. β-Protein is coded for by chromosome 21, which is also the chromosome involved in Down syndrome (trisomy 21). The protein is converted to an amyloid protein that is toxic to cells in the brain, leading to Alzheimer's disease. Down syndrome patients who survive cardiovascular disease (endocardial cushion defects) early in their disease are more likely to die of complications related to Alzheimer's disease when they are older. Prealbumin is associated with amyloidosis producing restrictive cardiomyopathy. Calcitonin is the tumor marker and protein converted to amyloid in medullary carcinoma of the thyroid. Light chains in multiple myeloma may be converted to amyloid (primary amyloidosis). Serum-associated amyloid protein is an acute-phase reactant that may be the precursor for secondary amyloidosis, seen in chronic inflammatory conditions such as tuberculosis, leprosy, chronic osteomyelitis, and rheumatoid arthritis.

IMMUNOHEMATOLOGY AND

TRANSFUSION DISORDERS

SYNOPSIS

OBJECTIVES

1. To understand the clinical significance of the ABO blood group system.
2. To describe the Rh antigen system and non-Rh antigen systems of clinical importance.
3. To review blood transfusion and the indications for blood component therapy.
4. To understand ABO incompatibility and the prevention of Rh hemolytic disease of the newborn.

Objective 1: To understand the clinical significance of the ABO blood group system.

I. ABO blood group system
   A. The **ABO system** is the product of one gene locus having specific genes which code for transferases that attach antigenically different carbohydrate moieties to the terminal end of H antigen protruding from the surface of the RBC membrane.
      1. The **H gene** codes for a transferase that attaches fucose to the terminal end of a glycolipid to produce **H antigen**.
      2. The **A gene** codes for a transferase that attaches **N-acetylgalactosamine** to the H antigen, thereby producing A antigen (blood group A).
      3. The **B gene** codes for a transferase that attaches **galactose** to H antigen to produce **B antigen** (blood group B).
      4. The **O gene** is inactive, hence neither A nor B antigens are on the surface of blood group O RBCs.
      5. **Group AB** individuals have H antigen that carries either A or B active sugars.
      6. The A and B antigens are also located on cells other than RBCs (e.g., sperm, squamous cells, and neoplastic cells).
      7. An individual receives one blood group antigen from the mother and one from the father.
   B. In the laboratory, a **forward type** identifies the blood group antigen on the surface of RBCs by using anti-A and anti-B test serum, while a **back type** reacts A and B test RBCs against patient serum to identify the isohemagglutinins that correspond with the blood group (Table 14–1).
      1. A forward type does not determine the **geno-**

type (true genetic makeup) of the patient's blood group; for example, an AA or an AO individual is phenotypically (the phenotype is the physical expression of the genotype) blood group A.
      2. The genotype can be derived in families where the ABO status is available for parents and children; for example, if an A mother and a B father have an O child, then the parents must be genotypically AO and BO.

		B	O	Father
Mother	A	AB	AO	
	O	BO	OO	

   C. In **transfusion therapy**, the ABO system must be appropriately matched between recipient and donor.
      1. For example, a blood group A person, who has anti-B IgM isohemagglutinins, can receive only A or O blood.
      2. Individuals with blood group O can receive only O blood owing to the presence of anti-A IgM, anti-B IgM, and anti-A,B IgG in their serum, which would destroy cells with A or B antigen on their surface.
      3. Blood group O (universal donor) packed RBCs may be transfused into patients of any blood group owing to the lack of A and B antigens on the RBCs.
      4. Individuals with blood group AB (universal recipient) may receive blood from any group, since they have no isohemagglutinins to destroy the transfused cells.

Objective 2: To describe the Rh antigen system and non-Rh antigen systems of clinical importance.

II. Rh and non-Rh antigens
   A. The Rh antigen system has three adjoining gene loci, one locus coding for D antigen (no d antigen), another locus coding for C and/or c antigen, and the remaining locus coding for E and/or e antigen.
      1. If the D antigen locus on one or both chromosomes does not produce D antigen, d is used to designate this lack of production and should not be construed as representing the production of

TABLE 14–1. ABO Blood Groups

Phenotype	Isohemagglutinins	Whites	African Americans	Asians	Native Americans	Comments
O	Anti-A IgM Anti-B IgM Anti-A,B IgG	45%	49%	40%	79%	Universal donor (no antigens on the surface). Anti-A,B IgG is responsible for ABO incompatibility. Can only receive O blood (antibodies would destroy A, B, or AB blood). Predisposition for peptic ulcer disease.
A	Anti-B IgM	40%	27%	28%	16%	Predisposition for gastric carcinoma.
B	Anti-A IgM	11%	20%	27%	4%	
AB	None present	4%	4%	5%	<1%	Universal recipient (no antibodies).

d antigen, which does not exist; hence, possible genotypes are D/D, D/d, or d/d.

2. The C/c locus can produce individuals with the following antigen profile: C/C, C/c, or c/c (the E locus produces similar combinations).
3. An individual may have similar or different sets of these three Rh antigens on each chromosome; for example, CDE/cde, cde/cde, or CdE/cdE.
4. One of the sets of three Rh antigens from each parent is transmitted to each child in an **autosomal codominant fashion** (each antigen can express itself in dominant fashion similarly to HLA antigens).

		cde	CDE	Father
Mother	cDE	cDE/cde	cDE/CDE	
	CDE	CDE/cde	CDE/CDE	

5. An individual who is positive for D antigen is considered Rh positive (85% of the population).
6. Individuals with a weak variant of D antigen, called the **Du variant**, are considered Rh positive.

B. The complete Rh phenotype of an individual is determined by reacting the patient's RBCs with antisera against each of the Rh antigens; for example, a patient may have an Rh phenotype that is positive for C, c, D, and E antigens but negative for e antigen (CcDE).
C. **Alloimmunization** (formation of an antibody against an antigen) occurs if a person is exposed to an Rh or a non-Rh antigen (e.g., Kell antigen) that is not on the patient's RBCs (e.g., an Rh-negative person exposed to Rh-positive RBCs may develop anti-D antibodies).
   1. The majority of clinically important antibodies that may produce a transfusion reaction are warm-reacting (IgG) antibodies (e.g., anti-D, anti-Kell) rather than cold-reacting (IgM) antibodies.
   2. A patient with an antibody against a specific antigen should receive donor blood that is negative for that antigen in order to avoid a possible hemolytic transfusion reaction.
D. Kell antigen is a potent non-Rh antigen present in 10% of the population.
E. African Americans commonly lack **Duffy (Fy) antigens** on their RBCs, which protects their cells from *Plasmodium vivax* infestation, since these sporozoans require Duffy antigen as a receptor to bind to the RBCs.

F. The **I antigen system** may be associated with cold-reacting IgM antibodies against **i antigen** or **I antigens** leading to a cold autoimmune hemolytic anemia (e.g., **anti-i** is associated with infectious mononucleosis and **anti-I** with *Mycoplasma pneumoniae* infection).
G. **Lewis antigens** are closely related to ABH antigens and are produced in body secretions.
   1. Lewis antigens are absorbed onto the surface of RBCs.
   2. Naturally occurring IgM antibodies develop against these antigens, but they are generally weak antibodies of no clinical importance.

Objective 3. To review blood transfusion and the indications for blood component therapy.

III. Blood donors
A. **Autologous transfusion**, the safest form of transfusion, is the process of collection, storage, and reinfusion of the patient's own blood.
B. In the blood bank, donor blood is tested for group (ABO) and type (Rh), atypical antibodies (e.g., anti-D, anti-Kell) using the indirect Coombs' test (Chapter 12), syphilis (by serologic tests), hepatitis B surface antigen, antibodies against hepatitis C, antibodies for HIV-1 and 2 (ELISA test), and antibodies directed against HTLV-1.
C. Regardless of screening, there is still a 1:3300 chance per unit of contracting viral hepatitis (90% of cases are secondary to hepatitis C), 1:676,000 risk of AIDS, and a risk for contracting cytomegalovirus (CMV) and other infectious diseases.
IV. Blood storage
A. The goal in blood banking is to increase the shelf life of preserved blood and to maintain high intraerythrocyte **2,3-bisphosphoglycerate** (BPG) levels for the best oxygen exchange with tissue.
B. **CPDA-1** (citrate-phosphate-dextrose-adenine) preserves cells for 35 days owing to the action of citrate as an anticoagulant, phosphate and adenine as substrates for ATP synthesis, and dextrose as the fuel for anaerobic glycolysis in RBCs.
C. Components that increase in stored blood over time include plasma potassium, ammonia, and phosphate, while factors that decrease include RBC 2,3-BPG and plasma pH (acidosis).
V. Crossmatch
A. The **standard crossmatch** on the recipient consists

of ABO group and Rh type, an antibody screen for atypical antibodies (indirect Coombs' test), a direct Coombs' test (to identify IgG antibodies on RBCs), and a major crossmatch.
B. The **major crossmatch** is accomplished in a test tube by mixing a sample of the recipient's serum with a sample of RBCs from the donor unit.
1. The purpose of this crossmatch is to detect atypical (not naturally occurring) antibodies present in the recipient's serum that may be directed against foreign antigens on the RBCs in the donor unit.
2. A compatible crossmatch does not guarantee that donor RBCs will survive or that the recipient will not develop antibodies against a foreign antigen present on donor RBCs.
VI. Blood administration
A. All donor units have blood bank identification numbers that should be the same as those on a bracelet previously placed on the patient's wrist by laboratory personnel.
B. In bone marrow recipients and those with congenital immune deficiencies, blood must be irradiated to kill donor leukocytes in order to prevent graft-versus-host disease and CMV infection (Chapter 4).
VII. Blood component therapy
A. **RBCs** are transfused to increase the transport of oxygen to the tissues.
1. The decision to transfuse is based not only on the Hb concentration but also on other factors such as a clinical assessment of the patient, whether medical therapy is available to correct the anemia (e.g., iron in iron deficiency), and results of laboratory studies that evaluate oxygen reserve in the patient (oxygen consumption ratio and mixed venous oxygen content).
2. In general, an Hb of < 7 g/dL requires transfusion if bleeding persists, the patient is hemodynamically unstable, oxygen delivery reserves are poor, and other means of correcting the anemia are not available.
3. **Packed RBCs** are infused more frequently than whole blood in the treatment of anemia, since they have less volume (260 versus 520 mL) and a higher hematocrit (69% versus 45%) than whole blood.
4. Each unit of packed RBCs should raise the Hb by 1 g/dL and the Hct by 3%.
B. **Platelets** possess HLA antigens, ABO, and PL^{A1} antigens on their surface but not Rh antigens (Chapter 5).
1. Platelet transfusions (from random donors or single-donor pheresed) are generally indicated when patients have a platelet count < 50,000 cells/μL and have clinical evidence of bleeding or are candidates for a surgical or invasive procedure.
2. Each unit of platelets infused should raise the platelet count by 5000–10,000 cells/μL.
C. **Granulocyte transfusions** are reserved for patients who have severe sepsis associated with an absolute neutropenia < 500 cells/μL that has not responded appropriately to antibiotics within 48 hours.
D. **Fresh-frozen plasma** (FFP) contains all the coagulation factors and is the component of choice in bleeding associated with multiple (not single) factor deficiencies as commonly observed in severe

liver disease, over-anticoagulation with warfarin, and disseminated intravascular coagulation (DIC; Chapter 5).
E. **Cryoprecipitate** contains factor VIII, fibrinogen, factor XIII, and fibronectin (opsonizing protein) and is the component of choice in the treatment of mild von Willebrand's disease and fibrinogen deficiency (Chapter 5).
F. **Factor VIII concentrates** are primarily used in the treatment of hemophilia A.
G. **Albumin, plasma protein fraction** (PPF), **crystalloid solutions** (e.g., normal saline, Ringer's lactate [sodium, chloride, potassium, calcium, and lactate]), and **colloid substitutes** (e.g., dextran and hydroxyethyl starch) are utilized as volume expanders.
H. **Immune serum globulin** is useful in the treatment of hypogammaglobulinemia (e.g., Bruton's agammaglobulinemia) and the prevention of hepatitis A (possibly of hepatitis C).
VIII. Transfusion reactions
A. **Febrile reactions** (fever, chills, headache, and flushing) are the most common and are due to the presence of antibodies in the recipient that are directed against HLA antigens on donor leukocytes (type II cytotoxic antibody hypersensitivity reaction).
B. **Allergic reactions** (urticaria, fever, tachycardia, wheezing, dyspnea, and cyanosis) are secondary to antibodies directed against plasma proteins in the donor unit including IgA (type I IgE-mediated hypersensitivity reaction).
C. **Acute hemolytic transfusion reactions** (hypotension, burning at the site of infusion, fever, pain in the lower back or chest, bleeding from intravenous sites or surgical wounds [DIC], oliguria [renal failure], and hemoglobinuria) may be intravascular or extravascular.
1. **Intravascular hemolytic transfusion reactions** are due to an **ABO mismatch** (type II hypersensitivity reaction), in which a patient is infused with blood of a blood group that is incompatible with the ABO blood group of the patient (e.g., blood group A person receives B blood).
a. If a blood group A person receives B blood, the anti-B IgM antibodies in the recipient will attach to the donor group B RBCs, with subsequent activation of the complement system, leading to intravascular hemolysis.
b. Hypovolemic shock, DIC, and renal failure are common complications.
2. **Extravascular hemolytic transfusion reactions** are associated with the presence of an atypical antibody in the recipient (e.g., anti-Kell) that was undetectable (too low a titer) in the initial antibody screen.
a. The atypical antibody (usually IgG) will attach to the antigen on the donor RBCs, leaving the cells subject to macrophage phagocytosis and destruction (type II hypersensitivity reaction).
b. Results are a positive direct Coombs' test, a drop in the Hb, and jaundice.
3. **Delayed hemolytic transfusion reactions** occur 3–10 days after the infusion of blood and are most often due to extravascular hemolysis from an atypical antibody reaction against donor RBCs.

IX. ABO incompatibility and Rh hemolytic disease of the newborn

A. **ABO incompatibility** is the most common cause of HDN, anemia in the newborn, and jaundice in the first 24 hours after birth.

1. It occurs in ~25% of normal pregnancies and invariably involves an O mother with an A or B baby, since O individuals already have anti-A,B IgG in their plasma that is capable of crossing the placenta and attaching to fetal RBCs surfaced by A or B antigen.

2. The sensitized fetal RBCs are removed extravascularly by macrophages in the fetal spleen, liver, and bone marrow, resulting in anemia and an increase in unconjugated bilirubin, the latter metabolized by the mother's liver.

3. After delivery, the baby's immature liver enzymes are unable to handle the increased unconjugated bilirubin load, resulting in jaundice shortly after birth (not at birth).

4. ABO incompatibility may occur during the first or any other pregnancy involving a baby with blood group A or B antigens on its RBCs.

5. ABO incompatibility protects against Rh sensitization, since any fetal Rh-positive cells entering the maternal circulation are immediately destroyed by the O mother's anti-A IgM and anti-B IgM antibodies.

6. Abnormal laboratory tests in newborns with ABO incompatibility include spherocytes in the peripheral blood, a weakly positive direct Coombs' test, and a positive indirect Coombs' test secondary to maternally derived anti-A,B IgG antibodies in the newborn's serum.

7. Treatment usually utilizes phototherapy, with ultraviolet light oxidizing unconjugated bilirubin in the skin to harmless water-soluble dipyrroles that are eliminated in the urine.

8. Exchange transfusions are not usually required.

B. **Rh hemolytic disease of the newborn** is most commonly due to anti-D antibodies that have developed in a woman from exposure to Rh-positive RBCs in a previous pregnancy or blood transfusion.

1. An Rh-negative woman who is carrying an Rh-positive infant for the first time does not have to worry about her newborn developing HDN; however, if she becomes sensitized (develops anti-D) in that pregnancy, the risk for HDN and the severity of HDN increase with subsequent pregnancies.

2. Anti-D IgG antibodies in the mother in subsequent pregnancies will cross the placenta and attach to fetal Rh-positive RBCs, where they are removed by macrophages, leading to anemia and unconjugated hyperbilirubinemia.

3. If the degree of anemia is severe, extramedullary hematopoiesis (RBC production in the spleen, liver, etc.) may occur as compensation, as well as cardiac failure, resulting in generalized edema in the fetus (**hydrops fetalis**).

4. After delivery, the immature liver conjugation systems are overwhelmed, producing a rapid increase in unconjugated bilirubin in the blood.

5. Fetal albumin binding sites become fully saturated by the unconjugated bilirubin, hence increasing the **free (unbound) lipid-soluble unconjugated bilirubin**, which crosses the immature blood-brain barrier and deposits in the lipid-soluble brain to produce a condition called **kernicterus**.

6. During pregnancy, Rh-negative women without anti-D antibodies are given a standard dose of **Rh immunoglobulin** (RhIG) containing purified IgG anti-D antibodies at 28 weeks' gestation, thereby reducing the chance for sensitization by 90%.

7. Rh-negative and anti-D–negative women who have not received RhIG during their pregnancy and who deliver Rh-positive babies are still candidates for RhIG immunization (passive immunization).

a. The amount of fetal blood in the mother's circulation is determined by the **Kleihauer-Betke test**, which detects fetal Hb in fetal RBCs.

b. An estimate of the amount of fetal RBCs in the mother's circulation is calculated so that the appropriate amount of RhIG is administered intramuscularly within 72 hours following delivery.

c. RhIG may work because the anti-D antibodies attach to fetal Rh-positive cells, resulting in their premature destruction, or the antibody may cover the antigen, preventing its exposure to the mother's immune system.

QUESTIONS

DIRECTIONS. (Items 1–7): Each of the numbered items or incomplete statements in this section is followed by answers or by completions of the statement. Select the ONE lettered answer or completion that is BEST in each case. Correct answers and explanations are given at the end of the chapter.

1. A patient has the following blood bank profile:

Patient RBCs against anti-A test serum	Patient RBCs against anti-B test serum	Patient serum against blood group A test cells	Patient serum against blood group B test cells	Patient serum against Kell antigen-positive test cells
Negative	Negative	Positive	Positive	Negative

Patient RBCs against anti-D test sera	Patient RBCs against anti-C test sera	Patient RBCs against anti-c test sera	Patient RBCs against anti-E test sera	Patient RBCs against anti-e test sera
Negative	Positive	Negative	Positive	Positive

Which of the following statements is correct concerning this patient's profile?

(A) The patient's blood can be used as a universal donor.
(B) The patient is ABO compatible with transfused AB blood.
(C) The patient has the potential for developing antibodies against Rh-positive, C antigen–positive, and Kell antigen–positive blood.
(D) The patient's blood group imposes an increased risk for gastric adenocarcinoma.
(E) The patient's blood group has galactose attached to the terminal end of H antigen.

2. Which of the following components when infused into a patient imposes an increased risk for contracting hepatitis or other types of infectious disease?

(A) Crystalloid solution
(B) Immune serum globulin (ISG)
(C) Rh immunoglobulin (RhIG)
(D) Fresh-frozen plasma (FFP)
(E) Factor VIII (recombinant DNA)

3. Which of the following would be common to both ABO incompatibility and Rh hemolytic disease of the newborn (HDN)?

(A) Spherocytes in the peripheral blood of newborns
(B) Increased risk and severity of hemolysis in future pregnancies
(C) Positive direct Coombs' test on newborn RBCs
(D) Mother invariably blood group O
(E) Possible development of hemolytic anemia in the first pregnancy

4. A 65-year-old man with refractory anemia must be transfused every 3 months in order to maintain a stable Hb concentration. One hour after receiving his second unit of crossmatch-compatible blood, he develops fever, shaking chills, and hypotension. A posttransfusion blood sample shows negative indirect and direct Coombs' tests and the plasma is clear (no visible hemoglobin). A repeat major crossmatch on the pretransfusion sample as well as a repeat antibody screen (indirect Coombs' test) is unremarkable. A posttransfusion urine sample is negative for blood. The mechanism for this patient's reaction is most closely related to

(A) atypical antibodies reacting against donor RBCs
(B) naturally occurring anti-Lewis antibodies reacting against donor RBCs
(C) a host reaction against proteins in the donor unit
(D) the presence of anti-HLA antibodies directed against donor leukocytes
(E) an ABO mismatch with intravascular hemolysis

5. ABO incompatibility protects the mother from developing antibodies against fetal Rh-positive cells because

(A) fetal Rh-positive cells have a weaker D antigen than normal Rh-positive adult RBCs do
(B) the fetal cells are destroyed in the first trimester, hence preventing alloimmunization
(C) isohemagglutinins in the blood group A or B mother destroy Rh-positive fetal cells that have these antigens
(D) it is not possible to have both ABO and Rh incompatibility at the same time
(E) naturally occurring antibodies in the mother will destroy the Rh-positive fetal cells before alloimmunization occurs

6. Which of the following clinical disorder/component therapy relationships is correct?

(A) Severe hemophilia A: treat with cryoprecipitate
(B) Hb 8 g/dL in an asymptomatic patient with good oxygen reserve: transfuse packed RBCs
(C) Platelet count 60,000 cells/μL in an asymptomatic (nonbleeding) patient: do not give platelet transfusion
(D) Normal prothrombin and partial thromboplastin time in an asymptomatic (nonbleeding) patient with liver disease: give fresh-frozen plasma to prevent bleeding
(E) Hypovolemic shock secondary to fluid loss from diarrhea: give fresh-frozen plasma for volume repletion

7. A 35-year-old woman 4 days after a spontaneous abortion that required replacement of 5 units of blood develops fever and jaundice. Laboratory studies reveal an increase in unconjugated bilirubin, a drop in Hb concentration from that noted at discharge from the hospital 2 days ago, and a positive direct Coombs' test. The mechanism most likely responsible for her findings is

(A) an ABO mismatch that was undetected in the hospital
(B) an autoimmune hemolytic anemia unrelated to her blood transfusions
(C) an atypical antibody reacted against a foreign antigen in one or more units of blood
(D) a febrile reaction related to anti-HLA antibodies directed against RBCs in one or more of the donor units
(E) an allergic reaction directed against an RBC antigen in one or more of the donor units

ANSWERS AND EXPLANATIONS

1. The answer is A: The patient's blood can be used as a universal donor. The patient's RBCs do not react against anti-A or anti-B test sera (forward type = blood group O), and the serum reacts against both A and B test cells, indicating the presence of anti-A and anti-B (back type confirms blood group O). Blood group O patients are universal donors owing to the lack of A and B antigens on their RBCs, and they are at increased risk for peptic ulcer disease (blood group A has an increased incidence of gastric adenocarcinoma). Blood group A patients have N-acetylgalactosamine attached to the terminal end of H antigen, while blood group B patients have galactose attached to the terminal end of H antigen. Group O patients have an inactive O gene, hence no sugar moiety is added to H antigen (this antigen contains fucose on the terminal end). The patient is Rh negative (no D antigen), c antigen negative, and Kell antigen negative, hence antibodies could potentially develop against D, c, and Kell antigens but not against C antigen, since the patient is positive for this antigen.

2. The answer is D: fresh-frozen plasma (FFP). FFP can transmit any of the infectious diseases including hepatitis C and HIV. Crystalloid solutions (e.g., normal saline), immune serum globulin (in which viruses are destroyed in the manufacturing process), Rh immunoglobulin (purified anti-D), and factor VIII prepared by recombinant DNA techniques (lyophilized preparations, however, have a small risk) do not transmit infectious diseases. Packed RBCs, platelet concentrates, granulocyte infusions, and cryoprecipitate can transmit disease.

3. The answer is C: positive direct Coombs' test on newborn RBCs. ABO incompatibility differs from Rh incompatibility in that spherocytes are usually present in the peripheral blood of newborns, the risk and severity of hemolysis do not increase in subsequent pregnancies, hemolytic anemia may develop in the first pregnancy, and the mother is invariably blood group O and the baby blood group A or B. Both Rh HDN and ABO incompatibility have a positive direct Coombs' reaction on the baby's RBCs owing to the presence of anti-D IgG and anti-A,B IgG antibodies, respectively. In addition, both types of HDN have extravascular hemolysis by fetal macrophages, anemia, and unconjugated hyperbilirubinemia. Rh HDN does not occur in the first pregnancy, since sensitization to D antigen usually occurs at the time of delivery when Rh-positive fetal cells have access to the maternal circulation. There is an increase in the risk and severity of HDN with subsequent pregnancies.

4. The answer is D: the presence of anti-HLA antibodies directed against donor leukocytes. The antibodies most likely developed from previous transfusions the patient received for his refractory anemia. Negative indirect and direct Coombs' tests on a posttransfusion blood sample rule out atypical antibodies from a hemolytic transfusion reaction. No allergic signs are present in the patient (urticarial rash) to indicate a type I hypersensitivity reaction against donor proteins. The repeat major cross-match on the pretransfusion serum (patient serum against donor RBCs) and the antibody screen indicate that no atypical antibodies were missed prior to the transfusion. The absence of intravascular hemolysis (no hemoglobin in the plasma) and hemoglobin in the urine rules out an ABO mismatch. Naturally occurring anti-Lewis antibodies are not clinically significant.

5. The answer is E: naturally occurring antibodies in the mother will destroy the Rh-positive fetal cells before alloimmunization occurs. ABO incompatibility invariably occurs in an O mother who has a baby with A or B antigens on its RBCs. If an O-negative mother has an A or B antigen Rh-positive baby, when the baby's RBCs enter her circulation during delivery (very uncommon in the first trimester), her naturally occurring anti-A IgM, anti-B IgM antibodies will destroy the fetal cells within seconds, hence preventing alloimmunization. Fetal D antigen has similar antigenicity to adult D antigen and so is not a factor in the potential for alloimmunization in the mother upon exposure to fetal Rh-positive cells.

6. The answer is C: platelet count 60,000 cells/μL in an asymptomatic (nonbleeding) patient: do not give a platelet transfusion. In general, a platelet count > 50,000 cells/μL in a patient who is asymptomatic does not require platelet transfusion. Severe hemophilia A is normally treated with factor VIII lyophilized or recombinant DNA concentrates and not cryoprecipitate, which is primarily reserved for mild von Willebrand's disease. In general, patients with an Hb > 7 g/dL who are asymptomatic do not require packed RBC transfusions. An asymptomatic patient with liver disease who has a normal prothrombin and partial thromboplastin time does not require fresh-frozen plasma to prevent bleeding. Hypovolemic shock secondary to fluid loss from diarrhea is not an indication for FFP, since crystalloid solutions are a safer and less expensive way to restore plasma volume.

7. The answer is C: an atypical antibody reacting against a foreign antigen in one or more units of blood. The patient has a classic history for a delayed hemolytic transfusion reaction where a preexisting (but initially undetected) atypical antibody resurfaces secondary to reappearance of the antigen in one or more of the transfused donor units. Fever, drop in Hb, jaundice, and a positive direct Coombs' test are the key findings. An ABO mismatch would have resulted in immediate signs of intravascular hemolysis. An autoimmune hemolytic anemia unrelated to her blood transfusions is highly unlikely owing to the time relationship of her signs and previous blood transfusions. A febrile reaction is related to anti-HLA antibodies directed against donor leukocytes, not RBCs. An allergic reaction is directed against proteins in the donor unit and not RBC antigens.

CHAPTER FIFTEEN

DISORDERS OF THE

GASTROINTESTINAL TRACT

SYNOPSIS

OBJECTIVES

1. To be familiar with common benign and malignant disorders of the oral cavity.
2. To discuss nonneoplastic and neoplastic disorders involving the esophagus.
3. To understand the pathogenesis of pyloric stenosis, gastritis, peptic ulcer disease, and cancer of the stomach.
4. To outline the pathophysiology of malabsorption and diarrhea and their complications.
5. To discuss obstructive, vascular, and diverticular disorders of the small and large bowel.
6. To compare and contrast ulcerative colitis and Crohn's disease.
7. To outline the polyp types, polyposis syndromes, and common cancers of the small and large bowel.
8. To review common disorders associated with the appendix and anus.

Objective 1: To be familiar with common benign and malignant disorders of the oral cavity.

I. Benign disorders of the oral cavity
   A. **Cleft lip** (usually upper lip) and **palate** are the most common congenital disorders in the oral cavity.
   B. Viral, bacterial, and fungal infections may involve the mucosa in the oral cavity.
      1. **Coxsackievirus A** is associated with two vesicular diseases of the oral cavity: **herpangina** and **hand-foot-and-mouth disease**.
      2. **Herpes simplex type I** produces **gingivostomatitis** and **herpes labialis** (fever blisters).
      3. **Epstein-Barr virus** (EBV) causes **exudative pharyngitis** (infectious mononucleosis) and **hairy leukoplakia**, a white lesion located on the lateral border of the tongue and found in patients who are HIV positive.
      4. *Streptococcus pyogenes* accounts for ~20–35% of cases of **exudative pharyngitis/tonsillitis**, while ~50% are virus induced.
      5. *Candida albicans* produces **thrush** (white pseudomembrane) in neonates and a more chronic disease in immunocompromised patients (AIDS).

C. Complications associated with **dental caries** (*Streptococcus mutans*) include **gingivitis, periodontitis** (involvement of alveolar bone), and **pulpitis**.
D. Systemic diseases and skin disorders that may involve the mouth include the following:
   1. **Pemphigus vulgaris** is an immunologic vesicular disease with IgG antibodies directed against the intercellular attachment sites between keratinocytes.
   2. **Mucous membrane pemphigoid** is an immunologic vesicular disease with circulating IgG antibodies directed against antigens in the basement membrane.
   3. **Erythema multiforme** is a hypersensitivity reaction that develops against infectious agents (*Mycoplasma*) or drugs (sulfonamides) and may also involve the mouth (**Stevens-Johnson syndrome**).
   4. **Addison's disease** (oral pigmentation), **lead poisoning** (lead line), and **macroglossia** (e.g., due to hypothyroidism, amyloidosis) affect the mouth.
   5. **Lichen planus** produces fine, lacy white lines on the mucosal surface called **Wickham's striae**.
E. **Aphthous ulcers** (canker sores) are recurrent painful, localized ulcerations in the mouth that may or may not be associated with systemic disease (e.g., **Behçet's** and **Reiter's syndromes**).
F. **Leukoplakia** (white patch), **erythroleukoplakia** (red and white patch), and **erythroplakia** (red patch) are clinical terms describing mucosal lesions that predispose to squamous cell cancer if left untreated (particularly those with red patches).
   1. They do not wipe off of the mucosal surface.
   2. They are caused by use of tobacco products and excessive ingestion of alcohol.
   3. Biopsy is required to rule out squamous cell cancer.

II. Malignant disorders of the oral cavity
   A. **Squamous cell carcinoma** is the most common cancer (95%) in the oral cavity.
      1. It is more common in men over 50 years of age than in women.

2. Predisposing factors include smoking (most important factor), excessive alcohol consumption (cocarcinogen with tobacco), leukoplakia, and erythroplakia.
3. Sites of predilection, in descending order, are the lateral border of the tongue, lower lip, and floor of the mouth.
4. The majority are well-differentiated (low-grade) keratinizing cancers that locally metastasize to submental and jugular nodes.

B. A **verrucous carcinoma** is a low-grade, well-differentiated squamous carcinoma associated with smokeless tobacco.

C. **Kaposi's sarcoma** (due to herpesvirus 8) in the oral cavity is most frequently associated with AIDS and located on the palate.

III. Benign salivary gland disorders

A. **Mumps** causes bilateral parotitis (which increases serum amylase) most commonly in children < 14 years of age.
  1. The incubation period is 16–18 days.
  2. Complications include orchitis (unilateral; no sterility risk), oophoritis, aseptic meningitis (most common extrasalivary complication), and pancreatitis (also increases serum amylase).

B. The majority of **salivary gland tumors** are benign (pleomorphic adenoma), and most occur in the major salivary glands (usually the parotid).
  1. The ratio of benign to malignant tumors is largest in the parotid gland and smallest in the minor salivary glands.
  2. The **pleomorphic adenoma (mixed tumor)** is the most common benign tumor in both the major (parotid gland) and minor salivary glands.
    a. These are encapsulated tumors with an epithelial component surrounded by a myxomatous stroma often containing foci of bone or cartilage.
    b. In rare cases, the tumor may develop into a carcinoma (**carcinoma ex pleomorphic adenoma**).
  3. **Papillary cystadenoma lymphomatosum (Warthin's tumor)** is a multicentric tumor that arises from parotid duct epithelium within or immediately subjacent to a lymph node.

IV. Malignant salivary gland disorders

A. **Mucoepidermoid** (squamous and glandular component) **carcinoma** is the most common malignancy of the major (usually the parotid) and minor salivary glands.

B. **Adenoid cystic carcinomas** most commonly arise in the minor salivary glands located on the hard palate.

Objective 2: To discuss nonneoplastic and neoplastic disorders involving the esophagus.

V. Symptoms associated with esophageal disease
A. **Dysphagia** is difficulty in swallowing foods and may be limited to solids (sign of obstruction) or solids and liquids (implicates motor dysfunction).
B. **Odynophagia**, or pain on swallowing, is most commonly caused by gastric reflux or infectious esophagitis.

C. **Heartburn**, the most common manifestation of esophageal disease, is a burning sensation in the retrosternal area associated with gastric reflux.

VI. Benign disorders of the esophagus
A. A **tracheoesophageal fistula** is the most common congenital esophageal anomaly.
  1. The proximal end of the esophagus ends blindly, while the distal end arises from the trachea.
  2. Newborns may develop chemical pneumonia (from milk reflux into the lungs) and commonly have distention of the stomach by air.

B. **Plummer-Vinson syndrome** is associated with iron deficiency, an esophageal web (dysphagia for solids), glossitis, leukoplakia, koilonychia (spoon nails), and achlorhydria.

C. **Diverticula** are outpouchings of the GI wall and are analogous to aneurysms in the cardiovascular system or bronchiectasis in the respiratory tract.
  1. **True diverticula** are lined by mucosa, submucosa, muscularis propria, and adventitia (e.g., Meckel's diverticula).
  2. **False (pulsion) diverticula** are created by increased intraesophageal pressure herniating the mucosa, submucosa, and part of the muscularis propria though an area of weakness in the underlying muscle wall.
  3. The three most common pulsion diverticula in the upper, middle, and lower esophagus, respectively, are **Zenker's diverticulum** (most common; defect in the cricopharyngeus muscle), **traction diverticulum** (due to motor abnormalities), and **epiphrenic diverticulum** (in association with achalasia).

D. **Motor disorders** affecting normal peristalsis of food and emptying of food into the stomach (dysphagia for solids and liquids) include progressive systemic sclerosis (PSS) and achalasia.
  1. **PSS (scleroderma)** is an autoimmune disease associated with increased synthesis of collagen in organ systems throughout the body.
    a. The GI tract is most often involved, particularly the smooth muscle of the lower esophagus.
    b. Abnormalities include relaxation of the lower esophageal sphincter (LES) and dilatation and lack of peristalsis in the proximal esophagus.
    c. The **CREST syndrome**, a variant of PSS, is also associated with esophageal motility problems.
  2. **Achalasia** is a neuromuscular disorder with increased pressure and failure of relaxation of the LES as well as dilatation and absence of peristalsis in the proximal esophagus.
    a. The ganglion cells that normally secrete vasointestinal peptide (which relaxes the LES) are absent in the myenteric plexus of the LES (loss of ganglion cells is analogous to Hirschsprung's disease).
    b. Acquired achalasia (and Hirschsprung's disease) may occur in **Chagas' trypanosomiasis** (*Trypanosoma cruzi*).

E. **Sliding hiatal hernias** (most common type) are characterized by protrusion of the proximal stomach through a widened diaphragmatic hiatus.
  1. When symptomatic, they produce nocturnal epigastric distress owing to reflux esophagitis.

2. Complications include gastric reflux, ulceration, bleeding (hematemesis), stricture formation, and **Barrett's esophagus** (glandular metaplasia with a risk for adenocarcinoma in 5–10% of cases).

F. **Acute** and **chronic esophagitis** may be secondary to gastric reflux, infections, drug use, irradiation, trauma, and corrosive agents.

1. **Gastroesophageal reflux disease** (GERD) is due to relaxation of the LES with subsequent regurgitation of gastric juices (acid and bile), leading to inflammation of the distal esophagus.
   a. Predisposing factors include sliding hiatal hernias, pregnancy, peptic ulcer disease (PUD), and factors that lower the LES tone (β-adrenergics, alcohol, smoking, caffeine).
   b. Patients complain of heartburn (particularly at night when reflux is worse), nocturnal cough, and nocturnal asthma.
   c. Complications are similar to those of sliding hiatal hernias.
2. **Viruses** (HSV type I [25% of all cases], CMV, HIV) and **fungi** (*Candida*), the most frequent causes of **infectious esophagitis**, usually occur in the setting of an immunocompromised host (e.g., in AIDS).
3. **Corrosive esophagitis**, due to ingestion of strong alkaline agents (which produce liquefactive necrosis) or acids (which produce coagulative necrosis), usually heals with stricture formation.

G. **Esophageal varices** are a complication of portal hypertension, which is most commonly caused by alcoholic cirrhosis.

1. Increased pressure leads to rupture (left gastric and azygous veins) and massive hematemesis (vomiting of blood).
2. Endoscopy is the primary tool for confirming and treating varices (by sclerotherapy).

H. Vomiting or retching (forceful vomiting) may lead to tears (**Mallory-Weiss syndrome**) or rupture (**Boerhaave's syndrome**) of the esophagus and/or proximal stomach.

VII. Malignant disorders of the esophagus

A. The most common malignant tumor of the esophagus is a **squamous cell carcinoma** (60%).

1. It frequents the 50- to 60-year-old age group and is more common in men than in women and in African Americans than in whites.
   a. Predisposing factors include smoking, alcohol (a cocarcinogen), nitrosamines, lye strictures, Plummer-Vinson syndrome, and achalasia.
   b. Most cancers are located in the mid-esophagus and have a polypoid appearance.
   c. Patients initially present with dysphagia for solids and weight loss.
   d. It first spreads beneath the mucosa, then locally by lymphatics that drain into regional lymph nodes before finally spreading systemically to distant sites (liver, lungs, and adrenals).
   e. The 5-year survival is < 5%.

B. **Adenocarcinoma** of the distal esophagus is the second most common esophageal tumor (40%) and generally arises from Barrett's esophagus.

Objective 3: To understand the pathogenesis of pyloric stenosis, gastritis, peptic ulcer disease, and cancer of the stomach.

VIII. Benign disorders of the stomach

A. Congenital pyloric stenosis (hypertrophy of the circular muscles) is a male-dominant disorder that presents with projectile vomiting of non–bile-stained fluid 2–4 weeks after birth.

B. **Acute (erosive) gastritis** is most commonly caused by NSAID use, which inhibits prostaglandin synthesis and its ability to produce and maintain the bicarbonate-rich mucous barrier.

1. Erosions do not extend beyond the muscularis mucosa.
2. Other causes include infection (e.g., CMV in AIDS patients), direct chemical toxicity (e.g., alcohol), uremia, smoking, CNS injury (**Cushing's ulcers**), and burns (**Curling's ulcers**).

C. **Chronic gastritis** is characterized by gland and mucosal atrophy secondary to chronic inflammation.

1. **Type A chronic atrophic gastritis** involves the body and fundus (acid-secreting portion of the stomach) and is most commonly associated with **pernicious anemia**.
   a. Autoantibodies directed against parietal cells or intrinsic factor lead to achlorhydria and macrocytic anemia.
   b. There is an increased incidence of adenocarcinoma (10%) and carcinoid tumors (G cell hyperplasia leads to cancer secondary to loss of acid inhibition of gastrin secreted in the antrum).
2. **Type B chronic atrophic gastritis** (most common type) primarily involves the antrum and is associated with *Helicobacter pylori*.
   a. *H. pylori* is a gram-negative, S-shaped rod that produces urease.
      (1) It is transmitted by the fecal-oral route and is found within the mucous layer lining the surface of the antrum or lining the pits.
      (2) The organism is identified in gastric biopsy specimens with silver stains or by its ability to produce urease (clofazimine [CLO] test); serologic tests are also available.
      (3) The virulence of *H. pylori* is secondary to the toxic effects of ammonia produced by urease, the release of cytotoxins that destroy tight junctions between the epithelial cells, and the induction of an inflammatory/immune response.
   b. Complications include gastric ulcers (most common), carcinoma, and malignant lymphomas.
3. **Type AB** (**environmental gastritis**), the most common type outside the United States, is due to a combination of *H. pylori* and dietary factors; it predisposes to adenocarcinoma.

D. **Ménétrier's disease** (hypertrophic gastritis) is associated with giant rugal folds, achlorhydria, and hypoalbuminemia secondary to protein loss (protein-losing enteropathy).

E. **Peptic ulcer disease** (PUD) is most commonly due to gastric and duodenal ulcers, which in turn are caused by *H. pylori*.

1. The pathogenesis of PUD involves acid injury resulting from a defective mucosal barrier (gastric ulcer) or hypersecretion of acid (duodenal ulcer).

2. The ulcers are clean, sharply demarcated, and slightly elevated around the edges and have four layers, which, in sequence, are necrotic debris, granulation tissue, inflammation, and fibrosis.

3. **Duodenal ulcers** when compared with gastric ulcers have the following characteristics:
   a. Epidemiology: most common PUD, male/female ratio of 2/1, blood group O, AD inheritance pattern (some cases), greater association with *H. pylori*.
   b. Pathogenesis: excess acid production, increased parietal cell mass, decreased bicarbonate in the mucous barrier (possible *H. pylori* effect), smoking, cirrhosis, chronic renal disease.
   c. Location: anterior portion of the first part of the duodenum (most common) and the posterior portion (danger of perforation into pancreas).
   d. Complications: most common cause of hematemesis, melenemesis (vomiting of coffee ground material), melena (black tarry stools), and perforation (air under the diaphragm).
   e. Clinical findings: burning epigastric pain 1–3 hours after a meal, frequently relieved by antacids or food; pain may wake the patient at night.

4. **Gastric ulcers** when compared with duodenal ulcers are characterized by the following:
   a. Epidemiology: male/female ratio of 1/1, blood group A.
   b. Pathogenesis: defective mucosal barrier due to *H. pylori*, mucosal ischemia (reduced prostaglandin), bile reflux, smoking, COPD.
   c. Location: single ulcer on the lesser curvature of the antrum.
   d. Complications: cancer association with a benign ulcer in 1–3% (no cancer relationship with duodenal ulcers).
   e. Clinical findings: burning epigastric pain soon after eating that is relieved by antacids but aggravated by food.

F. **Pancreatic heterotopic rests (choristomas)** most commonly occur in the wall of the stomach.

G. **Hyperplastic (regenerative) polyps** are nonneoplastic polyps that may be associated with chronic blood loss.

H. **Adenomas** are neoplastic polyps that increase with age and pose a risk for transformation into a gastric adenocarcinoma.

I. **Leiomyomas**, the most common benign soft tissue tumors in the GI tract, are most commonly located in the stomach; they may ulcerate and bleed.

IX. Malignant disorders of the stomach
A. **Gastric adenocarcinomas** account for 90–95% of malignant tumors arising in the stomach but are declining in the United States owing to increased use of vitamin C and refrigeration, both of which block nitrosamine formation.
   1. The incidence of cancer parallels the presence of chronic gastritis secondary to *H. pylori*.
   2. Predisposing factors include nitrosamines, achlorhydria, blood group A, chronic atrophic gastritis (types A, B, and AB), and gastric adenomas.

3. The majority are located in the pyloroantrum (50%) with a predilection for the lesser curvature, while the remainder occur in the cardia (25%) and body and fundus (25%).
4. **Early gastric cancer** is confined to the mucosa or submucosa regardless of the lymph node status of the patient; the superficial type has an excellent prognosis.
5. **Invasive carcinoma** is **intestinal** (has an association with *H. pylori* and arises from intestinal metaplasia) or **diffuse** (linitis plastica type, or "leather bottle" stomach, has signet-ring cells and no relation to *H. pylori*).
6. Weight loss and epigastric pain are the most common symptoms.
7. Adenocarcinomas metastasize to local lymph nodes first and then to distant sites (e.g., Virchow's node, liver, lungs, and ovaries [**Krukenberg's tumor**]).
8. The 5-year survival rate is < 20% with lymph node involvement.

B. The stomach is the most common extranodal site for **primary malignant lymphomas**.
   1. They arise from *mucosa-associated lymphoid tissue* (MALT).
   2. The majority are high-grade, large-cell immunoblastic lymphomas of B-cell origin; low-grade B-cell lymphomas (MALTomas) are more likely to be associated with *H. pylori*.

C. **Carcinoid tumors** may be associated with type A chronic atrophic gastritis.

Objective 4: To outline the pathophysiology of malabsorption and diarrhea and their complications.

X. Pathophysiology of malabsorption
A. **Malabsorption** is defined as increased fecal excretion of fat with concurrent deficiencies of vitamins, minerals, carbohydrates, and proteins.
B. Characteristic findings include weight loss, diarrhea, and malnutrition.
C. **Steatorrhea** is excessive, large, sticky stools that float as a result of maldigestion of fats by pancreatic lipase or malassimilation of the fat by the small bowel.
D. **Pancreatic insufficiency** (e.g., chronic pancreatitis), **bile salt deficiency** (e.g., cirrhosis, cholestasis), and **small bowel disease** (e.g., celiac disease) are the three most common causes of malabsorption.
E. The gold standard test to document fat malabsorption is the **quantitative 72-hour stool for fat**.
F. The D-xylose test is useful in identifying assimilation problems in the small bowel (decreased uptake of the pentose sugar).
G. Complications associated with malabsorption include the following:
   1. Multiple fat- and water-soluble vitamin deficiencies.
   2. Hypoproteinemia leading to pitting edema, ascites, hypogammaglobulinemia (infections), and fatty liver (decreased apolipoproteins).
   3. Anemia from iron and/or folate/B_{12} deficiency.
   4. Failure to thrive (in children).
H. **Celiac disease** is an autoimmune disease (HLA-B8, -Dr3, -DQ2 associations) that begins in infancy with exposure to wheat gluten in the diet.

1. Antibodies develop against **gliadin** (a component of gluten), leading to immune destruction (atrophy) of the villi in the distal ileum and jejunum and hyperplasia of the intestinal crypts.
2. Children present with failure to thrive, abdominal distention, and diarrhea, while adults present with weight loss, diarrhea, and malnutrition (there is also a risk for T-cell lymphoma of the small bowel).
3. A gluten-free diet is the cornerstone of therapy.

I. **Whipple's disease** is a male-dominant systemic disease due to infection by *Tropheryma whippelii*.
   1. There is blunting of the villi in the jejunum and ileum and a heavy infiltrate of foamy macrophages (containing the organisms; seen only with EM) in the lamina propria that blocks lymphatic uptake of fat (malabsorption).
   2. Patients present with fever, diarrhea, joint pain, gray-brown skin pigmentation, and generalized lymphadenopathy; antibiotics are curative.

J. **Tropical sprue** (infectious disease in the Far East), **giardiasis** (*Giardia lamblia*), and **intestinal lymphangiectasia** (abnormal dilated lymphatics) are additional causes of malabsorption.

XI. Pathophysiology of diarrhea
   A. **Diarrhea** is the passage of more than 250 g of stool per day (normal, 100 g/d).
   B. **Osmotic types** (e.g., due to lactase deficiency) are large-volume diarrheas that draw water into the lumen, resulting in a hypotonic diarrhea without mucosal inflammation.
   C. **Secretory types** are large-volume diarrheas secondary to stimulation of the cyclic AMP mechanism for chloride secretion (e.g., cholera toxin, toxin of enterotoxigenic *Escherichia coli*), leading to the loss of a chloride-rich isotonic fluid without mucosal inflammation.
   D. **Invasive diarrhea** (e.g., shigellosis) is a low-volume diarrhea with invasion of the intestinal mucosa and production of an inflammatory exudate (detected by fecal smear for leukocytes).
   E. **Microbial pathogens** associated with diarrhea are summarized below.
      1. **Rotavirus**, the most common childhood cause of diarrhea, is transmitted by the fecal-oral route; it produces a watery, nonbloody diarrhea.
      2. The **Norwalk virus** is a common cause of both adult and childhood gastroenteritis.
      3. **Food poisoning** (gastroenteritis) from ingestion of preformed toxin in food is associated with *Staphylococcus aureus*, *Bacillus cereus* (contaminated fried rice), and adult *Clostridium botulinum* (in canned foods; toxin blocks cholinergic nerves).
      4. *Clostridium perfringens*, *C. botulinum* (in infants), and *Salmonella enteritidis* produce food poisoning after first colonizing the bowel and then releasing their toxins.
      5. *Clostridium difficile*, the organism associated with antibiotic-induced (most commonly ampicillin and clindamycin) **pseudomembranous colitis**, is best diagnosed by toxin assay of stool; it is treated with metronidazole.
      6. *Shigella sonnei*, the most common cause of shigellosis, is transmitted by the oral-fecal route; it produces bloody diarrhea and pseudomembranous inflammation in the ileum and colon.
      7. Most *Salmonella* species producing enterocolitis (*S. typhimurium* most commonly) have animal reservoirs (poultry, turtles) and are transmitted by the oral-fecal route.
      8. **Typhoid fever** (enteric fever), caused by *S. typhi* (human reservoir), invades Peyer's patches and produces septicemia (blood is the best culture medium for isolation) during the first week.
         a. The second week of infection is marked by diarrhea and the classic triad of bradycardia, absolute neutropenia, and hepatosplenomegaly.
         b. It may produce a chronic carrier state (persistence of the organism 1 year postinfection), usually in the gallbladder.
      9. *Campylobacter jejuni*, the most common invasive bacterial enterocolitis in the United States, is contracted by eating contaminated poultry or drinking contaminated milk; it produces a bloody diarrhea with crypt abscesses and ulcers resembling ulcerative colitis.
      10. *E. coli* produces toxin-induced and invasive diarrheas.
         a. The **enteropathogenic strain** produces a nontoxin type of mild diarrhea in infants and young children.
         b. The **enterotoxigenic strains** produce a heat-labile toxin (LT) stimulating cyclic AMP (secretory diarrhea) or a heat-stable toxin (ST) stimulating guanylate cyclase and producing a secretory diarrhea (most common cause of traveler's diarrhea).
         c. The **enteroinvasive strain** is associated with an invasive enterocolitis.
         d. The **enterohemorrhagic strain**, associated with the O157:H7 serotype contaminating raw ground beef, may produce hemolytic uremic syndrome and hemorrhagic or pseudomembranous colitis.
      11. *Vibrio cholerae* produces a powerful enterotoxin that stimulates adenylate cyclase in the small bowel, leading to a severe secretory diarrhea ("ricewater stools"); it is best treated with a glucose/electrolyte solution.
      12. *Cryptosporidium parvum* (acid-fast positive) and *Microsporidia* species are two protozoans associated with diarrhea in the gay bowel syndrome.

Objective 5: To discuss obstructive, vascular, and diverticular disorders of the small and large bowel.

XII. Obstructive disorders of the small and large bowel
   A. **Duodenal atresia**, most commonly associated with Down syndrome, is characterized by vomiting of bile-stained material at birth and an abdominal radiograph with the "**double bubble**" **sign**.
   B. **Hirschsprung's disease** (**congenital megacolon**) is associated with Down syndrome and Chagas' disease (acquired).
      1. It is due to a deficiency of ganglion cells in

Meissner's submucosal plexus and Auerbach's myenteric plexus; it primarily afflicts boys.

2. In most cases, it is restricted to the distal sigmoid colon and rectum.

3. The proximal bowel is dilated (ganglion cells are present), since peristalsis is not able to move stool beyond the contracted aganglionic segment.

4. Complications include constipation (initial presentation), enterocolitis, toxic megacolon, and perforation.

C. **Adhesions**, the most common cause of obstruction in the GI tract, are most commonly acquired from previous abdominal surgery.

D. **Indirect inguinal hernias**, the second most common cause of bowel obstruction, are the only hernias in which the small bowel extends into the scrotal sac (lateral to the triangle of Hesselbach).

E. **Direct inguinal hernias** occur through the posterior wall of the inguinal canal (center of the triangle of Hesselbach).

F. **Umbilical hernias** occur in children and in adults, the latter often precipitated by ascites or pregnancy.

G. **Ventral hernias** (incisional hernia) occur in previous surgical incision sites.

H. **Intussusception** is the telescoping of one segment of proximal bowel (usually the terminal ileum) into the distal bowel (usually the cecum).

1. It primarily occurs in children, who present with signs of obstruction (colicky pain) and rectal bleeding ("currant jelly stools") from bowel infarction.

2. In adults, intussusceptions are more commonly due to organic disease in which polyps or cancer serve as the nidus.

I. **Volvulus** is twisting of the bowel (usually the sigmoid colon) around the mesenteric root with subsequent obstruction and infarction.

J. **Gallstone ileus** occurs when a chronically inflamed gallbladder forms a fistula with the small bowel, resulting in passage of a stone that produces obstruction at the ileocecal valve.

K. **Meconium ileus** is a potential complication of a newborn with cystic fibrosis.

XIII. Vascular disorders of the small and large bowel

A. Ischemic injury to the bowel may be secondary to thrombosis over an atherosclerotic plaque (thrombosis of the proximal superior mesenteric artery most commonly), embolism (left heart thrombus), shock (hypovolemia), vasospasm (digitalis), venous thrombosis (polycythemia), or mechanical obstruction (volvulus).

B. **Small bowel infarction** is more likely to be transmural (full thickness) owing to only one major blood supply (superior mesenteric artery), while the **large bowel**, with more than one blood supply, most commonly presents with ischemic colitis involving the splenic flexure (junction of the superior and inferior mesenteric arteries).

1. In **transmural infarctions**, the bowel undergoes hemorrhagic infarction (danger of peritonitis) with mucosal ulcerations and pseudomembrane formation.

2. **Ischemic colitis** initially presents with abdominal pain and bloody diarrhea; repair by fibrosis may eventuate in ischemic strictures.

C. **Angiodysplasia** is a common cause of (often massive) lower GI bleeding in the elderly.

1. It is most commonly located in the cecum and right colon, where dilated submucosal vessels are noted in the submucosa; these are best identified by mesenteric angiography.

2. There is an unexplained association with aortic stenosis and von Willebrand's disease.

3. Diverticulosis and angiodysplasia are the first and second most common causes of massive hematochezia (bright red blood in the stool).

XIV. Diverticular disease of the small and large bowel

A. **Meckel's diverticulum**, representing persistence of the vitelline duct, most commonly presents with bleeding owing to the presence of heterotopic rests of gastric or pancreatic mucosa.

B. **Small bowel diverticula** (with the exception of Meckel's diverticulum) are of the pulsion type and may be associated with B_{12} deficiency and bile salt deficiency (malabsorption) owing to bacterial overgrowth.

C. Most diverticula in the GI tract occur in the **sigmoid colon**.

1. They are pulsion diverticula that form two rows along the antimesenteric taeniae coli at the site where the arteries perforate the muscularis propria.

2. Under increased intraluminal pressure (presumably from a low-fiber diet), the mucosa and an attenuated portion of submucosa protrude through the defect in close proximity to vessels.

3. Complications include **diverticulitis** (most common), perforation with peritonitis, fistula formation, and massive hematochezia (most common cause), the last occurring in diverticula without inflammation. *bright red blood in stool*

Objective 6: To compare and contrast ulcerative colitis and Crohn's disease.

XV. Comparison between ulcerative colitis (UC) and Crohn's disease (CD)

A. Both UC and CD are of unknown etiology (psychological, infectious, and autoimmune factors have been implicated).

B. UC is restricted to the mucosa and submucosa of the rectum and colon (the anus is not commonly involved), while CD involves all layers of the small or large bowel.

C. UC begins in the rectum (friable, red mucosa) and extends in continuity to involve part or all of the colon, whereas CD locates in the terminal ileum (that area alone, 30%, colon and small bowel 50%, colon alone 20%) and has discontinuous involvement of the bowel.

D. UC produces ulceration with pseudopolyp formation, while CD produces linear ulcers, cobblestoning, luminal narrowing (string sign on barium studies), and fistula formation.

E. UC produces crypt abscesses and crypt atrophy, whereas CD is associated with noncaseating granulomas, lymphoid aggregates, and aphthoid mucosal ulcers.

F. UC is more likely to result in adenocarcinoma (increased risk with duration), HLA-B27–positive

CD – skip lesions

ankylosing spondylitis, toxic megacolon, and sclerosing pericholangitis, while CD is more likely to involve other areas of the GI tract from mouth to anus (fissures, fistulas).

G. UC presents with abdominal cramping, diarrhea with blood and mucus, rectal bleeding, and tenesmus (ineffectual and painful straining at stool), whereas CD presents with right lower quadrant colicky pain (obstruction) with diarrhea and anal bleeding.

Objective 7: To outline the polyp types, polyposis syndromes, and common cancers of the small and large bowel.

XVI. Polyps of the small and large bowel

A. **Hyperplastic polyps** (**hamartomatous**), the most common polyp in the colon (rectosigmoid), have an epithelium with a "sawtooth" appearance; there is no malignant potential.

B. **Juvenile polyps** are solitary hamartomatous polyps in children that most commonly locate in the rectum; they may be associated with the juvenile polyposis syndrome (AD variant has a 10% risk of malignancy).

C. **Peutz-Jeghers syndrome** is an AD disease associated with hamartomatous polyps (in the small bowel, stomach, and colon, in descending order of frequency) and pigmentation of the lips.

D. **Adenomas** are premalignant dysplastic polyps that are subdivided into tubular (most common; "raspberry on a stalk"), tubulovillous, and villous types.

1. The risk for malignant transformation parallels the percentage of the villous component (finger-like projections) in the polyp and size (> 2 cm increases the risk).

2. The villous adenoma (rectosigmoid location) has the greatest risk for malignant transformation.

XVII. Polyposis syndromes

A. **Familial polyposis coli** (FPC), the most common polyposis syndrome (> 100 tubular adenomas), is an AD condition associated with inactivation of the APC suppressor gene on chromosome 5.

1. By 40 years of age, 100% of patients with FPC will have cancer, hence the need for a prophylactic total colectomy.

2. **Gardner's syndrome**, a variant of FPC (AD inheritance) is associated with benign osteomas in the mandible and abdominal desmoid tumors.

3. **Turcot's syndrome**, a possible variant (AR inheritance) of Gardner's syndrome, is associated with malignant brain tumors.

B. Progression from an adenoma to cancer involves a series of steps involving the deletion in the long arm of the APA gene in chromosome 5, a point mutation in the *ras* oncogene, and other mutations involving the *p53* suppressor gene on chromosome 17.

XVIII. Malignant tumors of the small and large bowel

A. **Carcinoid tumors** are malignant neuroendocrine tumors whose potential for metastasis is based on size (> 2 cm) and depth of intramural invasion.

1. They are slightly more common in the appendix (tip of the appendix; rarely metastasize)

than in the terminal ileum (commonly metastasize).

2. The **carcinoid syndrome** (flushing, diarrhea, right heart valvular disease) is characterized by the elaboration of neuroendocrine compounds by tumors that have metastasized to the liver; there is an increase in 5-hydroxyindoleacetic acid (5-HIAA) in the urine.

B. **Colorectal adenocarcinomas** represent the second most common cancer killer in both men and women.

1. Predisposing conditions include age (> 50 years old); low-fiber, high-fat diet; first-degree relative with colorectal cancer; hereditary polyposis syndromes; hereditary nonpolyposis syndrome (Lynch syndrome); and UC (CD to a lesser extent).

2. Most are located in the rectosigmoid (napkin ring configuration with obstruction), while on the right side, they have a polypoid appearance and most commonly present with bleeding.

3. The grade and stage of the tumor (Astler-Coller staging system) determine the prognosis; the overall 5-year survival regardless of stage is 35%.

4. The liver is the most common site of metastasis; CEA is an excellent marker to detect recurrent disease.

C. The most common **primary cancers in the small bowel**, in decreasing order of frequency, are the carcinoid tumor, adenocarcinoma, and malignant lymphoma; metastasis is the most common cancer.

Objective 8: To review common disorders associated with the appendix and anus.

XIX. Acute appendicitis

A. Acute appendicitis is primarily a disease of adolescents and young adults and has no sex predilection.

1. Greater than 60% of cases are associated with proximal obstruction of the lumen by a fecalith, leading to an increase in intraluminal pressure, ischemic mucosal injury, and secondary bacterial invasion.

2. Complications include a periappendiceal abscess (most common; often associated with perforation), peritonitis, pylephlebitis (inflammation of the portal vein; air is present in the portal vein on x-ray), septicemia, and subphrenic abscess.

XX. Disorders of the anus

A. **Hemorrhoids** are dilated venous plexuses derived from the superior hemorrhoidal vein (internal hemorrhoids) or inferior hemorrhoidal veins (external hemorrhoids).

B. **Epidermoid carcinomas** are most frequently encountered in the anus and the anorectal junction (most common site).

C. In the male homosexual population, HPV-induced squamous cell cancer may occur (HPV types 16 and 18).

D. **Transitional cell** or **basaloid cell tumors** may occur at the squamocolumnar junction or transitional zone (sometimes called **cloacogenic carcinomas**).

QUESTIONS

DIRECTIONS. (Items 1–17): Each of the numbered items or incomplete statements in this section is followed by answers or by completions of the statement. Select the ONE lettered answer or completion that is BEST in each case. Correct answers and explanations are given at the end of the chapter.

1. This is a gross specimen removed at autopsy from a 62-year-old woman with weight loss and epigastric pain. A barium study prior to death was unusual in that the stomach did not distend properly with the contrast material. You would expect that the histologic sections revealed

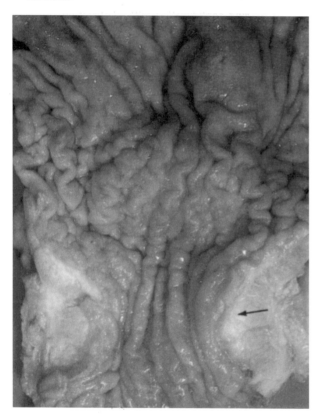

   (A) ulceration of the mucosal surface
   (B) hypertrophic gastritis (Ménétrier's disease)
   (C) signet-ring cells in the wall of the stomach
   (D) fibrosis secondary to duodenal ulcer disease
   (E) granulomatous inflammation

2. The gross specimen in this photograph is a partial resection of bowel from a 65-year-old man with weight loss, a positive stool guaiac, and alternating bouts of constipation and diarrhea. The arrows point to additional lesions. Which of the following best describes this patient's disease?

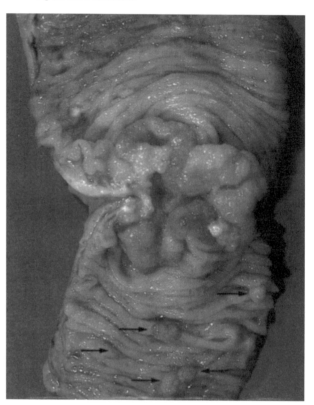

   (A) Diverticular disease involving the sigmoid colon
   (B) Inflammatory bowel disease with obstruction
   (C) Ischemic stricture most likely at the splenic flexure
   (D) Annular stenosing lesion consistent with adenocarcinoma
   (E) Inflammatory bowel disease with pseudopolyp formation

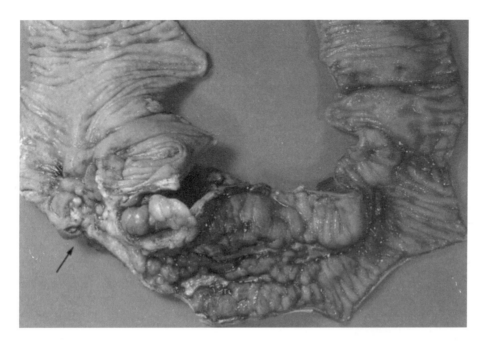

3. The photograph is of a partial resection of the terminal ileum and cecum (arrow at the ileocecal valve) from a 35-year-old man with a long history of colicky right lower quadrant pain, diarrhea, and rectal bleeding. You would expect sections of the bowel to reveal

   (A) a lymphoid infiltrate and noncaseating granulomas
   (B) crypt abscesses and inflammation limited to the mucosa and submucosa
   (C) a diffuse infiltrate of malignant lymphocytes with mucosal ulceration
   (D) nests of cells that contain neurosecretory granules on ultrastructural examination
   (E) a diffuse infiltrate of malignant cells with gland formation

4. This gross specimen of esophagus was removed at autopsy from a 42-year-old man who was found dead under a bridge. The pathogenesis of the lesion noted in the photograph is most closely related to

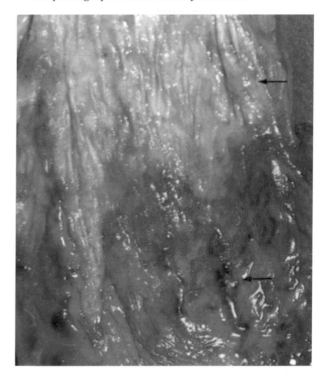

   (A) gastroesophageal reflux disease
   (B) failure of relaxation of the lower esophageal sphincter
   (C) a collagen vascular disease with increased production of collagen
   (D) portal hypertension secondary to cirrhosis
   (E) neoplastic transformation of glandular epithelium

5. This is a colectomy specimen from a 37-year-old man with a family history of gastrointestinal disease. A biopsy of one of the mucosal lesions in the gross specimen would most likely reveal

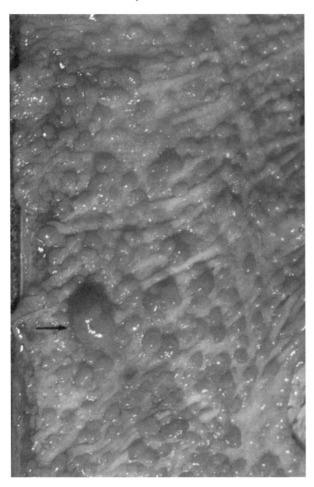

   (A) a hyperplastic polyp
   (B) a juvenile polyp
   (C) a hamartomatous polyp
   (D) a pseudopolyp
   (E) an adenoma

6. Diverticulosis and angiodysplasia both predispose to

   (A) colorectal cancer
   (B) infection
   (C) hematochezia
   (D) fistula formation
   (E) bowel obstruction

7. Achalasia and Hirschsprung's disease are both associated with

   (A) Down syndrome
   (B) absence of ganglion cells
   (C) a predisposition for cancer
   (D) aperistalsis of the proximal dilated segment
   (E) transmural inflammation

8. A 65-year-old man has a 4-month history of severe, steady pain in the left mid-abdomen that develops approximately 30 minutes after eating. He has lost 20 pounds for fear of eating. He now presents with similar pain, bloody diarrhea, abdominal distention, and hypotension. His serum amylase is markedly elevated, and there is an absolute neutrophilic leukocytosis with a shift to the left. The pathogenesis of his condition most closely relates to

   (A) ischemic injury to bowel
   (B) a neoplastic process
   (C) an infectious process
   (D) mechanical obstruction
   (E) inflammatory bowel disease

9. A 32-year-old man with flushing, diarrhea, and multiple lesions in the liver on CT scan would most likely have a primary disorder located in the

   (A) esophagus
   (B) stomach
   (C) small bowel
   (D) appendix
   (E) rectosigmoid

10. An afebrile 28-year-old woman with long-standing diarrhea has a positive quantitative stool for fat and an abnormal D-xylose test. You would expect this patient to most likely have a

   (A) long history of recurrent pancreatitis
   (B) small bowel biopsy showing foamy macrophages in the lamina propria
   (C) small bowel biopsy showing dilated lymphatic channels in the submucosa
   (D) small bowel biopsy showing flattened villi and hyperplastic crypts
   (E) bacterial overgrowth syndrome with bile salt deficiency

11. Weight loss and dysphagia for solids in a 62-year-old man with a long history of alcoholism would most likely be secondary to

   (A) an esophageal web
   (B) a squamous carcinoma
   (C) esophageal varices
   (D) a motor disorder of the esophagus
   (E) infectious esophagitis

12. A nonsmoking 29-year-old homosexual male has non-painful white patches located on the lateral borders of his tongue. The patches do not wipe off with gauze. You suspect that the pathogenesis of these lesions is most closely related to

   (A) a neoplastic process
   (B) a fungal infection
   (C) a dysplastic process
   (D) a viral infection
   (E) an autoimmune disease

13. The pathogenesis of both diverticulitis and acute appendicitis is most often associated with

   (A) a previous history of viral gastroenteritis
   (B) luminal obstruction by a fecalith
   (C) hematogenous spread of infection
   (D) submucosal lymphoid hyperplasia
   (E) luminal obstruction by parasites

14. The most common site for polyps and adenocarcinoma in the gastrointestinal tract is the

    (A) esophagus
    (B) stomach
    (C) small bowel
    (D) right colon
    (E) rectosigmoid

15. Which of the following is more commonly associated with a gastric rather than a duodenal ulcer?

    (A) *Helicobacter pylori* infection
    (B) Perforation
    (C) Hematemesis
    (D) Male sex
    (E) Defective mucosal barrier

16. Which of the following is more likely associated with ulcerative colitis than with Crohn's disease?

    (A) Risk for adenocarcinoma
    (B) Obstruction
    (C) Fistula formation
    (D) Transmural inflammation
    (E) Aphthoid ulcers

17. Which of the following infectious disease relationships is correctly matched?

    (A) Shigellosis: bradycardia, neutropenia, splenomegaly
    (B) *Campylobacter jejuni*: secretory diarrhea
    (C) Enterohemorrhagic *Escherichia coli*: hemolytic uremic syndrome
    (D) *Vibrio cholerae*: mucosal ulceration
    (E) *Salmonella typhi*: positive stool culture in the first week

---

ANSWERS AND EXPLANATIONS

---

1. The answer is C: signet-ring cells in the wall of the stomach. There is no visible ulceration on the mucosal surface; however, the wall is markedly thickened by white tissue causing constriction of the stomach. Along with the history of weight loss, pain, and lack of distensibility of the stomach by barium, linitis plastica ("leather bottle" stomach) is the most likely diagnosis. Malignant signet-ring cells would likely be present in the thickened wall. The other choices listed would not be associated with the history or the gross abnormalities noted on the slide. (Photograph reproduced, with permission, from B.C. Morson. *Color Atlas of Gastrointestinal Pathology.* London, Harvey Miller Publishers, W.B. Saunders Co., 1988, p. 67.)

2. The answer is D: annular stenosing lesion consistent with adenocarcinoma. This lesion exhibits a napkin ring (annular) configuration with mucosal ulceration and stenosis of the lumen. Five adenomas are noted as incidental findings. The obstructive findings in the history (constipation and diarrhea), weight loss, blood in the stool of a patient >50 years old, and the gross findings are consistent with an adenocarcinoma, most likely in the left colon. Diverticular disease, inflammatory bowel disease, and ischemia would not present with this history or have the gross findings noted in this specimen. (Photograph reproduced, with permission, from B.C. Morson. *Color Atlas of Gastrointestinal Pathology.* London, W.B. Saunders Co., 1988, p. 244.)

3. The answer is A: a lymphoid infiltrate and noncaseating granulomas. The specimen shows cobblestoning and longitudinal ulceration of the mucosal surface (serpiginous ulcers) and stenosis at the ileocecal valve. The history and gross findings are consistent with Crohn's disease involving the terminal ileum and ileocecal valve. A lymphoid infiltrate and noncaseating granulomas would very likely be present in the wall of the bowel. Although carcinoid tumors (nests of cells with neurosecretory granules) and malignant lymphomas (malignant lymphocytes) most commonly occur in the terminal ileum, they do not produce the gross findings noted in this specimen. An adenocarcinoma (malignant

cells with gland formation) would be unlikely in this age bracket. Ulcerative colitis (crypt abscesses) is more likely to involve the left colon and would not have the gross findings noted above. (Photograph reproduced, with permission, from B.C. Morson. *Color Atlas of Gastrointestinal Pathology.* London, W.B. Saunders Co., 1988, p. 122.)

4. The answer is D: portal hypertension secondary to cirrhosis. The photograph depicts dilated and tortuous veins (arrow) in the submucosa consistent with esophageal varices. Varices are most commonly secondary to portal hypertension from alcoholic cirrhosis. Gastroesophageal reflux disease would be associated with mucosal ulceration. Achalasia (failure of relaxation of the LES) produces tapering of the distal esophagus at the esophagogastric junction. PSS, a collagen vascular disease with increased production of collagen, is not associated with vessel dilatation. An adenocarcinoma arising from Barrett's esophagus (neoplastic transformation of glandular epithelium) would likely be polypoid or ulcerative in its gross appearance. (Photograph reproduced, with permission, from B.C. Morson. *Color Atlas of Gastrointestinal Pathology.* London, W.B. Saunders Co., 1988, p. 33.)

5. The answer is E: an adenoma. The patient has familial polyposis coli (FPC), an AD type of polyposis syndrome. The majority of the polyps (>100 in this photograph) are tubular adenomas. All patients with FPC will develop adenocarcinoma by 40 years of age, hence the requirement for a prophylactic colectomy. Hyperplastic polyps are hamartomatous polyps that are rarely associated with a polyposis syndrome. Juvenile polyps are solitary hamartomatous polyps that commonly locate in the rectum in children. Pseudopolyps are noted in UC (there is no mucosal ulceration in the specimen). Peutz-Jeghers polyps are also hamartomatous; however, they are not commonly located in the colon. (Photograph reproduced, with permission, from B.C. Morson. *Color Atlas of Gastrointestinal Pathology.* London, W.B. Saunders Co., 1988, p. 240.)

6. The answer is C: hematochezia. Diverticulosis and an-

giodysplasia (vascular lesions in the right colon), in descending order, are the most common causes of profuse rectal bleeding (hematochezia). Neither disorder predisposes to colorectal cancer or bowel obstruction. Diverticular disease is associated with infection (diverticulitis) and fistula formation.

7. The answer is B: absence of ganglion cells. Both achalasia and Hirschsprung's disease have absence of ganglion cells, the former in the myenteric plexus and the latter in both the myenteric and Meissner's submucosal plexus. Neither condition is associated with transmural inflammation. Achalasia predisposes to esophageal cancer and has aperistalsis of the proximal dilated segment. Hirschsprung's disease is associated with Down syndrome.

8. The answer is A: ischemic injury to bowel. The patient most likely had mesenteric angina owing to atherosclerosis of the superior mesenteric artery to explain his history of pain after eating. He now has an infarct in his small bowel (bloody diarrhea, increased amylase of bowel origin), most likely due to thrombus over an atherosclerotic plaque in the same artery. The chronicity of his complaints argues against an infectious process. Mechanical obstruction produces colicky pain and absence of stool and gas (obstipation). Inflammatory bowel disease does not have this type of history, and his age argues against that diagnosis as well. A neoplastic process usually has alternating bouts of constipation and nonbloody diarrhea in left-sided lesions and is not associated with leukocytosis and hyperamylasemia.

9. The answer is C: small bowel. The history of flushing and diarrhea is compatible with the carcinoid syndrome, which is most commonly due to a carcinoid tumor of the terminal ileum that has metastasized to the liver. Carcinoid tumors in the small bowel synthesize neuroendocrine products (e.g., serotonin), which normally are metabolized in the liver. Metastasis to the liver bypasses metabolism of serotonin and other compounds and allows their access to the systemic circulation. There is an increase in 5-hydroxyindoleacetic acid in the urine of people with the syndrome. All carcinoid tumors are malignant; however, only those that are > 2 cm or have significant intramural invasion are potentially capable of metastasizing. Hence, the appendiceal carcinoids rarely metastasize, unlike those located in the small bowel. Carcinoid tumors in the stomach and rectum do not usually produce the carcinoid syndrome. The esophagus is not normally a primary site for carcinoid tumors.

10. The answer is D: small bowel biopsy showing flattened villi and hyperplastic crypts. The patient has malabsorption due to small bowel disease based on the positive quantitative stool for fat and abnormal D-xylose test. The most common small bowel disease associated with malabsorption is celiac disease, an autoimmune disease with antibodies directed against the gliadin component in gluten, which is found in wheat products. The immune destruction is primarily of the villi (villous atrophy), while the underlying crypts are hyperplastic. Chronic pancreatitis yields a normal D-xylose test, since amylase is not necessary to break down xylose (pentose sugar) for absorption. A small bowel biopsy with foamy macrophages (containing *Tropheryma whippelii*) or dilated lymphatic channels represents Whipple's disease (systemic disease) and intestinal lymphangiectasia, respectively. Both are uncommon causes of malabsorption. A bacterial overgrowth syndrome with bile

salt deficiency could produce a false positive D-xylose; however, it is an uncommon cause of malabsorption.

11. The answer is B: a squamous carcinoma. Weight loss and dysphagia for solids (sign of obstruction) in a person with alcoholism most likely represents a squamous cell carcinoma of the esophagus. Esophageal webs are part of the Plummer-Vinson syndrome, which is a female-dominant disorder associated with iron deficiency. Esophageal varices do not produce dysphagia. Infectious esophagitis produces odynophagia (painful swallowing) and not dysphagia for solids. Motor disorders (PSS and achalasia) produce dysphagia for solids and liquids.

12. The answer is D: a viral infection. The patient most likely has hairy leukoplakia due to Epstein-Barr virus. This is most commonly seen in HIV-positive individuals and predates the onset of AIDS. The virus induces squamous hyperplasia of the epithelium. Most white patches that do not wipe off with gauze are called leukoplakia (clinical diagnosis). They are most often associated with the use of tobacco products with or without alcohol abuse. Unlike hairy leukoplakia, this type of leukoplakia is considered a precursor for squamous cancer, and there should be a biopsy to rule out dysplasia or overt cancer. White patches associated with *Candida* infection of the tongue will wipe off and leave a bleeding surface. Autoimmune diseases in the mouth (pemphigus vulgaris, pemphigoid, SLE) are not associated with leukoplakia.

13. The answer is B: luminal obstruction by a fecalith. Fecaliths commonly obstruct the lumen in both diverticular sacs and the appendix. In some cases, they obstruct the egress of mucous secretions by the mucosal cells with subsequent increase in intraluminal pressure and compression of venous channels, leading to ischemia. Ischemia disrupts the mucosal barrier, hence allowing access of bacteria into the wall of the diverticula and appendix, resulting in acute inflammation. Luminal obstruction by parasites and submucosal lymphoid hyperplasia (viral infection) are less common associations with acute appendicitis. Neither condition is produced by hematogenous spread of infection. Viral gastroenteritis may occasionally produce lymphoid hyperplasia in the appendix but not in diverticula.

14. The answer is E: rectosigmoid. The most common polyps in the GI tract are hyperplastic polyps and adenomas, both of which are most commonly located in the rectosigmoid. The location of adenomas (premalignant polyps) parallels the location of colorectal cancer, the third most common cancer in men and women and the second most common cause of death due to cancer. The next best answer is the right colon (cecum and ascending colon), which also is a common site for polyps and adenocarcinoma. Polyps are uncommon in the other sites listed.

15. The answer is E: defective mucosal barrier. *H. pylori* infection, perforation, hematemesis, male dominance, and increased production of acid are more characteristic of duodenal than gastric ulcers. Gastric ulcers are more often associated with normal to reduced acid production; however, a defective mucous barrier (*H. pylori*–related) renders the mucosa more susceptible to acid injury.

16. The answer is A: risk for adenocarcinoma. Obstruction, fistula formation, transmural inflammation, and aphthoid ulcers (mucosal ulcerations; early finding) all characterize Crohn's disease. UC has a greater risk for adenocarcinoma particularly, if there is pancolitis and

the duration of disease is > 10 years. UC is also more likely to have toxic megacolon, crypt abscesses, rectal involvement, sclerosing pericholangitis, and HLA-B27–positive ankylosing spondylitis.

17. The answer is C: enterohemorrhagic *Escherichia coli*: hemolytic uremic syndrome. *E. coli* serotype O157:H7 (which often contaminates raw ground beef) is associated with a toxin that produces hemolytic uremic syndrome and hemorrhagic colitis. *C. jejuni* is the most common invasive enterocolitis in the United States. *S. typhi* is associated with the classic triad of bradycardia, neutropenia, and splenomegaly. Blood is more likely to isolate the organism in the first week (septicemic phase) than stool (diarrhea occurs in the second week). *V. cholerae* is a secretory diarrhea (toxin stimulates cAMP) and is not associated with mucosal inflammation.

CHAPTER SIXTEEN

DISORDERS OF THE LIVER, GALLBLADDER, PANCREAS, AND PERITONEUM

SYNOPSIS

OBJECTIVES

1. To discuss laboratory tests available to diagnose liver disease.
2. To outline the classic hexagonal lobule in the liver and the zones of hepatocytes that extend from the portal triad to the terminal hepatic venule.
3. To understand bilirubin metabolism as it relates to the classification of jaundice.
4. To be familiar with the five most common types of viral hepatitis and some less common infectious diseases involving the liver.
5. To understand the pathophysiology of common vascular disorders involving the liver.
6. To discuss the pathogenesis and morphologic features of alcohol-related liver disease.
7. To be familiar with autoimmune hepatitis.
8. To review the pathophysiology and morphologic features of cholestatic liver disease.
9. To be familiar with the morphologic patterns of drug- and chemical-induced liver disease.
10. To outline the liver diseases associated with an accumulation of iron, copper, glycogen, and α_1-antitrypsin.
11. To understand liver disease associated with pregnancy and childhood.
12. To review the complications associated with alcoholic and other types of cirrhosis.
13. To be familiar with tumors in the liver, biliary tree, and pancreas.
14. To be conversant with inflammatory conditions involving the peritoneal cavity.
15. To understand the pathogenesis of gallstones and the relationship to acute and chronic cholecystitis.
16. To outline the pathophysiology of cystic fibrosis as it relates to pancreatic function.
17. To review the pathogenesis of acute and chronic pancreatitis.

Objective 1: To discuss laboratory tests available to diagnose liver disease.

I. Liver function tests

A. After the history and physical examination, liver function tests help delineate the cause of liver disease.
B. Table 16–1 summarizes the key liver function tests.

Objective 2: To outline the classic hexagonal lobule in the liver and the zones of hepatocytes that extend from the portal triad to the terminal hepatic venule.

II. Morphology of the liver
A. The classic **hexagonal lobule** in the liver centers around the **terminal hepatic venule** (THV), with the **portal triads** located at three of the six angles.
1. The **portal triads** contain tributaries from the hepatic artery, portal vein, and bile ducts.
2. Blood from the triad vessels empties into the **sinusoids**, which drain into the **THV**, which eventually drains into the vena cava and right heart.
B. From a metabolic standpoint, the hepatic parenchyma is subdivided into **zone I** (periportal; greatest amount of oxygen and nutrients), **zone II** (midzonal), and **zone III** (around the THV; least amount of oxygen and nutrients).

Objective 3: To understand bilirubin metabolism as it relates to the classification of jaundice.

III. Normal and abnormal bilirubin metabolism
A. Figure 16–1 outlines **normal bilirubin metabolism**.
1. Fixed macrophages in sinusoidal tissue produce **unconjugated bilirubin** (UCB), which is taken up and conjugated in the liver to form water-soluble **conjugated bilirubin** (CB).
2. CB is actively transported to the bile canaliculi and subsequently drains into the bile ducts, which empty bile into the small intestine.

TABLE 16–1. Liver Function Tests (LFTs)*

Index	Test	Comments
Necrosis index	Transaminases: Alanine transaminase (ALT) Aspartate transaminase (AST)	**AST** (formerly SGOT) is primarily a mitochondrial enzyme. **ALT** (formerly SGPT) is located in the cytosol. ALT is more specific than AST for liver disease. AST and ALT are released only by hepatocyte injury/necrosis. **Alcoholic liver disease:** AST > ALT since alcohol is a mitochondrial poison. Enzyme levels are rarely >200–300 U/L. **Viral hepatitis:** ALT > AST. ALT is the last enzyme to return to normal. Enzyme levels are often >1000 U/L in acute hepatitis.
Cholestasis index	Alkaline phosphatase (AP) γ-Glutamyl transferase (GGT)	Obstructive jaundice is called cholestasis (intrahepatic or extrahepatic). Enzymes increase secondary to synthesis (not cell damage) owing to obstruction or compression of bile ducts by a parenchymal mass. GGT synthesis increases when drugs enhance the cytochrome P-450 system (e.g., alcohol, phenobarbital, rifampin). AP is present in many tissues (liver, bone, placenta, WBCs), while GGT is primarily located in the liver. **Obstructive jaundice:** AP and GGT are markedly increased (↑↑↑), while transaminases are mildly increased (↑). **Alcoholic liver disease:** AST > ALT and GGT is disproportionately increased (↑↑↑) (induced synthesis by alcohol). **Focal benign liver disease (granulomas):** bilirubin, LDH, and transaminases are normal, while AP and GGT are slightly increased (↑). **Focal metastatic liver disease:** same as above except LDH is also increased (↑). **AP of liver versus bone or other tissue origin:** AP and GGT are increased if AP is of liver origin. AP is increased only if it is not of liver origin.
Excretory index	Total bilirubin (TB) with fractionation into conjugated (CB) and unconjugated bilirubin (UCB)	**CB/TB × 100 = CB fractionation <20%:** primary increase in UCB (extravascular hemolysis, problem with uptake or conjugation). **20–50%:** mixed CB and UCB (hepatitis). **>50%:** primarily CB (obstructive jaundice).
Severity index	Serum albumin Prothrombin time (PT)	Hypoalbuminemia and a prolonged PT indicate severe functional impairment of the liver.
Immune index	Autoantibodies	**Autoantibodies:** increase in antimitochondrial antibody in primary biliary cirrhosis. Increase in anti–smooth muscle antibody, anti–liver/kidney microsome antibody, and antinuclear antibody in autoimmune hepatitis.
Tumor marker index	Carcinoembryonic antigen (CEA) α-Fetoprotein (AFP) α₁-Antitrypsin (AAT)	**Metastatic disease:** metastasis to the liver from a primary in the stomach, pancreas, or bowel increases CEA. **Hepatocellular carcinoma (adults) and hepatoblastoma (children):** increase in AFP and AAT.

	Urine bilirubin	Urine urobilinogen:
Normal	Absent	Trace
CB <20%	Absent	↑↑↑
CB 20–50%	↑↑	↑↑
CB >50%	↑↑↑	Absent

* The number of arrows correlates with the degree of magnitude.

3. In the **terminal ileum** and **colon**, CB is reduced by **bacterial β-glucuronidases** back into UCB (and a small amount reabsorbed), which is further reduced to **colorless urobilinogens**.
   a. Approximately 20% of **urobilinogen** is recycled back to the liver (**enterohepatic circulation**).
   b. Urobilinogen entering the colon is oxidized to **colored urobilins** that provide the color to stool.
B. **Jaundice** (yellowish discoloration of skin and mucous membranes) is subdivided into unconjugated (< 20% CB) and conjugated (> 50% CB) types of hyperbilirubinemia (see Table 16–1).
   1. **UCB hyperbilirubinemia** is secondary to increased production, impaired uptake, or defective conjugation of bilirubin.
   2. **CB hyperbilirubinemia** is associated with **intrahepatic** or **extrahepatic** obstruction to bile flow, which is designated **cholestasis**.

3. **Hereditary hyperbilirubinemias** that are **predominantly UCB** (CB < 20%) include the following:
   a. Extravascular hemolytic anemia (e.g., congenital spherocytosis [AD inheritance]).
   b. **Gilbert syndrome**, a benign AD disease with mild hemolysis and defects in uptake and conjugation.
   c. **Crigler-Najjar syndrome type I** (incompatible with life) and **type II** with conjugating enzyme deficiencies.
4. **Hereditary hyperbilirubinemias that are predominantly CB** (CB > 50%) consist of Dubin-Johnson syndrome (AR disease with a secretion defect and black liver) and **Rotor's syndrome** (AR disease similar to Dubin-Johnson but without a black liver).
5. **Acquired UCB hyperbilirubinemias** include **physiologic jaundice of the newborn** (uptake and conjugation defects), **ABO incompatibility**

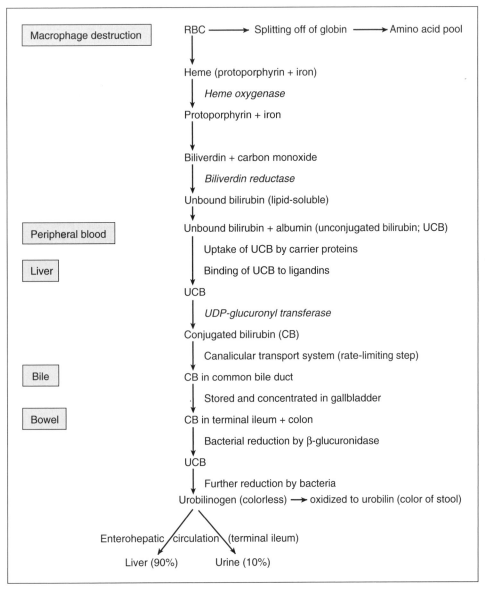

FIGURE 16–1. Normal bilirubin metabolism. CB, conjugated bilirubin; UCB, unconjugated bilirubin.

(increased production), and **breast milk jaundice** (conjugation defect).

6. **Acquired CB hyperbilirubinemias** consist of drug-induced cholestasis (e.g., from oral contraceptive use), biliary atresia, primary biliary cirrhosis (PBC), and choledocholithiasis (stone in common bile duct).

7. A **mixed type** of hyperbilirubinemia (CB 20–50%) is characteristic of viral and alcoholic hepatitis.

Objective 4: To be familiar with the five most common types of viral hepatitis and some less common infectious diseases involving the liver.

IV. Viral hepatitis

A. Viral hepatitis, the most common infectious disease involving the liver, has a **prodrome**, **icteric** or **nonicteric phase**, and **recovery phase**.

B. Table 16–2 lists key differences among viral hepa-

titis A (HAV), B (HBV), C (HCV), D (HDV), and E (HEV).

C. A **marked transaminasemia** with ALT > AST and a mixed hyperbilirubinemia are the most common laboratory abnormalities in all the viral hepatitis types (see Table 16–1).

D. Figure 16–2 summarizes the serologic diagnosis of HBV infections.

E. The **histopathology** of **acute viral hepatitis** consists of focal ballooning degeneration, apoptosis (Councilman bodies are seen), a lymphocytic infiltrate, hypertrophy/hyperplasia of Kupffer's cells, and portal tract inflammation.

F. **Chronic viral hepatitis** can be **chronic persistent hepatitis** (CPH); **chronic lobular hepatitis** (CLH), a less inflammatory variant of CPH; or **chronic aggressive (active) hepatitis** (CAH).

1. **CPH** is characterized by a mild portal triaditis and "ground glass" hepatocytes (HBsAg in HBV infections) and rarely progresses to CAH.

TABLE 16–2.   Summary of Common Causes of Viral Hepatitis

	HAV	HBV	HCV	HDV	HEV
Type of virus	RNA (picornavirus)	DNA (hepadnavirus)	RNA (flavivirus)	Incomplete RNA virus (requires HBsAg)	RNA (calicivirus)
Prevalence	40%	35%	20%	5%	<1%
Transmission	Fecal-oral, food, water, anal intercourse. In children, 10% of infections occur in day-care centers.	Parenteral, close contact with an infected patient. Present in blood, semen, saliva.	Same as HBV.	Same as HBV. Coinfection (same needle contains both viruses). Superinfection (exposure to HDV at later date). Superinfection is more severe than coinfection.	Same as HAV.
Incubation	2–6 weeks	2–6 months	5–7 weeks	Same as HBV.	2–9 weeks
Clinical associations	Traveler's hepatitis (80%), intravenous drug abusers (20%), male homosexuals (35%).	Serum sickness picture (5–10%): polyarthritis, urticaria, nephritis, vasculitis. Virus is not cytolytic, but CD8 cytotoxic T cells destroy the hepatocyte.	Most common cause of posttransfusion hepatitis (1:3300 chance). Common in alcoholic liver disease (25–60%).	Cytolytic to hepatocytes (rapid deterioration with superinfections). Intravenous drug abusers and male homosexuals.	Poor prognosis in pregnant women (20% mortality).
Chronic carrier state/chronic hepatitis	None	Yes (10% in adults, 90% in newborns left untreated)	Yes (40–60%)	Yes (10–40%)	None
Laboratory diagnosis	Anti-HAV-IgM: indicates active disease. Anti-HAV-IgG: indicates inactive disease, protective.	See Figure 16–2.	Anti-HCV: indicates infection, not protective. ELISA test positive in 2–6 weeks. Recombinant immunoblot assay (RIBA) is a confirmatory test along with polymerase chain reaction (PCR) testing.	Anti-HDV-IgM or IgG: indicates infection, not protective.	Anti-HEV-IgM or IgG: IgM indicates current infection. IgG indicates recovery and protection.

2. **CAH** is associated with piecemeal necrosis (disruption of the limiting plate), bridging fibrosis, and a tendency to progress to cirrhosis.

G. Parasitic diseases in the liver include the following:
   1. **Amebiasis**, due to *Entamoeba histolytica* and characterized by flask-shaped ulcers in the cecum and an abscess in the liver.
   2. **Echinococcosis** (sheepherder's disease), due to *Echinococcus granulosis* and associated with single or multiple hydatid cysts in the liver.
   3. **Schistosomiasis**, due to *Schistosoma mansoni* and associated with "pipe stem" cirrhosis owing to portal vein fibrosis.
   4. **Clonorchiasis**, secondary to *Clonorchis sinensis*, which predisposes to carcinoma of the bile ducts (cholangiocarcinoma).

H. **Tuberculosis** and **sarcoidosis** are the most common cause of infectious and noninfectious granulomatous hepatitis, respectively.

I. In **tertiary syphilis**, there is a granulomatous hepatitis, extensive scarring, and gummas, resulting in a contracted liver called **hepar lobatum**.

J. **Yellow fever** is a viral infection transmitted by *Aedes aegypti* that produces zone II mid-zonal necrosis.

K. **Q fever** caused by *Coxiella burnetii* produces an interstitial pneumonia and ring (doughnut) granulomas in the bone marrow and liver.

Objective 5: To understand the pathophysiology of common vascular disorders involving the liver.

V. Vascular disorders of the liver
   A. **Acute** and **chronic hepatic congestion** ("nutmeg" liver) are most commonly due to right heart failure.
   B. **Hepatic vein thrombosis (Budd-Chiari syndrome)**, which produces painful hepatomegaly, portal hypertension, and ascites is most commonly due to polycythemia vera (less commonly to oral contraceptive use and paroxysmal nocturnal hemoglobinuria).
   C. **Venoocclusive disease** of the small- to medium-sized hepatic veins may be associated with pyrrolizidine alkaloids in *Crotalaria* and *Senecio* species of plants.
   D. **Portal vein thrombosis** producing portal hypertension and ascites may be secondary to pylephlebitis (appendicitis is the most common pre-

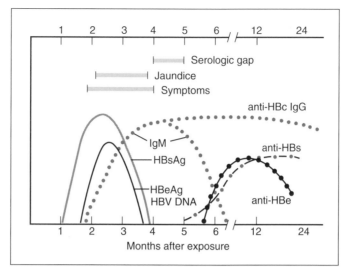

FIGURE 16–2. Serology of acute and chronic hepatitis B. Hepatitis B surface antigen (HBsAg) is in the envelope of the virus (noninfective) and first appears in the plasma 2–8 weeks before symptoms develop (even before transaminase elevation) and persists for up to 4 months. It is the first marker to arrive and the last to leave if the patient is going to recover. Persistence beyond 6 months is chronic HBV. HBeAg, HBV, DNA, and HBV DNA, and HBV DNA polymerase arrive shortly after HBsAg and leave before HBsAg if the patient is going to recover. Both HBe and HBV DNA are excellent markers of infectivity; however, HBV DNA is the best overall marker. Anti-HBV core antibody IgM (anti-HBc-IgM) is a nonprotective antibody that arrives shortly after HBsAG. It is positive in all acute infections and is the only marker of infection during the serologic gap, or window, when all the antigens have disappeared and anti-HBV surface antibody (anti-HBs) has not appeared. Anti-HBc-IgM persists for 3–6 months before converting to anti-HBc-IgG, which is a good marker of old infection. Persistence of anti-HBc-IgM beyond 6 months occurs in 70% of patients with chronic hepatitis (correlates with severity of disease as well as ongoing replication of the virus). Anti-HBs is detected 1–4 months after disappearance of HBsAg and is protective against future infections. It is the only marker of immunization after HBV vaccination. Anti-HBe indicates that HBeAg is either absent or dropping in titer, hence it is an indicator of possible recovery in HBsAg and HBeAg-positive chronic hepatitis. The presence of HBsAg beyond 6 months is synonymous with chronic hepatitis. In patients with normal immune function, chronic HBV occurs in ~10% of cases, whereas ~90% of immunocompromised patients will develop chronic disease. A "healthy carrier" is one who is HBsAg positive and negative for HBeAg/HBV-DNA. This poses only a small risk for transmitting the virus to another person. An "infective carrier" is one who is HBsAg and HBeAg/HBV DNA positive. These people are at high risk for transmitting disease to others and have a poor outcome. Pregnant women who are HBsAg positive and HBeAg/HBV DNA negative have a 20% chance of transmitting the disease to their baby (usually by blood contamination during delivery, less commonly transplacentally), while those who are HBsAg and HBeAg/HBV DNA positive will transmit disease to >90% of their newborns. Hence, newborns must be actively immunized (vaccine) and passively immunized (immunoglobulin) to prevent the disease (85% recovery rate). Patients who receive hepatitis B vaccine or recombinant hepatitis B vaccine develop only anti-HBs antibodies (90% of cases). Active immunization protects the recipient for 3–8 years. Universal childhood vaccination is recommended. Vaccination protects against contracting HBV, HDV, and hepatocellular carcinoma, which may be the outcome of HBV infection.

hepatic cause) and cirrhosis (most common intrahepatic cause).

E. **Peliosis hepatis**, most often due to use of oral contraceptives and anabolic steroids, is the accumulation of RBCs in cavities located in the space of Disse (between the hepatocyte and the sinusoids).

Objective 6: To discuss the pathogenesis and morphologic features of alcohol-related liver disease.

VI. Alcohol-related liver disease
   A. Alcohol-related liver disease is classified as **fatty liver disease** (most common), **alcoholic hepatitis** (inflammatory hepatitis with neutrophils and Mallory's bodies), and **cirrhosis**.
   B. Risk factors include the duration and amount of alcohol consumed, sex (women are more susceptible than men), nutritional status (alcohol provides "empty calories"), and genetic factors.
   C. **Alcohol metabolism** results in the production of substrates that contribute to the pathology of liver disease and laboratory abnormalities associated with alcoholic liver disease, as shown below:

$$\text{Alcohol} \xrightarrow{\text{Alcohol dehydrogenase}} \text{acetaldehyde} +$$

$$\text{NADH} + \text{H}^+ \xrightarrow{\text{Aldehyde dehydrogenase}} \text{acetate} +$$

$$\text{NADH} + \text{H}^+ \rightarrow \text{acetyl-CoA}$$

1. **Acetaldehyde** complexed with protein has the following adverse effects:
   a. It interferes with the normal hepatocyte secretion of protein (cellular swelling) and VLDL (fatty change).
   b. It disrupts microtubular function in the hepatocyte.
   c. It stimulates collagen synthesis by myofibroblasts around the THV (**perivenular fibrosis**) and lipocytes (Ito cells) in the space of Disse (fibrosis blocks nutrient movement to hepatocytes), which may eventuate in cirrhosis.
   d. It acts as a neoantigen that leads to immunologic injury to hepatocytes.
2. When bands of fibrosis develop around islands

of regenerating hepatocytes, cirrhosis becomes the final stage of alcoholic liver disease.
3. The **increase in NADH** in alcohol metabolism reverses the NAD$^+$/NADH ratio, hence favoring the production of **lactic acid** (pyruvate to lactate) and **triglycerides** (DHAP to glycerol 3-phosphate to TG).
4. The **increase in acetyl-CoA** leads to ketogenesis in the liver with a predilection for β-hydroxybutyric acid (the increase in NADH favors this reaction over acetoacetic acid).

Objective 7: To be familiar with autoimmune hepatitis.

VII. Autoimmune ("lupoid") hepatitis
   A. Autoimmune hepatitis is a progressive type of chronic active hepatitis that is most commonly seen in young women.
   B. It is commonly associated with autoantibodies against smooth muscle and liver/kidney/microsome antigens.

Objective 8: To review the pathophysiology and morphologic features of cholestatic liver disease.

VIII. Cholestatic liver disease
   A. Exclusion of bile from the intestine due to intra- or extrahepatic obstruction leads to **malabsorption of fat and fat-soluble vitamins**.
   B. **Primary bile acids (cholic and chenodeoxycholic acids)** derive from CH, which is the major route of elimination of CH.
      1. Primary bile acids are conjugated into **primary bile salts (glycocholic and taurochenodeoxycholic acids)**.
      2. Approximately 95% of bile salts are actively reabsorbed in the terminal ileum (**enterohepatic circulation**) to maintain the bile salt pool.
      3. **Bile salts** entering the colon are deconjugated by anaerobic bacteria into **secondary bile salts (deoxycholic and lithocholic acids)**, which are passively reabsorbed in the colon.
      4. **Deficiency of bile acids/salts** may be due to liver disease (e.g., cirrhosis), intra- or extrahepatic cholestasis, bacterial overgrowth in the small bowel, bile salt–binding resins, and terminal ileal disease (e.g., Crohn's disease).
   C. Patients with cholestatic liver disease commonly have hypercholesterolemia (cannot excrete CH), pruritus (bile salt deposition in skin), dark urine (CB), and clay-colored stools (absence of urobilin pigment).
   D. The **cholestasis enzymes** alkaline phosphatase (AP) and γ-glutamyltransferase (GGT) are primarily elevated rather than the transaminases.
   E. **Primary sclerosing cholangitis** (PSC) is a patchy obliterative inflammatory fibrosis of the large bile ducts that leads to strictures and cholestasis.
      1. PSC is primarily associated with ulcerative colitis.
      2. Endoscopic retrograde cholangiopancreatography (ERCP) is the gold standard diagnostic test.
   F. **Primary biliary cirrhosis** (PBC) is a female-dominant progressive disease characterized by autoimmune destruction of small interlobular bile ducts and bile duct radicals in the portal triads.
      1. **Antimitochondrial antibodies** (present in 90% of cases) are directed against epithelial antigens in the bile duct epithelium.
      2. **Pruritus without jaundice** (jaundice is a late manifestation) is the earliest sign.
      3. The **cholestasis enzymes** are markedly elevated, and IgM levels are increased (95%).
   G. **Secondary biliary cirrhosis** occurs in response to chronic obstruction of the bile ducts (e.g., in cystic fibrosis).

Objective 9: To be familiar with the morphologic patterns of drug- and chemical-induced liver disease.

IX. Drug- and chemical-induced liver disease
   A. Drug-related injury is **predictable (with intrinsic hepatotoxins)** when severity is related to the dose of the drug or **unpredictable (idiosyncratic hepatotoxins)** when the reaction is not dose related.
      1. **Predictable reactions** involve conversion of the parent compound into a more toxic metabolite by the cytochrome P-450 system (e.g., carbon tetrachloride to CCl$_3$ free radicals or acetaminophen to its free radical).
      2. **Idiosyncratic reactions** commonly present with fever, rash, arthralgias, and eosinophilia (a type I drug hypersensitivity reaction).
   B. Morphologic patterns of disease include the following:
      1. **Acute/chronic hepatitis** (e.g., isoniazid, methyldopa, acetaminophen).
      2. **Granulomas** (e.g., allopurinol, phenylbutazone, sulfonamides).
      3. **Fatty change with nucleus peripheralization** (e.g., amiodarone, corticosteroids, ethanol).
      4. **Fatty change with a microvesicular pattern**, in which the nucleus remains centrally located (e.g., tetracycline, valproic acid).
      5. **Cholestasis** (e.g., oral contraceptives, anabolic steroids, chlorpromazine, erythromycin estolate, amoxicillin–clavulanic acid).
      6. **Fibrosis** (e.g., methotrexate, hypervitaminosis A).
      7. **Tumors** (see below).

Objective 10: To outline the liver diseases associated with an accumulation of iron, copper, glycogen, and α$_1$-antitrypsin.

X. Liver accumulations
   A. **Hemochromatosis** is a male predominant AR disease with an HLA-A3 inheritance pattern (70%).
      1. An increase in **membrane iron-binding protein** on the mucosal cells of the small intestine leads to an excessive absorption of iron and deposition in parenchymal tissue.
      2. Organs and associated pathology include the following:
         a. **Liver** (main target organ; pigment cirrhosis, hepatocellular carcinoma in 30%).
         b. **Pancreas** (malabsorption, diabetes mellitus).
         c. **Heart** (restrictive cardiomyopathy).
         d. **Hypothalamus** (hypogonadism).

e. **Skin** (bronzing due to melanin stimulation and iron).

f. **Joints** (degenerative arthritis).

3. Laboratory abnormalities consist of the following:

   a. An **increase in serum iron**, **percent saturation**, and **ferritin** and a **decrease in total iron-binding capacity** (increased iron stores decreases liver synthesis of transferrin).

   b. Increased iron in a liver biopsy (confirmatory test).

4. Phlebotomy is the mainstay of treatment.

B. **Hemosiderosis** is an acquired iron overload disease (e.g., from multiple transfusions), and deposits occur primarily in fixed macrophages rather than parenchymal tissue until late in the disease.

C. **Wilson's disease** (**hepatolenticular degeneration**) is an AR disease characterized by a defect in the excretion of copper into the bile.

1. It produces acute hepatitis, which progresses to chronic active hepatitis and **postnecrotic cirrhosis**.

2. The combination of a low ceruloplasmin level plus **Kayser-Fleischer ring** in the eye is diagnostic.

3. Degeneration of the lenticular nuclei produces signs of spasticity, dysarthria, and tremors.

4. The total copper concentration is decreased, owing to decreased ceruloplasmin, while the free copper level is increased.

5. The confirmatory test is a liver biopsy with quantitation of copper.

6. Treatment is with penicillamine, a copper-chelating agent.

D. In **von Gierke's glycogen storage disease** (AR), absence of the gluconeogenic enzyme glucose-6-phosphatase leads to fasting hypoglycemia and deposition of normal glycogen in the liver (nuclear localization of glycogen) and kidneys.

E. α_1-Antitrypsin (AAT) deficiency is an AR disease (inherited in codominant fashion) characterized by either abnormally low AAT levels in the plasma or defective secretion of AAT by the liver.

1. AAT is a **protease inhibitor** that is synthesized in the liver.

2. The protease inhibitor (Pi) phenotype PiMM is the normal phenotype.

3. The most common abnormal alleles are S and Z.

4. Patients with the PiZZ variant almost have no AAT in the plasma.

5. **Liver disease in children** (PiZZ variant) ranges from neonatal cholestasis, to cirrhosis, to hepatocellular carcinoma in 2–3% of patients.

6. Globules of AAT in hepatocytes (AAT cannot be secreted) are visualized with PAS stains.

Objective 11: To understand liver disease associated with pregnancy and childhood.

XI. Liver disease in pregnancy

A. **Acute viral hepatitis** is the most common liver disease in pregnancy.

B. **Benign intrahepatic cholestasis** occurs during the second and third trimesters and is primarily due to estrogen inhibition of bile secretion.

C. **Acute fatty liver of pregnancy** (microvesicular pattern of fat) is a frequently fatal disease that occurs in the third trimester unless the baby is promptly delivered.

D. The liver in **preeclampsia/eclampsia** (pregnancy-induced hypertension) is associated with hepatocellular necrosis around zone I in the portal triad, fibrin deposition in the sinusoids, and the HELLP syndrome in a small percentage of cases.

XII. Liver disease in children

A. **Neonatal cholestasis** refers to prolonged hyperbilirubinemia secondary to an increase in CB.

1. It may be idiopathic or secondary to neonatal hepatitis (most common cause), biliary atresia (one-third of cases), metabolic disease (e.g., galactosemia), infection (e.g., CMV), AAT deficiency, or cystic fibrosis.

2. **Neonatal hepatitis** is an idiopathic disease in low-birth-weight infants that is associated with a "giant cell" hepatitis, bile plugs in the canaliculi, and inflammation.

3. **Biliary atresia** may be intrahepatic (rare) or extrahepatic.

   a. **Extrahepatic biliary atresia** is associated with atresia involving all or parts of the extrahepatic biliary tree.

   b. A proliferation of bile duct radicals in the portal triads and cholestasis is characteristically seen on biopsy.

B. **Reye's syndrome** is a childhood disease that may occur after an influenza or chickenpox infection, usually with a history of ingestion of aspirin.

1. It primarily targets the brain and the liver.

2. There is an abnormality in mitochondrial β-oxidation of fatty acids.

3. Liver biopsies reveal a microvesicular type of fatty liver without inflammation, and megamitochondria are noted on electron microscopy.

4. The urea cycle is interrupted owing to mitochondrial abnormalities, and ammonia levels are increased.

5. Neuropsychological sequelae are severe, but liver abnormalities are reversible.

6. Cerebral edema with encephalopathy is the usual cause of death (10% mortality).

Objective 12: To review the complications associated with alcoholic and other types of cirrhosis.

XIII. Complications of cirrhosis

A. Cirrhosis refers to the presence of irreversible diffuse fibrosis (the key criterion) in the liver with or without the formation of regenerative nodules.

1. Morphologic patterns include **micronodular** (< 3 mm nodules), **macronodular** (> 3 mm nodules), and **mixed types**.

2. Alcoholic liver disease is the most common cause of cirrhosis (~65%) in the United States, followed by macronodular (postnecrotic) cirrhosis secondary to HBV.

3. The most common cause of death in cirrhosis is rupture of **esophageal varices**.

B. Complications associated with cirrhosis in general relate to the following:

1. **Portal hypertension** (due to fibrotic obliteration of the intrasinusoidal bed) resulting in as-

cites, esophageal varices, hemorrhoids, and dilated cutaneous veins around the umbilicus (caput medusae).

2. **Dysfunction of the detoxifying capabilities** of the liver, which may result in hepatic encephalopathy (reversible alteration in mental status), hyperestrinism (e.g., gynecomastia), and secondary aldosteronism (salt and water retention).

3. **Decreased synthesis of proteins**, which may produce hypoalbuminemia (which reduces oncotic pressure) and a bleeding diathesis (due to multiple coagulation factor defects).

4. **Hepatorenal syndrome**, defined as acute renal failure with no visible gross or microscopic abnormalities.

5. **Ascites**, or the collection of fluid within the peritoneal cavity.
   a. It is most commonly due to **alcoholic cirrhosis**.
   b. It is caused by portal hypertension, decreased oncotic pressure (hypoalbuminemia), an increase in hepatic lymph formation, and secondary hyperaldosteronism (salt and water retention).

Objective 13: To be familiar with tumors in the liver, biliary tree, and pancreas.

XIV. Tumors of the liver
   A. **Cavernous hemangiomas** are the most common overall benign tumor of the liver.
   B. **Liver cell (hepatic) adenomas** are vascular tumors (that have a tendency to rupture) associated with the use of oral contraceptives and anabolic steroids.
   C. **Metastasis** is the most common cancer of the liver.
      1. Common metastatic tumors include primary carcinomas located in the lung (most common cause), gastrointestinal tract (second most common cause; esophagus, stomach, pancreas, and colon), and breast.
      2. The CT scan is the most accurate imaging technique for detecting metastasis.
   D. **Hepatocellular carcinoma** (HCC) is the most common primary cancer of the liver.
      1. Cirrhosis is the most common cause, specifically, postnecrotic cirrhosis secondary to HBV (aflatoxins are cocarcinogens).
      2. HCC commonly invades portal and hepatic veins.
      3. Clinical deterioration in a known cirrhotic, increasing abdominal girth (ascites), bloody ascitic fluid, and a sudden rise in serum GGT and AP are highly predictive of HCC.
      4. Patients have an increase in α-fetoprotein (75–90%; usually > 500 ng/mL) and AAT.
      5. Secondary polycythemia (erythropoietin production by the tumor) and hypoglycemia related to production of an insulin-like factor are also noted.
      6. Vaccination against HBV should decrease the incidence of HCC.
   E. **Angiosarcomas** are associated with exposure to vinyl chloride, arsenic, or Thorotrast (mnemonic: VAT).

XV. Tumors of the biliary tract
   A. **Gallbladder cancer** is the most common cancer of the biliary tree and has a well-established relationship with cholelithiasis and porcelain gallbladder.
   B. **Cholangiocarcinomas** are malignancies of the bile ducts and are increased in patients with clonorchiasis, PSC, and previous exposure to Thorotrast.

XVI. Tumors of the pancreas
   A. Approximately 90% of pancreatic tumors involve the pancreatic ducts, while the remaining 10% are tumors involving the islet cells.
   B. **Pancreatic adenocarcinoma** is increasing in incidence in the United States.
      1. Risk factors include cigarette smoking, chronic pancreatitis (> 9-fold risk), and a family history of the nonpolyposis colon cancer syndrome.
      2. Mutations involving the *ras* oncogene (75% of cases) have been clearly identified.
      3. The head of the pancreas is the most common location and accounts for jaundice, clay-colored stools, hepatomegaly, and a palpable gallbladder.

Objective 14: To be conversant with inflammatory conditions involving the peritoneal cavity.

XVII. Peritoneal inflammation
   A. **Acute peritonitis** is most commonly due to a ruptured viscus (e.g., duodenal ulcer), bacterial infection (e.g., acute appendicitis, acute diverticulitis), or ischemic bowel disease.
      1. Mixed aerobic (*Escherichia coli*) and anaerobic bacteria (*Bacteroides fragilis*) are frequently cultured.
      2. It produces diffuse abdominal wall pain with rebound tenderness and paralytic ileus.
   B. **Spontaneous bacterial peritonitis** (no evidence of rupture of a viscus) most commonly develops in the setting of ascites.
      1. In **hepatocellular failure** accompanying cirrhosis in adults, *E. coli* is the most common organism isolated.
      2. In ascites associated with the **nephrotic syndrome** in children, *Streptococcus pneumoniae* is most commonly isolated.

Objective 15: To understand the pathogenesis of gallstones and the relationship to acute and chronic cholecystitis.

XVIII. Gallstones and acute and chronic cholecystitis
   A. An increased incidence of **gallstones** is noted in women, Native Americans, and African Americans and people with diabetes, cirrhosis, and chronic extravascular hemolysis.
      1. Risk factors for stone formation are decreased bile acids/salts with or without increased cholesterol solubilized in bile (90% of cases).
      2. **CH stones** (80%) are most commonly mixed and usually radiolucent.
      3. **Pigment stones** (20%) that are **black** are associated with extravascular hemolytic anemias, while those which are **brown** are more com-

monly associated with infection of bile and bile stasis.

4. Complications associated with stone formation consist of obstruction (e.g., common bile duct), acute cholecystitis, acute pancreatitis, and gallbladder cancer.

5. Ultrasonography is the gold standard test for the diagnosis of stones and duct dilatation.

B. **Acute cholecystitis** is a female-dominant disease that is most commonly the result of an impacted stone (90%) in the cystic duct.

1. Obstruction predisposes to bacterial invasion as a secondary event (*E. coli*).

2. Clinically, patients develop an acute onset of a constant, dull aching right upper quadrant pain (which may radiate to the right scapula and shoulder) within 15–30 minutes of eating.

C. **Chronic cholecystitis** is the most common symptomatic disorder of the gallbladder.

1. It may result from previous attacks of acute cholecystitis and the presence of stones (in > 90%) or it may arise without preexisting acute cholecystitis.

2. Chemical inflammation has been implicated, since most cases do not involve a bacterial infection.

3. **Porcelain gallbladder** refers to a chronically inflamed gallbladder with dystrophic calcification that is well visualized on x-ray.

Objective 16: To outline the pathophysiology of cystic fibrosis as it relates to pancreatic function.

XIX. Cystic fibrosis (CF)

A. CF is an AR disease that affects ~1:3000 live births.

B. **Recurrent pulmonary infections** and **pancreatic insufficiency** leading to failure to thrive and malnutrition are the primary abnormalities.

C. The **gene for CF** is located on **chromosome 7**.

1. The fundamental defect involves the transport of chloride ions through certain epithelial cells.

a. In sweat glands, neither sodium nor chloride can be reabsorbed.

b. In respiratory epithelium, chloride ions cannot be secreted, but sodium and water are easily reabsorbed, leading to thick mucous secretions.

2. The gene on chromosome 7 that codes for a **CF transmembrane regulator** (CFTR) **protein** is defective.

D. **Pancreatic abnormalities** occur in 90% of cases (e.g., exocrine insufficiency leading to malabsorption).

E. In newborns, **meconium ileus** with intestinal obstruction (20%) is pathognomonic for CF.

F. The **pulmonary system** is most affected in CF, and progressive respiratory failure is the most common cause of death.

G. In the **reproductive system**, sterility in the male occurs in 95% of cases (absence or atresia of the vas deferens), and fertility is also impaired in women.

H. The **sweat chloride test** is the gold standard test for diagnosis.

Objective 17: To review the pathogenesis of acute and chronic pancreatitis.

XX. Acute and chronic pancreatitis

A. **Acute pancreatitis** is an acute inflammatory process that commonly spreads to other sites owing to the retroperitoneal location of the pancreas.

1. Most cases are due to **gallstones** impacted at the distal end of the CBD where it connects with the pancreatic duct of Wirsung and as a **complication of alcoholism**.

2. The pathogenesis involves the activation of zymogens within the pancreas by trypsin and increasing pancreatic duct permeability.

a. **Zymogen activation** occurs by intraacinar activation of trypsin from trypsinogen (autoactivation), which is the key initiating event, since trypsin activates zymogens.

b. **Pancreatic duct permeability** may be increased by increasing intraductal pressure due to thick protein secretions induced by alcohol or an impacted gallstone in the duct.

3. Laboratory abnormalities include elevation of serum amylase (80–90% of cases) and an elevated serum lipase.

4. CT scanning is the imaging method of choice in assessing the pancreas (e.g., detecting stippled calcification) and pancreatic complications.

5. Complications may be local (e.g., pseudocyst, abscess) or systemic (e.g., hypovolemic shock, DIC, ARDS).

B. **Chronic pancreatitis** is a continuing inflammatory disease of the pancreas that is irreversible and causes pain and permanent functional impairment.

1. Approximately 70–80% of cases are due to **alcoholism**, and 40–50% of these patients also have alcoholic liver disease.

2. It is further subclassified as **chronic calcifying pancreatitis** (more common) due to protein-calcium concretions obstructing the ducts or **obstructive chronic pancreatitis**.

3. Chronic pancreatitis predisposes to pancreatic carcinoma.

4. The triad of pancreatic calcifications, steatorrhea, and diabetes mellitus is highly predictive for the diagnosis.

QUESTIONS

DIRECTIONS. (Items 1–12): Each of the numbered items or incomplete statements in this section is followed by answers or by completions of the statement. Select the ONE lettered answer or completion that is BEST in each case. Correct answers and explanations are given at the end of the chapter.

1. The photograph is representative of a liver biopsy from a 42-year-old man with fever, tender hepatomegaly, and jaundice. You would expect this patient to have

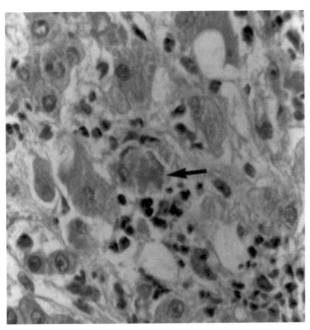

   (A) a positive antimitochondrial antibody
   (B) a positive HBsAg
   (C) AST greater than ALT
   (D) anti–smooth muscle antibody
   (E) conjugated bilirubin fraction <20%

2. The photograph is a close-up view of the surface of the liver removed at autopsy from a 52-year-old man who was found dead beneath a bridge. You would least expect the man to have had

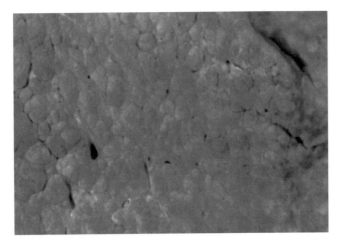

   (A) a prolonged prothrombin time
   (B) hypoalbuminemia
   (C) secondary aldosteronism
   (D) hyperestrinism
   (E) an elevated α-fetoprotein

3. The photograph represents a liver biopsy from a 30-year-old woman who died in a car accident 3 days after returning from Naples, Italy, where she had spent 1 month with her grandparents. Scleral icterus was noted. There were no needle tracks to indicate intravenous drug abuse. Her medical history supplied by her husband was unremarkable. He stated that she had been feeling tired and had abdominal discomfort prior to leaving Naples. Based on the history, physical findings, and biopsy, you would expect the serologic tests for the patient to be positive for

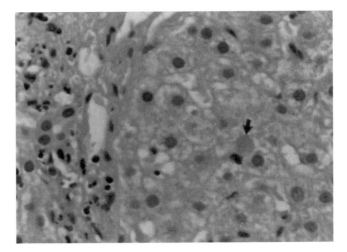

   (A) anti-HAV-IgM antibody
   (B) HBsAg
   (C) antinuclear antibodies
   (D) anti-HCV antibody
   (E) antimitochondrial antibody

4. Which of the following laboratory tests would best differentiate a patient who has been vaccinated against HBV versus one with a previous history of HBV and an uneventful recovery?

   (A) HBsAg
   (B) Anti-HBc-IgG antibody
   (C) Anti-HBs antibody
   (D) HBV DNA antigen
   (E) Anti-HBc-IgM antibody

5. In which of the following groups of liver disorders are both disorders an unconjugated hyperbilirubinemia?

   (A) ABO incompatibility and Dubin-Johnson syndrome
   (B) Acute viral hepatitis and alcoholic hepatitis
   (C) Crigler-Najjar syndrome and primary biliary cirrhosis
   (D) Physiologic jaundice of the newborn and Gilbert syndrome
   (E) Breast milk jaundice and primary sclerosing cholangitis

6. A 22-year-old man with a history of recurrent respiratory infections, malabsorption, and infertility would most likely have a

   (A) positive sweat chloride test
   (B) high serum ferritin concentration
   (C) low serum ceruloplasmin concentration
   (D) low serum α_1-antitrypsin level
   (E) liver biopsy exhibiting amyloid deposition

7. In which of the following groups of complications related to alcoholic cirrhosis is one of the complications a byproduct of portal hypertension and the other related to dysfunctional metabolism of hormones?

   (A) Hepatic encephalopathy and palmar erythema
   (B) Esophageal varices and gynecomastia
   (C) Ascites and hepatorenal syndrome
   (D) Asterixis and periumbilical caput medusae
   (E) Reduced free testosterone levels and a bleeding diathesis

8. An afebrile 71-year-old man with a history of chronic alcoholism and steatorrhea presents with weight loss, a slow onset of jaundice, and normocytic anemia. Physical examination reveals a palpable gallbladder, nodular liver, splenomegaly by percussion, shifting dullness, and light-colored stool on rectal examination. Based on the history and physical findings, you would expect

   (A) an increase in α-fetoprotein concentration
   (B) serum albumin minus ascitic fluid albumin difference < 1.1
   (C) conjugated bilirubin fractionation > 50% of the total bilirubin
   (D) urine strongly positive for bilirubin and urobilinogen
   (E) a greater overall increase in transaminases than in the cholestasis enzymes

9. A 58-year-old woman with a history of rheumatoid arthritis presents with severe pruritus, hepatomegaly, and marked elevation of her cholestasis enzymes without elevation of bilirubin. Based on this history and her physical and laboratory abnormalities, you would expect that her disease is associated with

   (A) mid-zonal liver cell necrosis with Councilman bodies
   (B) perivenular fibrosis of the terminal hepatic venules
   (C) "pipe stem" cirrhosis
   (D) ring (doughnut) granulomas
   (E) granulomatous destruction of bile duct radicals

10. You would least expect gallstones to complicate

    (A) metastatic liver disease
    (B) Crohn's disease
    (C) oral contraceptive use
    (D) alcoholic cirrhosis
    (E) cystic fibrosis

11. Which of the following drugs produces a type of liver disease that is morphologically different from the other drugs listed?

    (A) Oral contraceptives
    (B) Isoniazid
    (C) Acetaminophen
    (D) Methyldopa
    (E) Halothane

12. Which of the following liver–biliary tract tumor/pathogenesis relationships is correct?

    (A) Gallbladder cancer: *Clonorchis sinensis* infestation
    (B) Hepatocellular carcinoma: HBV postnecrotic cirrhosis
    (C) Cholangiocarcinoma: vinyl chloride
    (D) Angiosarcoma: anabolic steroids
    (E) Cavernous hemangiomas: oral contraceptives

DIRECTIONS. (Items 13–17): Each set of matching questions in this section consists of a list of lettered options followed by several numbered items. For each numbered item, select the ONE option that is most closely associated with it. Each lettered option may be selected once, more than once, or not at all.

(A) Hepatic vein thrombosis (Budd-Chiari syndrome)
(B) Venoocclusive disease
(C) Cardiac sclerosis (cirrhosis)
(D) Secondary biliary cirrhosis
(E) Extrahepatic biliary atresia
(F) Intrahepatic biliary atresia
(G) Neonatal hepatitis
(H) Amebiasis
(I) Echinococcosis
(J) Tertiary syphilis
(K) Congenital syphilis
(L) Ascending cholangitis

13. Most common cause of neonatal cholestasis in the first week of life

14. Painful hepatomegaly, jaundice, ascites, and portal hypertension in a patient with polycythemia vera

15. Immigrant from Mexico with a space-occupying mass in the right lobe of the liver and bloody diarrhea with mucus.

16. Neonatal jaundice, bile duct proliferation in the portal triads, and normal uptake of radionuclide but absence of radionuclide in the small intestine 24 hours later

17. Triad of fever, right upper quadrant pain, and jaundice

ANSWERS AND EXPLANATIONS

1. The answer is C: AST greater than ALT. The liver biopsy exhibits fatty change, a neutrophilic infiltrate, and an arrow pointing to a Mallory body, all of which point to alcoholic hepatitis as the most likely diagnosis. You would expect AST to be greater than ALT, since alcohol is a mitochondrial poison (produces megamitochondria on electron microscopy) and AST is a mitochondrial enzyme. Antimitochondrial antibodies are diagnostic of primary biliary cirrhosis. A positive HBsAg indicates HBV hepatitis, which is unlikely in this case owing to fatty change, the Mallory bodies, and a neutrophilic rather than a lymphocytic infiltrate. Anti–smooth muscle antibodies are common in autoimmune hepatitis, which is more likely to afflict young women. The conjugated bilirubin in alcoholic hepatitis has a mixed pattern (conjugated bilirubin between 20% and 50% of the total bilirubin) rather than a predominant increase in unconjugated bilirubin. (Photomicrograph reproduced, with permission, from N. Gitlin and R.M. Strauss. *Atlas of Clinical Hepatology*. Philadelphia, W.B. Saunders Co., 1995, p. 30.)

2. The answer is E: an elevated α-fetoprotein. The liver exhibits a micronodular cirrhosis with evenly spaced regenerative nodules. There is no evidence of hepatocellular carcinoma (mass lesion, vessel invasion), hence the α-fetoprotein should not be elevated. The patient most likely had alcoholism, since this is the most common cirrhosis and has a micronodular pattern. You would expect a prolonged prothrombin time (decreased synthesis of coagulation factors), hypoalbuminemia (decreased synthesis of albumin), secondary aldosteronism (reduced metabolism and activation of the renin-angiotensin-aldosterone system due to reduced cardiac output), and hyperestrinism (reduced metabolism and aromatization of 17-ketosteroids). (Photomicrograph reproduced, with permission, from N. Gitlin and R.M. Strauss. *Atlas of Clinical Hepatology*. Philadelphia, W.B. Saunders Co., 1995, p. 19.)

3. The answer is A: anti-HAV-IgM antibody. The biopsy shows ballooning degeneration and regeneration of hepatocytes, an arrow pointing to an acidophilic body (sign of apoptosis), and a mild infiltrate of lymphocytes consistent with acute viral hepatitis. The most likely cause of traveler's hepatitis is HAV, which is particularly common in Naples, Italy. Thus, you would expect a positive anti-HAV-IgM antibody. A positive HBsAg, representing HBV hepatitis, would be unlikely based on her negative medical history and parenteral transmission of the disease. The same is true for HCV hepatitis, hence anti-HCV antibodies would not be expected. A positive serum antinuclear antibody test indicating autoimmune hepatitis or a positive antimitochondrial antibody suggesting primary biliary cirrhosis (PBC) are highly unlikely based on the histopathology of the liver. The patient is also too young for PBC. (Photomicrograph reproduced, with permission, from N. Gitlin and R.M. Strauss. *Atlas of Clinical Hepatology*. Philadelphia, W.B. Saunders Co., 1995, p. 56.)

4. The answer is B: anti-HBc-IgG antibody. Patients who have been actively immunized with recombinant HBV vaccine develop anti-HBs antibodies in 90% of cases, since the antigen in the vaccine is HBsAg. Patients who have recovered from HBV will have both anti-HBs and anti-HBc-IgG antibodies, the former antibody having a protective function and the latter no protective function. The presence of HBsAg, anti-HBc-IgM, and HBV DNA indicates active infection.

5. The answer is D: Physiologic jaundice of the newborn and Gilbert syndrome. Physiologic jaundice is the most common jaundice in the newborn and is due to defects in uptake and conjugation, increased uptake of unconjugated bilirubin in the bowel, and increased production of bilirubin from the breakdown of fetal RBCs. Gilbert syndrome is the second most common cause of jaundice in the United States (viral hepatitis is first). It is a benign AD disorder involving RBC hemolysis, uptake, and conjugation abnormalities. ABO incompatibility (increased production of bilirubin from extravascular hemolysis), breast milk jaundice (defect in conjugation), and Crigler-Najjar syndrome (defect in conjugation) are all unconjugated hyperbilirubinemias. Dubin-Johnson syndrome (AR disease with a defect in secretion of CB), acute viral and alcoholic hepatitis (defect in uptake, conjugation, and secretion of bilirubin), primary biliary cirrhosis (bile duct destruction with an increase in CB), and primary sclerosing cholangitis (fibrosis around large bile ducts) are all CB hyperbilirubinemias.

6. The answer is A: positive sweat chloride test. A young man with a history of recurrent respiratory infections, malabsorption most likely related to pancreatic insufficiency, and infertility (probable absence or atresia of the vas deferens) most likely has cystic fibrosis (CF). A sweat chloride > 60 mEq/L is confirmatory. A high serum ferritin concentration is associated with hemochromatosis (AR disease) or hemosiderosis (acquired iron overload), neither one of which is associated with respiratory problems. A low serum ceruloplasmin concentration is associated with Wilson's disease, which is an AR disease with an inability to excrete copper into the bile. Liver disease, lenticular degeneration in the CNS, and Kayser-Fleischer rings in the eyes are characteristic findings. A low serum α1-antitrypsin (AAT) level is present in AAT deficiency, which is an AR disease that can produce severe liver disease or lung disease (panacinar emphysema). Infertility is not a feature. Amyloidosis would not be expected in this young an individual and is not associated with recurrent respiratory problems.

7. The answer is B: esophageal varices and gynecomastia. Portal hypertension (PH) is most commonly due to alcoholic cirrhosis. It is the result of obliteration of the intrasinusoidal system of the liver from fibrosis, compression of residual sinusoids by regenerative nodules, and portosystemic shunts connecting the venous with the arterial system. Esophageal varices, caput medusae, ascites, and hemorrhoids are possible complications of PH. Hyperestrinism secondary to dysfunctional metabolism of estrogen and 17-ketosteroids (aromatized in adipose tissue to estrogen) may produce gynecomastia, palmar erythema, secondary female sex characteristics in males (sparse axillary and pubic hair, soft skin), spider angiomas, and reduced free testosterone levels (owing to increased synthesis of sex hormone–binding globulin, which has a high affinity for testosterone). Hepatic encephalopathy is a reversible disorder characterized by asterixis (inability to sustain posture), mental status abnormalities, abnormal sleep patterns,

and coma. An increase in false neurotransmitters (γ-aminobenzoic acid, octopamine) and ammonia have been implicated. The hepatorenal syndrome refers to acute renal failure associated with liver disease. The kidneys are grossly and microscopically normal, and tubular function is intact (UNa$^+$ < 20 mEq/L). A bleeding diathesis is associated with reduced synthesis of coagulation factors, defective synthesis of fibrinogen (dysfibrinogenemia), and defective macrophage clearance of fibrin and fibrinogen degradation products, which interferes with platelet function.

8. The answer is C: conjugated bilirubin fractionation > 50% of the total bilirubin. The patient has carcinoma of the head of the pancreas based on obstructive signs of a palpable gallbladder (Courvoisier's sign) and light-colored stools (absence of urobilin pigment). He also has evidence of alcoholic cirrhosis (nodular liver, ascites [shifting dullness], and splenomegaly). It is likely that the cancer developed from chronic pancreatitis owing to the history of steatorrhea. One would expect bilirubin in the urine but not urobilinogen, owing to obstruction of bile flow. The physical findings do not suggest development of hepatocellular carcinoma, which is associated with an increase in α-fetoprotein. The serum albumin minus ascitic fluid albumin difference would be >1.1, since the ascitic fluid is a transudate with a much lower albumin concentration than serum. The cholestasis enzymes alkaline phosphatase and γ-glutamyltransferase show a much greater increase in activity than the transaminases in cholestatic disease.

9. The answer is E: granulomatous destruction of bile duct radicals. With a history of rheumatoid arthritis (autoimmune disease), pruritus (bile salt deposition in the skin), normal bilirubin levels, and elevation of the cholestasis enzymes in a middle-aged woman, primary biliary cirrhosis is the most likely diagnosis. It is characterized by the development of antimitochondrial antibodies that attack antigens in the bile duct epithelium. Granulomatous inflammation is commonly present in the triads. Jaundice is a late feature of the disease. Mid-zonal liver cell necrosis with Councilman bodies represents yellow fever. Perivenular fibrosis of the terminal hepatic venules is a characteristic finding in alcoholic liver disease owing to acetaldehyde-protein complex stimulation of myofibroblasts to synthesize collagen. "Pipe stem" cirrhosis is the classic finding of schistosomiasis (*Schistosoma mansoni*) involving the portal vein radicals, which leads to fibrosis of the vessels. Ring (doughnut) granulomas are a feature of Q fever due to *Coxiella burnetii*. Interstitial pneumonia and granulomatous hepatitis are two consistent features of the disease.

10. The answer is A: metastatic liver disease. Metastatic liver disease is the most common cancer of the liver. Since it does not produce diffuse liver cell disease, disruption of bile acid/salt synthesis, one of the factors responsible for stone formation, is highly unlikely. Crohn's disease and alcoholic cirrhosis both have bile salt abnormalities, the former owing to inadequate reabsorption of bile salts in the terminal ileum and the latter from reduced synthesis of bile salts. Oral contra-

ceptives decrease the secretion of bile into the canaliculi and also increase serum cholesterol levels (progesterone effect). Inspissated bile is produced in cystic fibrosis, leading to problems with bile secretion and focal secondary biliary cirrhosis.

11. The answer is A: oral contraceptives. Oral contraceptives produce noninflammatory cholestatic liver disease, peliosis hepatis, liver cell adenomas (having a tendency to spontaneously rupture), and hepatocellular carcinoma. Isoniazid (an acetylhydrazine metabolite is responsible for damage), acetaminophen (free radical injury), methyldopa, and halothane (metabolites are responsible for damage) all produce a viral hepatitis type of liver damage.

12. The answer is B: hepatocellular carcinoma: HBV postnecrotic cirrhosis. Hepatocellular carcinoma most commonly develops in a background of cirrhosis most commonly secondary to HBV postnecrotic cirrhosis. Other causes include HCV-related liver disease, pigment cirrhosis, and alcoholic cirrhosis. Gallbladder cancer is most commonly associated with gallstones and porcelain gallbladder; cholangiocarcinoma with *Clonorchis sinensis* infestation; and angiosarcoma with exposure to vinyl chloride, arsenic, or Thorotrast. Cavernous hemangiomas have no specific pathogenetic relationships.

13. The answer is G: neonatal hepatitis. Neonatal hepatitis is idiopathic and is most likely to occur in premature infants. Other causes of neonatal cholestasis must be excluded (biliary atresia, metabolic disease, congenital infections). Liver biopsies reveal a giant cell hepatitis with intracanalicular bile plugs.

14. The answer is A: hepatic vein thrombosis (Budd-Chiari syndrome). Hypercoagulable states (e.g., polycythemia vera [most common], oral contraceptives) predispose to hepatic vein thrombosis. Thrombi develop in the hepatic vein and smaller venous tributaries, producing painful hepatomegaly and portal hypertension, leading to ascites.

15. The answer is H: amebiasis. The trophozoites of *Entamoeba histolytica* predominantly localize in the cecum and right colon. In this location, they produce flask-shaped ulcers in the mucosa and gain access to the portal system, which drains into the liver, producing an abscess. The mucosal inflammation in the colon produces bloody diarrhea with mucus.

16. The answer is E: extrahepatic biliary atresia. Approximately one-third of cases of neonatal cholestasis is due to biliary atresia, the most common cause of which is extrahepatic biliary atresia. Intrahepatic biliary atresia has a paucity of bile duct radicals in the portal triads, whereas extrahepatic biliary atresia has bile duct proliferation. Uptake of radionuclide material in both types of atresia is normal, but excretion of the material into the small intestine is absent.

17. The answer is L: ascending cholangitis. Ascending cholangitis is usually associated with acute cholecystitis complicated by a stone in the common bile duct. The infection extends up the common bile duct into the portal triads of the liver and out into the parenchyma, where it produces multiple liver abscesses. The triad of fever, jaundice, and right upper quadrant pain (Charcot's triad) is useful in alerting the clinician to a potential cause of death.

CHAPTER SEVENTEEN

DISORDERS OF THE KIDNEY,

LOWER URINARY TRACT, AND

MALE GENITALIA

SYNOPSIS

OBJECTIVES

1. To understand the congenital and cystic diseases of the kidneys.
2. To be familiar with the pathogenesis of glomerular diseases and those which commonly present with the nephritic, nephrotic, or mixed syndromes.
3. To discuss prerenal, renal, and postrenal causes of acute renal failure.
4. To be conversant with the causes and complications of chronic renal failure.
5. To discuss acute and chronic interstitial nephritis.
6. To outline the vascular disorders involving the kidneys.
7. To review the obstructive disorders of the urinary tract.
8. To understand the benign nonneoplastic disorders of the lower urinary tract, and male reproductive system.
9. To outline the neoplastic disorders of the kidney, lower urinary tract, and male reproductive system.
10. To be conversant with causes of male hypogonadism and impotence.

Objective 1: To understand the congenital and cystic diseases of the kidneys.

I. Congenital and cystic diseases of the kidneys
  A. **Horseshoe kidneys** are fused at the lower poles in 90% of cases and may predispose to infection and stone formation.
  B. Renal cystic diseases in **children** are associated with oligohydramnios in the mother (if fetal renal disease is bilateral), Potter facies (low-set ears, "parrot beak" nose, hypoplasia of the lungs), and palpable abdominal or flank masses.
    1. They are the most common cause of a palpable abdominal or flank mass in a newborn.
    2. **Autosomal recessive polycystic kidney disease** (infantile polycystic kidney disease) occurs in early infancy.
      a. Both kidneys are enlarged owing to the presence of small cysts originating from collecting tubules that are oriented at right angles to the cortical surface.

b. It is also associated with bile duct cysts and congenital hepatic fibrosis (portal hypertension).
  3. **Familial juvenile nephronophthisis** (AR inheritance) is associated with small, cystic kidneys; salt wasting; defects in renal concentration (polyuria); and progressive renal failure leading to death at an early age.
  4. **Medullary sponge kidney** is a nonhereditary disease with cysts in the medullary pyramids that have a "Swiss cheese" appearance.
    a. It may be associated with hematuria, recurrent urinary tract infection, or recurrent urinary stones.
    b. It pursues a benign course.
  5. **Renal dysplasia** is the most common cystic disease in children.
    a. It has no inheritance pattern and is associated with abnormal development of the metanephric structures, resulting in urinary tract obstruction and malformed kidneys.
    b. It may be unilateral or bilateral and affect either all or part of a kidney.
    c. Histologic sections reveal embryonal tissues, primitive glomerular structures, cartilage, and mesenchymal tissue.
    d. Most cases present as a unilateral flank mass in an otherwise asymptomatic infant.
  6. **Adult polycystic kidney disease** (APKD) is an AD disease that is most often associated with the APKD-1 gene located on chromosome 16.
    a. Cysts are not present at birth but develop over time.
    b. Renal function is retained until the third and fourth decades.
    c. It may be associated with hypertension, abdominal pain, extrarenal cysts (liver most common, pancreas), intracranial berry aneurysms (10%–30%), and mitral valve prolapse.
    d. Both kidneys are enlarged owing to large cysts distributed throughout both cortex and medulla, which are easily visualized by ultrasound.

e. Approximately 50% of patients die of renal failure by 50–60 years of age, and another third die of complications related to hypertension.

7. **Simple renal retention cysts**, the most common cysts in adults, are acquired cysts that derive from tubular obstruction and dilatation.

Objective 2: To be familiar with the pathogenesis of glomerular diseases and those which commonly present with the nephritic, nephrotic, or mixed syndromes.

II. Overview of glomerular structure

  A. **Glomerular capillaries** derive from the afferent arterioles and empty into the efferent arterioles, which become the peritubular capillaries.

  B. The capillaries are lined by **fenestrated endothelial cells** and reside in Bowman's capsule.

  C. The capsule contains **parietal epithelium** that is continuous with the proximal tubules.

  D. **Visceral epithelium** (podocytes) covers the outer aspect of the glomerular capillaries.

  E. The **glomerular basement membrane** (GBM) is composed of type IV collagen and negatively charged heparan sulfate proteoglycans to repel negatively charged proteins such as albumin.

  F. **Podocytes** have interdigitating processes called foot processes with spaces between each process called **filtration slits**.

  G. The **mesangium** has modified smooth muscle cells that support the capillary tuft, control intraglomerular blood flow, have phagocytic properties, and produce an extracellular matrix when stimulated.

III. Terminology of glomerular disease

  A. Cells normally present in a glomerulus consist of epithelial (parietal and visceral), endothelial, and mesangial cells.

  B. Cellular proliferations are designated **proliferative** if > 100 cells are present.

    1. Proliferations are **diffuse** if they involve all or most of the glomeruli, **focal** if they involve < 50% of the glomeruli, and **segmental** if they involve only portions of individual glomeruli.

    2. **Crescents** are proliferations of the parietal epithelial cells, which fill Bowman's capsular space.

    3. The term **membranous** is applied to just thickening of the GBM, while **membranoproliferative** is used if both thickening and hypercellularity are present.

    4. **Glomerulosclerosis** refers to an increase in extracellular matrix (hyalinization) within the mesangium.

    5. **Inflammatory cells** are not normally present in the glomerulus.

      a. Their presence correlates with immunocomplex deposition in the glomerulus and subsequent activation of the complement system with generation of chemotactic complement components (e.g., C5a) that attract neutrophils to the area.

      b. Neutrophils damage glomerular structures by means of their enzymes and generation of free radicals.

IV. Workup of glomerular disease

  A. A **renal biopsy** specimen is subdivided for routine H and E and specialized staining, immunofluorescence (IF) studies, and ultrastructural examination by electron microscopy (EM).

  B. Routine and specialized stains help classify the glomerular disease as diffuse, focal, membranous, proliferative, etc.

  C. IF studies identify patterns of deposition of IgG, IgA, IgM, fibrin, light chains, C1q, C3, and albumin.

    1. **Linear patterns** mainly occur in disorders associated with **anti-GBM antibodies** (e.g., Goodpasture's syndrome).

    2. **Granular patterns** ("lumpy bumpy") represent the deposition of immunocomplexes in the glomerulus.

      a. Their distribution is less uniform owing to differences in their charge, size, and solubility.

      b. EM identifies immunocomplexes as electron dense material in a subendothelial, intramembranous, subepithelial, or mesangial location.

      c. EM also identifies structural abnormalities (e.g., fusion of the foot processes in the nephrotic syndrome).

V. Pathogenesis of glomerular disease

  A. The majority of the glomerular disorders are immunologic diseases.

  B. Antibodies may combine with antigens in the serum (e.g., DNA, viral products) to form circulating immunocomplexes (type III hypersensitivity) that deposit in the glomeruli.

  C. Antibodies may also be directed against antigens that are normally present (e.g., collagen in the GBM; type II hypersensitivity) or have been "planted" in the glomerulus (e.g., bacterial products, DNA, drugs), hence forming in situ immunocomplexes.

VI. Nephritic syndrome

  A. This group of diseases (Table 17–1 and Figure 17–1) is characterized by abrupt onset of oliguria, salt retention with hypertension, periorbital edema, and urinary findings of mild to moderate proteinuria (< 3.5 g/24 h), RBC casts, hematuria (with dysmorphic RBCs), and WBCs.

  B. Reactive cellular proliferation with neutrophilic infiltration (which damages the glomeruli) marks the glomerular histology.

  C. A disease is classified as **primary** if it originates in the kidneys (e.g., IgA nephropathy) or **secondary** if it is a part of a systemic disease (e.g., SLE, poststreptococcal glomerulonephritis).

  D. A glomerular disease may begin as a nephritic syndrome and progress to a nephrotic syndrome or be a combination of the two.

VII. Nephrotic syndrome

  A. The **nephrotic syndrome** (Table 17–2 and Figure 17–1) is characterized by massive proteinuria > 3.5 g/24 h in association with lipiduria and fatty casts (which contain cholesterol and triglyceride).

  B. Glomerular disease results in loss of the normal negative charge of the GBM (polyanion loss) and alteration in the permeability of the matrix to proteins.

  C. Complications associated with massive proteinuria include the following:

    1. Generalized pitting edema (loss of oncotic pressure).

TABLE 17–2. Glomerular Diseases Commonly Associated with the Nephrotic Syndrome

Disease	Microscopic Findings	Pathogenesis	Immunofluorescence Pattern	Electron Micrographic Findings	Clinical/Laboratory Findings	Prognosis
Minimal change disease (lipoid nephrosis, nil disease)	Positive fat stains in the glomerulus and tubules. Glomeruli otherwise normal.	Probable cellular immune reaction with T cell production of a lymphokine that destroys the negative charge barrier (polyanion loss). Selective proteinuria (albumin).	No pattern.	Fusion of the podocytes (see Figure 17–1D).	Most common cause of nephrotic syndrome in children (65%). Most common in boys from 6 to 8 years of age usually after an upper respiratory infection. Normal blood pressure. Renal biopsies usually not done if the presentation is classic. Association with atopic history, nodular sclerosing Hodgkin's disease (HD), non-HD chronic lymphocytic leukemia.	Patients respond dramatically to corticosteroids in 90% of cases.
Membranous glomerulonephritis (GN)	Diffuse thickening of membranes but no cell proliferation. Epimembranous spikes with a hair-on-end appearance noted with special stains (correspond with subepithelial deposits of IgG and C3).	In situ IC deposition (resembles Heymann's GN in rats with antibody directed against epithelial antigen). Most cases idiopathic (85%). **Secondary causes:** drugs (captopril, penicillamine, gold, mercury, trimethadione), infections (malaria, leprosy, schistosomiasis, syphilis, hepatitis B, filariasis), malignancy (carcinoma of lung, colon cancer, lymphoma, melanoma), SLE (type V), sarcoidosis, diabetes, thyroiditis (thyroglobulin), sickle cell anemia.	Granular; IgG, C3.	Subepithelial deposits; fusion of podocytes (see Figure 17–1E).	Most common cause of nephrotic syndrome in adults (30–40%). Occurs in males more often than in females. Most patients >30 years of age. Normotensive early but hypertensive late. Laboratory: Normal C3.	About 40–50% progress to end-stage disease.
Focal segmental glomerulosclerosis (FSG)	Focal segmental disease with sclerotic areas. Vacuolization of visceral epithelial cells. Detachment of epithelial cells from GBM (hallmark of disease).	May be part of minimal change disease spectrum in adults. No IC deposits. Association with HIV, renal transplantation, intravenous heroin abuse, reflux nephropathy. Nonselective proteinuria.	IgM, C3 in some cases.	Fusion of podocytes; no electron-dense deposits.	About 80% of patients have nephrotic syndrome. Mild hypertension in 50%. Laboratory: normal C3.	Poor prognosis (50–80% develop end-stage renal disease within 10 years). Recurrence after renal transplantation.

Type I membranoproliferative GN Type II membranoproliferative GN (dense deposit disease)	Both types have diffuse thickening of membranes and cell proliferation. In type I, special stains reveal double contour of GBM ("tram tracks") due to ingrowth of mesangium between endothelial cell and GBM. Not prominent in type II.	Type I: IC disease. Strong association with hepatitis C. Other associations: cryoglobulins, neoplasms. Type II: C3 nephritic factor (autoantibody against alternative pathway C3 convertase [C3bBb]; stabilizes convertase, leading to sustained activation of C3). Intramembranous deposits are C3.	Type I: granular; IgG, IgM, C3, C1q, C4. Type II: granular; C3 and absent IgG, C1q, C4.	Type I: subendothelial deposits. Type II: intramembranous deposits (see Figure 17-1F).	Affects patients between 5 and 30 years of age. Slightly favors females over males. Type I accounts for 90% of cases and type II for 10% (rarely after 30 years of age). HCV serology should always be obtained in type I MPGN. Most patients have hypertension. Laboratory: Low C3 in both types. C3 nephritic factor in type II.	Poor prognosis (50% develop chronic renal failure within 10 years).
Systemic lupus erythematosus (SLE)					See Table 17-1. Types III, IV, and V may sometimes produce nephrotic syndrome.	
Kimmelstiel-Wilson syndrome (diabetic glomerulosclerosis)	Focal areas of glomerulosclerosis, afferent and efferent hyaline arteriolosclerosis. Initially diffuse glomerulosclerosis with thickening of the mesangium and capillary loops; eventually becomes nodular. Capsular drops of protein seen on inside of Bowman's capsule. Nodular glomerulosclerosis, or the Kimmelstiel-Wilson kidney, has "Christmas ball-like" deposits in the mesangium along with afferent and efferent hyaline arteriolosclerosis.	Nonenzymatic glycosylation GBM and tubule basement membranes, glomerular hypertrophy (from cytokine release from leukocytes), osmotic damage (sorbitol toxic to endothelial cells and GBM), hyperfiltration damage to mesangium (increased GFR early in disease). Efferent arteriole first involved with vessel change; leads to increased GFR.	Trapping of proteins.	Fusion of podocytes, thick membranes. No electron-dense deposits.	Most common overall disease involving the glomerulus. Develops in ~20–40% of cases of type I, insulin-dependent diabetes mellitus (DM) in 17 ± 6 years; ~15–20% of cases of type II DM develop renal disease. Microalbuminuria is first sign of nephropathy (begins after 10 years). Captopril slows onset of nephropathy by decreasing angiotensin II, which normally vasoconstricts the efferent arteriole (this releases pressure on the glomerulus). Hypertension occurs when proteinuria is present. Retinopathy parallels nephropathy.	Diabetes is most common cause of end-stage renal disease (55%) in United States. Other problems: renal papillary necrosis, acute and chronic pyelonephritis.
Amyloidosis	Thickening of GBM, mesangial deposits. A Congo red stain under polarized light reveals apple-green birefringence (color of a Granny Smith apple).	Deposition of amyloid (derived from light chains in multiple myeloma, serum associated amyloid in reactive amyloidosis [90% of cases]) in mesangium and GBM (increases permeability to proteins).	Nonspecific trapping of proteins.	Demonstrates amyloid fibrils in mesangium, GBM, renal tubule BM.	Kidneys commonly involved in systemic amyloidosis in 80% of cases (Chapter 13).	Renal failure is a common cause of death in amyloidosis.
Pregnancy-induced hypertension (preeclampsia/eclampsia)	Diffuse disease; bloodless glomerular capillaries; swollen endothelial cells ("endotheliosis").	Abnormal placentation, resulting in decrease in perfusion. Vasoconstriction overrides vasodilation of vessels. Damage to endothelial cells.	Nonspecific deposits of IgG, IgM, fibrin.	Vacuolated endothelial cells; widened subendothelial spaces.	Patients present with hypertension, proteinuria, and edema (convulsion is called eclampsia) usually in the third trimester.	Reversible.

IC, immunocomplexes; GBM, glomerular basement membrane; BM, basement membrane.

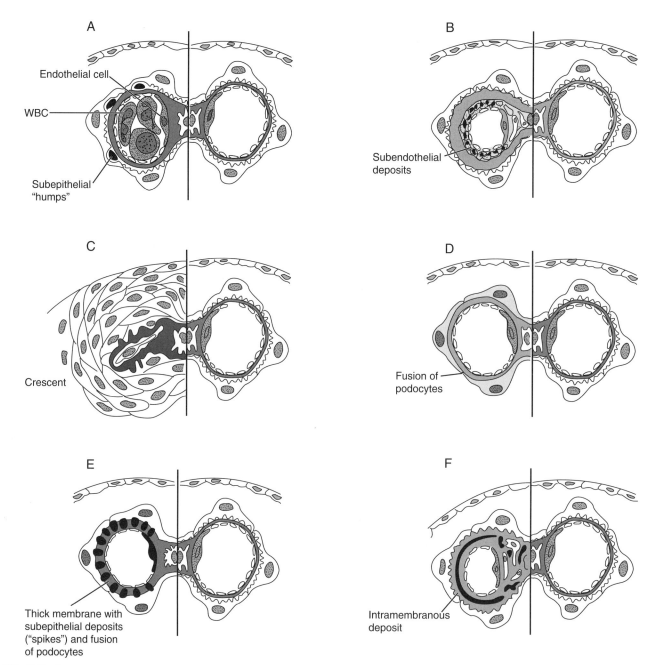

FIGURE 17–1. Ultrastructure of glomerular diseases. (A) Poststreptococcal glomerulonephritis with cell proliferation, neutrophilic infiltration, and subepithelial "humps," representing immunocomplexes. **(B)** Subendothelial deposits in type IV diffuse proliferative glomerulonephritis in systemic lupus erythematosus. **(C)** Crescent formation from proliferation of parietal cells in Bowman's capsule in a patient with Goodpasture's disease and rapidly progressive crescentic glomerulonephritis. **(D)** Fusion of the podocytes in a patient with minimal change disease. **(E)** Diffuse thickening of the glomerular basement membrane, subepithelial immunocomplexes ("spikes"), and fusion of the podocytes in diffuse membranous glomerulonephritis. **(F)** Intramembranous dense deposit representing C3 in type II membranoproliferative glomerulonephritis (dense deposit disease). (Slightly modified and reproduced, with permission, from L. J. Striker, J. L. Olson, and G. L. Striker. *The Renal Biopsy,* 2nd ed. Philadelphia, W. B. Saunders Co., 1990.)

2. Infection (loss of immunoglobulins, leading to hypogammaglobulinemia).
3. Hypercoagulability (loss of antithrombin III, leading to venous clots and renal vein thrombosis).
4. Hypercholesterolemia (stimulus for increased liver synthesis of LDL), resulting in accelerated atherosclerosis and loss of lipid in the urine (fatty casts, oval fat bodies [tubular cells or macrophages with lipid]).

    D. Primary diseases exhibit fusion of the podocytes.

VIII. Chronic glomerulonephritis

    A. Glomerulonephritis (GN) accounts for ~14% of cases of chronic renal failure.

    B. In descending order of frequency, rapidly progressive crescentic GN, focal segmental glomerulosclerosis, and membranoproliferative GN most commonly progress to chronic GN.

Objective 3: To discuss prerenal, renal, and postrenal causes of acute renal failure.

IX. Acute renal failure and acute tubular necrosis
- A. **Acute renal failure** (ARF) is failure in renal function resulting in inability of the kidneys to excrete urea and maintain normal fluid and electrolyte homeostasis.
- B. Causes of ARF may be prerenal, renal, or postrenal.
  1. **Prerenal azotemia** implies a reduction in the glomerular filtration rate (GFR) in the presence of normal renal function.
     - a. It is the most common setting for subsequent development of ARF.
     - b. It may be secondary to dehydration (e.g., diarrhea, vomiting, diuretics), congestive heart failure, and septic shock.
     - c. If left uncorrected, prerenal azotemia most frequently progresses to **ischemic acute tubular necrosis** (ATN), which is the most common cause of ARF.
  2. **Renal azotemia**, or uremia, refers to intrinsic renal disease.
     - a. Intrinsic renal diseases target the glomeruli (e.g., rapidly progressive crescentic GN), tubules (e.g., ischemia, toxins), interstitium (e.g., acute interstitial nephritis from drug use), or vessels (e.g., malignant hypertension).
     - b. After ischemic ATN, nephrotoxic ATN is the second most common cause of ARF.
  3. **Postrenal azotemia** is secondary to urinary tract obstruction (e.g., obstruction of the urethra in prostatic hyperplasia, retroperitoneal fibrosis) and back-diffusion of urine urea into the blood stream.
  4. The serum BUN is often expressed with the serum creatinine as a **BUN/creatinine ratio**.
     - a. The serum BUN/creatinine ratio is normally 10/1.
     - b. In both **prerenal** and **postrenal azotemia**, there is a disproportionate increase in the reabsorption of BUN in the proximal tubule, while the serum creatinine is only mildly increased (less is excreted in the urine), hence the BUN/creatinine ratio increases to 15/1 or greater.
     - c. In **renal azotemia**, intrinsic disease in the kidneys equally affects the excretion of BUN and creatinine, hence both analytes increase proportionately and the ratio remains 10/1.
- C. ATN is the most common cause of ARF.
  1. About 70% of cases are **oliguric** (urine output < 400 mL/d), and the remaining 30% are **non-oliguric** (polyuric ATN).
  2. The **reduced GFR** associated with the oliguric type of ATN is secondary to the following:
     - a. Tubular injury triggering vasoconstriction of afferent arterioles (increase in endothelin [vasoconstrictor], thromboxane A_2 [vasoconstrictor], decrease in nitric oxide [vasodilator]).
     - b. Intraluminal obstruction by sloughed-off renal tubular cells.
     - c. Increased interstitial pressure from back flow of fluids through damaged cells and disrupted basement membranes.
  3. The clinical course for the oliguric type of ATN, in order of sequence, is as follows:
     - a. Stage of onset (36 hours).
     - b. Oliguric stage (few days to 3 weeks) with azotemia (increased serum BUN), metabolic acidosis, and hyperkalemia.
     - c. Early diuretic phase (about third week).
     - d. Late diuretic phase, leading to recovery.
  4. Two patterns of ATN are **ischemic** (80%) and **nephrotoxic**.
     - a. Ischemic ATN is the most common overall cause of ARF.
     - b. Aminoglycosides and radiocontrast agents are the most common causes of nephrotoxic ATN.
     - c. In either type, the kidneys are enlarged, the cortex is pale, and the medulla is congested.
     - d. Ischemic ATN damages tubular cells from all parts of the nephron and focally disrupts basement membranes (**tubulorrhexis**), particularly the ascending thick limb of the loop of Henle.
     - e. Nephrotoxic ATN primarily targets the first part of the nephron, since that is the part the nephrotoxic agent first comes in contact with after filtration; there is no tubulorrhexis.
     - f. In either type, tubular cells undergo a combination of coagulation necrosis and apoptosis with subsequent sloughing of the cells into the lumen, resulting in the formation of pigmented renal tubular cell casts.
     - g. Nephrotoxic ATN has a more favorable prognosis than the ischemic type, since the basement membrane is intact for tubular cell regeneration and fewer tubules are destroyed.
     - h. Sepsis and cardiovascular and pulmonary dysfunction are the most common causes of death in ATN.
X. Differentiation of the oliguric states
- A. The four causes of oliguria are **prerenal azotemia** (most common cause), **acute GN**, **ATN**, and **postrenal azotemia**.
- B. Laboratory manifestations of tubular dysfunction are loss of concentration of urine (urine osmolality < 350 mOsm/kg [normal, > 500 mOsm/kg]) and inability to reabsorb sodium (urine sodium > 40 mEq/L [normal, < 40 mEq/L]), fractional excretion of sodium [FENa*] > 1 [normal, < 1]).
- C. **Prerenal azotemia** and **acute GN** demonstrate preservation of tubular function (Uosm > 500 mOsm/kg, UNa < 40 mEq/L, FENa < 1); hematuria and RBC casts occur in acute GN but not prerenal azotemia.
- D. **ATN** and **postrenal azotemia** (long-standing obstruction; early obstruction shows normal tubular function) exhibit tubular dysfunction (Uosm < 350 mOsm/kg, UNa > 40 mEq/L, FENa > 1); ATN

---

*FENa = [(UNa) × (PCr)/(PNa) × (UCr)] × 100, where UNa = urine sodium, UCr = urine creatinine, PNa = plasma sodium, PCr = plasma creatinine.

demonstrates renal tubular casts and postrenal azotemia does not.

Objective 4: To be conversant with the causes and complications of chronic renal failure.

XI. Chronic renal failure
  A. Chronic renal failure (CRF) is most frequently caused by the following disorders, in descending order of frequency: diabetes mellitus, hypertension, glomerulonephritis, unknown causes, and interstitial nephritis.
  B. **Electrolyte abnormalities** include either sodium loss (early) or sodium retention (late), hyperkalemia (potassium cannot be excreted, transcellular shift related to pH), and increased anion gap metabolic acidosis (retention of organic acids).
  C. **Hypocalcemia** occurs owing to hypovitaminosis D (loss of the 1α-hydroxylating enzyme) and hyperphosphatemia (due to decreased excretion), which drives calcium into tissue.
  D. **Bone alterations** include osteomalacia (decreased bone mineralization), osteoporosis (decreased bone matrix; due to buffering action of metabolic acidosis), and osteitis fibrosa cystica from secondary hyperparathyroidism.
  E. **Cardiopulmonary disorders** consist of accelerated atherosclerosis (increased VLDL from decreased catabolism), congestive heart failure with pulmonary edema (volume overload), hypertension (salt retention, volume overload) and uremic pericarditis (fibrinous type, often with hemorrhage).
  F. **Normocytic anemias** are most frequently due to a deficiency of erythropoietin and **platelet abnormalities** to interference of uremic toxic metabolites with platelet aggregation (prolonged bleeding time).
  G. **Gastrointestinal disturbances** consist of hemorrhagic gastritis, peptic ulcer disease, and intractable hiccups.
  H. There is an increased susceptibility to **infection** (hepatitis C, CMV, hepatitis B, HIV) owing to functional leukocyte abnormalities and the hazards of hemodialysis.
  I. **Urinalysis** demonstrates isosthenuria (fixed specific gravity; loss of both concentration and dilution), proteinuria, and the presence of waxy and broad cell casts.

Objective 5: To discuss acute and chronic interstitial nephritis.

XII. Acute and chronic interstitial nephritis
  A. Acute and chronic interstitial nephritis may be due to infection, drug use, toxins (e.g., heavy metals), physical agents (e.g., irradiation), immunologic reactions (e.g., SLE, Sjögren's syndrome), and metabolic diseases (e.g., hypercalcemia).
  B. **Acute interstitial nephritis** is most frequently secondary to infection (e.g., acute pyelonephritis) and drug use.
  C. **Chronic interstitial nephritis** is most often associated with drug use and less commonly with chronic pyelonephritis.
  D. **Acute pyelonephritis** (PN) is most commonly secondary to ascending infection by *Escherichia coli* and less commonly to hematogenous spread.
    1. **Predisposing causes** include urinary tract obstruction, cystic diseases, diabetes mellitus, vesicoureteral reflux (VUR), previous instrumentation of the urinary tract, and pregnancy.
    2. **Ascending infection** (distal colonization in the urethra by *E. coli*) is the most common cause of pyelonephritis and of all urinary tract infections.
    3. Microabscesses develop in the tubules (producing the characteristic WBC cast) and interstitium.
    4. Acute PN usually occurs in young women, who present with sudden onset of spiking fever, flank pain, chills, nausea and vomiting, and lower urinary tract signs of dysuria and increased frequency of urination.
    5. Complications of acute PN consist of chronic PN, perinephric abscess, pyonephrosis (pus in the renal pelvis), renal papillary necrosis, septicemia, and endotoxic shock.
    6. Urinalysis findings include pyuria (WBCs in the urine), bacteriuria (positive urine dipstick for nitrite), WBCs (positive urine dipstick for leukocyte esterase), WBC casts (key finding), and hematuria (positive urine dipstick for blood).
  E. **Chronic PN** is secondary to reflux (most common) or obstruction.
    1. The **reflux type** targets children under 5 years old and is associated with **VUR** due to an incompetent ureterovesical junction.
    2. **Obstructive disease** due to tumors, prostatic hyperplasia, or renal stones is associated with dilatation of the ureter and renal pelvis (hydronephrosis).
    3. The kidney in reflux disease is associated with U-shaped cortical scars overlying a blunt calyx that has been destroyed by inflammation and replaced by scar tissue.
    4. The obstructive type is associated with uniform dilatation of the calyces and diffuse thinning of the cortical tissue owing to **hydronephrosis**.
    5. Histologically, both types have a chronic inflammatory infiltrate, fibrosis, tubular atrophy (tubules contain eosinophilic material resembling thyroid tissue), and secondary scarring of the glomeruli.
  F. **Acute drug-induced interstitial nephritis** presents with abrupt onset of azotemia, oliguria, fever, eosinophilia, rash, mild to moderate proteinuria, hematuria, and eosinophiluria (eosinophils in the urine).
    1. Pathogenesis is attributed to cellular immunity related to the delayed type of T-cell hypersensitivity reaction or to cytotoxic T-cell injury.
    2. The most frequently implicated drugs include penicillin (particularly methicillin), rifampin, sulfonamides, NSAIDs, allopurinol, and diuretics (thiazides, furosemide).
    3. Withdrawal of the drug usually results in reversal of the disease.
  G. **Analgesic nephropathy** is a common cause of chronic drug-induced interstitial nephritis.
    1. The combination of **acetaminophen** (a metabolite of phenacetin) and **aspirin** in the setting of a patient (usually a woman) with chronic

headache or chronic pain is responsible for most cases.
2. Renal papillary necrosis, hypertension, accelerated atherosclerosis, renal pelvic and bladder transitional cell carcinomas (very high risk), and end-stage renal disease are potential complications.
3. A cumulative ingestion of ≥ 3 kg or daily consumption of ≥ 1 g/d for 3 or more years is sufficient to produce renal damage.
4. Acetaminophen causes cellular injury owing to the formation of acetaminophen free radicals, while aspirin inhibits prostaglandin synthesis, hence eliminating the vasodilator effects of prostaglandin and adding an element of ischemic injury (coagulation necrosis) in the renal medulla.
    a. Sloughing of the renal papillae (renal papillary necrosis) is associated with gross hematuria, proteinuria, and colicky flank pain.
    b. An intravenous pyelogram reveals a "ring defect" where one or more papillae used to reside.
    c. Other causes of renal papillary necrosis include diabetes mellitus, sickle cell trait or disease, acute pyelonephritis, and obstructive uropathy.
H. **Nephrocalcinosis** is the deposition of calcium in the tubular basement membranes secondary to metastatic calcification resulting from hypercalcemia (e.g., primary hyperparathyroidism) or hyperphosphatemia; it is associated with tubular dysfunction and subsequent progression to renal failure if left untreated.
I. **Urate nephropathy** is associated with the deposition of urate crystals in the tubules and interstitium owing to a massive release of purines (precursor of uric acid) resulting from aggressive treatment of disseminated cancer (e.g., leukemia).
J. **Chronic lead poisoning** is associated with interstitial nephritis, an increase in the reabsorption of uric acid (urate nephropathy), and nephrotoxic damage to the tubules.
K. **Multiple myeloma** produces renal insufficiency owing to toxic tubular injury from Bence Jones proteinuria ("**myeloma kidney**") or hypercalcemia, leading to nephrocalcinosis.

Objective 6: To outline the vascular disorders involving the kidneys.

XIII. Vascular disorders of the kidneys
A. The kidney disease of essential hypertension is called **benign nephrosclerosis** (BNS) and is primarily due to vascular changes located within the cortex of both kidneys.
1. The interlobar and arcuate arteries exhibit intimal fibrosis, reduplication of the internal elastic lamina, and smooth muscle hypertrophy with narrowing of the lumen, leading to ischemia.
2. The afferent arterioles reveal classic hyaline arteriolosclerosis, the small-vessel disease of hypertension.
3. The ischemic changes induced by these vascular changes lead to secondary atrophy of the

tubules in the renal cortex, interstitial fibrosis, and glomerular sclerosis.
4. The kidneys are symmetrically diminished in size owing to atrophy of the cortical surface (resembling the surface of a football), and V-shaped scars are noted secondary to cortical infarctions.
5. Laboratory manifestations include proteinuria, hematuria, and an increase in the serum BUN (azotemia) and serum creatinine.
6. BNS may progress to renal failure (it is the third most common cause of death in hypertension) and, in some cases, malignant hypertension.
B. **Malignant hypertension** most commonly arises from preexisting BNS.
1. It is also associated with hemolytic uremic syndrome, thrombotic thrombocytopenic purpura, and the kidney disease of progressive systemic sclerosis.
2. Patients present with diastolic pressures > 130 mm Hg, high plasma renin activity, papilledema, cerebral edema, headache, and visual impairment.
3. The kidneys are edematous and have petechial hemorrhages on the surface ("flea-bitten" appearance).
4. Histologic findings include hyperplastic arteriolosclerosis ("onion skinning"), fibrinoid necrosis in the wall of small and large vessels, necrotizing arteriolitis of the afferent arterioles (source of the "flea bitten" appearance), and segmental tuft necrosis of glomerular capillaries.
5. The most common cause of death is ARF, followed by intracerebral hemorrhage.
C. **Renal infarctions** (pale, wedge-shaped infarcts) are most commonly secondary to thromboembolization from the left heart (90%), embolization of vegetations or atherosclerotic plaque, vasculitis (e.g., polyarteritis nodosa), and sickle cell disease.
D. **Diffuse cortical necrosis**, a type of infarction limited to the renal cortex, most commonly occurs in pregnant women (70%) with preeclampsia, eclampsia, or abruptio placentae.
E. In **disseminated intravascular coagulation** (DIC), the renal glomerular capillaries are filled with fibrin/platelet clots.

Objective 7: To review the obstructive disorders of the urinary tract.

XIV. Obstructive disorders of the urinary tract
A. Urinary tract obstruction may be secondary to obstruction within the upper (renal tubules, renal pelvis, ureters) or lower urinary tract (urethra, prostate, bladder).
B. Obstruction is usually associated with **hydronephrosis**, which refers to dilatation of the renal pelvis, flattening of the calyces, and variable degrees of compression atrophy of the cortex and medulla.
C. Causes of hydronephrosis include congenital anomalies, calculi (most common cause in the ureters), cervical cancer (most common cause of death), benign prostatic hyperplasia, bladder cancer, and a gravid uterus.

D. Increased intratubular hydrostatic pressure initially drops the GFR and the medullary blood flow, and as tubular injury progresses, renal concentration and other tubular functions are compromised.

E. Incomplete obstruction presents with polyuria, while complete obstruction presents with anuria.

F. Complications include flank pain, palpable flank mass (common in children), hematuria (usually associated with stones), infection, hypertension, and ARF.

   1. Renal ultrasound is most useful for the initial evaluation of obstruction.

   2. Obstruction due to stones is evaluated with plain films of the kidneys, ureters, and bladder (KUB film) or intravenous pyelography.

G. **Nephrolithiasis** is three times more common in men than in women.

   1. The majority of stones are unilateral, and ~90% of stones are radiodense on KUB films.

   2. Factors predisposing to stones consist of the following:

      a. Low urine volume.

      b. Increased concentration of urinary solutes (e.g., calcium, uric acid, oxalates).

      c. Decreased urine citrate concentration (reduced chelation of the stone constituent or constituents by citrate).

      d. Hypercalciuria, which is the most common metabolic abnormality in calcium stone formers.

   3. Approximately 75% of stones contain calcium oxalate, either alone (35%) or in combination with hydroxyapatite or carbonate.

      a. Calcium phosphate stones are seen in children with recurrent infections or certain types of distal renal tubular acidosis.

      b. Excess oxalate may derive from certain foods (e.g., spinach, chocolate) or increased reabsorption from the small intestine in patients with Crohn's disease where malabsorption of bile salts and fatty acids nonselectively increases the mucosal absorption of oxalates.

   4. **Non–calcium-containing stones** include magnesium ammonium phosphate (struvite stones, which form staghorn calculus), uric acid, cystine, and xanthine.

      a. Uric acid and xanthine stones are radiolucent, struvite stones are radiolucent unless they contain calcium, and cystine stones may or may not be visualized with plain films.

      b. Staghorn calculi in the renal pelvis derive from recurrent urinary tract infections secondary to urease-producing organisms (e.g., *Proteus, Pseudomonas*).

   5. Stones present with an abrupt onset of severe, colicky pain in the flank radiating into the groin; they are associated with either microscopic or macroscopic hematuria.

   6. The first step in management of renal colic is urinalysis (UA), followed by a KUB abdominal film.

   7. Stone analysis by x-ray diffraction is mandatory (urine must be strained), since treatment is often tailored to the composition of the stone.

   8. Treatment for stones is increased water intake, hydrochlorothiazide for calcium stone formers (to increase calcium reabsorption), and dietary and urine pH modifications depending on the type of stone (e.g., uric acid stones precipitate at an acid pH, so the urine should be alkalinized).

Objective 8: To understand the benign nonneoplastic disorders of the lower urinary tract and male reproductive system.

XV. Benign disorders of the bladder

A. **Exstrophy** of the bladder is absence of the anterior part of the bladder and abdominal wall; there is an increased risk for adenocarcinoma.

B. **Diverticula** most commonly develop in elderly men with prostatic hyperplasia and obstruction.

C. **Malacoplakia** is associated with yellow-brown plaques on the mucosal surface.

   1. Histologic sections reveal numerous histiocytes within which are the pathognomonic **Michaelis-Gutmann bodies**, which are spheroidal structures composed of calcium phosphate.

   2. There is a defect in the bactericidal activity of monocytes and an association with *E. coli* infection.

D. **Acute cystitis** is most commonly secondary to bacterial infection, with *E. coli* accounting for 80–90% of cases.

   1. *Staphylococcus saprophyticus*, a coagulase-negative bacterium, is associated with 10–20% of cases in young, sexually active females.

   2. Other causes of cystitis include adenovirus infection (hemorrhagic cystitis), instrumentation, and cyclophosphamide therapy (hemorrhagic cystitis).

   3. Ascending infection from the urethra is the most common route of infection.

   4. Up to 1 year of age, boys with underlying urinary tract abnormalities (renal ultrasound examination should be performed) are most commonly affected, while after 1 year of age it is a female-dominant disease owing to the shorter urethra.

   5. Patients present with dysuria, increased frequency of urination, a sense of urgency, and discomfort over the bladder.

   6. Urinalysis findings include pyuria, hematuria, and positive dipstick reactions for nitrite and leukocyte esterase.

XVI. Benign disorders of the prostate

A. The prostate is subdivided into peripheral (70%), central (25%), and transitional zones.

   1. The **peripheral zone** is the part that is palpated on rectal examination and is the primary site for prostate cancer.

   2. The **central zone** contains the heaviest concentration of glands.

   3. The **transitional zone** enlarges in benign prostatic hyperplasia (BPH).

   4. **Dihydrotestosterone** (DHT) is the primary androgen responsible for stimulation of glands and stroma in the prostate.

   5. **Estrogen** inhibits prostatic growth by inhibiting the release of luteinizing hormone, which normally stimulates Leydig's cells to synthesize androgens.

B. **Acute prostatitis** is most commonly linked with infections of the urethra or bladder or is a complication of urethral catheterization; *E. coli* is the most common microbial pathogen (80%).

C. The majority of cases of **chronic prostatitis** are abacterial and present with pain and painful ejaculation.

D. **Prostatic infarcts** are most commonly secondary to vascular insufficiency in a previously enlarged gland or as a sequela of instrumentation.

E. **Benign prostatic hyperplasia** (BPH) is a normal age-dependent process.
   1. African Americans are more likely to develop symptomatic BPH than whites owing to higher levels of DHT.
   2. In concert with estrogen, which sensitizes the tissue to androgens, DHT induces the proliferation of glands and fibromuscular stroma, primarily in the transition zone of the prostate.
   3. There is diffuse or nodular enlargement of glandular tissue and stroma.
   4. It may be associated with periurethral obstruction, difficulty in initiating the urinary stream, incomplete emptying of the bladder, dribbling after urination, frequency, nocturia, and hematuria on occasion.
   5. It does not predispose to prostate cancer although prostate cancer commonly occurs in glands with BPH.
   6. Prostate-specific antigen (PSA) is increased in 25% of patients but is rarely > 10 ng/mL (normal, 0–4 ng/mL).

XVII. Other benign disorders of the male reproductive system
   A. **Varicoceles** are proliferations of venous channels within the spermatic cord, most commonly located on the left side, that are an important cause of male infertility.
   B. **Torsion of the testis** around the spermatic cord may result in a hemorrhagic infarction of the testis.
   C. A **hydrocele** is an accumulation of fluid in the tunica vaginalis of the scrotum; it is the most common cause of scrotal enlargement.
   D. A **spermatocele** is a cyst arising from the epididymis or testis that bulges into the tunica vaginalis; it contains spermatozoa.
   E. **Acute epididymitis** is usually sexually transmitted in patients < 35 years of age (*Neisseria gonorrhoeae, Chlamydia trachomatis, Ureaplasma urealyticum*), whereas in patients > 35 years, *E. coli* or *Pseudomonas aeruginosa* is usually implicated.
   F. **Tuberculous epididymitis** may occur from direct hematogenous spread from the lungs (most common) or by extension from renal TB, which is the most common extrapulmonary site for TB.
   G. **Cryptorchidism** is due to a combination of genetic, hormonal, neural, and mechanical factors.
   1. It is bilateral in 75% of children and unilateral in 80% of adults.
   2. The most common location is in the inguinal canal.
   3. Complete descent into the scrotum usually occurs during the first year of life.
   4. If left untreated, undescended testicles may undergo atrophy with the potential for infertility.
   5. There is also an increased risk for developing

a seminoma in untreated undescended testicles or in those which have been repositioned to the scrotum (by orchiopexy); the risk extends to the normal testis as well.

H. **Primary orchitis** may be associated with syphilis, mumps, or HIV.

I. **Phimosis** refers to inability to retract the prepuce over the glans; if not corrected, it may be associated with secondary bacterial infection of the glans (**balanitis**) or glans and prepuce (**balanoposthitis**).

J. **Hypospadias** is an opening of the urethra located on the ventral surface (most common congenital anomaly) of the penis, while in **epispadias** the opening is on the dorsal surface.

K. **Peyronie's disease** is fibromatosis involving Buck's fascia of the penis and the sheath of one or both corpora cavernosa.

L. **Urethral caruncles** are small, red, painful masses of granulation tissue that occur around the orifice or the external urethral meatus in females.

Objective 9: To outline the neoplastic disorders of the kidney, lower urinary tract, and male reproductive system.

XVIII. Neoplastic disorders of the kidneys
   A. **Angiomyolipomas** are mesenchymal tumors (hamartomas) that are associated with tuberous sclerosis in ~50% of cases.
   B. **Renal adenomas** and adenocarcinomas are tumors that occur in the renal cortex and derive from the proximal tubular cells.
   1. In the absence of metastasis, it may be impossible to histologically differentiate a benign from a malignant tumor.
   2. A general rule of thumb is that any tumor < 3 cm is considered benign (renal adenoma), while those > 3 cm are considered renal adenocarcinomas and are treated as malignant.
   C. **Renal adenocarcinomas** (Grawitz's tumor, hypernephroma) are the most common primary kidney cancer in adults.
   1. Males are two times more often affected than females, and the tumors usually occur during the sixth and seventh decades of life.
   2. Risk factors include smoking (most important), obesity, phenacetin analgesic abuse, Lindau–von Hippel disease (50–60% of cases; most are bilateral), acquired renal cystic disease, and adult polycystic kidney disease.
   3. They are solitary, > 3 cm well-circumscribed, yellow to tan tumors exhibiting hemorrhage, necrosis, and cyst formation; renal vein invasion is grossly present in 50% of patients.
   4. The tumors are composed of bland cells with a clear cytoplasm.
   5. The triad of hematuria (most consistent finding), pain, and a palpable mass occurs in < 10% of cases.
   6. Common sites of metastasis (often occurring after a long disease-free interval), in order of decreasing frequency, include the lungs, bone (lytic lesions), skin (it is one of the few cancers that metastasize to skin), liver, and brain.
   7. They can ectopically secrete parathormone-like peptide (hypercalcemia), erythropoietin

(polycythemia), renin (hypertension), gonadotropins (feminization or masculinization), or cortisol (ectopic Cushing's syndrome).

8. The average 5-year survival is 45%.

D. **Transitional cell carcinomas** account for ~90% of the tumors of the renal pelvis; risk factors are smoking, exposure to aromatic amines (e.g., 2-naphthylamine, benzidine), phenacetin (high risk), and cyclophosphamide.

E. **Squamous cell cancers** are frequently associated with calculi and chronic infections of the renal pelvis.

F. **Wilms' tumor (nephroblastoma)** is a common childhood cancer (second or third most common solid tumor) and the most common cancer (80%) involving the kidney.
1. The tumors derive from nephrogenic rests (mesonephric mesoderm).
2. Boys and girls are equally affected, and over 90% of cases are discovered in the first 4–5 years of life.
3. Patients present with a unilateral palpable mass in the abdomen, abdominal pain, hematuria, hypertension, and fever.
4. In 15–20% of cases, they are inherited as an AD trait with a deletion on chromosome 11.
5. There is an association with aniridia (congenital absence of the iris), cryptorchidism, hemihypertrophy of an extremity, and Beckwith-Wiedemann syndrome (omphalocele, macrosomia, and hypoglycemia).
6. They are large, well-demarcated gray-white tumors demonstrating hemorrhage, necrosis, and invasion of the renal vein in 50% of cases.
7. Microscopically, they are composed of small round cells (blastema) within a spindle cell stroma containing rhabdomyoblasts and primitive-appearing glomeruli.
8. They metastasize to the lungs, lymph nodes, liver, and bones.
9. The cure rate is 85% owing to new chemotherapy techniques, irradiation, and surgery.

XIX. Neoplastic disorders of the bladder
A. **Transitional cell carcinoma** is the most common primary cancer of the bladder (also the ureter and renal pelvis).
1. It is three times more common in men than in women and frequents people > 50 years of age.
2. Predisposing factors include smoking (most important risk factor), 2-naphthylamine (used in the dye industry), benzidine, phenacetin abuse, and cyclophosphamide.
3. They may be papillary (75–90%), which tend to be low-grade cancers that remain in situ, or flat, which are more likely to be high grade and invade the wall of the bladder.
4. Multifocality and recurrences are commonly observed.
5. Common metastatic sites are regional lymph nodes, liver, lung, and bones.
6. The most frequent clinical presentation is painless hematuria (70%).
7. The 5-year survival in papillary types of tumors is ~90%, dropping to 20–50% in solid tumors that infiltrate the muscle wall.

B. **Squamous cell carcinomas** most often compli-

cate *Schistosoma haematobium* infections involving the bladder wall.

C. **Embryonal rhabdomyosarcomas** (sarcoma botryoides) are the most common sarcoma in children and present as grape-like masses protruding from the urethra in males (primary lesion in the bladder).

XX. Neoplastic disorders of the male reproductive system
A. **Prostate adenocarcinoma** is the most common cancer in men and the second most common cause of death in men due to cancer.
1. It is an age-dependent cancer that is uncommon before age 40.
2. It is more common in African Americans than in whites, and detection has been increasing owing to the use of PSA and digital rectal examination (DRE) as annual screening procedures for males aged 50 years and older.
3. Testosterone and DHT are essential for tumor growth (castrated males do not develop cancer).
4. Risk factors include age (most important), African American ethnicity, and family history (twofold increase with an affected first-degree relative).
5. The majority are located in the peripheral zone of the prostate, which is amenable to DRE.
6. The tumors are multifocal, have a characteristic yellow-white appearance, and exhibit small glands infiltrating the stroma and around nerves on microscopic sections.
7. Metastatic spread is both lymphatic (first) and hematogenous (later), the former affecting the obturator and iliac nodes first, while the latter route is generally to bone, where the tumor produces an osteoblastic response (increased bone density and an elevated alkaline phosphatase).
8. The **Gleason grading system** correlates with tumor progression.
9. Early prostate cancer is asymptomatic and is discovered as an indurated area on DRE; transrectal ultrasound and needle biopsy of suspicious areas confirm the diagnosis of cancer in ~50% of cases detected by DRE.
10. Advanced prostate cancer may present with urinary obstruction and bone pain, usually in the lower lumbosacral vertebral column.
11. PSA is highly sensitive but not specific for prostate cancer owing to an increase in false positives from hyperplasia; it is also useful for staging prostate cancer, detecting recurrences, evaluating cancer volume, and monitoring response to therapy.
12. Treatment ranges from "watchful waiting" in stage I cancers to radical prostatectomy, irradiation, or hormone manipulation aimed at blocking the effect of androgens on tumor growth.

B. The **adenomatoid tumor** is the most common tumor of the epididymis; it is benign and derives from mesothelial cells.

C. Most **testicular tumors** are malignant and of **germ cell origin** (95%).
1. They are more common in whites than in African Americans, and in the age range of 20–35

years, they are the most common cancer in men.
2. Cryptorchidism is the most important risk factor.
3. They are subclassified as **seminomatous** or **nonseminomatous**.
4. Greater than 50% of germ cell tumors have more than one germ cell component.
5. **Seminomas** are the most frequent testicular cancers (35–45%) and occur from 30 to 50 years of age.
   a. They have the greatest association with cryptorchid testes.
   b. They contain a uniform population of large, clear cells with centrally located nuclei having prominent nucleoli and a characteristic lymphoid infiltrate.
   c. Approximately 10% of patients are positive for β-hCG because of trophoblastic tissue within the tumor.
   d. They spread by lymphatics to retroperitoneal, mediastinal, and supraclavicular lymph nodes and are highly radiosensitive.
   e. A much less common **spermatocytic variant** occurs in older men and pursues a benign course.
6. **Embryonal carcinomas** are usually mixed with other germ cell tumors (40%) and less commonly are pure cancers.
   a. They occur in a younger age group (20–30 years) than do seminomas.
   b. When combined with teratomas, they are called **teratocarcinomas**.
   c. Teratocarcinomas show an increase in both β-hCG and α-fetoprotein (AFP) in 90% of cases.
7. **Choriocarcinomas** are the most aggressive and lethal of the germ cell tumors; they secrete β-hCG.
8. **Yolk sac tumors** (endodermal sinus tumors) are the most common testicular tumors in infants and children under 4 years of age; they secrete AFP.
9. **Metastatic malignant lymphomas** are the most common testicular tumors in men over 50 years of age.
10. Most testicular cancers present as a painless enlargement of the testicle.
11. The majority of nonseminomatous germ cell tumors spread by both lymphatic and hematogenous routes (lungs and liver) and are not radiosensitive, hence their natural history is markedly different from that of seminomas.
12. Seminomas have an 80–95% cure rate, while nonseminomatous tumors are associated with a long-term remission in 50–90% of patients.
13. The most common non–germ cell tumors of the testis are Leydig cell tumors (which may cause precocious puberty by secreting androgens or produce feminization) and Sertoli cell tumors.

D. **Squamous cell carcinoma** is the most common cancer of the penis.
   1. Predisposing factors for squamous carcinoma of the penis are Bowen's disease (develops on the shaft of the penis), erythroplasia of Queyrat (red lesions that develop on the glans), and lack of circumcision.
   2. There is a link with human papillomaviruses types 16 and 18 in over two-thirds of cases.

Objective 10: To be conversant with causes of male hypogonadism and impotence.

XXI. Male hypogonadism
   A. Male hypogonadism refers to failure of the Leydig cells to produce testosterone, failure of seminiferous cells to generate sperm, or an abnormality in androgen receptors.
   B. **Primary hypogonadism** involves testicular problems in synthesizing testosterone in the Leydig cells (increased LH levels, decreased sperm count, normal FSH) or generating spermatozoa in the seminiferous tubules (increased FSH [decreased inhibin], low sperm count, normal LH and testosterone).
   C. **Secondary hypogonadism** refers to disorders in the pituitary or hypothalamic axis or to receptor deficiencies.
   D. Approximately 90% of male infertility is due to hypogonadism resulting in impaired spermatogenesis in the presence of normal production of testosterone (seminiferous tubule dysfunction).

XXII. Male impotence
   A. Male impotence is defined as persistent inability to obtain an erection during attempted sexual intercourse; it occurs in ~10–35% of adult men.
   B. It may be due to psychological problems, vascular disease (e.g., severe atherosclerosis), neurologic disease (e.g., autonomic neuropathy), drug effects (e.g., alcohol, methyldopa, psychotropics, cimetidine, spironolactone), and endocrine disease (e.g., hypothyroidism, hypopituitarism).
   C. **Testosterone deficiency** accounts for ~15–20% of cases.
   D. The most useful finding that excludes an organic cause of impotence is the presence of nocturnal penile tumescence (erections that normally occur during sleep).

QUESTIONS

DIRECTIONS. (Items 1–14): Each of the numbered items or incomplete statements in this section is followed by answers or by completions of the statement. Select the ONE lettered answer or completion that is BEST in each case. Correct answers and explanations are given at the end of the chapter.

1. The photomicrograph represents a finding in the urinary sediment (×100) from a normotensive 10-year-old boy with an upper respiratory infection and low-grade fever. His urinalysis is otherwise unremarkable including a dipstick test for protein. Which of the following best describes your evaluation of this patient?

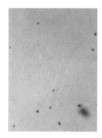

   (A) Minimal change disease
   (B) Urinary tract infection
   (C) Nephritic syndrome
   (D) Nephrotic syndrome
   (E) No follow-up necessary

2. The photomicrograph is from a urinary sediment (×200) in a 55-year-old man. His specific gravity is 1.010 on his first morning void and 1.010 in the late afternoon. The most likely disorder based on this limited information is

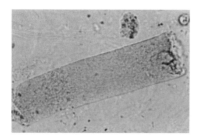

   (A) chronic renal failure
   (B) chronic prostatitis
   (C) benign prostatic hyperplasia
   (D) acute tubular necrosis
   (E) acute interstitial nephritis

3. The photomicrograph is of a urinary sediment finding (×200) in a 10-year-old boy who recovered from impetigo 3 weeks ago. He now presents with hypertension, periorbital edema, and oliguria. His urinalysis reveals a specific gravity > 1.020, an acid pH, a 2+ protein (sulfosalicylic acid method 2+), a positive dipstick test for blood, and negative dipstick results for nitrites and leukocyte esterase. You would expect ultrastructural examination of the glomeruli in this patient to reveal

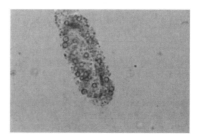

   (A) intramembranous electron-dense deposits
   (B) fusion of the podocytes
   (C) subendothelial electron-dense deposits
   (D) subepithelial electron-dense deposits
   (E) absence of electron-dense deposits

4. The photomicrograph is of a urinary sediment finding (×200) in a 25-year-old man with a history of sudden onset of colicky right flank pain with radiation to the right groin. His work is located outdoors, and he has been working in a hot environment for the past week. Urinalysis reveals an acid pH, 1+ protein, and a 4+ dipstick result for blood, while the remaining dipstick parameters are all negative. You strongly suspect the patient has

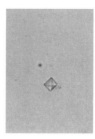

   (A) a struvite renal stone
   (B) a uric acid stone
   (C) hemorrhagic cystitis
   (D) a calcium oxalate stone
   (E) nephrotoxic acute tubular necrosis

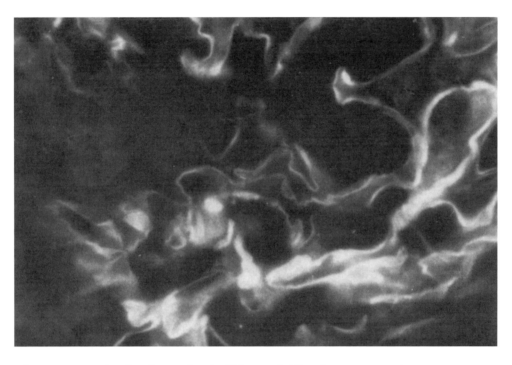

5. This immunofluorescent study of a glomerulus (×300) is from a renal biopsy performed on a 26-year-old man with a serum blood urea nitrogen of 80 mg/dL (normal, 7–18 mg/dL) and a serum creatinine of 8 mg/dL (normal, 0.6–1.2 mg/dL). His urinalysis on admission to the hospital revealed a 2+ dipstick protein (sulfosalicylic acid method 2+), 3+ dipstick result for blood, and negative nitrite and esterase results. The sediment examination exhibited RBCs and RBC casts. On the basis of this limited information, you would expect the H and E biopsy specimen to reveal

(A) focal segmental glomerulosclerosis
(B) diffuse proliferative glomerulonephritis
(C) diffuse membranous glomerulonephritis
(D) diffuse membranoproliferative glomerulonephritis
(E) rapidly progressive crescentic glomerulonephritis

6. The photomicrograph is representative of the majority of glomeruli (×300) in a renal biopsy performed on a 58-year-old man with a non-Hodgkin's malignant lymphoma. He has generalized pitting edema and hypertension, and urinalysis revealed a 4+ dipstick protein (sulfosalicylic acid method 4+) and a sediment with refractile casts that demonstrate Maltese crosses on polarization. On the basis of these findings, which of the following glomerular abnormalities would you expect?

(A) Linear immunofluorescence pattern - Good pastures
(B) Double-contoured glomerular basement membranes Membranoproliferative
(C) Epimembranous "spikes" - subepithelium
(D) Subendothelial electron-dense deposits - SLE
(E) "Wire-looping" in the glomerular capillaries SLE

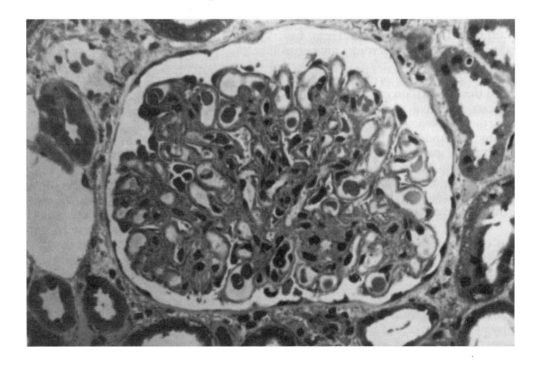

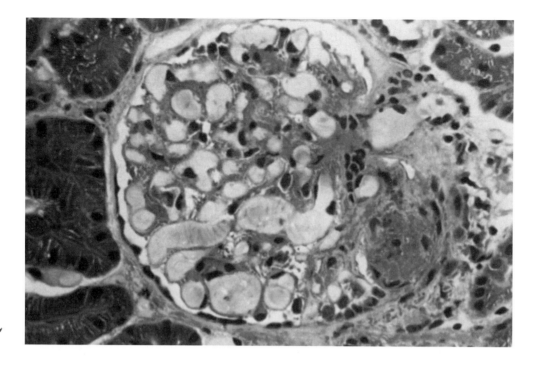

7. The photomicrograph is representative of 30% of the glomeruli (×300) in a renal biopsy specimen from a hypertensive 28-year-old man in chronic renal failure. His 24-hour urine for protein was 8.2 g. Immunofluorescence studies revealed no distinctive pattern, and electron micrograph studies were negative for electron-dense deposits. On the basis of this limited history, you expect the patient to have which of the following clinical profiles?

(A) History of a positive ELISA for HIV antibody
(B) Past history of Henoch-Schönlein purpura
(C) Five-year history of type I diabetes mellitus

(D) Family history of glomerulonephritis and nerve deafness
(E) History of chronic hepatitis C infection

— Membranoproliferative glomerulonephritis

8. The ultrastructural findings in this photograph of a glomerulus (×6000) would most likely be expected in a patient with

(A) Kimmelstiel-Wilson syndrome
(B) diffuse membranous glomerulonephritis
(C) Goodpasture's syndrome
(D) minimal change disease
(E) type IV lupus glomerulonephritis

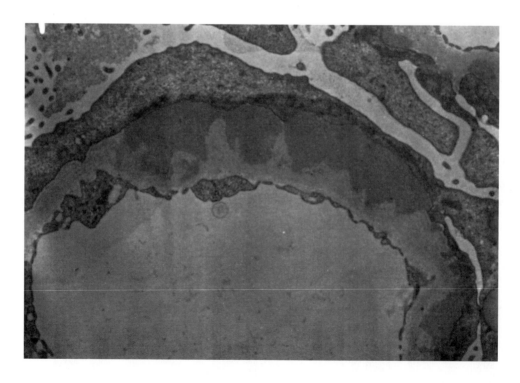

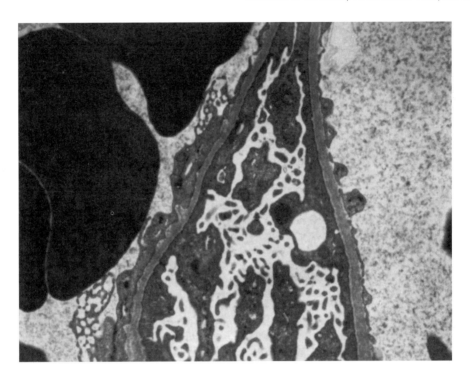

9. The ultrastructural findings in this glomerulus are most consistent with which of the following histologic or laboratory abnormalities?

(A) Normal-appearing glomeruli with routine stains
(B) Crescent formation in Bowman's capsule
(C) C3 nephritic factor in the serum
(D) Low C3 complement levels in the serum
(E) Positive ASO titer in the serum

10. A patient who is taking hydrochlorothiazide abruptly develops fever, rash, and oliguria. Additional studies reveal an increase in the serum BUN and creatinine, eosinophilia, and a urinalysis with positive dipstick tests for protein (2+) and blood (2+). No casts are present. The mechanism for this patient's disease is most closely related to

(A) immunocomplex deposition in the glomeruli
(B) a type I IgE-mediated hypersensitivity reaction
(C) obstructive uropathy
(D) a type IV cellular immune reaction
(E) antiglomerular basement membrane antibodies

11. A 52-year-old man with congestive heart failure develops oliguria. He takes an angiotensin converting enzyme inhibitor. His random urine sodium is 10 mEq/L, urine osmolality is 600 mOsm/kg, and fractional excretion of sodium (FENa) is 0.6, and the urinalysis contains a few hyaline casts. The serum blood urea nitrogen is 60 mg/dL (normal, 7–18 mg/dL), and the serum creatinine is 2 mg/dL (normal, 0.6–1.2 mg/dL). The mechanism for this patient's oliguria is most closely related to

(A) ischemic acute tubular necrosis
(B) nephrotoxic acute tubular necrosis
(C) prerenal reduction in the glomerular filtration rate
(D) acute primary glomerular disease
(E) acute drug-induced interstitial nephritis

12. Which of the following disorders is most frequently associated with obstruction to urine flow at an early stage in its development?

(A) Prostate cancer
(B) Renal adenocarcinoma
(C) Benign prostatic hyperplasia
(D) Carcinoma of the penis
(E) Transitional cell carcinoma of the bladder

13. In chronic renal failure, you would expect
(A) low parathormone levels
(B) macrocytic anemia
(C) hypercalcemia
(D) urine osmolality >500 mOsm/kg
(E) low arterial pH and low bicarbonate level

	Patient A	Patient B	Patient C	Patient D	Patient E
Protein	+1	+4	+2	+2	+2
Glucose	Negative	Negative	Negative	Negative	Negative
Blood	Positive	Negative	Positive	Negative	Positive
Nitrite	Positive	Negative	Negative	Negative	Positive
Esterase	Positive	Negative	Negative	Negative	Positive
Crystals	None	Negative	Negative	Calcium oxalate	Negative
Casts	WBC casts	Fatty casts	RBC casts	Renal tubular cells	None
Cells/bacteria	WBCs, RBCs, bacteria	Oval fat bodies	Dysmorphic RBCs	Renal tubular cells	WBCs, RBCs, bacteria

14. Which interpretation of the urine profiles listed above is correct?

   (A) Patient A most likely ingested ethylene glycol and progressed to renal failure.
   (B) Patient B most likely has Kimmelstiel-Wilson syndrome.
   (C) Patient C most likely has a lower urinary tract infection.
   (D) Patient D most likely has a nephritic type of glomerular disease.
   (E) Patient E most likely has an upper urinary tract infection.

   Directions. (Items 15–17): Each set of matching questions in this section consists of a list of lettered options followed by several numbered items. For each numbered item, select the ONE option that is most closely associated with it. Each lettered option may be selected once, more than once, or not at all.

   (A) Varicocele
   (B) Hydrocele
   (C) Malacoplakia
   (D) Epididymitis
   (E) Renal dysplasia
   (F) Adult polycystic kidney disease
   (G) Prostate adenocarcinoma
   (H) Squamous cancer of penis
   (I) Squamous cancer of bladder
   (J) Transitional carcinoma of bladder
   (K) Seminoma
   (L) Embryonal carcinoma
   (M) Teratocarcinoma
   (N) Yolk sac tumor
   (O) Choriocarcinoma
   (P) Malignant lymphoma
   (Q) Renal adenocarcinoma
   (R) Wilms' tumor

15. Painless enlargement of the testicle in a 35-year-old man.

16. Metastatic disease in the lung and bilateral gynecomastia in a 35-year-old man with a normal renal ultrasound examination.

17. Hypertension in a 5-year-old boy with aniridia and a unilateral abdominal mass.

ANSWERS AND EXPLANATIONS

1. The answer is E: no follow-up necessary. The sediment finding is a typical hyaline cast with smooth contours and no cellular material. These casts are commonly found in patients with fever. Since no other urine abnormalities are present, the potential for glomerular disease is highly unlikely, especially without proteinuria. (Photomicrograph reproduced, with permission, from J.B. Henry. *Clinical Diagnosis and Management by Laboratory Methods,* 19th ed. Philadelphia, W.B. Saunders Co., 1996.)

2. The answer is A: chronic renal failure. The sediment exhibits a waxy cast with sharp, refractile borders. These casts are commonly present in chronic renal failure secondary to end-stage diabetic nephropathy, hypertensive nephropathy, or glomerulonephritis. They are the final breakdown product of a cellular cast (renal tubular, WBC) and require at least 3 months to develop in the tubules, hence their association with chronic disease. Casts are not a feature of chronic prostatitis or BPH, which are not intrinsic renal diseases, nor would they be expected in acute tubular necrosis (renal tubular casts) or acute interstitial nephritis (WBC cast). (Photomicrograph reproduced, with permission, from

J.B. Henry. *Clinical Diagnosis and Management by Laboratory Methods,* 19th ed. Philadelphia, W.B. Saunders Co., 1996.)

3. The answer is D: subepithelial electron-dense deposits. The sediment finding is an RBC cast, which, although the photograph is black and white, can be deduced by the positive dipstick test for blood and the classic history of a group A streptococcal infection (impetigo) followed by a nephritic pattern of glomerular disease. The patient most likely has poststreptococcal GN, which characteristically exhibits subepithelial "humps" representing either in situ or circulating immunocomplexes of antibody and bacterial antigens. Intramembranous electron-dense deposits are noted in type II membranoproliferative GN and fusion of the podocytes in the nephrotic syndrome, and subendothelial electron-dense deposits in SLE type IV disease or type I membranoproliferative GN. (Photomicrograph reproduced, with permission, from J.B. Henry. *Clinical Diagnosis and Management by Laboratory Methods,* 19th ed. Philadelphia, W.B. Saunders Co., 1996.)

4. The answer is D: a calcium oxalate stone. The sediment finding is a calcium oxalate crystal, which looks like the

back of an envelope, hence the patient most likely has a stone composed of the same material. Inadequate intake of water while working outdoors was instrumental in producing the stone. A struvite renal stone (magnesium ammonium phosphate) develops in an alkaline urine owing to chronic infection by urease producers that split ammonium from urea (e.g., *Proteus*). Uric acid stones are uncommon, and the crystal does not have a fan-shaped appearance. Hemorrhagic cystitis is not associated with colicky pain, which is characteristic of ureteral obstruction. Nephrotoxic acute tubular necrosis, presumably from myoglobinuria induced by working outdoors, would not present with colicky pain, and renal tubular casts would be present in the sediment. (Photomicrograph reproduced, with permission, from J.B. Henry. *Clinical Diagnosis and Management by Laboratory Methods,* 19th ed. Philadelphia, W.B. Saunders Co., 1996.)

5. The answer is E: rapidly progressive crescentic glomerulonephritis. The immunofluorescent pattern is linear, indicating the presence of anti-GBM antibodies and the likelihood of Goodpasture's syndrome. The patient has renal failure owing to retention of the 10/1 BUN/creatinine ratio, and the urinalysis findings are compatible with a nephritic syndrome. Rapidly progressive crescentic glomerulonephritis is the usual terminal renal event in patients with Goodpasture's syndrome and the most common cause of renal failure due to glomerular disease. Focal segmental glomerulosclerosis, diffuse membranous GN, and diffuse membranoproliferative GN most commonly present with a nephrotic syndrome and a granular IF pattern. Diffuse proliferative glomerulonephritis would most likely have a granular pattern and a history compatible with postinfectious GN or SLE. (Photograph reproduced, with permission, from L.J. Striker, J.L. Olson, and G.L. Striker. *The Renal Biopsy,* 2nd ed. Philadelphia, W.B. Saunders Co., 1990, p. 27.)

6. The answer is C: epimembranous "spikes." The biopsy reveals thickening of the GBM without an increase in cellularity, and the urinalysis findings are consistent with the nephrotic syndrome (4+ protein, fatty casts with Maltese crosses), hence diffuse membranous GN secondary to malignant lymphoma is the most likely diagnosis. Membranous GN is associated with subepithelial deposits that produce "spikes" best visualized with silver stains. A granular IF pattern would be expected owing to the deposition of immunocomplexes. Double-contoured GBMs are associated with type I membranoproliferative GN, and "wire-looping" in the glomerular capillaries is noted in SLE-associated GN with subendothelial deposits. (Photomicrograph reproduced, with permission, from L.J. Striker, J.L. Olson, and G.L. Striker. *The Renal Biopsy,* 2nd ed. Philadelphia, W.B. Saunders Co., 1990, p. 58.)

7. The answer is A: history of a positive ELISA for HIV antibody. The patient has focal segmental glomerulosclerosis (sclerosis at 5 o'clock), which is the renal disease associated with HIV, intravenous drug abuse, and renal transplantation. It produces the nephrotic syndrome (patient has a 24-hour protein >3.5 g/24 h), is associated with hypertension, and rapidly progresses to chronic renal failure. There is no characteristic IF pattern or dense deposit on ultrastructural examination. An IgA type of GN may be associated with a past history of Henoch-Schönlein purpura. Diabetic glomerulosclerosis often produces a nephrotic syndrome; however, the time frame is too short. Alport's syndrome is a hereditary glomerulonephritis characterized by nerve

deafness and ocular abnormalities. It does not have a focal segmental pattern. A history of chronic hepatitis C infection would most likely be associated with type I membranoproliferative GN. (Photograph reproduced, with permission, from L.J. Striker, J.L. Olson, and G.L. Striker. *The Renal Biopsy,* 2nd ed. Philadelphia, W.B. Saunders Co., 1990, p. 121.)

8. The answer is B: diffuse membranous glomerulonephritis. The electron-dense deposits are in a subepithelial location, which, of the choices given, is most characteristic of diffuse membranous GN. Kimmelstiel-Wilson syndrome is diabetic glomerulosclerosis (no deposits), Goodpasture's syndrome is not associated with deposits (anti-GBM antibodies), minimal change disease does not have deposits, and type IV lupus glomerulonephritis has subendothelial deposits. (Photomicrograph reproduced, with permission, from L.J. Striker, J.L. Olson, and G.L. Striker. *The Renal Biopsy,* 2nd ed. Philadelphia, W.B. Saunders Co., 1990, p. 61.)

9. The answer is A: normal-appearing glomeruli with routine stains. The glomerulus exhibits extensive fusion of the podocytes (center of the photograph). The epithelial cells form a continuous sheet of cytoplasm. No electron-dense deposits are in the GBM. These findings are most consistent with minimal change disease, which is not associated with histologic changes in the glomeruli or immunocomplex formation. Fusion of the podocytes is noted in glomerular diseases associated with the nephrotic syndrome. Crescent formation in Bowman's capsule is associated with diseases that present with a nephritic type of syndrome. The C3 nephritic factor is an autoantibody against C3 convertase in the alternative complement pathway and is a feature of type II membranoproliferative GN, which has intramembranous dense deposits. A low C3 is associated with immunocomplex diseases that activate the alternative (e.g., poststreptococcal GN, type II membranoproliferative GN) or classical pathway (type IV lupus GN). A positive ASO titer is associated with poststreptococcal GN, which has subepithelial deposits and presents as a nephritic syndrome. (Photograph reproduced, with permission, from L.J. Striker, J.L. Olson, and G.L. Striker. *The Renal Biopsy,* 2nd ed. Philadelphia, W.B. Saunders Co., 1990, p. 47.)

10. The answer is D: a type IV cellular immune reaction. The abrupt onset of fever, rash, oliguria, azotemia, eosinophilia, proteinuria, and hematuria in a patient taking a drug is most likely a drug-induced acute interstitial nephritis. Thiazides are one of the more common causes of this reaction. Delayed-reaction hypersensitivity and cytotoxic T-cell destruction have been implicated in the pathogenesis of the interstitial reaction, which simulates acute tubular necrosis. Withdrawal of the drug reverses the disease. The other choices do not have this causal relationship of signs and symptoms developing abruptly after starting a drug.

11. The answer is C: prerenal reduction in the glomerular filtration rate. The oliguria workup reveals preservation of tubular function (Uosm > 500 mOsm/kg, UNa < 40 mEq/L, FENa < 1) and a few hyaline casts. The BUN/creatinine ratio is 30/1 (60/2), indicating a disproportionate increase in urea reabsorption in the proximal tubule owing to a decrease in the GFR. All findings are consistent with prerenal azotemia from congestive heart failure (decreased cardiac output leading to decreased GFR). Left untreated, this patient would likely progress to ischemic ATN with evidence of tubular dysfunction (Uosm < 350 mOsm/kg, UNa > 40 mEq/L, FENa

>1, and renal tubular casts). Nephrotoxic ATN and acute drug-induced interstitial nephritis would exhibit tubular dysfunction in the laboratory data. An acute primary glomerular disease would show preservation of tubular function; however, the urine sediment would contain abnormal casts (e.g., RBC casts, fatty casts) depending on the type of syndrome (nephritic or nephrotic).

12. The answer is C: benign prostatic hyperplasia. BPH develops in the transitional area of the prostate, hence affecting the periurethral tissue at an early stage with subsequent alterations in urine flow (e.g., in initiating the stream, dribbling, retaining urine). Prostate cancer, carcinoma of the penis, and transitional cell carcinoma of the bladder are associated with obstructive signs late in their natural history. Renal adenocarcinoma is not associated with obstruction and most commonly presents with hematuria.

13. The answer is E: low arterial pH and low bicarbonate level. In chronic renal failure, the kidney cannot excrete organic acids, hence an increased anion gap metabolic acidosis is commonly present (low arterial pH and low bicarbonate). Owing to a loss of 1α-hydroxylase, the second hydroxylation for vitamin D is disrupted, leading to hypovitaminosis D and hypocalcemia. Hypocalcemia is a stimulus for secondary hyperparathyroidism. Erythropoietin is also decreased, which produces a normocytic anemia. Tubular function is destroyed, and urine cannot be concentrated or diluted (fixed specific gravity), hence the urine osmolality would be < 350 mOsm/kg.

14. The answer is B: patient B most likely has Kimmelstiel-Wilson syndrome. Patients with Kimmelstiel-Wilson syndrome, or diabetic glomerulosclerosis, commonly have the nephrotic syndrome. Note that patient B has a 4+ protein and fatty casts in the urine, which are characteristic of the nephrotic syndrome. Patient A has acute pyelonephritis, an upper urinary tract infection, owing to the presence of WBC casts. Patient C has a nephritic pattern of glomerulonephritis with RBC casts. Patient D has acute tubular necrosis (renal tubular casts) and would most likely have ingested ethylene glycol (which produces calcium oxalate crystals) and progressed to renal failure. Patient E has the classic findings of a lower urinary tract infection.

15. The answer is K: seminoma. Painless enlargement of the testicle is cancer until proved otherwise. In a 35-year-old man, it would most likely represent a seminoma, the most common overall testicular cancer and the most common type in his particular age bracket.

16. The answer is O: choriocarcinoma. Choriocarcinoma of the testicle secretes β-hCG, which is an LH analogue that can produce gynecomastia. Choriocarcinoma is the most aggressive testicular cancer and commonly metastasizes to the lungs. A renal adenocarcinoma can secrete gonadotropins; however, the patient's renal ultrasound examination is normal.

17. The answer is R: Wilms' tumor. Wilms' tumor may be associated with other congenital abnormalities including aniridia (absence of the iris). It produces hypertension by secreting renin and presents as a palpable abdominal mass. Renal dysplasia may also produce hypertension and a unilateral mass, but it is not associated with aniridia.

CHAPTER EIGHTEEN

DISORDERS OF THE

FEMALE REPRODUCTIVE

TRACT AND BREAST

SYNOPSIS

OBJECTIVES

1. To differentiate the different types of sexually transmitted diseases.
2. To be familiar with the nonneoplastic disorders of the vulva, vagina, cervix, uterus, fallopian tubes, ovaries, and placenta.
3. To discuss the neoplastic disorders of the vulva, vagina, cervix, uterus, ovaries, and placenta.
4. To understand hormone-related disorders associated with the uterus.
5. To be conversant with the workup of hirsutism and virilization.
6. To be familiar with the nonneoplastic and neoplastic disorders of the female breast.

Objective 1: To differentiate the different types of sexually transmitted diseases.

I. See Table 18–1.

Objective 2: To be familiar with the nonneoplastic disorders of the vulva, vagina, cervix, uterus, fallopian tubes, ovaries, and placenta.

II. Nonneoplastic disorders of the vulva
   A. Vulvar dermatoses commonly present as **leukoplakia** (white, parchment-like patch) on the labia in postmenopausal women.
   B. **Lichen sclerosus** shows thinning of the squamous epithelium (atrophy) overlying a broad band of hypocellular collagenous tissue in the dermis.
   C. **Squamous hyperplasia** (**lichen simplex chronicus**) has a thickened epithelium, which, when atypical, may progress to dysplasia and squamous cell cancer.

III. Nonneoplastic disorders of the vagina
   A. A **Gartner duct cyst** is of wolffian (mesonephric) duct origin and is located along the anterolateral aspect of the vulva or lateral wall of the vagina.
   B. **Vaginal adenosis** is the most common manifesta-

tion of maternal exposure to **diethylstilbestrol** (DES).
   1. DES inhibits müllerian differentiation.
   2. It is the precursor lesion for **clear cell adenocarcinoma** (0.14% risk).

IV. Nonneoplastic disorders of the cervix
   A. A **cervical Pap** (i.e., Papanicolaou) **test** must contain endocervical cells, since the transformation zone between the cervix and endocervix is the primary site for cervical dysplasia and cancer.
      1. **Superficial squamous cells** (SSCs) in the vagina and cervix mature with estrogen stimulation and **intermediate squamous cells** (ISCs) with progesterone.
      2. Unstimulated squamous cells are called **parabasal cells** (PBCs).
      3. In a 100-cell count (called a **maturation index**), a normal adult female has 70% SSCs, 30% ISCs, and no PBCs.
      4. A predominance of SSCs represents excessive exposure to estrogen (e.g., from unopposed estrogen therapy, ovarian tumor), while a predominance of PBCs represents atrophy.
   B. **Endocervical polyps** are the most common nonneoplastic cervical growth and cause of postcoital bleeding.
   C. **Acute** and **chronic cervicitis** are present in most adult women and frequently cause cervical discharge (leukorrhea).
   D. Squamous metaplasia may block the opening of endocervical glands resulting in the formation of **nabothian cysts** (large, dilated endocervical glands filled with inspissated mucus).
   E. **Microglandular hyperplasia** may occur in women taking birth control pills.

V. Nonneoplastic disorders of the uterus
   A. **Chronic endometritis** (due to *Chlamydia trachomatis*, *Neisseria gonorrhoeae*, *Actinomyces israelii* [from use of intrauterine devices]) is characterized by the presence of **plasma cells** in the stroma (plasma cells are not normally in the endometrial mucosa).

TABLE 18–1. Sexually Transmitted Diseases (STDs)

Organism	Epidemiology and Clinical Findings	Laboratory Diagnosis and Treatment
Herpesvirus type 2	**Genital herpes** is most commonly due to herpes simplex virus type 2 (HSV-2; 70–80%) and is transmitted by sexual contact. Primary infection due to HSV-2 is associated with systemic signs and symptoms and painful vesicles that ulcerate. In the male, vesicles are located on the penis; in the female, lesions are on the labia, vulva, and cervix (erosive cervicitis with discharge). Herpes proctitis is noted in those practicing anal intercourse. Vesicles heal within 3 weeks and may recur every 4–6 weeks without systemic signs or symptoms.	Scrapings at the base of the vesicles (Tzanck preparation) reveal multinucleated squamous cells with intranuclear inclusions. Acyclovir decreases the frequency of recurrences. In pregnancy, viral shedding may occur without visible lesions. In the presence of viral shedding, babies must be delivered by cesarean section.
Human papillomavirus	**Human papillomavirus** (HPV) types 6 and 11 are associated with condyloma acuminatum (venereal warts) located in moist areas in the anogenital region and on the cervix. They have a fern-like appearance and may be confused with condyloma latum of secondary syphilis. HPV types 16 (most common), 18, and 31 are associated with cervical, vulvar, vaginal, and anal squamous cell carcinoma (in homosexual males).	Histologic sections reveal koilocytic change in squamous epithelium characterized by wrinkled pyknotic nuclei surrounded by a halo. Topical podophyllin is the treatment of choice.
Chlamydia trachomatis	*Chlamydia trachomatis* is responsible for genitourinary disease in both males and females. It is the most common cause of STD. Chlamydial and gonococcal infections frequently coexist. In males, it is responsible for 50% of nonspecific urethritis (NSU). The incubation period is 2–3 weeks following sexual exposure. Patients present with dysuria (painful urination) and a thin, watery exudate containing numerous neutrophils without bacteria on gram staining. *Chlamydia* also causes epididymitis in men <35 years of age. Chlamydial urethritis in women is a common cause of the acute urethral syndrome. Mucopurulent cervicitis is most commonly due to *Chlamydia* often coexisting with gonorrhea. Cervical involvement is the source of conjunctivitis in newborns (most common cause of ophthalmia neonatorum). Approximately 50% of pelvic inflammatory disease (PID) is due to *Chlamydia* (see Gonorrhea).	Doxycycline is the treatment of choice of NSU. Erythromycin eye drops have reduced ophthalmia neonatorum, which usually occurs after 1 week. In a cervical Pap test, the presence of *Chlamydia* is suggested by red inclusions in endocervical cells.
Lymphogranuloma venereum	**Lymphogranuloma venereum** (LGV; *Chlamydia trachomatis* subspecies) is characterized by the development of tiny papules in the genital region associated with reactive lymphadenitis. Fibrous stricture formation may block lymphatics, producing localized lymphedema of the scrotum or vulva. Women may have strictures around the rectum.	A fluctuant lymph node should be aspirated and cultured. Lymph nodes exhibit granulomatous microabscesses with multiple draining sinuses. Treatment is with doxycycline.
Neisseria gonorrhoeae	**Gonorrhea** is due to the gram-negative diplococcus *Neisseria gonorrhoeae*. Women are more likely to be asymptomatic carriers than men; however, men are more likely to transmit the disease to women after each sexual exposure. Chromosomal mutations and β-lactamase production (plasmid-mediated) are responsible for drug resistance. Gonococcal urethritis is the most common presentation in men. It presents with a creamy, purulent penile exudate within 2–5 days of exposure. Gonorrhea may result in stricture, epididymitis, proctitis (in male homosexuals), and prostatitis. In women, gonorrhea primarily infects glandular epithelium rather than squamous epithelium (estrogen is protective), except in the prepubescent female, where it may produce vulvovaginitis. Other infections include urethritis (dysuria), cervicitis (most common site; cervical discharge), Bartholin's gland abscess (most common cause of an abscess), and PID (see below). Complications include sterility, ectopic pregnancy from tubal scarring (most common cause), and disseminated gonococcemia (dermatitis, tenosynovitis, septic arthritis). Birth control pills protect against gonorrhea but not *Chlamydia*. PID occurs in 10–15% of untreated women with gonorrhea. It most often occurs during or shortly after menses. Other pathogens include *Chlamydia* and mixed aerobes and anaerobes (*Bacteroides*). Patients present with lower abdominal pain, adnexal tenderness on movement of the cervix, fever, and an elevated neutrophil count. Pus may collect under the diaphragm and on top of the liver, producing perihepatitis (Fitz-Hugh–Curtis syndrome) with adhesions. Other gonococcal infections include pharyngitis (result of fellatio), proctitis (from anal intercourse), and ophthalmia neonatorum (bilateral conjunctivitis in the first week).	Gram staining of urethral exudate is performed in men and endocervical smear in women. Thayer-Martin medium is used for culture. Urethral or endocervical gonorrhea is treated with doxycycline. PID is treated with ceftriaxone (for gonorrhea) and doxycycline (for *Chlamydia*). Spectinomycin is reserved for treatment failures.

TABLE 18–1. Sexually Transmitted Diseases (STDs) *Continued*

Organism	Epidemiology and Clinical Findings	Laboratory Diagnosis and Treatment
Haemophilus ducreyi	**Chancroid** is caused by the gram-negative rod *Haemophilus ducreyi*. It is characterized by painful (whereas the syphilis chancre is painless) genital and perianal ulcers with suppurative inguinal nodes.	A smear and/or biopsy specimen is obtained from the edge of the ulcer or a fluctuant lymph node is aspirated. Gram staining shows the classic "school of fish" orientation of the bacteria. Culture. Treat with ceftriaxone.
Calymmatobacterium granulomatis (Donovan's bacillus)	**Granuloma inguinale** is caused by *Calymmatobacterium granulomatis* (Donovan's bacillus), which is a gram-negative coccobacillus. The organism is encapsulated and is phagocytized by macrophages (Donovan's bodies). The disease is characterized by a creeping, raised sore that heals by scarring.	Scrapings or smears are stained to demonstrate the intracellular Donovan's bodies. Treatment is with tetracycline or sulfisoxazole.
Gardnerella vaginalis	**Bacterial vaginosis** is caused by the gram negative rod *Gardnerella vaginalis*. It is often associated with other anaerobes such as *Mobiluncus* and some *Bacteroides* species. It does not produce an inflammatory exudate (no neutrophils or erythema) and is commonly noted when the vaginal pH is between 5 and 5.5 owing to a reduction in lactobacilli.	*Gardnerella* adheres to the surface of squamous cells, producing characteristic "clue cells." Potassium hydroxide produces a fishy, amine-like odor when added to vaginal material containing the organism. It is treated with metronidazole.
Treponema pallidum	**Syphilis** is caused by *Treponema pallidum*. It is primarily contracted by sexual contact. The organism produces a vasculitis called endarteritis obliterans, which produces localized ischemic necrosis of tissue. The disease has primary, secondary, latent, and tertiary stages. Primary syphilis is characterized by a solitary, painless, indurated chancre (3–4 weeks after exposure), most commonly located on the shaft of the penis in a male or the labia of a female. The chancre persists for 1–5 weeks and spontaneously resolves. Secondary syphilis occurs 6 weeks to 6 months later. It is the most contagious stage. Characteristic findings include (1) diffuse maculopapular rash frequently involving the palms and soles, (2) generalized lymphadenopathy, and (3) condyloma latum, which are raised lesions located around moist areas of the anogenital region. Less common complications include pericholangitis, meningitis, and the nephrotic syndrome. The lesions heal in 4–12 weeks, and the disease may enter the latent phase. Latent syphilis, usually asymptomatic, is associated with positive serology. It is considered noninfective when the duration is >4 years except in pregnancy, where the disease can be transmitted to the fetus. Overall, approximately one-third of patients left untreated will enter the tertiary phase. This phase is associated with cardiovascular disease (most common; Chapter 10), CNS disease (Chapter 22), and locally destructive disease due to gummas. Congenital syphilis is discussed in Chapter 7.	Laboratory diagnosis includes darkfield microscopy (gold standard for primary and secondary syphilis) and serologic tests that measure nonspecific and specific treponemal antibodies. The nonspecific antibodies react with cardiolipin antigens from beef heart, which is the basis for the RPR (rapid plasma reagin) and VDRL (Venereal Disease Research Laboratory) tests. These tests have a sensitivity of 75% in primary syphilis, 99% in secondary syphilis, 70% in latent syphilis, and ~50% in tertiary syphilis. False positives may occur in SLE owing to the presence of anticardiolipin antibodies. False negatives occur in secondary syphilis owing to antibody excess (prozone), hence the need to dilute the serum until an agglutination reaction occurs. RPR/VDRL become nonreactive after 1 year in primary syphilis, 2 years in secondary syphilis, and 2–5 years in latent syphilis. The fluorescent treponemal antibody absorption test (FTA-ABS) has the highest sensitivity and specificity for diagnosing syphilis in all stages of the disease. It remains positive even after treatment. Hence, a positive FTA-ABS represents either active or inactive syphilis. Syphilis is the only bacterial STD that has not changed its antibiotic susceptibility. It is exquisitely sensitive to penicillin. The Jarisch-Herxheimer reaction commonly occurs within a few hours of treatment of secondary syphilis owing to the increase in number of treponemes (fever, headache, intensification of the rash).
Candida albicans	*Candida* vaginitis can be transmitted sexually, but this is uncommon. Vaginal candidiasis is common in women with diabetes, women taking systemic antibiotics, and pregnancy. It produces an intensely pruritic vaginitis with a cottage-cheese discharge.	A KOH preparation reveals budding yeast with pseudohyphae.
Trichomonas vaginalis	**Trichomoniasis** is due to the flagellated protozoan *Trichomonas vaginalis*. The organism locates in the urethra (males and females), prostate, seminal vesicles, and vagina. It produces a vaginitis characterized by intense pruritus, strawberry-colored mucosa, leukorrhea (discharge), and urethritis with increased frequency and dysuria.	Laboratory diagnosis is made by noting tumbling motility of the trophozoites in a hanging drop preparation of the discharge. Patient and partner are treated with metronidazole.

B. **Endometrial polyps** are a common cause of **menorrhagia** (excessive menstrual flow).
C. **Endometrial hyperplasia** is the result of prolonged estrogenic stimulation of the endometrial mucosa (e.g., from unopposed estrogen therapy, polycystic ovary syndrome) and is the precursor lesion for endometrial adenocarcinoma.
   1. It can be **simple** (**cystic hyperplasia**) or **complex**, with or without atypia.
   2. In **cystic hyperplasia** (simple hyperplasia), there are large, dilated glands that are widely separated from each other.
   3. In **complex hyperplasia**, there is crowding of the glands and branching of the glands with papillary infolding or outpouching.
D. **Adenomyosis** is a type of "diverticulosis" of the stratum basalis into the myometrium and may produce enlargement of the uterus and menstrual irregularities.
E. **Endometriosis** refers to endometrial glands and stroma in abnormal locations outside the uterus (most commonly the ovaries, where they are called "chocolate cysts").
   1. Reverse menses through the fallopian tube is the most popular theory for peritoneal involvement, but transplantation to other sites via lymphatic or vascular means and metaplasia may also be responsible.
   2. The majority of endometrial implants bleed during the menstrual cycle.
   3. Chronic pelvic pain is the most common symptom.
   4. Laparoscopy is the gold standard for securing the diagnosis.
   5. The diagnosis rests on finding endometrial glands, stroma, and hemosiderin in the stroma on microscopy of biopsy tissue.

VI. Disorders of the fallopian (uterine) tube
   A. **Ectopic pregnancy** (EP) most commonly occurs in the fallopian tube.
      1. **Pelvic inflammatory disease** (PID) is the most important predisposing condition.
      2. It produces **hematosalpinx**, or blood in the tube, owing to the presence of trophoblastic tissue implanted in the mucosa with extension into the muscle.
      3. Patients most commonly present with a sudden onset of hypogastric pain (90–100%), and rupture is a frequent complication and cause of death in early pregnancy.
      4. Serum β-hCG is the most important diagnostic test, while transvaginal ultrasound is useful in identifying the amniotic sac.
   B. **Hydatids of Morgagni** are pedunculated cysts located near the fimbriated end of the tube.

VII. Nonneoplastic disorders of the ovary
   A. **Tubo-ovarian abscess** is most commonly due to PID.
   B. Nonneoplastic ovarian **cysts**, most of which are **follicular cysts**, are the most common cause of ovarian enlargement.
   C. A **corpus luteum cyst** is the most common cause of ovarian enlargement in pregnancy.
   D. **Polycystic ovary syndrome** (POS), or **Stein-Leventhal syndrome**, is characterized by multiple subcortical cysts of the ovaries.
      1. It is associated with a clinical syndrome of obe-

sity, menstrual irregularities (oligomenorrhea), hirsutism, and infertility.
   2. There is a defect in the hypothalamic-pituitary axis, leading to excessive release of LH.
      a. LH stimulates the synthesis of excessive androstenedione (17-ketosteroid; cause of hirsutism) in the ovarian stroma, with subsequent aromatization into estrone (cause of endometrial hyperplasia).
      b. Estrogen suppresses the release of FSH; thus, there is no follicle development (cyst formation).
      c. Estrogen has a positive feedback on LH, hence continuing the cycle of excessive LH stimulation and suppression of FSH.
      d. Laboratory findings include an increased LH, a normal to low FSH, an increased plasma androstenedione and testosterone, and an increased serum estrone (from peripheral conversion of androstenedione).

VIII. Nonneoplastic disorders of the placenta
   A. A **normal chorionic villus** is lined by an outer layer of **syncytiotrophoblast**, which synthesizes β-hCG and human placental lactogen, and an inner layer of **cytotrophoblast**.
   B. **Placenta previa**, in which implantation occurs over the cervical os, presents with **painless vaginal bleeding**.
   C. **Placenta accreta** is adherence of the placenta directly to the myometrium with no intervening decidua.
   D. **Abruptio placentae** is due to premature separation of the placenta, with a resultant retroplacental clot.
      1. It may be associated with maternal hypertension, preeclampsia, smoking, and cocaine abuse.
      2. It presents with **painful vaginal bleeding**.
   E. **Twin placentas** may house identical or fraternal twins.
      1. **Monozygous twins** (identical) arise from the division of a single fertilized egg, while **dizygous twins** (fraternal) arise from fertilization of two separate ova by two sperm.
      2. **Identical twins** always arise from a **monochorionic placenta**, whether they are **monoamniotic** (and share one cavity) or **diamniotic** (and have separate cavities).
         a. **Fetus-to-fetus transfusion** is a potential complication in monochorionic placentas, since both share the same blood supply.
         b. **Conjoined (Siamese) twins** are most commonly in a monoamniotic monochorionic placenta.
         c. Twin placentas that are dichorionic may represent either identical or fraternal twinning.
   F. **Chorioamnionitis** is infection of the fetal membranes and is most often the result of ascending infection from the vaginal tract by group B streptococci (*Streptococcus agalactiae*).
   G. Pregnancy-induced hypertension (PIH) usually occurs after the 32nd week of gestation.
      1. It is the sudden development of **maternal hypertension**, **edema**, and **proteinuria**; the addition of generalized convulsions is designated **eclampsia**. ⌐→ seizures
      2. **Risk factors** include nulliparity, previous medical problems (e.g., diabetes mellitus, hypertension), twin gestation, and hydatidiform mole.
      3. The **pathogenesis** of PIH favors an abnormal

placentation, resulting in a decrease in perfusion (**uteroplacental ischemia**).

4. Eclampsia is treated with magnesium sulfate.

H. **Polyhydramnios** is defined as excessive amniotic fluid (AF) due to abnormalities that interfere with swallowing and reabsorption of the AF (tracheo-esophageal fistula, duodenal atresia), diabetes mellitus, and open neural tube defects.

I. **Oligohydramnios** is most commonly related to fetal renal abnormalities, such as renal agenesis or urinary tract obstruction.

IX. Tests performed on amniotic fluid

A. **Fetal lung maturity** is evaluated by measuring **surfactant** in AF.

1. Cortisol and thyroxine enhance its synthesis by type II pneumocytes, while insulin has an inhibitory effect.

2. The gold standard test is thin-layer chromatography with measurement of the **ratio of lecithin to sphingomyelin** (L/S ratio > 2 indicates lung maturity).

B. **Increased levels of α-fetoprotein** (AFP) in either maternal serum or AF may indicate an open neural tube defect, while a **low level** may represent Down syndrome.

Objective 3: To discuss the neoplastic disorders of the vulva, vagina, cervix, uterus, ovaries, and placenta.

X. Neoplastic disorders of the vulva

A. **Vulvar dysplasia** may progress to **squamous cell carcinoma** (SCC), the most common primary cancer of the vulva.

B. SCC usually occurs on the labia (most common site).

1. Predisposing causes include HPV type 16, atypical squamous hyperplasia, smoking, diabetes mellitus, and immunosuppression.

2. In elderly women (> 70 years old), SCC is rarely associated with HPV, whereas in younger women (mean age of 55), HPV is present in 75% of cases.

3. Vulvar SCC metastasizes early to the regional lymph nodes and then to distant sites (e.g., lung, liver).

C. **Verrucous carcinoma** of the vulva is also associated with HPV; it rarely metastasizes but is locally invasive.

D. **Extramammary Paget's disease** of the vulva primarily occurs in elderly women.

1. It presents as an eczematoid rash (erythroleukoplakia) located in the vulvar, perianal, or perineal areas.

2. Unlike Paget's disease of the breast, which is due to invasion of the overlying epidermis by an underlying ductal adenocarcinoma, extramammary Paget's is primarily an adenocarcinoma that is usually limited to the epidermis.

XI. Neoplastic disorders of the vagina

A. **Vaginal SCC** is more commonly an extension of a cervical cancer than a primary cancer arising in the vagina.

B. **Embryonal rhabdomyosarcoma** (sarcoma botryoides) of the vagina is the most common sarcoma in children and presents as a bleeding, grape-like mass that projects from the vagina.

XII. Neoplastic disorders of the cervix

A. **Cervical dysplasia** is a precursor lesion for cervical SCC.

1. Predisposing causes for both cervical dysplasia and cancer are the following:
   a. Early age of first intercourse.
   b. Multiple sexual partners.
   c. Cigarette smoking, oral contraceptive use, and immunosuppression.
   d. Infection with HSV-2 (an initiator) and HPV type 16 (most common; a promoter).

2. Activation of the *ras* oncogene and inactivation of the *p53* suppressor oncogene play an important role in cervical oncogenesis.

3. Cervical intraepithelial neoplasia (CIN) has the following subclassifications:
   a. CIN I (mild dysplasia) involves the innermost one-third of the cervical epithelium.
   b. CIN II (moderate dysplasia) involves two-thirds of the thickness of the epithelium.
   c. CIN III (severe to CIS) involves the full thickness of the epithelium without invasion through the basement membrane. *no BM*

4. **Koilocytic atypia** (HPV effect) is frequently noted in cytologic preparations and biopsy specimens.

5. Most low-grade cervical dysplasias are reversible if the irritating factor is removed.

6. CIN I usually occurs in 20- to 30-year-olds, CIN II and III in 30- to 40-year-olds, and invasive cancer in 40- to 60-year-olds.

7. It takes ~10 years to progress from CIN I to CIN III and an additional 10 years to progress to invasive cancer.

B. **Cervical SCC** (least common of the gynecologic cancers) is decreasing in incidence in the United States because of Pap smear detection of cervical dysplasia.

1. **Microinvasive cancer** invades the cervical stroma to a maximum depth of 3 mm beneath the basement membrane without evidence of lymphatic or vascular involvement (metastasis rarely occurs).

2. **Invasive SCC** is subclassified histologically as **large-cell nonkeratinizing** (most common), **large-cell keratinizing**, and **small-cell types**.

3. Invasive SCC most commonly extends into contiguous structures such as retroperitoneal tissue, leading to ureteral obstruction, renal failure, and death (most common cause of death due to cervical cancer).

4. The clinical stage is the most important prognostic factor for survival.

5. The 5-year survival for stage I cancer is 80% but only 10–15% for stage IV disease.

XIII. Neoplastic disorders of the uterus

A. **Leiomyomas** ("fibroids") of the uterus are the most common overall tumor in women (25–30%) and are more common in African Americans than in whites.

1. They are nonencapsulated, estrogen-sensitive, smooth muscle tumors.

2. They may be subserosal, intramural, or submucosal (causing menorrhagia) in location.

3. They rarely, if ever, transform into leiomyosarcomas.

4. Clinical abnormalities include menorrhagia,

secondary dysmenorrhea, infertility, and recurrent abortions.

B. **Endometrial adenocarcinoma** is the most common invasive cancer of the female genital tract followed, in descending order, by ovarian and cervical cancer.
   1. The overall incidence is slightly decreasing in the United States.
   2. It has a peak age of onset between 55 and 65 years of age.
   3. The following are risk factors:
      a. Unopposed estrogen stimulation (due to obesity; nulliparity; infertility; use of estrogen alone or tamoxifen [a weak estrogen]; granulosa cell tumor; low-fiber, high-fat diet; early menarche; or late menopause).
      b. Diabetes mellitus.
      c. Hypertension.
      d. History of breast cancer, endometrioid cancer, or clear cell carcinoma of the ovary.
   4. They have a fungating, polypoid appearance and have two microscopic variants: **endometrioid** and **papillary**.
   5. **Adenoacanthomas** are endometrial carcinomas with benign squamous metaplasia, while **adenosquamous carcinomas** are a mixture of adenocarcinoma and squamous carcinoma.
      a. Most patients are postmenopausal women who present with vaginal bleeding (90%).
      b. The lungs are the most common site for distant metastasis.
      c. It has the best prognosis of all gynecologic cancers (90% 5-year survival), followed by cervical and ovarian cancer (worst prognosis).

C. **Leiomyosarcomas** are the most common uterine sarcomas and are primarily differentiated from benign leiomyomas by counting mitoses ($\geq$ 5 per 10 high-power fields).

XIV. Neoplastic disorders of the ovary

A. Tumors are more likely to be benign in women < 45 years old (1:15 are malignant) and malignant in women > 45 years old (1:3 are malignant).

B. They have the highest mortality of all gynecologic tumors and are the second most common gynecologic malignancy.

C. Risk factors include nulliparity; high-fat, low-fiber diet; late menopause; history of a hereditary ovarian cancer syndrome; and gonadal dysgenesis.

D. *Ras* oncogene activation (50%) and *p53* suppressor oncogene inactivation (80%) assume a pivotal role in development.

E. Oral contraceptive use reduces the risk for cancer.

F. It most commonly spreads by seeding.

G. It presents with abdominal distention and bowel obstruction (most common complication).

H. **Surface epithelial tumors** (65–70%) replicate the epithelial lining of the fallopian tube (serous tumors), endometrium (endometrioid carcinomas), endocervical mucosa (mucinous tumors), and transitional epithelium (Brenner tumor).
   1. Most benign and malignant ovarian tumors are of surface epithelial origin (serous cystadenoma and cystadenocarcinoma, respectively).
   2. **Serous tumors** are benign (serous cystadenoma), intermediate (borderline serous cystadenocarcinoma), and malignant tumors (serous cystadenocarcinoma).
      a. They have the greatest incidence of **bilaterality**.
      b. **Serous cystadenocarcinomas** have **psammoma bodies** (calcification of necrotic tumor cells) and are present in ~30% of cases.
   3. **Mucinous tumors** have endocervix-like epithelium.
      a. They are the largest ovarian tumor.
      b. **Mucinous cystadenomas** are commonly associated with Brenner tumors (see below) and cystic teratomas.
      c. Mucinous cystadenocarcinomas commonly present with pronounced abdominal distention resembling ascites or pregnancy.
      d. A complication associated with mucinous tumors is **pseudomyxoma peritonei**, which is due to rupture of the tumor, leading to tumor implants scattered over the peritoneal and bowel serosa.
   4. **Endometrioid carcinomas** and **clear cell carcinomas** are associated with endometriosis and endometrial carcinoma.
   5. **Brenner tumors** are benign surface epithelial tumors characterized by nests of transitional epithelium called **Walthard's rests**.

I. **Germ cell tumors** (15–20%) include teratomas (most common), dysgerminomas (most common malignant tumor), choriocarcinomas, embryonal tumors, and yolk sac tumors (endodermal sinus tumors) of the ovary.
   1. **Cystic teratomas** may be mature, immature, or highly specialized.
      a. **Mature cystic teratomas (dermoid cysts)** primarily occur in young women (50% of ovarian tumors in children) and contain material derived from ectoderm (skin; most commonly sebaceous glands), endoderm (glandular tissue), and mesoderm (bone, cartilage, muscle).
      b. They often show **calcifications** on an abdominal film representing bone or teeth (30%).
      c. They most commonly present with torsion and subsequent hemorrhagic infarction, leading to abdominal pain.
      d. **Immature teratomas** (immature tissue elements or the presence of immature neuroepithelium) are malignant.
      e. A **struma ovarii** is composed of mature functional thyroid tissue.
   2. **Dysgerminomas** are the female counterpart of seminomas in the testicle.
      a. They are increased in Turner's syndrome.
      b. They are extremely radiosensitive.
   3. The endodermal sinus, or yolk sac, tumor, a highly malignant tumor, predominates in patients under 20 years of age, secretes α-fetoprotein, and has papillary projections into cystic cavities called **Schiller-Duval bodies**.

J. **Sex cord–stromal tumors** (5–10%) are the most common tumors that secrete sex hormones.
   1. **Ovarian fibromas** (most common) may be associated with **Meigs' syndrome** (ovarian fibroma, ascites, and a right-sided pleural effusion).
   2. **Granulosa cell tumors** are best considered as potentially malignant ovarian tumors that are

All 3 Mesoderm + Ectoderm + Endoderm

Serous cystadenoma - benign, cystadenocarcinoma - malignant

more common in postmenopausal women than in children.

  a. They are the most common ovarian tumor associated with **estrogen production** (75%).

  b. A key histologic feature is the **Call-Exner body**, which is a rosette-like structure resembling an ovarian follicle.

3. **Thecomas** are benign tumors that secrete estrogen.

4. **Sertoli-Leydig cell tumors** (**arrhenoblastoma, androblastoma**) are benign tumors most commonly found during the reproductive years.

  a. They may virilize the patient owing to excess secretion of androgens.

  b. **Hilar cell, or Leydig cell, tumors** are benign, androgen-secreting tumors that contain **crystalloids of Reinke**.

5. **Gonadoblastomas** are a combination of a germ cell tumor plus a sex cord–stromal tumor and are most commonly associated with **gonadal dysgenesis**, particularly Turner's syndrome with a Y chromosome.

K. Most **metastases** (5% of all ovarian tumors) are bilateral, and the breast is the most common primary site.

1. **Krukenberg's tumors** of the ovary are most frequently derived from metastatic, signet-ring carcinomas of the stomach.

2. **Burkitt's lymphoma** (B-cell malignancy), the most common malignant lymphoma in children, commonly involves the ovaries.

L. **CA125** tumor antigen is elevated in 80% of advanced nonmucinous ovarian epithelial carcinomas (e.g., serous cystadenocarcinoma and endometrioid carcinoma).

XV. Neoplastic disorders of the placenta

A. The three gestational neoplasms are **hydatidiform mole**, **invasive mole**, and **choriocarcinoma**, the last being the only malignant type.

B. They all secrete **β-hCG**, which is an excellent tumor marker.

C. **Hydatidiform moles** can be complete (most common) or partial.

1. **Complete moles** have a 46,XX genotype (90%) and do not contain an embryo.

  a. Both X chromosomes are of paternal origin (**androgenesis**).

  b. They may progress to choriocarcinoma.

2. **Partial moles** are trisomies, may contain an embryo, and rarely progress to choriocarcinoma.

3. The chorionic villi in hydatidiform moles are swollen (resembling grapes), avascular, and covered by trophoblastic tissue in varying proportions.

4. Preeclampsia in the first trimester is commonly associated with moles.

D. An **invasive mole** has the ability to invade the myometrium and to metastasize; however, it is considered a benign tumor.

E. **Choriocarcinomas** arise from hydatidiform moles in 50% of cases, previous abortions in 25%, and normal pregnancy in the remainder.

1. They are composed only of trophoblastic tissue and lack villous structures.

2. They most frequently metastasize to the lungs ("cannonball metastasis") and to the vagina (second most common metastatic site).

3. They are sensitive to chemotherapy (e.g., actinomycin D, methotrexate) and have close to 100% survival rates.

Objective 4: To understand hormone-related disorders associated with the uterus.

XVI. Hormone disorders

A. The sequence of events leading up to **menarche** is breast development (thelarche), growth spurt, development of pubic hair and axillary hair, and menarche.

B. The **menstrual cycle** (normally 28 days) is subdivided into the proliferative phase (variable phase), ovulation, and the secretory phase (most constant phase).

1. The **proliferative phase** is associated with gland proliferation and mitoses secondary to estrogen stimulation.

  a. Estrogen is derived from aromatization of testosterone in the granulosa cells.

  b. Testosterone and the 17-ketosteroids (DHEA and androstenedione) are synthesized in the theca interna under LH stimulation.

  c. Estrogen has a negative feedback on FSH and a positive feedback on LH, the latter resulting at midcycle in the LH surge and the induction of ovulation.

2. **Ovulation** on day 14 is associated with subnuclear vacuoles in the endometrial glands.

3. The **secretory phase** is controlled by progesterone (produced in the theca interna under LH stimulation) and is characterized by gland tortuosity and secretions and stromal edema.

  a. Progesterone increases the body temperature (useful in documenting ovulation).

  b. Progesterone increases salt and water retention and inhibits LH.

4. Estrogen eventually declines, the corpus luteum involutes, and progesterone drops, resulting in menses.

C. **Fertilization** occurs in the ampullary portion of the fallopian tube.

1. It requires ~3 days for the embryo to move through the tube and another 2–3 days to implant in the endometrium (day 21).

2. Syncytiotrophoblastic tissue from the developing placenta synthesizes β-hCG, an LH analogue that maintains the production of progesterone by the corpus luteum for 8–10 weeks, after which the placenta takes over hormone production.

D. **Androgens** in a woman derive from the ovaries and adrenals and from peripheral conversion in the adipose.

1. Approximately 50% of **serum testosterone** is derived from the peripheral conversion of androstenedione in the adipose, and the remaining 50% is synthesized in the ovaries (25%) and adrenals (25%).

2. Approximately 50% of the circulating **androstenedione** is synthesized by the adrenals and the other half by the ovaries.

3. The adrenal glands primarily synthesize **DHEA** (80%) and **DHEA sulfate** (95%).

4. **Sex hormone–binding globulin** (SHBG) binds both estrogens and testosterone.

a. It is an estrogen amplifier, since it has a higher binding affinity for testosterone.

b. An increase in estrogen increases the synthesis of SHBG, hence hyperestrinism automatically lowers the free testosterone levels in both men and women.

c. In obesity and hypothyroidism, there may be a decrease in SHBG levels that causes an increase in free testosterone levels, leading to hirsutism.

E. Presumptive evidence of **menopause** is the presence of elevated gonadotropins (FSH and LH), secondary amenorrhea, hot flushes (75%), decreased vaginal secretions, and night sweats.

F. **Dysfunctional uterine bleeding** (DUB) is hormonal imbalance that results in abnormal bleeding at irregular intervals which is either too excessive or too scanty.

1. It does not refer to bleeding associated with a pathologic lesion such as a polyp or cancer.

2. **Anovulatory cycles** are most common at the extremes of reproductive life, namely, menarche and the perimenopausal period.

G. **Amenorrhea** is subdivided into **primary** (absence of bleeding by 16 years of age) and **secondary types** (no bleeding for > 3 months).

1. It is the hallmark of hypogonadism (hypoestrinism), assuming no end-organ disease is preventing the exit of menstrual flow.

2. **Hypoestrinism** may be secondary to a hypothalamic-pituitary disturbance (low FSH and LH; hypopituitarism), hence the term **hypogonadotropic hypogonadism**, or a primary ovarian disorder (increased FSH and LH; Turner's syndrome), which is called **hypergonadotropic hypogonadism**.

1° pit problem

2°

3. If the gonadotropins are normal and secondary sex characteristics are normal, then an **end-organ abnormality** (e.g., imperforate hymen) may be present.

4. A normal delay in puberty and end-organ disease (e.g., imperforate hymen) are the most common causes of primary amenorrhea, while pregnancy and menopause are the most common cause of secondary amenorrhea.

5. **Turner's syndrome** is the most common genetic cause of prepubertal ovarian failure.

XO
female

H. **Primary dysmenorrhea** (painful menses) is due to increased production of prostaglandin F, which increases uterine contractions, while endometriosis is the most common cause of **secondary dysmenorrhea**.

Objective 5: To be conversant with the workup of hirsutism and virilization.

XVII. Hirsutism and virilization

A. **Hirsutism** is the presence of excess hair in normal androgen-sensitive areas of the body.

B. **Virilization** occurs when a female develops male secondary sex characteristics and clitorimegaly.

C. **Hyperandrogenic states** originate from problems related to the **ovaries** (e.g., polycystic ovary syndrome), **adrenals** (e.g., congenital adrenal hyperplasia), or exposure to drugs having androgenic side effects (e.g. progestins).

D. A markedly elevated serum testosterone (total and free testosterone fractions) usually indicates an ovarian cause, while an increase in DHEA sulfate indicates an adrenal cause of hyperandrogenicity.

E. **Spironolactone** is a general treatment for hirsutism and inhibits androgen receptors on hair follicles.

Objective 6: To be familiar with the nonneoplastic and neoplastic disorders of the female breast.

XVIII. Overview

A. Most glandular tissue is located beneath the nipple and in the upper outer quadrant; thus, cancer is most commonly located in this quadrant.

B. **Breast disease** can present as a painless mass lesion, nipple discharge, pain localized to one or both breasts, or a skin abnormality involving the nipple or underlying subcutaneous tissue.

C. A **breast mass** in a woman is likely to be due, in order of decreasing frequency, to fibrocystic change (40%), no disease (30%), other benign disease (13%), cancer (10%), or a fibroadenoma (7%).

D. Breast lesions localize to different areas of the breast.

1. The **nipple** may be the site of Paget's disease or a breast abscess.

2. The **lactiferous ducts** and **sinuses** commonly house benign intraductal papilloma, galactocele (blocked lactiferous duct in a lactating woman), breast abscess, or plasma cell mastitis.

3. **Large ducts** are the most common site for fibrocystic change and most ductal cancers.

4. The **terminal lobules** are involved in sclerosing adenosis (a variant of fibrocystic change) and lobular and tubular carcinomas.

5. The **breast stroma** is the source of a benign fibroadenoma or a malignant cystosarcoma phyllodes.

XIX. Nonneoplastic disorders of the breast

A. **Fibrocystic change** (FCC) is an example of hormonal imbalance that leads to distortions in the ducts, lobules, and stroma.

1. It frequents women from 20 to 50 years of age.

2. The morphologic changes involve the glands or stroma and include cysts, fibrosis, ductal hyperplasia (most important risk factor for ductal cancer), and sclerosing adenosis.

B. **Acute mastitis** is limited to the lactating period, when bacteria (Staphylococcus aureus) can enter the tissue through cracks and fissures in the nipple.

C. **Traumatic fat necrosis** is a unilateral, localized process characterized by necrotic fat cells, foamy macrophages, granulation tissue formation, and dystrophic calcification, often simulating cancer.

XX. Neoplastic disorders of the breast

A. **Fibroadenomas** are the most common benign tumors of the female breast in women under 35 years of age.

1. They arise from stromal cells, with the epithelial component representing the secondary effect of stromal proliferation compressing the

ducts into slit-like spaces (intracanalicular pattern).

2. Fibroadenomas are freely moveable masses and are treated by excision.

B. **Intraductal papillomas** are benign tumors located in the lactiferous duct or sinus that most commonly present as a bloody nipple discharge in women under 50 years of age.

C. **Breast cancer** is the second most common cause of a mass lesion in the 35- to 50-year-old age bracket and the most common cause of a mass lesion in women over age 50 in the United States.

1. The incidence of breast cancer increases significantly with age.

2. The incidence is steadily increasing owing to screening mammography.

3. The major risk factors are increasing age (most important), family history, excessive exposure to estrogen, preexisting breast disease, and environmental factors.

   a. Increasing age, family history (first-degree relative), atypical ductal hyperplasia, and previous breast cancer in the contralateral breast have the highest risk.

   b. **Excessive exposure to estrogen** can be due to menarche, late menopause, nulliparity, postmenopausal estrogen therapy, history of endometrial cancer, and oral contraceptive use.

   c. **Preexisting breast diseases** that increase risk include atypical ductal hyperplasia, atypical lobular hyperplasia, and previous history of breast cancer in the contralateral breast.

   d. **Environmental factors** that increase risk include a high-fat, low-fiber diet; radiation exposure; obesity; and alcohol abuse.

4. Most breast cancers present as a **painless breast mass** (70–90%).

5. **Mammography** is most useful in detecting nonpalpable breast masses.

   a. Early detection of tumor has been documented to decrease mortality, hence the importance of screening.

   b. Most organizations recommend an annual mammogram beginning at 40 years of age.

6. **Intraductal carcinomas** have a cribriform (noncomedo) and a comedo type, the latter containing necrotic debris in the duct lumen resembling a comedo.

7. **Infiltrating ductal adenocarcinoma** is the most common breast cancer.

   a. Grossly, it has a stellate appearance, reflecting its invasive nature.

   b. The cut surface is indurated (scirrhous) and gritty.

c. The overall 5-year survival is 60%.

8. **Medullary carcinomas** tend to be bulky, soft, well-circumscribed tumors with large cells and a lymphoid infiltrate.

9. **Colloid (mucinous) carcinomas** are primarily seen in elderly women.

10. **Paget's disease** of the breast presents as a scaly, eczematous rash usually involving the nipple in elderly women (see ¶IX.D.2).

11. **Inflammatory carcinoma** is a clinical diagnosis associated with erythematous, warm, edematous skin (plugs of tumor in the dermal lymphatics) exhibiting peau d'orange overlying an infiltrating ductal carcinoma.

12. **Lobular carcinomas** are the most common cancer in the terminal lobule and have a high degree of bilaterality (20–50%).

    a. Lobular carcinoma in situ is characterized by distention of the terminal lobules by small to intermediate-sized cells with very few mitoses.

    b. Invasive lobular cancer commonly has a single-file pattern.

13. **Cystosarcoma phyllodes** is the most common stromal malignancy of the breast.

    a. The term cystosarcoma phyllodes indicates cyst-like spaces within which are leaf-like projections.

    b. It is considered as a low-grade malignancy and has a cellular-appearing stroma within which are cystic spaces occupied by benign glandular epithelium.

    c. Whether of low or high grade, it rarely metastasizes to lymph nodes or distant sites (lung most commonly).

14. In tumors < 1 cm in diameter, size is the important **prognostic factor**; in tumors between 1 and 2 cm, grade is the most important prognostic factor; and in tumors > 2 cm, the status of the lymph nodes is the most important prognostic factor.

    a. Other important prognostic factors include the grade and lymph node status.

    b. Patients who are **ERA/PRA receptor positive** (more likely in postmenopausal than premenopausal women) have a better remission rate (60–80% response rate).

15. A **modified radical mastectomy** removes all ipsilateral breast tissue, the pectoralis minor muscle, the nipple-areola complex, and axillary lymph nodes below the axillary vein.

16. A **lumpectomy** is a segmental mastectomy plus low axillary node dissection (breast-conserving therapy) that is followed by radiation therapy.

QUESTIONS

DIRECTIONS. (Items 1–17): Each of the numbered items or incomplete statements in this section is followed by answers or by completions of the statement. Select the ONE lettered answer or completion that is BEST in each case. Correct answers and explanations are given at the end of the chapter.

1. The photograph (×1000) is of a Papanicolaou-stained slide of a vaginal discharge in a 25-year-old pregnant woman. She most likely has

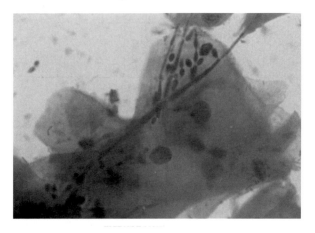

  (A) trichomoniasis
  (B) bacterial vaginosis
  (C) herpes genitalis
  (D) candidiasis
  (E) chlamydial cervicitis

2. The photograph is of a routine Papanicolaou-stained slide (×1000) of a cervical/vaginal smear in an asymptomatic woman. She should be treated with

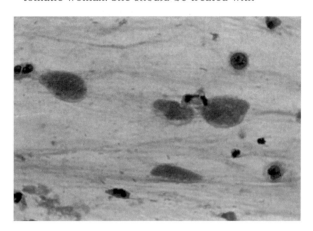

  (A) metronidazole
  (B) penicillin
  (C) doxycycline
  (D) an imidazole derivative
  (E) podophyllin

3. The photograph (×1000) represents a Papanicolaou-stained scraping from a cervical erosion in a woman with erosive cervicitis with leukorrhea. A potential treatment for this patient is

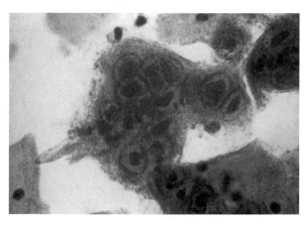

  (A) podophyllin
  (B) acyclovir
  (C) cervical conization
  (D) penicillin
  (E) metronidazole

4. Which of the following is a possible precursor lesion for cancer?

  (A) Endometrial polyp
  (B) Complete mole
  (C) Lichen sclerosus
  (D) Intraductal papilloma
  (E) Traumatic fat necrosis

5. Which of the following ovarian tumors has a different origin (derivation) from the others listed?

  (A) Mucinous cystadenoma
  (B) Brenner tumor
  (C) Serous cystadenocarcinoma
  (D) Endometrioid carcinoma
  (E) Endodermal sinus tumor

6. Which of the following breast location/disease relationships is correctly matched?

  (A) Nipple: medullary carcinoma
  (B) Lactiferous duct: lobular carcinoma
  (C) Major duct: sclerosing adenosis
  (D) Terminal duct: comedocarcinoma
  (E) Stroma: fibroadenoma

7. The lesion listed below that would most likely pursue a benign course is

   (A) vaginal adenosis
   (B) adenomyosis
   (C) extramammary Paget's disease
   (D) endometrial hyperplasia
   (E) adenoacanthoma

8. A 68-year-old woman presents with abdominal distention and pain. Physical examination reveals an absence of shifting dullness and the presence of induration in the rectal pouch on rectal examination and bilateral adnexal masses. Her breast examination and recent mammogram are normal. She most likely has

   (A) serous cystadenocarcinomas of both ovaries
   (B) Krukenberg's tumors of the ovaries
   (C) malignant ascites
   (D) Meigs' syndrome
   (E) dysgerminomas of both ovaries

9. An obese 24-year-old woman presents with a long history of oligomenorrhea and hirsutism. She has palpable bilateral ovarian masses. An ultrasound of her ovaries would likely reveal

   (A) serous cystadenomas
   (B) cystic teratomas
   (C) subcortical cysts in both ovaries
   (D) bilateral endometriomas
   (E) solid masses consistent with ovarian fibromas

10. A 33-year-old African American woman presents with severe iron deficiency, a long history of menorrhagia, and an enlarged, nodular uterus on physical examination. The most likely cause of her bleeding is

    (A) endometriosis
    (B) adenomyosis
    (C) endometrial carcinoma
    (D) leiomyomas of the uterus
    (E) cervical cancer

11. A 16-year-old female has not yet started having menstrual cycles. Her secondary sex characteristics appear normal as does external examination of her genitalia. She is given an intramuscular injection of progesterone and 5 days later she has her first period. The mechanism responsible for the delay in menses is

    (A) hypoestrinism
    (B) hypopituitarism
    (C) an end-organ abnormality
    (D) lack of an estrogen-primed endometrium
    (E) a normal constitutional delay in menarche

12. A cervical Pap smear report stating that "koilocytic atypia is present" indicates the

    (A) presence of high-grade cervical intraepithelial neoplasia
    (B) cytologic effect of herpesvirus type 2
    (C) cytologic effect of human papillomavirus
    (D) presence of a chlamydial infection
    (E) presence of an invasive squamous cancer

13. Cigarette smoking and long-term use of oral contraceptives in a woman would most likely predispose to primary cancer in which of the following sites?

    (A) Breast
    (B) Ovary
    (C) Endometrium
    (D) Cervix
    (E) Vulva

14. Nulliparity and late menopause are risk factors for which of the following groups of diseases?

    (A) Cervical cancer and endometrial hyperplasia
    (B) Ovarian cancer and endometrial polyp
    (C) Vulvar cancer and endometrial cancer
    (D) Endometrial cancer and breast cancer
    (E) Cervical cancer and ovarian cancer

15. Hypertension, proteinuria, and pitting edema are noted in the second month of the first pregnancy in a 25-year-old woman. The pathogenesis of her presenting complaints is most closely associated with

    (A) a benign tumor of the chorionic villi
    (B) gestational diabetes mellitus
    (C) primary endometrial cancer
    (D) a malignant trophoblastic tumor
    (E) a tumor arising from the myometrium

16. In a 60-year-old woman with a painless lump in the right upper outer quadrant of her breast, the greatest risk factor for it representing a malignant tumor would be

    (A) its location in the upper outer quadrant
    (B) the fact that she is 60 years old
    (C) a history of a sister with breast cancer
    (D) a history of a mother with breast cancer
    (E) a history of breast cancer in the contralateral breast

17. Cancer is the least common and infection the most common disease in the

    (A) cervix
    (B) endometrium
    (C) fallopian tube
    (D) ovary
    (E) breast

ANSWERS AND EXPLANATIONS

1. The answer is D: candidiasis. The photograph depicts yeast forms budding from pseudohyphae consistent with *Candida* species. Vaginal candidiasis is commonly seen in pregnancy and diabetes and in women taking antibiotics. It produces a cottage-cheese discharge and intense pruritus and erythema of the vaginal mucosa. *Trichomonas* is a pear-shaped organism, bacterial vaginosis (*Gardnerella vaginalis*) has clue cells, herpes genitalis has multinucleated squamous cells with intranuclear inclusions, and *Chlamydia* has vacuoles with red inclusions in glandular cells. (Photomicrograph reproduced, with permission, from B.F. Atkinson. *Atlas of Diagnostic Cytopathology.* Philadelphia, W.B. Saunders Co., 1993, p. 76.)

2. The answer is A: metronidazole. The smear shows pear-shaped organisms with indistinct nuclei consistent with *Trichomonas vaginalis.* Not all patients are symptomatic with a vaginal discharge. Both this patient and her partner should be treated with metronidazole. Penicillin would be used for syphilis, doxycycline for chlamydial infection, imidazole derivatives for candidiasis, and podophyllin for condyloma acuminatum (HPV). (Photomicrograph reproduced, with permission, from B.F. Atkinson. *Atlas of Diagnostic Cytopathology.* Philadelphia, W.B. Saunders Co., 1993, p. 79.)

3. The answer is B: acyclovir. A multinucleated squamous cell with intranuclear inclusions is seen. It is consistent with herpes genitalis due to HSV-2. Acyclovir does not cure the disease but reduces viral shedding and decreases recurrences. Podophyllin is used for treating condyloma acuminatum (HPV), cervical conization for severe cervical dysplasia/carcinoma in situ, penicillin for syphilis, and metronidazole for bacterial vaginosis and trichomoniasis. (Photomicrograph reproduced, with permission, from B.F. Atkinson. *Atlas of Diagnostic Cytopathology.* Philadelphia, W.B. Saunders Co., 1993, p. 80.)

4. The answer is B: complete mole. Complete moles are benign neoplasms of the chorionic villi that are responsible for up to 50% of cases of choriocarcinoma, which is a malignant disease of trophoblastic tissue (syncytiotrophoblast and cytotrophoblast). Endometrial polyps are a common cause of menorrhagia but are not precancerous. Lichen sclerosus is a benign vulvar dermatosis presenting as leukoplakia. It has no malignant potential. An intraductal papilloma is a benign tumor that is the most common cause of bloody nipple discharge in a woman < 50 years old. It is not precancerous. Traumatic fat necrosis simulates a breast cancer but is not precancerous.

5. The answer is E: endodermal sinus tumor. Endodermal sinus tumors derive from germ cells, whereas all the others listed are surface epithelium–derived tumors of the ovary. An endodermal sinus, or yolk sac, tumor is a highly malignant tumor that predominates in women < 20 years old and secretes α-fetoprotein as a tumor marker. It contains glomerulus-like Schiller-Duval bodies.

6. The answer is E: stroma: fibroadenoma. Fibroadenomas are the most common benign tumor and stromal tumor of breast. The stroma compresses the ducts into slit-like spaces. They occur in women < 35 years of age. Paget's disease most commonly involves the nipple (eczema-like rash from tumor invasion), while medullary

carcinoma arises from the major ducts. An intraductal papilloma most commonly derives from the lactiferous ducts, whereas a lobular carcinoma primarily involves the terminal lobules. Most ductal cancers (comedocarcinoma) arise from the major ducts, while sclerosing adenosis (variant of FCC) involves the terminal lobules and ducts.

7. The answer is B: adenomyosis. Adenomyosis is the presence of benign glands and stroma within the myometrium. It is a common cause of diffuse uterine enlargement and menstrual irregularities; however, it is not a precancerous lesion. Vaginal adenosis is a DES-related precursor lesion for clear cell adenocarcinoma of the vagina. Extramammary Paget's disease is an intraepithelial adenocarcinoma. Endometrial hyperplasia is a precursor lesion of endometrial carcinoma. An adenoacanthoma is an endometrial adenocarcinoma with a benign component of mature squamous cells.

8. The answer is A: serous cystadenocarcinomas of both ovaries. These tumors are the most common malignant tumors of ovaries and the most common tumors associated with bilaterality. The absence of shifting dullness excludes malignant ascites. Krukenberg's tumors are metastatic lesions to the ovaries from a primary stomach cancer. Meigs' syndrome is unilateral fibromas associated with ascites and a right-sided pleural effusion. Dysgerminomas are malignant germ cell tumors that are not commonly bilateral nor common to this woman's age bracket.

9. The answer is C: subcortical cysts in both ovaries. The patient has polycystic ovary syndrome. This is due to excessive stimulation of the ovaries by LH, with subsequent production of androstenedione (hirsutism) and aromatization of androstenedione into estrone. Estrone has a negative feedback on FSH (follicles die, leaving subcortical cysts) and a positive feedback on LH. Serous cystadenomas, cystic teratomas, ovarian fibromas, and endometriomas (endometrial implants of endometriosis) are not associated with menstrual irregularities or hirsutism.

10. The answer is D: leiomyomas of the uterus. Submucosal leiomyomas may produce severe menorrhagia, leading to iron deficiency. An enlarged, nodular uterus is not characteristic of endometriosis, adenomyosis, or cervical cancer. She is too young for endometrial adenocarcinoma.

11. The answer is E: a normal constitutional delay in menarche. The patient has primary amenorrhea. Her secondary sex characteristics are normal, indicating an adequate exposure to estrogen, hence ruling out hypoestrinism and hypopituitarism. Although her external genitalia examination is normal, the proof of the lack of an end-organ abnormality is that she was able to bleed after being given progesterone. This also proves that her endometrial mucosa was primed with estrogen.

12. The answer is C: cytologic effect of human papillomavirus. HPV infection of squamous cells produces wrinkled nuclei surrounded by a clear halo. This is called koilocytosis. Whether it is indicative of a low- or high-grade lesion in the cervix requires tissue documentation, which is usually obtained during colposcopy.

13. The answer is D: cervix. Smoking and long-term use of oral contraceptives predisposes to cervical cancer. Oral

contraceptives are protective against ovarian cancer. Oral contraceptives are thought to be a risk factor for breast cancer; however, there is no association between breast cancer and smoking. Smoking increases the risk for vulvar cancer. Neither smoking nor oral contraceptives are a risk factor for endometrial cancer.

14. The answer is D: endometrial cancer: breast cancer. Nulliparity and late menopause are factors associated with increased exposure to estrogen, hence they are operative in endometrial, breast, and ovarian cancer and endometrial hyperplasia. Unopposed estrogen stimulation is not operative in endometrial polyps, cervical cancer, or vulvar cancer.

15. The answer is A: a benign tumor of the chorionic villi. Preeclampsia (hypertension, proteinuria, pitting edema) in the first trimester is most often secondary to a hydatidiform mole, which is a benign neoplasm of the chorionic villi. The uterus is frequently too large for gestational age, and fetal heart sounds are absent.

It is too early in this patient's pregnancy for gestational diabetes, and she is too young for endometrial cancer. Choriocarcinomas are malignant trophoblastic tumors that most commonly develop from a preexisting complete mole. A tumor arising from the myometrium (leiomyoma) is not associated with preeclampsia.

16. The answer is E: a history of breast cancer in the contralateral breast. Although age and a family history of breast cancer in first-degree relatives are major risk factors, the history of a previous cancer in the contralateral breast supersedes those risk factors. Location of the tumor is not a major risk factor.

17. The answer is C: fallopian tube. Cancer is the least common and infection (pelvic inflammatory disease) the most common disorder in the fallopian tubes. Cancer is common in the cervix (even though it has decreased in incidence), endometrium, ovary, and breast. Acute and chronic cervicitis are the most common nonneoplastic disorders of the cervix.

C H A P T E R   N I N E T E E N

DISORDERS OF THE

ENDOCRINE SYSTEM

SYNOPSIS

OBJECTIVES

1. To understand the nomenclature of endocrine disease, negative and positive feedback, and the use of stimulation and suppression tests.
2. To discuss the most common causes of hypopituitarism and pituitary hormone excess states.
3. To be familiar with thyroid function tests.
4. To understand the nonneoplastic and neoplastic conditions affecting the thyroid gland.
5. To review primary, secondary, and tertiary hyperparathyroidism and the differential diagnosis of hypercalcemia.
6. To be familiar with the causes of primary hypoparathyroidism and the differential diagnosis of hypocalcemia.
7. To review the causes of hypercortisolism, mineralocorticoid excess, catecholamine excess, and hypocortisolism.
8. To define the islet cell tumors.
9. To be conversant with the pathophysiology of diabetes mellitus, impaired glucose tolerance, and gestational diabetes mellitus.
10. To discuss the causes of hypoglycemia.

Objective 1: To understand the nomenclature of endocrine disease, negative and positive feedback, and the use of stimulation and suppression tests.

I. Overview of endocrine disease
   A. **Primary disorders** involve the target organ, **secondary disorders** the anterior pituitary, and **tertiary disorders** the hypothalamus.
   B. Since hormones affect target organs at a distance from their site of origin, negative feedback loops exist to control an increase or decrease in hormone production.
      1. For example, an increase in serum T_4 inhibits (**negative feedback**) the release of both thyroid-stimulating hormone (TSH) and thyrotropin-releasing hormone (TRH).
      2. Conversely, a decrease in serum T_4 increases the release of TSH and TRH.
      3. In some cases, an increase in a hormone has a **positive feedback** (e.g., an increase in estrogen increases luteinizing hormone).
      4. Examples of **negative feedback loops** are calcium and parathormone (hypocalcemia stimulates, hypercalcemia suppresses PTH), glucose and insulin (hyperglycemia stimulates, hypoglycemia suppresses insulin), and cortisol and ACTH (hypocortisolism stimulates, hypercortisolism suppresses ACTH).
   C. **Stimulation tests** are performed when a hypofunctioning endocrine disorder is suspected (e.g., ACTH stimulation test for hypocortisolism).
   D. **Suppression tests** are utilized in the diagnosis of hyperfunction disorders (e.g., dexamethasone [a cortisol analogue] suppression test for Cushing's syndrome).
      1. The majority of hyperfunctioning endocrine diseases cannot be suppressed and therefore are autonomous (e.g., a pituitary adenoma producing acromegaly).
      2. Hyperfunction disorders that can be suppressed are prolactinomas and pituitary adenomas that produce Cushing's syndrome.

Objective 2: To discuss the most common causes of hypopituitarism and pituitary hormone excess states.

II. Pituitary hypofunction disorders
   A. **Hypopituitarism** may be secondary to hypothalamic or pituitary disease (most common).
      1. A **nonfunctioning pituitary adenoma** is the most common cause of adult hypopituitarism.
         a. It may be associated with the autosomal dominant **multiple endocrine neoplasia** (MEN) **I syndrome**.
         b. An expanding tumor destroys uninvolved portions of the pituitary gland, leading to the following trophic hormone deficiencies (in descending order of frequency): FSH and LH (secondary amenorrhea, impotence in the male), GH (hypoglycemia), TSH (hypothyroidism), ACTH (hypocortisolism), and prolactin (cessation of lactation).
         c. With the exception of secondary hypocortisolism (minimal electrolyte abnormalities), the clinical findings are similar to those arising from primary disease involving the target organs.
      2. **Sheehan's syndrome (postpartum pituitary ne-**

crosis, coagulation necrosis), the second most common cause of hypopituitarism in adults, presents with a sudden cessation of lactation.
3. **Craniopharyngiomas**, the most common cause of hypopituitarism in children, are benign pituitary tumors derived from **Rathke's pouch** remnants (ectoderm).
   a. Most have a suprasellar location and extend caudally into the sella turcica to destroy the gland as well as anteriorly (causing visual field defects) or superiorly into the hypothalamus (increasing intracranial pressure).
   b. They are cystic tumors with hemorrhage and dystrophic calcification that is apparent on x-rays.
B. **Diabetes insipidus** (DI) may be central (lack of ADH) or nephrogenic (resistance to ADH).
   1. **Central DI** may be secondary to transection of the pituitary stalk (usually posttraumatic), infiltrative disease to the posterior pituitary (e.g., metastasis, sarcoidosis), and hypothalamic disease (e.g., histiocytosis X).
   2. **Nephrogenic DI** may be secondary to drug use (e.g., lithium), severe hypokalemia (vacuolar nephropathy), and genetic disease.
   3. DI presents with polyuria and polydipsia and an associated inability to reabsorb free water in the kidneys leading to hypernatremia (increased plasma osmolality [Posm]) and a low urine osmolality (Uosm).
   4. In the **water deprivation test**, the Posm is high and the Uosm is low in both types; the administration of vasopressin results in an increase in Uosm > 50% in central DI and < 45% in nephrogenic DI.
III. Pituitary hyperfunction disorders
A. **Excess growth hormone** (GH) from a functioning pituitary adenoma leads to gigantism in children (whose epiphyses have not closed) and acromegaly in adults.
   1. **GH** increases muscle mass, has an antiinsulin effect, and stimulates the synthesis and release of somatomedin C (SMC; insulin-like growth factor) in the liver.
   2. **SMC** enhances chondrogenesis as well as soft tissue and linear growth of bones.
   3. **Acromegaly** is characterized by generalized enlargement of bones in the extremities owing to lateral growth of the bone and soft tissue.
      a. Enlargement of the hands and feet, skull, jaw (teeth are separated), tongue (macroglossia), and viscera (heart, liver) is seen.
      b. There is diastolic hypertension (~30%) and diabetes mellitus (~20%).

due to anti-insulin effect

      c. **Laboratory abnormalities** include an increase in GH and SMC, lack of suppression of GH and SMC with the oral glucose tolerance test, and hyperglycemia.
      d. Heart failure due to cardiomegaly and hypertension is the most common cause of death.
B. A **prolactinoma** is the most common pituitary tumor and is inhibited by bromocriptine, a dopamine analogue.
   1. Prolactinomas produce secondary amenorrhea (prolactin inhibits GnRH) and galactorrhea in women and impotence in men.
   2. Other causes of hyperprolactinemia include drugs (e.g., chlorpromazine, tricyclic antide-

pressants), hypothalamic/pituitary disease (e.g., stalk transection), and primary hypothyroidism (low T_4 increases both TSH and TRH, the latter being a potent prolactin stimulator).

Objective 3: To be familiar with thyroid function tests.

IV. Thyroid function tests
A. The measured **total serum T_4** (and T_3) reflects hormone that is both bound to thyroid-binding globulin (TBG) and hormone that is free (metabolically active).
   1. Changes in either the free hormone level (hypo- or hyperthyroidism) or the concentration of TBG (estrogen increases, androgens decrease TBG synthesis) alter the total serum T_4.
   2. Since TBG alterations do not affect the free hormone level, a patient would be asymptomatic (TSH is normal).
B. The **resin T_3 uptake** (RTU) reflects the TBG concentration and is reported as a percentage (25–35%).
   1. A preset amount of radioactive T_3 is added to a sample of patient serum.
   2. Radioactive T_3 binds to all available binding sites on TBG, and the leftover is bound to a resin and measured.
   3. The RTU is converted to a **T_4 binding ratio** (T_4 BR) by dividing the measured RTU by the reference serum mean RTU, which is 30% (e.g., patient RTU 30%, T_4 BR = 1 [30/30]).
   4. The RTU and T_4 BR are low and high in hypo- and hyperthyroidism, respectively.
   5. The RTU and T_4 BR are both increased when TBG is decreased (fewer binding sites mean more is left over) and decreased when TBG is increased (more binding sites mean less is left over).
C. The **free T_4 index** (FT$_4$-I) represents a calculated free T_4 hormone concentration.
   1. It is calculated by multiplying the total serum T_4 by the T_4 BR.
   2. The FT$_4$-I is low and high in hypo- and hyperthyroidism, respectively.
   3. The FT$_4$-I is normal when the TBG is high or low, since the T_4 BR is decreased when the TBG is high and increased when the TBG is low, hence "normalizing" the FT$_4$-I.
D. The **serum TSH** has a negative feedback relationship with circulating T_4 and T_3.
   1. It is the single best test for diagnosing primary hypothyroidism (increased TSH) and hyperthyroidism (decreased TSH).
   2. It is normal when there are alterations in the TBG concentration, since the free T_4 hormone levels are normal.
E. The **radioactive ^{131}I** uptake may be used as a radionuclide scan of the thyroid to detect nodules or as an index of thyroid activity.
   1. Since thyroid hormones represent tyrosine with iodides attached to it, true hyperfunctioning of the gland (e.g., Graves' disease) increases the uptake of ^{131}I, whereas a hypofunctioning gland demonstrates decreased uptake.
   2. Nodules in the thyroid that are functionally active ("**hot**" nodules) preferentially take up ^{131}I

(the remainder of the gland is not visualized), while those that are inactive ("**cold**" **nodules**) do not take up ^{131}I (there are clear spaces).

Objective 4: To understand the nonneoplastic and neoplastic conditions affecting the thyroid gland.

V. Nonneoplastic disorders
  A. Remnants of the thyroglossal duct may fill up with cyst fluid (**thyroglossal duct cyst**) and present as a midline cystic mass.
  B. **Thyroiditis**, or inflammation of the thyroid gland, may be secondary to microbial pathogens or autoimmune disease.
    1. **Acute thyroiditis** is secondary to a bacterial infection caused by *Staphylococcus aureus, Streptococcus pneumoniae,* or *Streptococcus pyogenes.*
      a. The gland is enlarged and tender, and reactive cervical lymphadenopathy and fever are present.
      b. Signs of thyrotoxicosis may occur.
    2. **Subacute granulomatous thyroiditis** (**de Quervain's thyroiditis**) is the most common cause of a painful thyroid gland.
      a. It may follow a viral infection (e.g., coxsackievirus).
      b. The gland is enlarged, and granulomatous inflammation with multinucleated giant cells is present on microscopic examination.
    3. **Hashimoto's thyroiditis** is an autoimmune thyroiditis that predominates in women between 30 and 50 years of age.
      a. Its pathogenesis is associated with the development of antibodies against peroxidase (**antimicrosomal antibodies**) and thyroglobulin (**antithyroglobulin antibodies**) and with cytotoxic T-cell damage to the gland.
      b. There are **autoantibodies** against the **TSH receptor** that prevent TSH stimulation of the gland (most common cause of hypothyroidism).
      c. There is an increased incidence of other autoimmune diseases (e.g., Sjögren's syndrome, pernicious anemia).
      d. The enlarged gland has a heavy lymphocytic

[handwritten: Predisposes to malignancy]

infiltrate, germinal follicles, and oncocytic change in follicular cells (degenerative change) on microscopic sections.
      e. It predisposes to primary malignant lymphoma of the thyroid.
      f. **Laboratory findings** are those of hypothyroidism (Table 19–1), and antimicrosomal and antithyroglobulin antibodies are elevated in 90% and 50% of patients, respectively.
    4. **Reidel's thyroiditis** is characterized by an intense fibrous tissue replacement of the gland and surrounding tissue that may eventuate in respiratory embarrassment.
  C. **Hyperthyroidism** connotes excess production of thyroid hormone (e.g., Graves' disease), while **thyrotoxicosis** describes the end-organ effects of an excess of thyroid hormone, regardless of the etiology.
    1. **Graves' disease** is the most common cause of hyperthyroidism (60–90% of cases) and thyrotoxicosis.
      a. It is a female-dominant autoimmune disease that is due to synthesis of an autoantibody against the TSH receptor called **thyroid-stimulating antibody** (TSI).
      b. There is diffuse, symmetric, nontender thyromegaly with microscopic features of overactivity (e.g., scanty colloid, papillary infolding of the glands).
      c. **Clinical features** unique to Graves' disease are **infiltrative ophthalmopathy** often associated with exophthalmos and **pretibial myxedema** (excess glycosaminoglycan deposition).
      d. Other features of thyrotoxicosis include sinus tachycardia (also atrial fibrillation), systolic hypertension, nervousness, weight loss, heat intolerance, muscle weakness, and diarrhea.
      e. Laboratory findings are given in Table 19–1.
    2. **Toxic nodular goiter** (**Plummer's disease**) develops in the setting of a multinodular goiter (see ¶E, on following page).
    3. **Less common causes of thyrotoxicosis** include choriocarcinoma (which has TSH-like qualities), struma ovarii (functioning thyroid tissue in an

TABLE 19–1. Summary of Thyroid Profile and ^{131}I Uptake Results in Disorders Associated with Thyrotoxicosis, Hypothyroidism, or Alterations in Thyroid-binding Globulin*

Disorder	Total Serum T_4	RTU	FT_4-I	TSH	^{131}I
Graves' disease	Increased	Increased	Increased	Suppressed	Increased
Factitious thyrotoxicosis	Increased	Increased	Increased	Suppressed	Decreased
Thyroiditis (acute, subacute)	Increased	Increased	Increased	Suppressed	Decreased
Primary hypothyroidism (Hashimoto's)	Decreased	Decreased	Decreased	Increased	Decreased
Secondary hypothyroidism (hypopituitarism/ hypothalamic cause)	Decreased	Decreased	Decreased	Decreased	Decreased
Increased TBG (increased estrogen)	Increased	Decreased	Normal	Normal	Normal
Decreased TBG (increased androgens)	Decreased	Increased	Normal	Normal	Normal

* RTU, resin T_3 uptake; FT_4-I, free T_4 index; TSH, thyroid-stimulating hormone; ^{131}I, radioactive iodine-131 uptake; TBG, thyroid-binding globulin.

ovarian teratoma), and factitious hyperthyroidism.
D. **Hypothyroidism** is a reduction in the secretion of thyroid hormone due to primary disease or an abnormality in the pituitary or hypothalamus.
1. It is most commonly caused by **Hashimoto's thyroiditis**.
2. **Clinical findings** include weakness (myopathy with increased serum creatine kinase), coarse skin, periorbital puffiness, pretibial myxedema, brittle hair, constipation, cold intolerance, weight gain, delayed recovery of the Achilles reflex, and diastolic hypertension.
3. Laboratory findings are given in Table 19–1.
E. A **goiter** is an enlargement of thyroid gland due to an absolute or relative deficiency of thyroid hormone (frequently associated with iodide deficiency).
1. Owing to recurrent episodes of TSH stimulation (hyperplasia) and involution (colloid stage), the gland is initially diffusely enlarged but eventually becomes multinodular.
2. Hemorrhage into a cyst is the most common cause of sudden enlargement of the gland.
F. A **solitary thyroid nodule** is benign in most cases (~85%) and is commonly a "cold" nodule on a radionuclide scan.
VI. Neoplastic disorders
A. A **follicular adenoma**, the most common benign thyroid tumor, is surrounded by a complete capsule without evidence of capsular or vessel invasion.
B. Factors that suggest thyroid cancer are a history of irradiation to the head and neck area, any solitary nodule in a man or a child, and any irregular nodule associated with palpable cervical lymphadenopathy.
1. **Papillary adenocarcinoma** is the most common thyroid cancer in adults and children.
a. The tumors are multifocal, are associated with papillary fronds lined by empty-appearing nuclei ("**Orphan Annie nuclei**"), and contain **psammoma bodies** (dystrophic calcification of necrotic tumor cells).
b. Lymphatic invasion with focal cervical lymph node involvement is the rule; however, distant metastasis is uncommon.
2. **Follicular carcinoma** may present as a well-circumscribed encapsulated tumor with capsular or blood vessel invasion or as an invasive cancer without a capsule.
a. Blood vessel invasion without lymph node metastasis is the rule.
b. It is more likely to have distant spread than papillary cancer (e.g., lungs, bone, brain, and liver).
3. **Medullary carcinomas** may be sporadic (80%) or familial (20%), the latter being associated with the autosomal dominant **MEN IIa and IIb syndromes**.
a. They derive from the **parafollicular C cells** that synthesize calcitonin.
b. Calcitonin is a tumor marker for the cancer and also is changed into **amyloid**, which is present in the tumor.
c. The familial **MEN IIa** syndrome consists of medullary carcinoma, primary hyperpara-

thyroidism (parathyroid adenoma), and pheochromocytoma (usually bilateral).
d. The **MEN IIb** variant is associated with medullary carcinoma, mucosal neuromas involving the lips and tongue, pheochromocytoma (usually bilateral), and a marfanoid habitus.

Objective 5: To review primary, secondary, and tertiary hyperparathyroidism and the differential diagnosis of hypercalcemia.

VII. Hyperparathyroidism
A. **Primary hyperparathyroidism** (HPTH), the most common cause of hypercalcemia in the ambulatory population, is most commonly due to a benign parathyroid adenoma (primary hyperplasia and carcinoma are uncommon).
1. Adenomas are composed of sheets of chief cells with no intervening fat.
2. Most cases are discovered as an **incidental finding** on a biochemical profile.
3. **Renal stones** are the most common symptomatic presentation.
4. **Other clinical findings** include peptic ulcer disease, acute pancreatitis, constipation, polyuria (metastatic calcification of kidney tubules, nephrocalcinosis), short QT interval, diastolic hypertension, and bone disease (**osteitis fibrosa cystica**).
5. **Laboratory findings** consist of an elevated serum PTH, hypercalcemia, hypophosphatemia, normal anion gap metabolic acidosis (loss of bicarbonate in the urine is counterbalanced by an equal gain in chloride), increase in serum alkaline phosphatase (bone formation counteracts bone resorption), hypercalciuria, and hyperphosphaturia.
B. **Malignancy-induced hypercalcemia** may be secondary to bone metastasis with activation of osteoclasts (from secretion of interleukin-1 or prostaglandins) or due to ectopic secretion of a **PTH-like peptide** from a primary squamous cell carcinoma of the lung, renal adenocarcinoma, or breast cancer.
1. **PTH-like peptide** increases calcium reabsorption in the kidneys (hypercalcemia) and decreases phosphorus reabsorption (hypophosphatemia).
2. Hypercalcemia suppresses the patient's own PTH as it does in all other causes of hypercalcemia not related to primary HPTH.
C. Other causes of hypercalcemia are **sarcoidosis, thiazides, vitamin D toxicity**, and **multiple myeloma**.
D. **Secondary HPTH** is hyperplasia of all the parathyroid glands as compensation for hypocalcemia and is most commonly caused by hypovitaminosis D due to chronic renal failure.
E. **Tertiary HPTH** is hypercalcemia that has developed from secondary HPTH usually associated with chronic renal failure.

Objective 6: To be familiar with the causes of primary hypoparathyroidism and the differential diagnosis of hypocalcemia.

VIII. Hypoparathyroidism and hypocalcemia

A. **Primary hypoparathyroidism** is hypofunction of the parathyroid glands that leads to hypocalcemia.
   1. It is most commonly due to previous thyroid surgery.
   2. **Autoimmune hypoparathyroidism**, the second most common type of hypoparathyroidism, is usually associated with **polyendocrine deficiency syndromes (multiple endocrine gland deficiencies)**.
      a. A reduction in the ionized calcium level results in **tetany**.
      b. Tetany is manifested by circumoral paresthesia (numbness and tingling), **Chvostek's sign** (facial twitching elicited by tapping over cranial nerve VII), and **carpal spasm** due to muscle spasms (**Trousseau's sign**) when the blood pressure is taken.
      c. **Laboratory abnormalities** include a low PTH, hypocalcemia, a prolonged QT interval, and hyperphosphatemia.
B. **Pseudohypoparathyroidism** is a sex-linked dominant disease characterized by end-organ resistance to PTH.
   1. **Type I** disease has a defect proximal to the generation of cAMP (receptor problem: cAMP does not increase after infusion of PTH), while **type II** disease has a defect distal to the generation of cAMP (postreceptor problem: cAMP increases after infusion of PTH).
   2. **Laboratory findings** include hypocalcemia, hyperphosphatemia, and a normal to high PTH.
C. Other causes of hypocalcemia include the following:
   1. **Alkalotic conditions** (increased pH increases the number of negative charges on albumin, hence favoring further binding of ionized calcium to albumin and leading to tetany without altering the total calcium concentration).
   2. **Hypomagnesemia** (magnesium is a cofactor for adenylate cyclase, which generates cAMP, hence inhibiting PTH activity).
   3. **Acute pancreatitis** (calcium is used up in enzymatic fat necrosis).
   4. **Hypoalbuminemia** (most common cause, since it binds 40% of calcium; correction for hypoalbuminemia = total calcium − serum albumin + 4).

Objective 7: To review the causes of hypercortisolism, mineralocorticoid excess, catecholamine excess, and hypocortisolism.

IX. Adrenal hyperfunction disorders
   A. The **zona glomerulosa** produces aldosterone (derived from activation of the renin-angiotensin-aldosterone system), while the **zona fasciculata** and **zona reticularis** synthesize glucocorticoids (e.g., deoxycortisol, cortisol), sex hormones (e.g., estrogen, androgens), and weak mineralocorticoids (e.g., deoxycorticosterone, corticosterone).
      1. A **urine collection for 17-hydroxycorticoids** (17-OH) contains metabolites of 11-deoxycortisol (compound S) and cortisol.
      2. A **urine collection for 17-ketosteroids** (17-KS) contains **dehydroandrosterone** (DHEA) and **androstenedione**, which are weak androgens.
   B. The **adrenal medulla** (of neural crest origin) synthesizes the catecholamines **epinephrine** (EPI) and **norepinephrine** (NOR).
      1. EPI and NOR are metabolized into biologically inactive metabolites by monoamine oxidase (MAO) and catechol-O-methyltransferase (COMT), respectively, into **metanephrine** and **vanillylmandelic acid** (VMA), respectively.
      2. The metabolite of dopamine is **homovanillic acid** (HVA).
   C. **Cushing's syndrome** is a manifestation of hypercortisolism from any cause, the most common of which is long-term glucocorticoid therapy.
      1. Excluding exogenous glucocorticoids, it is subdivided into **pituitary Cushing's** (also called **Cushing's disease**), **adrenal Cushing's**, and **ectopic Cushing's**.
         a. **Pituitary Cushing's** (most common type) is most often due to a benign adenoma that secretes ACTH.
         b. **Adrenal Cushing's** is associated with excessive production of cortisol secondary to neoplasia (adenoma, carcinoma) or hyperplasia, hence ACTH is suppressed.
         c. **Ectopic Cushing's** is most commonly due to a small-cell carcinoma of the lung and demonstrates the highest ACTH levels.
      2. Cushing's syndrome presents with the following:
         a. Weight gain (90%) with fat deposition in the face ("moon facies"), upper back ("buffalo hump"), and trunk (truncal obesity) with sparing of the extremities.
         b. Diastolic hypertension (75%) due to increased synthesis of weak mineralocorticoids.
         c. Glucose intolerance (increased gluconeogenesis), hirsutism (increased 17-KS), purple abdominal striae, a plethoric face, and osteoporosis.
      3. **Screening laboratory tests** include the plasma ACTH, low-dose dexamethasone (cortisol analogue) test (cortisol is not suppressed), and a 24-hour urine collection for free cortisol (best screen; measures excess unbound cortisol).
      4. The **high-dose dexamethasone test** is a confirmatory test in which cortisol is suppressed in pituitary Cushing's (partially autonomous) but not in the other types.
   D. **Primary aldosteronism** (**Conn's syndrome**) is excessive production of mineralocorticoids most commonly from an adenoma.
      1. Patients have diastolic hypertension and severe muscle weakness (hypokalemia).
      2. Pitting edema is not present, owing to the loss of significant amounts of sodium in the urine.
      3. A **24-hour urine collection for potassium** is the best screening test (always increased), and a **saline infusion test** is confirmatory (aldosterone is not suppressed).
      4. Additional laboratory abnormalities include mild hypernatremia, hypokalemic metabolic alkalosis, and low plasma renin activity (suppressed by increased plasma volume).
   E. **Hyperfunctioning tumors** of the **adrenal medulla** include **pheochromocytoma** and **neuroblastoma**, both of which secrete excess amounts of catecholamines, leading to hypertension.
      1. **Pheochromocytomas** are increased in patients

with neurofibromatosis, MEN IIa and IIb, and Lindau–von Hippel disease.
  a. Most are unilateral, benign adenomas arising in the adrenal medulla unless they are associated with a MEN syndrome, when they tend to be bilateral.
  b. Highly predictive symptoms include hypertension with episodic palpitations, sweating (frequently drenching), and headache.
  c. The best **screening tests** are a 24-hour urine collection for VMA and metanephrine (the best overall screen).
  2. A **neuroblastoma** is a malignant tumor of neural crest origin.
  a. It is the third or fourth most common malignancy in children.
  b. A consistent defect is deletion or rearrangement of the short arm of chromosome 1, leading to amplification of the n-*myc* oncogene.
  c. It is a "small-cell" tumor composed of neuroblasts and **Homer Wright rosettes**, in which the cells are separated from connective tissue or a preformed vascular channel by pale fibrillary processes.
  d. The neuroblast is S100 antigen positive and contains dense-core neurosecretory granules, indicating its neural crest origin.
  e. It presents as a palpable abdominal mass with abdominal distention, diastolic hypertension, and metastasis (the most common site is bone).
  f. It demonstrates elevated urine VMA, metanephrine, and HVA.
  g. Patient age is the single most important factor determining prognosis (cure rate is 85–90% below 1 year of age and 15–40% in older children).
X. Adrenal hypofunction disorders
  A. **Primary adrenal insufficiency** refers to hypocortisolism resulting from disorders involving the adrenal glands.
  B. **Autoimmune destruction** of the adrenal is the most common cause of chronic insufficiency (**Addison's disease**).
  1. There are deficiencies of glucocorticoids, mineralocorticoids (including hypoaldosteronism), and 17-ketosteroids.
  2. Patients present with weakness, hypotension (due to salt loss in the urine), and diffuse hyperpigmentation in the mucous membranes of the mouth, on skin, and in scars resulting from an increase in plasma ACTH.
  3. **Laboratory abnormalities** include the following:
    a. No detectable increase in urine 17-OH in both short and prolonged ACTH stimulation tests.
    b. Elevated plasma ACTH.
    c. Hyponatremia (hypertonic loss of salt in the urine) and hyperkalemia (no exchange of sodium for potassium or hydrogen ions for potassium because of hypoaldosteronism).
    d. Fasting hypoglycemia (loss of gluconeogenic activity of cortisol).
    e. Eosinophilia (loss of the cortisol effect).
  C. Other causes of hypocortisolism are the following:

  1. Abrupt withdrawal of corticosteroids (most common cause of acute adrenal insufficiency).
  2. Tuberculosis (most common cause worldwide).
  3. Disseminated meningococcemia (**Waterhouse-Friderichsen syndrome**; DIC with bilateral adrenal hemorrhage).
  4. Congenital adrenal hyperplasia (Chapter 7).

Objective 8: To define the islet cell tumors.

XI. Islet cell tumors
  A. An **insulinoma**, the most common islet cell tumor, is a benign tumor arising from the β-islet cells that produces fasting hypoglycemia associated with high serum insulin and C-peptide levels.
  B. A **gastrinoma** (Zollinger-Ellison syndrome) is a malignant islet cell tumor arising from pancreatic G cells that produces an excess of gastrin, leading to hyperacidity and peptic ulcer disease.
  C. A **glucagonoma** is a malignant tumor of α-islet cells that secretes excessive glucagon and is associated with diabetes mellitus and a characteristic rash called necrolytic migratory erythema.
  D. A **somatostatinoma** is a malignant tumor of δ-islet cells secreting excessive somatostatin, resulting in achlorhydria (hormone inhibits gastrin), cholelithiasis (hormone inhibits cholecystokinin), diabetes mellitus (hormone inhibits gastric inhibitory peptide), and steatorrhea (hormone inhibits secretin and cholecystokinin).
  E. A **VIPoma** (pancreatic cholera, Verner-Morrison syndrome) is a malignant tumor associated with excessive secretion of vasoactive intestinal peptide (VIP) leading to severe secretory diarrhea and achlorhydria.

Objective 9: To be conversant with the pathophysiology of diabetes mellitus, impaired glucose tolerance, and gestational diabetes mellitus.

XII. Diabetes mellitus
  A. Diabetes mellitus (DM) is a metabolic disease that affects carbohydrate, fat, and protein metabolism.
  B. It may be the result of either an absolute deficiency of insulin (type I) or of inadequate insulin secretion coupled with resistance to insulin in the peripheral tissue (type II).
  C. **Primary DM** is subclassified as **type I insulin-dependent DM** and **type II non–insulin-dependent DM** (more common type).
  1. Type II DM is further subclassified into obese (80%) and nonobese (20%) types.
  2. Distinctions between types I and II are summarized in Table 19–2.
  D. **Secondary DM** may be due to pancreatic disease (e.g., chronic pancreatitis), drug use (e.g., thiazides), or endocrine disease (e.g., pheochromocytoma).
  E. The **pathologic abnormalities** associated with DM are the result of **nonenzymatic glycosylation** (NEG) and **osmotic damage**.
  1. In NEG, glucose combines with amino groups in proteins (e.g., glycosylated HbA$_{IC}$ [glycohemoglobin]), which forms **advanced glycosylation end products** (AGEs) that alter vessel permeability and increase atherogenesis.

TABLE 19-2.   Summary of Types I and II Diabetes Mellitus

Factor	Type I Diabetes Mellitus	Type II Diabetes Mellitus
Prevalence	5–10%.	90–95%.
Age	<20 years (80%), mean of 11 years.	>30 years.
Body habitus	Usually thin.	Obese (80%).
Family history	Family history uncommon (10%). About 50% concordance rate in identical twins.	Family history common. About 90% concordance rate in identical twins.
Pathogenesis	Insulin lack. HLA-DR3 and -DR4 association (90–95%). Mechanisms of insulin deficiency: viruses, autoimmunity, environmental factors. Pancreas devoid of β-cells. Islet cell antibodies in 80%.	No HLA relationship. Relative insulin deficiency and peripheral tissue insulin resistance secondary to receptor deficiency and postreceptor defects (glucose transporter abnormalities).
Initial symptoms	Rapid onset of polydipsia, polyuria, and weight loss.	Insidious onset, symptomatic or asymptomatic.
Ketoacidosis	May occur owing to insulin lack.	Hyperosmolar nonketotic coma.
Treatment	Insulin.	Diet most important factor. Oral glucose lowering agents. Insulin necessary in some cases.

    a. **Hyaline arteriolosclerosis,** which is the main cause of microvascular disease in DM and is particularly prominent in diabetic nephropathy and small-vessel disease throughout the body, is a complication of NEG.

    b. **Macrovascular disease** due to increased atherosclerosis and an increased incidence of coronary artery disease (predisposing to acute myocardial infarction), peripheral vascular disease (e.g., gangrene in the lower extremities), and cerebrovascular disease (e.g., atherosclerotic stroke) is another complication of NEG.

2. **Osmotic damage** is due to conversion of glucose to sorbitol and fructose by aldolase reductase and sorbitol dehydrogenase, respectively.

    a. Both **sorbitol** and **fructose** are osmotically active and draw water into tissue, leading to permanent damage.

    b. Complications primarily associated with osmotic damage include peripheral neuropathy (destruction of Schwann cells), cataracts, and microaneurysms in diabetic retinopathy (damage to pericytes weakens the vessel wall).

F. **Duration** and **severity** of disease are key factors underlying the clinical presentation of DM, with tight control of glucose reducing the onset and severity of complications related to retinopathy, neuropathy, and nephropathy.

G. **Diabetic ketoacidosis** (DKA) is primarily a complication of type I DM, since there is enough insulin in type II DM to prevent ketogenesis.

1. Hyperglycemia and ketogenesis are the two key abnormalities.

    a. The pathogenesis of **hyperglycemia** is related to reduced uptake of glucose by adipose and muscle, an increase in glycogenolysis (glucagon and the counterregulatory hormones), and an increase in gluconeogenesis (primarily a glucagon effect), which is the single most important cause of hyperglycemia.

    b. The pathogenesis of **ketone bodies** is related to increased β-oxidation of fatty acids leading to an excess of acetyl-CoA, which is con-

verted to **acetoacetate** (AcAc; also forms acetone, giving a fruity odor to the breath) and β-hydroxybutyrate (BHB).

2. Other abnormalities include the following:

    a. **Severe volume depletion** (from osmotic diuresis).

    b. **Dilutional hyponatremia** (osmotic effect of hyperglycemia; Chapter 5).

    c. **Potassium** and **phosphate ion loss** in the urine (from osmotic diuresis).

    d. **Hyperlipidemia** (from reduced capillary lipoprotein lipase degradation of chylomicrons and VLDL).

H. **Hyperosmolar nonketotic coma** (HNKC) is primarily seen in type II DM owing to the presence of sufficient insulin to prevent ketogenesis.

I. **Accelerated atherosclerosis** in DM is responsible for ischemic injury to the extremities (most common cause of nontraumatic amputation of limbs) and an increased incidence of abdominal aortic aneurysm, acute myocardial infarction (most common cause of death), and atherosclerotic stroke.

J. **Diabetic nephropathy** is discussed in Chapter 17.

K. Retinopathy in DM is the leading cause of blindness in the United States.

L. **Distal symmetric polyneuropathy** from osmotic damage of Schwann cells affecting both sensory and motor nerves is commonly seen in DM.

M. **Autonomic neuropathy** may occur (cardiac arrhythmias, gastroparesis, impotence).

N. Two unusual relationships associated with increased susceptibility to infection are **mucormycosis** of the **frontal sinuses**, leading to frontal lobe brain abscesses, and **malignant external otitis** from *Pseudomonas aeruginosa*.

O. **Laboratory diagnosis** of DM has been altered to reflect greater specificity than sensitivity.

1. Home monitoring of blood glucose is mandatory.

2. Glycohemoglobin is useful in evaluating long-term glycemic control, since it represents the mean glucose value for the last 4–8 weeks.

P. **Impaired glucose tolerance** describes a patient who does not fit the established criteria for DM but who does have an increased risk for macrovascular disease and neuropathy.

Q. **Gestational diabetes** (GDM) refers to glucose intolerance that first develops during pregnancy.
   1. It is due to increased placental size and the antiinsulin effect of human placental lactogen.
   2. Pregnant women at 24–28 weeks of gestation are screened by a 50-g glucose challenge followed by 1-hour glucose level (> 140 mg/dL is positive).
   3. The confirmatory test is a 3-hour, 100-g glucose tolerance test in which the glucose values are set at highest sensitivity.
   4. Newborns are at risk for macrosomia (insulin increases adipose stores of fat and muscle mass), respiratory distress syndrome (insulin inhibits surfactant production), open neural tube defects, and transposition of the great vessels.

Objective 10: To discuss the causes of hypoglycemia.

XIII. Hypoglycemia
   A. Hypoglycemia is defined as a low blood glucose, and insulin-induced hypoglycemia in a diabetic is the most common cause.

B. Clinical signs and symptoms are **adrenergic** (sweating, trembling, anxiety) or **neuroglycopenic** (dizziness, confusion, headache, inability to concentrate in a brain without glucose).
C. The 5- to 6-hour glucose tolerance test is no longer recommended.
D. Examples of disorders associated with hypoglycemia are listed below.
   1. **Alcoholism** produces fasting hypoglycemia owing to increased NADH production in alcohol metabolism, which converts pyruvate to lactate, hence inhibiting gluconeogenesis.
   2. Carnitine is a cofactor in the transport of fatty acids (carnitine acyltransferase) into the mitochondria, hence **carnitine deficiency** renders all tissues dependent on glucose for fuel (there is no β-oxidation of fatty acids or ketone body synthesis).
   3. Factitious hypoglycemia (surreptitious self-injection of insulin) is characterized by high serum insulin and low C peptide levels due to suppression of the patient's endogenous insulin release.

QUESTIONS

DIRECTIONS. (Items 1–12): Each of the numbered items or incomplete statements in this section is followed by answers or by completions of the statement. Select the ONE lettered answer or completion that is BEST in each case. Correct answers and explanations are given at the end of the chapter.

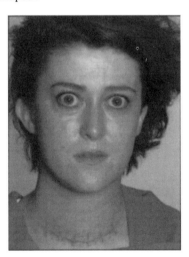

1. Which one of the following test results would be expected in this patient?

   (A) Hypercholesterolemia
   (B) Hypoglycemia
   (C) Hypocalcemia
   (D) Low serum TSH
   (E) Low urine calcium

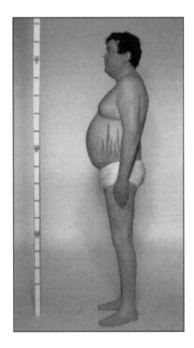

2. You would expect this 38-year-old man to have

   (A) hypoglycemia
   (B) hypotension
   (C) an increase in urine free cortisol
   (D) suppression of cortisol with a low-dose dexamethasone test
   (E) normal urine 17-ketosteroids

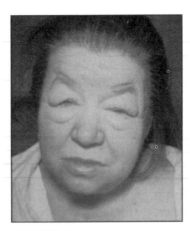

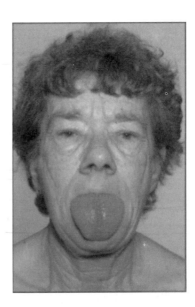

3. You would expect this elderly patient to have

   (A) a delayed Achilles tendon reflex
   (B) episodic bouts of diarrhea
   (C) systolic hypertension
   (D) truncal obesity
   (E) heat intolerance

4. This patient has noticed a gradual increase in hat size and headaches. She has recently been diagnosed with diabetes mellitus. You would also expect her to have

   (A) a high serum TSH
   (B) enlarged hands and feet
   (C) yellowish discoloration of the skin
   (D) a "buffalo hump"
   (E) carpal spasm

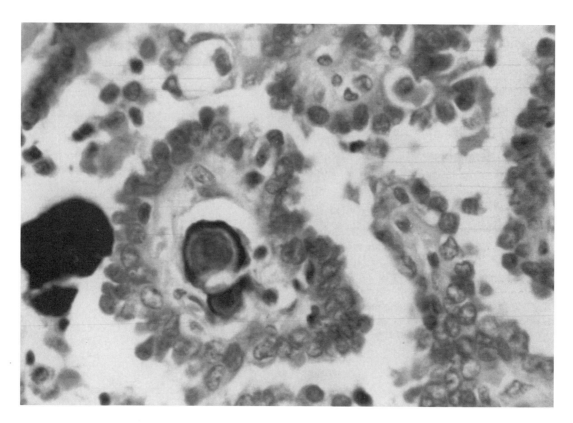

5. This is a representative microscopic section of thyroid tissue from a total thyroidectomy that was performed on a 32-year-old man. He had received irradiation to his face for control of severe acne when he was a teenager. The process represented in the slide is an example of

(A) autoimmune destruction of the gland
(B) a neoplastic transformation of the gland parenchyma
(C) an inflammatory condition with destruction of the gland
(D) a growth alteration secondary to deficiency of iodide
(E) a malignancy arising from parafollicular cells

6. A 62-year-old woman who presents with colicky right flank pain is noted to have a renal stone in the right ureter. A biochemical profile shows abnormalities in her serum calcium, phosphorus, and electrolytes. Which of the following tests would most likely confirm the cause of her renal stone?

(A) Bone marrow examination
(B) 24-hour urine collection for calcium
(C) 24-hour urine collection for phosphorus
(D) Bone scan
(E) Serum parathormone level

7. The most common cause of a low total calcium and a normal ionized calcium level is

(A) hypomagnesemia
(B) hypovitaminosis D
(C) hypoparathyroidism
(D) hypoalbuminemia
(E) respiratory alkalosis

8. A thin, 48-year-old man presents with diastolic hypertension, extreme muscle weakness, a U wave on an ECG and a positive Chvostek sign. Serum electrolytes reveal the following:

Serum sodium	151	mEq/L (normal, 135–147 mEq/L)
Serum chloride	110	mEq/L (normal, 95–105 mEq/L)
Serum potassium	2.0	mEq/L (normal, 3.5–5.0 mEq/L)
Serum bicarbonate	36	mEq/L (normal, 22–28 mEq/L)

The patient most likely has

(A) a pheochromocytoma
(B) primary aldosteronism
(C) diabetes insipidus
(D) Addison's disease
(E) inappropriate ADH syndrome

9. Which of the following would occur in a neuroblastoma rather than a pheochromocytoma?

(A) Metastasis
(B) Location in the adrenal medulla
(C) Increased 24-hour urine collection for metanephrines
(D) Increased 24-hour urine collection for vanillylmandelic acid (VMA)
(E) Hypertension

10. Which of the following is present in both Addison's disease and secondary hypocortisolism?

(A) Low ACTH
(B) Low urine 17-hydroxycorticoids
(C) Hypernatremia
(D) Hyperkalemia
(E) Hyperpigmentation

11. The pathogenesis of ketoacidosis in type I diabetes mellitus is most closely related to an increase in

    (A) β-oxidation of fatty acids
    (B) glycogenolysis
    (C) glycolysis
    (D) synthesis of VLDL
    (E) glycerol

12. In diabetes mellitus, nonenzymatic glycosylation is most likely operative in the pathogenesis of
    (A) peripheral neuropathy
    (B) microaneurysms in the retina
    (C) cataracts
    (D) hyaline arteriolosclerosis
    (E) osmotic diuresis

DIRECTIONS. (Items 13–17): Each set of matching questions in this section consists of a list of lettered options followed by several numbered items. For each numbered item, select the ONE option that is most closely associated with it. Each lettered option may be selected once, more than once, or not at all.

Item 13

The following laboratory test results are from a water deprivation test in three patients who presented with excessive thirst and polyuria.

	Posm Post–Water Deprivation	Uosm Post–Water Deprivation	Uosm Post–Intramuscular Injection of Vasopressin (ADH)
(A)	Increased	Decreased (<100)	Increased 80% over baseline Uosm
(B)	Normal	Increased (>500)	No change over baseline Uosm
(C)	Increased	Decreased (<100)	Increased 30% over baseline Uosm

13. A 4-year-old patient with bitemporal hemianopsia and a suprasellar, cystic mass with calcification.

Items 14–15

Match the following thyroid profile findings with the appropriate clinical condition.

	Serum T$_4$	T$_4$ BR*	FT$_4$-I†	TSH‡	^{131}I Uptake§
(A)	Increased	Increased	Increased	Decreased	Increased
(B)	Decreased	Increased	Normal	Normal	Normal
(C)	Increased	Decreased	Normal	Normal	Normal
(D)	Decreased	Decreased	Decreased	Increased	Decreased
(E)	Increased	Increased	Increased	Decreased	Decreased
(F)	Decreased	Decreased	Decreased	Decreased	Decreased

* T$_4$ binding ratio, which is the patient's resin T$_3$ uptake divided by 30.
† Free T$_4$ index.
‡ Thyroid-stimulating hormone.
§ Radioactive iodine-131 uptake.

14. A 40-year-old woman with atrial fibrillation, systolic hypertension, and diarrhea. She was being treated with a number of medications in a weight loss clinic that guaranteed fast results. Her physical examination is otherwise unremarkable. The thyroid is nonpalpable.

15. A 35-year-old woman who is taking birth control pills. She has a normal thyroid examination.

Items 16–17

Study the following chart relating serum calcium to PTH. The square box represents normal values.

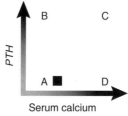

16. A patient with long-standing diabetes mellitus who now has chronic renal disease.

17. A 47-year-old woman with a history of a right radical mastectomy who complains of low back pain. An ECG reveals a short QT interval.

ANSWERS AND EXPLANATIONS

1. The answer is D: low serum TSH. The patient exhibits lid stare owing to retraction of the upper lid from increased sympathetic activity, which is consistent with Graves' disease. A suppressed serum TSH is the *sine qua non* of the diagnosis. Also note the recent surgical scar on the neck. You would also expect hypocholesterolemia (from increased synthesis of LDL receptors), hyperglycemia (from increased glycogenolysis), hypercalcemia (from increased bone turnover), and hypercalciuria (from increased bone turnover). (Photograph reproduced, with permission, from M.A. Mir. *Atlas of*

Clinical Diagnosis. Philadelphia, W.B. Saunders Co., 1995, p. 14.)

2. The answer is C: an increase in urine free cortisol. The patient exhibits truncal obesity with prominent striae on the lower abdomen consistent with Cushing's syndrome. Owing to excess production of cortisol, binding sites on transcortin are all filled and excess unbound (free) cortisol is filtered in the urine. An increase in urine free cortisol is the single best screening test for Cushing's. Additional findings would be hyperglycemia (from the gluconeogenic effect of cortisol), hyperten-

sion (from an increase in weak mineralocorticoids), lack of suppression of cortisol with the low-dose dexamethasone (cortisol analogue) suppression test, and elevated urine 17-ketosteroids due to increased production of dehydroepiandrosterone and androstenedione. (Photograph reproduced, with permission, from M.A. Mir. *Atlas of Clinical Diagnosis.* Philadelphia, W.B. Saunders Co., 1995, p. 10.)

3. The answer is A: a delayed Achilles tendon reflex. The patient has the classic facial puffiness of advanced hypothyroidism, which is most commonly caused by Hashimoto's autoimmune thyroiditis. Additional findings would likely be constipation, a history of cold intolerance (heat intolerance is present in thyrotoxicosis), diastolic hypertension (systolic hypertension is noted in thyrotoxicosis), and generalized obesity with pretibial myxedema (Cushing's syndrome exhibits truncal obesity). (Photograph reproduced, with permission, from M.A. Mir. *Atlas of Clinical Diagnosis.* Philadelphia, W.B. Saunders Co., 1995, p. 16.)

4. The answer is B: enlarged hands and feet. The patient has acromegaly, which is most often due to a functioning pituitary adenoma secreting excess growth hormone (GH). GH, in turn, stimulates the synthesis and release of somatomedin C from the liver, which is responsible for the enlargement of bones in her skull increasing her hat size. She would also have enlargement of her hands and feet. GH is responsible for diabetes mellitus because of its antiinsulin activity. Factors weighing against primary hypothyroidism are the increase in hat size and diabetes mellitus. Hence, one would not expect an elevated serum TSH or yellowish discoloration of the skin from lack of conversion of β-carotenes to vitamin A. A "buffalo hump" is characteristic of Cushing's syndrome, while carpal spasm indicates tetany, which is not a feature of acromegaly. (Photograph reproduced, with permission, from M.A. Mir. *Atlas of Clinical Diagnosis.* Philadelphia, W.B. Saunders Co., 1995, p. 78.)

5. The answer is B: a neoplastic transformation of the gland parenchyma. Given a history of irradiation to the head and neck area, a papillary adenocarcinoma is the most likely abnormality. This is confirmed by the presence of papillary structures and psammoma bodies (whorled concretions) in the microscopic section. Psammoma bodies are focal areas of dystrophic calcification in areas of tumor necrosis (from apoptosis). Regarding the other choices, (A) represents Hashimoto's thyroiditis, (C) thyroiditis (acute or subacute), (D) goiter, and (E) medullary carcinoma, which has no relationship to irradiation, papillary structures, or psammoma bodies. (Photomicrograph reproduced, with permission, from V.A. LiVolsi. *Surgical Pathology of the Thyroid.* Philadelphia, W.B. Saunders Co., 1995, p. 139.)

6. The answer is E: serum parathormone level. The patient most likely has primary hyperparathyroidism (HPTH). Renal stones are the most common symptomatic presentation. The laboratory abnormalities include an increase in serum PTH, hypercalcemia, hypophosphatemia, and a normal anion gap metabolic acidosis (PTH inhibits bicarbonate reabsorption in the kidneys). A bone marrow examination and bone scan are unnecessary in the workup of primary HPTH. A 24-hour urine collection for calcium (increased) and phosphorus (increased) are useful in the workup of any stone but would not confirm primary HPTH.

7. The answer is D: hypoalbuminemia. The total serum calcium represents calcium that is bound to albumin (40%) and other ions (13%) plus calcium that is free (ionized calcium), which is the metabolically active form. Hence, a decrease in albumin lowers the total calcium without affecting the ionized calcium level (no tetany). To correct for the effect of hypoalbuminemia, the following formula is used: corrected calcium = measured calcium − measured serum albumin + 4. Hypomagnesemia, the most common pathologic cause of hypocalcemia (magnesium is a cofactor in adenylate cyclase) in hospitalized patients, blocks the effect of PTH on calcium reabsorption, hence lowering the ionized calcium concentration. Hypovitaminosis D and hypoparathyroidism are uncommon causes of hypocalcemia. Respiratory alkalosis lowers the ionized calcium levels without altering the total serum calcium. Alkalosis increases negative charges on albumin, hence increasing the binding of calcium to the protein at the expense of lowering the ionized levels (tetany).

8. The answer is B: primary aldosteronism. Hypertension, muscle weakness, tetany (positive Chvostek's sign secondary to alkalosis), hypokalemia (U wave), hypernatremia, and metabolic alkalosis (increased bicarbonate) are characteristic of a mineralocorticoid excess state, most commonly primary aldosteronism (Conn's syndrome). Most cases are due to a benign adenoma arising from the zona glomerulosa. A pheochromocytoma is not associated with electrolyte abnormalities. Diabetes insipidus and Addison's disease demonstrate hypotension from hypovolemia. The inappropriate ADH syndrome is associated with severe hyponatremia.

9. The answer is A: metastasis. Both neuroblastomas and pheochromocytomas most commonly arise from the adrenal medulla. They are catecholamine-secreting tumors that produce hypertension and an increase in urine metanephrines and VMA. Neuroblastomas are malignant tumors that metastasize widely and are more common in children, whereas pheochromocytomas are benign and are more common in adults.

10. The answer is B: low urine 17-hydroxycorticoids. Addison's disease is primary hypocortisolism most commonly secondary to autoimmune destruction of the adrenal cortex, leading to glucocorticoid, mineralocorticoid, and sex hormone deficiencies. Secondary hypocortisolism is due to hypopituitarism, which results in deficiencies of glucocorticoids and sex hormones but not mineralocorticoids, since ACTH does not stimulate aldosterone release. Since both demonstrate glucocorticoid deficiency, the 17-OH are decreased in both (metabolites of deoxycortisol and cortisol). The plasma ACTH is high in Addison's and low in hypopituitarism. Hyponatremia rather than hypernatremia is present in both Addison's and hypopituitarism. Hyponatremia is most severe in Addison's (severe salt wasting in the urine) and less severe in hypopituitarism (mild inappropriate ADH syndrome). Hyperkalemia and hyperpigmentation (excess ACTH) are noted in Addison's and are not seen in hypopituitarism.

11. The answer is A: β-oxidation of fatty acids. The absence of insulin in DKA is counterbalanced by the presence of glucagon and other counterregulatory hormones. These latter hormones increase lipolysis of fat, leading to an increase in fatty acids and the β-oxidation of fatty acids in the mitochondria. One of the end products of β-oxidation is acetyl-CoA, which is converted in the liver to ketone bodies. Glycogenolysis and the conversion of glycerol to DHAP for use as a substrate in gluconeogenesis contribute to the hyperglycemia of

DKA. VLDL is often elevated in DKA owing to the absence of insulin, which normally degrades the lipoprotein by enhancing the synthesis of capillary lipoprotein lipase. Gluconeogenesis rather than glycolysis occurs in DKA; however, it does not contribute to ketoacidosis.

12. The answer is D: hyaline arteriolosclerosis. Nonenzymatic glycosylation (NEG) involves the combination of glucose with amino acids in proteins. This produces advanced glycosylation end products that increase vessel permeability to proteins in the plasma and enhance atherosclerosis. Hyaline arteriolosclerosis represents the effect of increased vessel permeability to proteins in arterioles. It is the most important vascular abnormality contributing to small-vessel disease in DM. Osmotic damage involves the conversion of glucose to sorbitol and fructose. Peripheral neuropathy (osmotic damage to Schwann cells), microaneurysms in the retina (damage to pericytes), and cataracts are all produced by osmotic damage. Osmotic diuresis is due to glucosuria.

13. The answer is A: Posm post–water deprivation increased, Uosm post–water deprivation decreased (< 100), Uosm post–intramuscular injection of vasopressin (ADH) increased 80% over baseline Uosm. The history in the child of a suprasellar mass with visual field defects and a cystic mass with calcification is indicative of a craniopharyngioma (which is of Rathke's pouch origin). Destruction of the posterior pituitary or invasion into the hypothalamus has produced a central diabetes insipidus (DI) with lack of antidiuretic hormone (ADH). The intramuscular administration of ADH has increased the baseline Uosm over 50% (80% in this case), hence qualifying the condition as a central DI. Patient B has psychogenic polydipsia, since the results indicate normal concentrating abilities. Patient C has nephrogenic DI, since the Uosm was < 45% from the baseline Uosm after ADH administration.

14. The answer is E: serum T_4 increased, T_4 BR increased, FT_4-I increased, TSH decreased, ^{131}I decreased. The patient has factitious hyperthyroidism from taking excess hormone. The key laboratory distinction from true hyperthyroidism (e.g., Graves' disease, choice A) is that the ^{131}I uptake is low because TSH is suppressed and the gland is atrophic. In Graves' disease, the ^{131}I uptake is increased owing to thyroid-stimulating immunoglobulin, which is an autoantibody against the receptor.

15. The answer is C: serum T_4 increased, T_4 BR decreased, FT_4-I normal, TSH normal, ^{131}I uptake normal. Estrogen in a birth control pill increases the synthesis of TBG, hence increasing the serum T_4. Since more binding sites are available with the extra TBG, the T_4 BR is decreased (less radioactive T_3 is left over), hence the FT_4-I is normal ($\uparrow$ serum $T_4 \times \downarrow T_4$ BR = normal FT_4-I). The TSH is normal because the free hormone level is normal. Patient B has a decrease in TBG (e.g., anabolic steroids), patient D has primary hypothyroidism, and patient F has secondary/tertiary hypothyroidism (pituitary/hypothalamic hypofunction).

16. The answer is B: increased PTH and decreased serum calcium. Chronic renal failure produces hypovitaminosis D (decreased second hydroxylation), leading to hypocalcemia, which is a stimulus for PTH and secondary hyperparathyroidism.

17. The answer is D: decreased PTH and increased serum calcium. The patient has metastatic breast cancer to the vertebral column, leading to hypercalcemia (short QT interval). Hypercalcemia lowers the patient's PTH. Patient A has primary hypoparathyroidism, and patient C has primary hyperparathyroidism.

CHAPTER TWENTY

DISORDERS OF

MUSCULOSKELETAL AND

SOFT TISSUE

SYNOPSIS

OBJECTIVES

1. To be conversant with synovial fluid analysis.
2. To be familiar with the most common arthritic conditions in group I to group III disorders of joint disease.
3. To understand the most common nonneoplastic and neoplastic diseases of bone.
4. To outline neurogenic, neuromuscular junction, and primary muscle disorders.
5. To review the nonneoplastic and neoplastic soft tissue tumors.

Objective 1: To discuss synovial fluid analysis.

I. Synovial fluid analysis
   A. Synovial fluid (SF) secreted by synoviocytes acts as a lubricant for joints (it is rich in hyaluronic acid) and nourishes articular cartilage.
   B. Routine studies performed on SF include gross appearance (e.g., normally pale yellow), WBC count and differential (normally < 200 cells/μL with neutrophils < 25% of the total count), crystal analysis, and culture and Gram's stain if infection is suspected.
   C. The most important crystals are **monosodium urate** (MSU) and **calcium pyrophosphate dihydrate** (CPPD) **crystals**, found in gout and pseudogout, respectively.
      1. MSU crystals are needle shaped (monoclinic), while CPPD crystals are either rhomboid (triclinic) or monoclinic.
      2. By using special filters (red compensator; background becomes red) and analyzers built into a microscope, the distinction between MSU and CPPD crystals can be made.
         a. When crystals are aligned parallel to the slow ray (axis) of the compensator, their color determines the type of crystal and indicates whether it is negatively or positively birefringent.
         b. If the crystal is **yellow** when parallel to the

slow ray, it is a **negatively birefringent MSU crystal**, whereas a **blue** color indicates a **positively birefringent CPPD crystal**.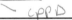

Objective 2: To be familiar with the most common arthritic conditions in group I to group III disorders of joint disease.

II. Group I joint disorders
   A. Osteoarthritis and neuropathic joint disease are examples of group I noninflammatory joint disease.
   B. **Osteoarthritis** (OA), the most common rheumatic disease and cause of joint disability in the United States, is characterized by progressive degeneration of articular cartilage.
      1. It is an age-dependent process that is universal after 65 years of age and is 10 times more common in women than in men.
      2. It primarily targets weight-bearing joints such as the hips and knees and the distal interphalangeal (DIP) joints of the hands.
      3. OA may be primary or secondary, the latter being a result of congenital hip dislocation in children, trauma, obesity, or other systemic disease (e.g., hemochromatosis).
      4. The most important factor that predisposes a joint to develop OA is the effect of an abnormal load placed on a weight-bearing joint.
         a. The articular surface reveals erosions and cleft formation, the latter occurring at right angles to the articular surface.
         b. The clefts penetrate the underlying subchondral bone in a process called **fibrillation**.
         c. Once articular cartilage is destroyed, bone rubs on bone, resulting in the formation of dense sclerotic bone resembling ivory (called **eburnation**).
         d. **Subchondral bone cysts** (visible on x-ray) develop beneath the articular surface.
         e. Reactive bone formation at the margins of the joints produce **osteophytes** (bony spurs).
            (1) Osteophytes are responsible for the "lipping"

269

found in the vertebral bodies on radiographs of the spine.

    (2) **Heberden's nodes** found at the base of the DIP joints of the fingers and **Bouchard's nodes** in the proximal interphalangeal (PIP) joints also represent osteophyte formation.

5. Clinically, patients with OA experience pain with passive motion of the joint (secondary synovitis) as well as joint stiffness and enlargement.

6. There are no specific laboratory alterations in OA.

C. **Neuropathic arthropathy** (**Charcot's joint**) is joint disease that develops secondary to a neurologic disease (e.g., diabetes mellitus [autonomic neuropathy], syringomyelia, tabes dorsalis).

II. Group II joint disorders

A. Group II joint disorders are characterized by noninfectious inflammation of the joints.

B. **Rheumatoid arthritis** (RA) and **juvenile rheumatoid arthritis** (JRA) are discussed in Chapter 4.

C. **Gouty arthritis** is male-dominant disease characterized by hyperuricemia, recurrent attacks of acute arthritis, and deposits of MSU (tophi) in soft tissue.

1. **Primary gout** is due to a disorder in the metabolism of uric acid (a by-product of purine metabolism), most commonly underexcretion of uric acid in the kidneys rather than overproduction.

2. **Secondary gout** may be due to diabetes mellitus, polycythemia vera, leukemia, diuretic therapy, or treatment of disseminated carcinoma.

3. The initial attack of **acute gouty arthritis** usually involves the metatarsophalangeal joint (big toe; called **podagra**).

    a. The inflammatory reaction is due to an interaction of MSU crystals with mononuclear phagocytes that stimulates their production of interleukin-1 (IL-1).

    b. IL-1 initiates the inflammatory reaction and is responsible for many of the systemic signs of the disease (e.g., fever).

    c. MSU crystals also lyse neutrophils, causing them to release lysosomal enzymes and free radicals, which contribute to the inflammatory reaction.

4. **Chronic gout** is defined by the presence of **tophi**, which usually develop after 10 years of the disease.

    a. Tophi represent deposits of MSU that occur in tissue most commonly around the affected joints.

    b. Sections through a tophus exhibit an exuberant granulomatous reaction complete with foreign body multinucleated giant cells surrounding a central core of amorphous MSU crystals.

5. Complications associated with gout include a deforming arthritis with erosion of cartilage and bone and renal disease (chronic interstitial nephritis, urolithiasis).

6. Laboratory diagnosis involves the demonstration of MSU crystals in SF rather than the presence of hyperuricemia.

7. The purpose of therapy (e.g., indomethacin, colchicine) in acute attacks is not to lower the uric acid level but to reduce inflammation.

    a. Colchicine inhibits the release of **leukocyte-derived crystal-induced chemotactic factor**, which initiates the inflammatory reaction in the joint when neutrophils phagocytose MSU crystals.

    b. Underexcretors of uric acid are treated with uricosuric agents such as probenecid or sulfinpyrazone.

    c. Overproducers of uric acid and patients with chronic gout (determined by the presence of tophi) are treated with allopurinol (which inhibits xanthine oxidase).

D. **Calcium pyrophosphate dihydrate crystal deposition arthropathy** (CPPD disease), or **pseudogout**, is a type of degenerative joint disease associated with the deposition of CPPD crystals in joints, most commonly the knee (> 50%).

1. The crystals deposit in articular cartilage (**chondrocalcinosis**), where they produce linear densities on radiographs.

2. Most patients experience progressive degeneration of the involved joints.

E. **Ankylosing spondylitis** (AS) is a seronegative (rheumatoid factor negative) spondyloarthropathy that targets young men between the ages of 15 and 30 years who are HLA-B27 positive (95% of cases).

1. It may also be associated with Reiter's syndrome, psoriasis, inflammatory bowel disease, and microbial pathogens.

2. It targets the sacroiliac joint (sacroiliitis is the first manifestation), vertebral column ("bamboo spine," or fusion of the vertebrae), aortic valves (aortic regurgitation), and uveal tract (uveitis).

F. **Reiter's syndrome** is a male-dominant seronegative spondyloarthropathy characterized by urethritis (usually due to *Chlamydia trachomatis*), conjunctivitis and an HLA-B27 positive arthritis.

G. **Psoriatic arthritis** is an HLA-B27 positive seronegative spondyloarthropathy that occurs in < 10% of patients with psoriasis.

H. **Enteropathic arthritis** refers to HLA-B27 positive arthritis associated with inflammatory bowel disease (e.g., ulcerative colitis [most common], Crohn's disease) or following gastroenteritis due to *Shigella, Campylobacter, Salmonella,* or *Yersinia* species.

IV. Group III joint disorders

A. These are inflammatory types of arthritis that are secondary to microbial pathogens (e.g., viruses [rubella], bacteria [*Staphylococcus aureus*], and fungi [coccidioidomycosis]).

B. **Infectious arthritis** may be secondary to hematogenous spread or osteomyelitis (particularly in children) or be a complication of intra-articular injection or surgery.

C. The majority of **nongonococcal** types of arthritis are due to *S. aureus,* most commonly in the knee.

D. **Gonococcal septic arthritis** is the most common overall cause of septic arthritis, particularly in urban populations.

1. It is usually associated with disseminated gonococcemia in asymptomatic young women, particularly those deficient in complement components C5 through C8.

2. Disseminated gonococcemia is associated with the following:

    a. Septic arthritis involving the knees, hands or feet.

    b. Tenosynovitis in the hands and feet.

    c. Dermatitis consisting of macules, papules, vesicles, or pustules on the hands and feet.

E. **Lyme disease** is a multisystem disease caused by a tick-borne (*Ixodes dammini*) spirochete called *Borrelia burgdorferi*.
1. In its early stages, there is a characteristic skin lesion called **erythema chronicum migrans**, which is a red, expanding lesion with concentric circles and a central area of clearing that develops at the site of the tick bite.
2. Later stages are associated with CNS disease (e.g., cranial nerve palsies, particularly bilateral Bell's palsy), cardiac abnormalities (e.g., myocarditis), or disabling joint disease (most commonly of the knee).
3. Serologic tests are available.
4. Tetracycline is the drug of choice in early stages, while ceftriaxone is utilized for later stages.

Objective 3: To understand the most common nonneoplastic and neoplastic diseases of bone.

V. Congenital disorders *[handwritten: brittle bone, blue sclera]*
A. **Osteogenesis imperfecta** (AD or AR inheritance), or brittle bone disease, is due to abnormal synthesis of type I collagen with resultant abnormalities in the skeleton (pathologic fractures), eyes (blue sclera), ears (deafness), joints, and teeth (defective dentine).
B. **Achondroplasia** (AD inheritance) is characterized by impaired enchondral ossification and premature closure of the epiphyseal plates of long bones, resulting in a normal-sized head and vertebral column but shortened arms and legs. *[handwritten: -dwarfism, -normal like span]*
C. **Osteopetrosis**, or "marble bone disease," is secondary to overgrowth and sclerosis of cortical bone ("too much bone") due to a defect in osteoclasts. *[handwritten: woven bone, white bone]*
1. There is gradual replacement of the marrow cavity by bone.
2. Pathologic fractures, anemia, cranial nerve compression (visual and hearing loss), and hydrocephalus are commonly present.
3. Bone marrow transplantation has been helpful owing to the introduction of normal osteoclasts.

VI. Osteoporosis
A. **Osteoporosis** is the most common metabolic abnormality of bone in the United States.
B. A reduction in normal mineralized bone (decreased bone mass) renders the bone subject to pathologic fractures.
C. It may be primary (e.g., postmenopausal) or secondary to an underlying disease (e.g., hypercortisolism) or medication (e.g., heparin).
D. **Postmenopausal osteoporosis** is secondary to estrogen deficiency.
1. Normally, estrogen serves to dampen the release of IL-1 (osteoclast-activating factor) from osteoblasts, hence its deficiency leads to greater breakdown of bone by osteoclasts than formation of bone by osteoblasts.
2. Patients may present with stress fractures of the vertebral bodies (most common fracture) or Colles' fractures of the distal radius (second most common fracture).
3. Diagnosis is confirmed by studies that evaluate bone density (e.g., **dual-photon absorptiometry**) and bone turnover (e.g., increased urinary concentration of **osteocalcin** and **pyridinium collagen cross-links**).

4. Estrogen therapy is the gold standard for prevention.
   a. Since unopposed estrogen increases the incidence of endometrial carcinoma, the addition of progesterone is recommended.
   b. An additional benefit is a 50% reduction in the incidence of ischemic heart disease.
   c. Additional preventive measures include calcium and vitamin D supplementation and weight-bearing exercise (this does not include swimming).
   d. Bisphosphonates (potent inhibitors of bone resorption) and calcitonin-salmon (which inhibits osteoclasts) are used in treatment.

VII. Infectious disorders
A. Infection of the bone marrow and bone is called **osteomyelitis**.
B. **Pyogenic osteomyelitis** most frequently targets children and young adults.
1. It is most commonly secondary to hematogenous spread of *S. aureus* to the metaphysis of bone (e.g., femur, tibia).
2. In **acute osteomyelitis**, neutrophils enzymatically destroy bone and leave behind devitalized portions of bone called **sequestra**.
3. **Chronic disease** is characterized by extensive reactive bone formation in the periosteum called **involucrum**.
4. **Brodie's abscess** is a type of osteomyelitis that becomes encapsulated and surrounded by dense sclerotic bone.
5. Complications of osteomyelitis include draining sinus tracts to the skin and squamous cell carcinoma within the sinus tract.
6. Patients with **sickle cell anemia** often develop osteomyelitis secondary to infection by *Salmonella* species, but *S. aureus* is the most common pathogen.
C. **Tuberculous osteomyelitis** is most commonly secondary to hematogenous extension from a primary focus in the lung and primarily targets the vertebral column (called **Pott's disease**).
D. *Pasteurella multocida* (a gram-negative rod) infection is associated with dog and cat bites; it may produce tendinitis, septic arthritis, and osteomyelitis.
E. Nail punctures through rubber footwear may be associated with *Pseudomonas aeruginosa* infection of the soft tissue and bone.

VIII. Avascular (aseptic) necrosis of bone
A. Avascular necrosis occurs when the microcirculation within bone is disrupted, leading to bone infarction.
B. The most common location is the femoral head in an elderly patient with a femoral head fracture.
C. Other disorders that predispose to aseptic necrosis of the femoral head include SLE, where patients are on long-term corticosteroid therapy, and sickle cell disease.
D. The bone has increased density on x-ray (MRI has highest sensitivity).
E. It may involve the ossification centers of various bones in children (called **osteochondrosis**) an example of which is **Legg-Calvé-Perthes disease** involving the femoral head.
1. It is more common in males than in females in the age range of 3 to 10 years.

benign—asymptomatic—resolves spon. (handwritten)

2. Secondary OA commonly occurs after many years.

IX. Nonneoplastic disorders of bone
  A. **Paget's disease of bone** (**osteitis deformans**) is an increased thickness of abnormal bone.
    1. It mainly occurs in elderly males and is of unknown etiology.
    2. It targets the pelvis, skull, and femur, in decreasing order of frequency.
    3. Initially, there is a phase of excessive osteoclastic resorption of bone, followed by a phase of excessive bone formation (increased alkaline phosphatase) with the production of thick, weak bone (mosaic bone) without a normal lamellar structure.
    4. The majority of patients are first recognized by the presence of an unexpectedly high serum alkaline phosphatase level on a biochemical profile. *↑ urinary hydroxyproline* (handwritten)
    5. Complications include pathologic fractures, head enlargement, and an increased risk for osteogenic sarcomas.
  B. **Fibrous dysplasia** is a benign, nonneoplastic process of bone that primarily targets children and young adults. *local dev't arrest* (handwritten)
    1. It may involve a single bone (monostotic) or many bones (polyostotic), the latter called *McCune* (handwritten) **Albright's syndrome** when associated with abnormal skin pigmentation and precocious sexual development.
    2. The ribs, femur, and cranial bones are primarily involved.
    3. There is a replacement of marrow by **woven bone** that lacks the normal lamellar pattern (and is subject to pathologic fractures).
  C. **Fibrous cortical defects** and **nonossifying fibromas** are essentially the same disease except for a difference in size (1–4 cm and 5–10 cm, respectively).
    1. Both lesions typically occur in children, and both involve the cortical aspect of the metaphysis of long bones, such as the femur, tibia, and fibula, in descending order of frequency.

    2. The lesion is recognized radiographically as an irregular, sharply demarcated radiolucent defect in the metaphyseal cortex.
  D. An **aneurysmal bone cyst** (ABC) is a benign condition that may arise *de novo* (primary ABC) or most commonly in association with another bone tumor (secondary ABC; e.g., giant cell tumor of bone).

X. Neoplastic disorders of bone
  A. The most common primary bone tumors, in order of increasing patient age, are Ewing's sarcoma, osteogenic sarcoma, chondrosarcoma, and multiple myeloma.
  B. The most common primary malignant tumors of bone, in descending order of frequency, are multiple myeloma, osteogenic sarcoma, chondrosarcoma, Ewing's sarcoma, and giant cell tumor of bone.
  C. Metastasis is the most common malignancy of bone, with breast cancer the most common primary site of origin.
  D. Tables 20–1 and 20–2 summarize the important cartilage and bone-forming tumors, respectively.
  E. **Ewing's sarcoma** is a highly malignant primary bone tumor of marrow origin that most frequently targets children in the first and second decades of life.
    1. It exhibits a primitive neural phenotype and is associated with a t(11;22) translocation.
    2. The femur, flat bones of the pelvis, and tibia are the most common locations.
    3. It is a "round cell" tumor like metastatic neuroblastoma, metastatic malignant lymphoma, and acute lymphoblastic leukemia.
    4. It presents as an infection with fever, localized heat over the tumor, anemia, and an increased erythrocyte sedimentation rate.
  F. **Giant cell tumors** are benign bone tumors that arise in the epiphysis and extend into the metaphysis.
    1. Favored locations are first the distal end of the femur and next the proximal end of the tibia.
    2. They have a nonneoplastic component consisting of multinucleated giant cells and a neoplastic mononuclear fibroblast-like cell that determines the biologic behavior of the tumor.

TABLE 20–1.   Cartilaginous Tumors of Bone

Name	Age/Sex	Location	Comments
Osteochondroma	Children and adolescents. Slight male dominance.	Metaphysis of long bones.	**Most common benign bone tumor.** Lobulated outgrowth of bone (exostoses) capped by benign proliferating cartilage. Solitary or multiple (osteochondromatosis; AD disease). Chondrosarcoma risk greatest with multiple tumors.
Enchondroma *Chondroma / Exostosis* (handwritten)	Children and adolescents. No sex difference.	Tubular bones in hand. Arises in medullary cavity.	Benign tumor. Solitary or multiple (enchondromatosis). Chondrosarcoma risk greatest with multiple tumors. **Ollier's disease:** multiple enchondromas. **Maffucci's syndrome:** multiple enchondromas plus angiomas of soft tissue.
Chondroblastoma	10–20 years old. Male dominant.	Epiphysis of distal end femur, proximal tibia, humerus.	Benign tumor. "Popcorn" appearance on radiographs. Extends into metaphysis.
Chondrosarcoma	>30 years old. Male dominant.	Pelvic bones (most common), upper end femur, humerus.	**Most common primary malignant cartilaginous tumor.** Arises *de novo* or secondary to osteochondromatosis or enchondromatosis. Grade determines biologic behavior. Low grade, 90% 10-year survival. High grade, <50% 10-year survival. Many different variants. Metastasizes to lungs.

TABLE 20–2. Bone-forming Tumors

Name	Age/Sex	Location	Comments
Osteoma	>40 years old. Male dominant.	Skull: sinuses (most common), jaws, facial bones.	Benign tumor. Association with **Gardner's syndrome** (AD polyposis syndrome).
Osteoid osteoma	5–25 years old. Male dominant.	Proximal femur. Cortex of bone.	Benign tumor. Radiograph exhibits small radiolucent focus (nidus) surrounded by densely sclerotic bone. **Nocturnal pain relieved by aspirin.**
Osteoblastoma	<30 years old. Male dominant.	Vertebra (most common), long bone.	Benign tumor. "Giant osteoid osteoma." Pain not worse at night and not relieved by aspirin.
Osteogenic sarcoma *(Osteosarcoma)*	10–25 years old. Male dominant.	Metaphysis of distal end femur (most common), upper end tibia.	**Second most common primary malignant tumor of bone.** Arises *de novo* or secondary to other conditions. **Risk factors:** Paget's disease of bone irradiation, bone infarct, retinoblastoma. In patient >40 years old usually secondary to above risk factors. Destruction of metaphysis and invasion of subjacent soft tissue with elevation of periosteum, producing **Codman's triangle** on x-ray. "**Sunburst**" appearance from calcified osteoid extending into soft tissue. Many different variants. Long-term survival in 65–80% with newer limb-saving techniques and chemotherapy. Metastasizes to lung (tumor frequently surgically removed).

Objective 4: To outline neurogenic, neuromuscular junction, and primary muscle disorders.

XI. Muscle disorders
  A. **Type I fibers** are slow-twitch fibers (red muscle) that are rich in mitochondria and oxidative enzymes and have a great capacity for long, sustained contraction without fatigue (e.g. soleus muscle).
  B. **Type II fibers** are fast-twitch fibers (white muscle) that are poor in mitochondria, are geared for anaerobic glycolysis, and respond to training with hypertrophy (e.g., biceps muscle).
  C. **Muscle weakness** may be secondary to diseases involving the motor neuron pathways (e.g., amyotrophic lateral sclerosis), neuromuscular synapse (e.g., myasthenia gravis), or the muscle itself (e.g., Duchenne's muscular dystrophy).
  D. **Neurogenic atrophy** occurs when a motor neuron or its axon degenerates, leading to atrophy of both type I and II fibers.
  E. **Muscular dystrophy** (MD) is an inherited progressive primary muscle disease that most commonly presents in early childhood.
    1. Duchenne's MD is the most common type in children, while myotonic dystrophy is most frequent in adults.
    2. The dystrophies are summarized in Table 20–3.
  F. **Congenital myopathies** are rare primary nonprogressive muscle diseases that present at birth with poor muscle tone (e.g., central core disease, nemaline [rod] myopathy).
  G. **Polymyositis** and **dermatomyositis** are reviewed in Chapter 4.
  H. **Myasthenia gravis** (MG) is an autoimmune disease characterized by a reduction in acetylcholine receptors due to the presence of an autoantibody against the receptors (type II hypersensitivity reaction).
    1. It is more likely to afflict women in the second and third decades and men in the sixth and seventh decades of life.
    2. Acetylcholine receptor antibody accelerates degradation of the receptor, blocks receptor function, or destroys the receptor in unison with complement activation.
    3. Approximately 85% of patients have thymic hyperplasia with germinal follicles, representing B-cell proliferation (site of antibody synthesis), while another 15% may have thymomas.
    4. Ptosis and diplopia are the most common initial presentation.
    5. The diagnosis is made by performing the edrophonium (Tensilon) test (Tensilon inhibits acetylcholinesterase and reverses muscle weakness) and by ordering an antiacetylcholine receptor antibody assay.
    6. Treatment may include the use of anticholinesterase drugs (e.g., pyridostigmine), surgical thymectomy (which results in improvement in most cases), immunosuppression (via corticosteroids), and plasmapheresis (to remove the antibody).

Objective 5: To review the nonneoplastic and neoplastic soft tissue tumors.

XII. Soft tissue disorders
  A. **Fibromatosis** comprises a group of nonneoplastic, proliferative connective tissue disorders that infiltrate tissue (usually muscle) and commonly recur after surgical excision.
    1. **Dupuytren's contracture**, the most common fibromatosis, involves the palms of the hands, where it causes the contraction of the fingers (usually the fourth and fifth); it is commonly associated with alcoholism.
    2. A **desmoid tumor** is a fibromatosis of the anterior abdominal wall in females that may be associated with previous trauma, multiple pregnancy, or Gardner's syndrome (AD polyposis syndrome).
  B. The soft tissue tumors are summarized in Table 20–4.

TABLE 20–3.   Summary of Muscular Dystrophy (MD)

Type/ Inheritance	Pathogenesis	Pathologic Features	Clinical Findings	Laboratory Findings
Duchenne's SXR (70%) or new mutation	Defect in **dystrophin,** which anchors actin to the membrane glycoprotein. Severity of muscle disease relates to type of dystrophin defect: (1) no production (Duchenne type), (2) provides anchorage but defective elsewhere in the protein (mild disease: **Becker type**).	Progressive degeneration of type I and II fibers. Attempt at regeneration and repair (prominent nucleoli). Fiber necrosis and macrophage phagocytosis. Progressive fibrosis and infiltration of muscle tissue by fatty tissue **(pseudohypertrophy of calf muscle)**.	Most common and severe MD. Presents in second to fifth year of life as weakness and wasting of proximal pelvic muscles ("waddling gait"; difficulty in standing up; placing hand on the knee to help stand ([Gower's sign]) and of shoulder girdle muscles. Progressive disablement by 10 years of age. Death by 20 years of age. May affect cardiac muscle (common cause of death).	Antenatal diagnosis possible (dystrophin defect) using recombinant DNA technology. Serum CK increased at birth (no clinical signs of disease). Serum CK declines as muscle tissue is progressively replaced by fat and fibrous tissue. **Female carriers** have elevated serum CK activity (70% of cases), and dystrophin defect can be identified.
Myotonic AD	Triplet repeat of CTG on chromosome 19, which codes for a protein kinase.	Selective atrophy of type I fibers and hypertrophy of type II fibers. Internalization of nuclei in muscle.	Most common adult MD. Initial presentation in adolescence with facial weakness (mouth hangs open) and distal extremity muscle weakness. Myotonia (inability to relax muscles [sustained grip]), frontal balding, cataracts, testicular atrophy, facial muscle wasting, and cardiac involvement.	Increased serum CK.

TABLE 20–4. Summary of Soft Tissue Tumors

Type	Location	Comments
Lipomatous Tumors		
Lipoma	Trunk, neck, proximal extremities	**Most common benign soft tissue tumor.** Arises in subcutaneous tissue. No clinical significance. Most do not transform into sarcoma. **Generalized lipomatosis (Dercum's disease):** multiple lipomas in subcutaneous tissue which, on rare occasions, may transform into liposarcoma.
Liposarcoma	Thigh, retroperitoneum	Most commonly occurs in men (70%) >50 years of age. **Second most common sarcoma.** Lipoblasts can be identified with fat stains. Myxoid type is the most common variant. Low-grade cancers are slow to metastasize (75% 5-year survival), while high-grade cancers are more aggressive (20% 5-year survival).
Fibrous Tissue Tumors		
Fibrosarcoma	Thigh, upper limb	Most commonly occurs in men (60%). May arise after irradiation (5–15 years later). Malignant fibroblasts produce a "herringbone" (interlacing) pattern. Has 40–50% 5-year survival.
Fibrohistiocytic Tumors		
Dermatofibroma	Lower extremities	Elevated, red nodule that umbilicates (has a central dimple) when squeezed. Benign, nonencapsulated proliferation of spindle cells confined to the dermis.
Dermatofibrosarcoma protuberans	Chest wall, trunk	Low-grade malignant tumor that grows large and ulcerates. "Cartwheel" pattern of spindle cells with increased mitotic activity.
Malignant fibrous histiocytoma	Thigh, retroperitoneum	**Most common sarcoma and soft tissue sarcoma associated with radiation therapy or surgical scars.** Occurs in older adults, usually men (70%). Prognosis depends on grade.
Skeletal Muscle Tumors		
Rhabdomyoma	Heart	Association with tuberous sclerosis (AD inheritance).
Embryonal rhabdomyosarcoma	Vagina, bladder in males, head and neck area	**Most common sarcoma in children and most common striated muscle malignancy.** Botryoid type presents as grape-like masses protruding from vagina or male urethra. Rhabdomyoblasts have cross-striations and stain positive for desmin. Intermediate prognosis.
Alveolar rhabdomyosarcoma	Distal extremities	Occurs between 10 and 25 years of age. Second most common type of skeletal muscle malignancy and has the worst prognosis.
Pleomorphic rhabdomyosarcoma	Thigh	Least common type of skeletal muscle malignancy and has the best prognosis.
Smooth Muscle Tumors		
Leiomyoma	Extremities, retroperitoneum	Uncommon as a soft tissue tumor but very common in organ pathology. Most common tumor in women and most commonly located in myometrium of uterus. Most common benign GI tumor and most commonly located in the stomach. May also arise from subcutaneous tissue or the wall of blood vessels. Rarely, if ever, progresses to leiomyosarcoma.
Leiomyosarcoma	Extremities, retroperitoneum	Most commonly arises from wall of blood vessels. Atypical mitoses and increased mitotic count differentiate it from cellular leiomyoma. Majority eventually metastasize. **Most common sarcoma in the GI tract and uterus.**
Neural Tumors		
Neurofibroma		See Chapter 7.
Neurilemmoma (schwannoma, acoustic neuroma)		See Chapter 22.
Neurofibrosarcoma	Major nerve trunks (sciatic)	Most arise in conjunction with type I neurofibromatosis.
Vascular Tumors		See Chapter 10.
Tumors of Unknown Histogenesis		
Synovial sarcoma	Lower and upper extremities	Not derived from synovial tissue. Located around rather than in the joint. Male dominant tumor between 25 and 35 years of age. Biphasic pattern with a sarcomatous stroma (one pattern) and gland-like spaces (second pattern) mimicking a synovial membrane. About 50% 5-year survival.

QUESTIONS

DIRECTIONS. (Items 1–10): Each of the numbered items or incomplete statements in this section is followed by answers or by completions of the statement. Select the ONE lettered answer or completion that is BEST in each case. Correct answers and explanations are given at the end of the chapter.

1. The patient is a 55-year-old man who first noticed problems with facial weakness and handgrip as an adolescent. At present he has heart disease and blurry vision from cataracts. The pathogenesis of his disease most closely relates to

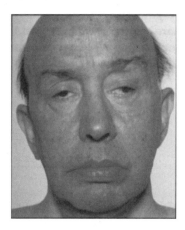

   (A) a defect in dystrophin
   (B) an inflammatory myopathy
   (C) autoantibodies against acetylcholine receptors
   (D) triplet repeats on chromosome 19
   (E) amyotrophic lateral sclerosis

2. The patient is a 35-year-old man who presented to his physician with a complaint of double vision, muscle weakness, and fatigue that improved with rest. A chest x-ray revealed a mass in the anterior mediastinum. The mechanism for this patient's disease most closely relates to

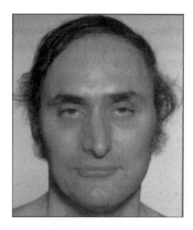

   (A) a defect in dystrophin
   (B) an inflammatory myopathy
   (C) autoantibodies against acetylcholine receptors
   (D) triplet repeats on chromosome 19
   (E) amyotrophic lateral sclerosis

3. The patient is a 50-year-old man who has had problems with his back since age 22. He states that the problem started with pain in his lower back when he got up in the morning, and over time the pain involved other parts of his spine. Which of the following best describes this patient's disease?

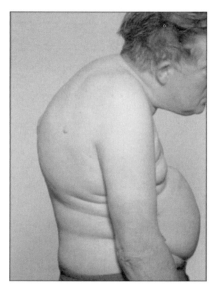

   (A) Spondyloarthropathy
   (B) Reduction in bone mass
   (C) Variant of rheumatoid arthritis
   (D) Noninflammatory joint disease
   (E) Defect in type I collagen synthesis

4. The photograph is of a finger of a 50-year-old woman who complains of tenderness around the distal joint. She also complains of problems with her right hip, which requires her to walk with a cane. The pathogenesis of this patient's disease is best described as

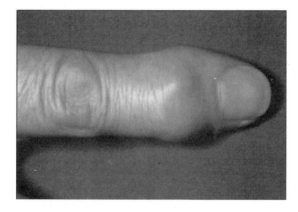

   (A) a defect in purine metabolism
   (B) degeneration of articular cartilage
   (C) destruction of articular cartilage by pannus
   (D) spondyloarthropathy associated with psoriasis
   (E) a defect in osteoclast function

5. These are the hands of a 55-year-old man with a history of alcohol abuse. The lesions in both hands are in the same group of disorders as

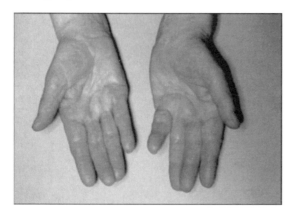

(A) Ehlers-Danlos syndrome
(B) rheumatoid arthritis
(C) fibrosarcoma
(D) fibrous dysplasia
(E) desmoid tumors

6. The patient is a 30-year-old man who presents with fever and pain in his foot. He has the smell of alcohol on his breath. His problem is most closely related to

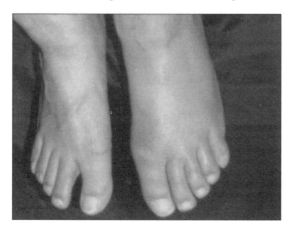

(A) joint inflammation secondary to a negatively birefringent crystal
(B) disseminated gonococcemia with septic arthritis
(C) a tick bite with subsequent development of infectious arthritis
(D) osteomyelitis secondary to hematogenous spread of *Staphylococcus aureus*
(E) an HLA-B27 positive spondyloarthropathy secondary to *Chlamydia trachomatis*

7. The photograph is of a wet preparation of synovial fluid aspirated from an inflamed right knee joint of a 60-year-old man. An x-ray of the joint exhibits linear densities in the articular cartilage. The pathogenesis of this patient's disease most closely relates to

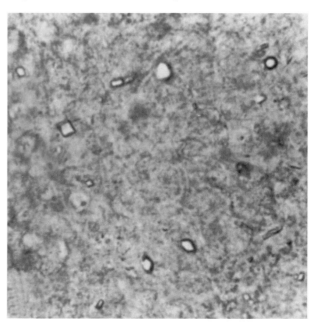

(A) deposition of monosodium urate in the articular cartilage
(B) synovial tissue proliferation with destruction of the articular cartilage
(C) deposition of a positively birefringent crystal in the articular cartilage
(D) septic arthritis secondary to *Staphylococcus aureus*
(E) age-dependent degeneration of articular cartilage

8. Which of the following characterizes the joint disease of rheumatoid arthritis rather than of osteoarthritis?

(A) Cartilage fibrillation
(B) Subchondral bone cysts
(C) Osteophytes
(D) Ankylosis of the joint
(E) Female dominance

9. The mechanism of postmenopausal osteoporosis is most closely associated with

(A) a reduction in the number of osteoblasts
(B) an increase in the number of osteoclasts
(C) decreased mineralization of bone
(D) greater osteoclastic than osteoblastic activity in bone
(E) lack of exercise and reduced remodeling of bone

10. A 3-year-old boy, who was normal at birth, is having difficulty in standing up and must push with his hands on his knees in order to stand. He has a peculiar duck-like walk. The pathogenesis of his disease is most closely related to

(A) an autosomal recessive disease
(B) triplet repeats on the X chromosome
(C) defective anchorage of actin to the membrane gly-coprotein
(D) a congenital myopathy
(E) a neuromuscular junction defect

DIRECTIONS (Items 11–13): Each set of matching questions in this section consists of a list of lettered options followed by several numbered items. For each numbered item, select the ONE option that is most closely associated with it. Each lettered option may be selected once, more than once, or not at all.

(A) Paget's disease
(B) Osteochondroma
(C) Enchondroma
(D) Chondroblastoma
(E) Chondrosarcoma
(F) Osteoma
(G) Osteoid osteoma
(H) Osteoblastoma
(I) Osteogenic sarcoma
(J) Ewing's sarcoma
(K) Giant cell tumor of bone
(L) Lipoma
(M) Liposarcoma
(N) Malignant fibrous his-tiocytoma
(O) Rhabdomyosarcoma
(P) Leiomyoma
(Q) Leiomyosarcoma
(R) Synovial sarcoma

11. An 18-year-old male complains of pain in the right knee. A radiograph reveals a mass in the metaphysis of the distal femur with extension into the soft tissue. The periosteum is raised, and calcifications are noted in the soft tissue component of the tumor.

12. A 60-year-old man complains of hip pain and head-aches. He states that his hat size has increased. A skull x-ray reveals increased thickening of bone. A biochemical profile reveals a markedly elevated serum alkaline phosphatase and a normal serum γ-glutamyltransferase.

13. A 65-year-old man with a history of pelvic irradiation for a non-Hodgkin's malignant lymphoma 10 years ago presents with bilateral hydronephrosis and renal failure. A CT scan reveals a large retroperitoneal mass. A CT-directed thin-needle biopsy of the mass reveals a malignant soft tissue tumor.

ANSWERS AND EXPLANATIONS

1. The answer is D: triplet repeats on chromosome 19. The patient has frontal balding, an expressionless face, bilateral ptosis, and a history of cataracts (blurry vision), cardiac disease, and difficulties with his handgrip (myotonia, or a sustained handgrip). These findings are compatible with myotonic dystrophy, an AD disease with a triplet repeat of CTG on chromosome 19. A defect in dystrophin is Duchenne's muscular dystrophy, which most commonly occurs in childhood. Inflammatory myopathy presents with muscle pain. Autoantibodies against acetylcholine receptors occur in myasthenia gravis, which is not associated with the other problems noted in the patient. Amyotrophic lateral sclerosis demonstrates both upper and lower motor neuron disease, which are not evident in this patient. (Photograph reproduced, with permission, from M.A. Mir. *Atlas of Clinical Diagnosis*. Philadelphia, W.B. Saunders Co., 1995, p. 29.)

2. The answer is C: autoantibodies against acetylcholine receptors. The history of diplopia, fatigue and muscle weakness that improves with resting, and radiographic evidence of an anterior mediastinal mass strongly suggests myasthenia gravis with either thymic hyperplasia (most common) or a thymoma (15% of cases). Note that the patient has drooping of both eyelids, which is the first muscle group to become involved. Eye muscle weakness is responsible for diplopia (double vision). MG is an autoimmune disease with antibodies directed against acetylcholine receptors. See question 1 regarding the other choices. (Photograph reproduced, with permission, from M.A. Mir. *Atlas of Clinical Diagnosis*. Philadelphia, W.B. Saunders Co., 1995, p. 29.)

3. The answer is A: spondyloarthropathy. The patient exhibits severe kyphosis (anterior flexion of the spine) secondary to ankylosing spondylitis, a rheumatoid factor negative, HLA-B27 positive spondyloarthropathy. The initial history of lower lumbar pain in the morning (sacroiliitis and muscle spasm) progressing to complete fusion of his vertebral column ("bamboo spine") is characteristic. This is not an example of osteoporosis (reduced bone mass), a defect in type I collagen synthesis (osteogenesis imperfecta), or a variant of rheumatoid arthritis. It is a group II inflammatory type of joint disease. (Photograph reproduced, with permission, from M.A. Mir. *Atlas of Clinical Diagnosis*. Philadelphia, W.B. Saunders Co., 1995, p. 143.)

4. The answer is B: degeneration of articular cartilage. The enlargement of the DIP joint is called Heberden's node, which is a characteristic finding in osteoarthritis (OA). The joint enlargement is secondary to secondary synovitis and the presence of osteophytes at the margins of the degenerating articular cartilage. The patient's history suggests involvement of the weight-bearing joint in her right hip as well. The characteristic location of the joint involvement argues against rheumatoid arthritis (choice C), which normally involves the MCP and PIP joints and also against gout (choice A). There is no evidence of nail pitting to suggest psoriatic arthritis (D). It is not an example of osteopetrosis (E), which is a AD or AR disease with a defect in osteoclastic function. (Photograph reproduced, with permission, from M.A. Mir. *Atlas of Clinical Diagnosis*. Philadelphia, W.B. Saunders Co., 1995, p. 166.)

5. The answer is E: desmoid tumors. The patient has bilat-

eral Dupuytren's contracture, which is a fibromatosis characterized by a nonneoplastic proliferation of connective tissue in the palmar fascia with subsequent contraction of the digits. It is commonly seen in patients with alcoholism, but may also occur in elderly patients and those with diabetes mellitus, gout or epilepsy. A desmoid tumor is also a fibromatosis; however, it most commonly involves the anterior abdominal wall in females. Ehlers-Danlos syndrome is associated with defects in collagen synthesis. Rheumatoid arthritis is an inflammatory joint disease. A fibrosarcoma is a malignancy that involves the thigh or deep tissue of the upper extremity. Fibrous dysplasia is a nonneoplastic disorder of bone and does not commonly involve the hands. (Photograph reproduced, with permission, from M.A. Mir. *Atlas of Clinical Diagnosis*. Philadelphia, W.B. Saunders Co., 1995, p. 192.)

6. The answer is A: joint inflammation secondary to a negatively birefringent crystal. The metatarsophalangeal joint of his left big toe is inflamed. It is the classic location for acute gouty arthritis, which may be triggered by drinking alcohol. MSU crystals are negatively birefringent, which means that they are yellow when they are aligned parallel to the slow ray (axis) of the compensator on a microscope. Although disseminated gonorrhea does affect the joints of the foot, the location of this joint involvement is more suggestive of gout. Lyme disease (choice C) does not usually localize to the big toe. Osteomyelitis most commonly targets the femur and tibia. Reiter's syndrome (choice E) is associated with urethritis, conjunctivitis, and an HLA-B27 positive spondylitis. (Photograph reproduced, with permission, from M.A. Mir. *Atlas of Clinical Diagnosis*. Philadelphia, W.B. Saunders Co., 1995, p. 232.)

7. The answer is C: deposition of a positively birefringent crystal in the articular cartilage. The history of linear densities in the articular cartilage of the knee (chondrocalcinosis) and the rhomboid-shaped crystals (triclinic crystals) in the wet preparation is compatible with calcium pyrophosphate dihydrate crystal deposition arthropathy (CPPD disease), or pseudogout. CPPD crystals are blue when they are aligned parallel to the slow axis of a compensator, which defines positive birefringence. These synovial fluid findings and crystals are not present in gouty arthritis (needle-shaped crystals; choice A), rheumatoid arthritis (choice B), septic arthritis (choice D), or osteoarthritis (choice E). (Photomicrograph reproduced, with permission, from J.B. Henry. *Clinical Diagnosis and Management by Laboratory Methods,* 18th ed. Philadelphia, W.B. Saunders Co., 1991, p. 461.)

8. The answer is D: ankylosis of the joint. Rheumatoid arthritis (RA) is an immunologic disorder characterized by the proliferation of inflamed synovial tissue that grows over articular cartilage (pannus) with subsequent release of enzymes that degrade bone and cartilage. Reactive fibrosis leads to fusion (ankylosis) of the joint and immobility. OA is a noninflammatory joint disease with progressive degeneration of articular cartilage associated with cartilage fibrillation, subchondral bone cysts, osteophytes, and a secondary synovitis leading to reduced joint mobility without fusion. Both RA and OA are female-dominant diseases.

9. The answer is D: greater osteoclastic than osteoblastic activity in bone. In osteoporosis, there is a reduction in normal mineralized bone (decreased bone mass) owing to a deficiency of estrogen. Normally, estrogen serves to dampen the release of interleukin-1 (osteoclast-activating factor) from osteoblasts, hence its deficiency leads to greater breakdown of bone by osteoclasts than formation of bone by osteoblasts. Decreased mineralization of bone describes osteomalacia, which results in an increased thickening of the osteoid seams. Although lack of exercise does reduce remodeling of bone, it is not the primary mechanism of postmenopausal osteoporosis. Alteration in the number of osteoblasts or osteoclasts is not the primary abnormality responsible for postmenopausal osteoporosis.

10. The answer is C: defective anchorage of actin to the membrane glycoprotein. The patient has the classic findings of Duchenne's muscular dystrophy, which is an SXR disease. There is a defect in dystrophin, which normally anchors actin to the membrane glycoprotein. The children are normal at birth but by 2–5 years of age they experience problems with standing up or walking owing to weakness in the pelvic girdle musculature. The genetic defect is not a triplet repeat abnormality as in myotonic dystrophy in adults. It is not a congenital myopathy, which comprises nonprogressive diseases that are evident at birth. It is not a neuromuscular junction defect like myasthenia gravis.

11. The answer is I: osteogenic sarcoma. The age of the patient, the location of the tumor in the distal end of the femur, elevation of the periosteum (Codman's triangle), and calcification in the soft tissue component (sunburst appearance) are most compatible with an osteogenic sarcoma. After multiple myeloma, it is the second most common primary malignancy of bone.

12. The answer is A: Paget's disease. Paget's disease of bone is associated with increased thickness of abnormal bone (mosaic bone) that does not have the structural integrity of lamellar bone. In decreasing order of frequency, it targets the pelvis, skull, and femur. The patient is in the osteoblastic phase of the disease, hence the elevation of serum alkaline phosphatase. The normal γ-glutamyltransferase indicates that the alkaline phosphatase is of bone rather than liver origin. The patient is at risk for pathologic fractures and osteogenic sarcoma.

13. The answer is N: malignant fibrous histiocytoma. Malignant fibrous histiocytoma is the most common adult sarcoma and the one most commonly associated with previous irradiation. The retroperitoneum is a favored location for the tumor.

CHAPTER TWENTY-ONE

DISORDERS OF THE SKIN

SYNOPSIS

OBJECTIVES

1. To understand the pathogenesis of eczema and dermatitis.
2. To review maculopapular and papulosquamous disorders of the skin.
3. To discuss vesiculobullous and pustular disorders of the skin.
4. To review skin disorders that present with urticaria, cellulitis, or atrophy.
5. To be familiar with nodular and cystic disorders of the skin.
6. To discuss melanocytic disorders of the skin.
7. To understand the pathogenesis of the most common porphyrias.

Objective 1: To understand the pathogenesis of eczema and dermatitis.

I. Normal skin
   A. The epidermis is composed of the following layers:
      1. **Stratum basale** contains actively dividing stem cells along the basement membrane.
      2. **Stratum spinosum** has prominent desmosome attachments.
      3. **Stratum granulosum** is a granular layer with keratohyaline granules.
      4. **Stratum corneum** contains anucleate cells with keratin.
   B. The **dermis** is subdivided into the **papillary** and **reticular** dermis.
II. Eczema and dermatitis
   A. **Eczema** comprises a large group of skin lesions characterized by pruritus and distinctive gross and microscopic features.
      1. Eczema has acute, subacute, and chronic stages.
         a. **Acute eczema** is characterized by a weeping, erythematous rash with vesicle formation and by spongiosis (intercellular edema) in the epidermis.
         b. **Subacute eczema** is associated with crusts developing over ruptured vesicles, erythema, and some scaling of the epidermis (hyperkeratosis, or increased thickness of the stratum corneum).
         c. **Chronic eczema** involves lichenification (thickening due to hyperkeratosis from constant scratching), scaling, and hyperpigmentation.
      2. Eczema may be secondary to immune reactions (IgE-mediated, cellular immunity), UV light, or microbial pathogens, or there may be no obvious offending agent.
   B. **Dermatitis** is a less specific term than eczema and indicates "inflammation of the skin."
      1. **Atopic dermatitis** is a type I IgE-mediated disease that presents in neonates as a rash on the cheeks, trunk, and extensor surfaces and then moves to the flexor creases as the child grows older.
      2. **Contact dermatitis** is an inflammatory disorder of skin that is associated with exposure to various antigens and irritating substances.
         a. **Allergic contact dermatitis** is a type IV cell-mediated hypersensitivity reaction against poison ivy, oak, and sumac; nickel; and chemicals found in household cleaners, cosmetics, fabrics, dyes, medications, and rubber products.
         b. **Irritant contact dermatitis,** the most common type, is a nonimmunologic reaction due to a local toxic effect of a chemical on the skin (e.g., detergents in soaps).
         c. **Contact photodermatitis** is a type of allergic contact dermatitis that is dependent on ultraviolet (UV) light reacting with drugs that have a photosensitizing effect (e.g., tetracycline, sulfonamides, thiazides).
         d. **Contact urticaria** is a wheal-and-flare reaction that may be secondary to an IgE-mediated or a nonimmunologic reaction.
      3. **Seborrheic dermatitis** is a scaly, often greasy type of dermatitis that is most commonly located on the scalp (dandruff, cradle cap in infants) and face (eyebrows, nasal creases); it is due to *Malassezia furfur.*
      4. The **superficial mycoses (dermatophytoses)** make up a group of fungi that are confined to the outermost layers of the skin or its appendages.
         a. **Tinea capitis** is most common in children, in whom it presents with circular or ring-shaped patches ("ringworm") of alopecia (hair loss) with erythema and scaling and usually is caused by *Trichophyton tonsurans.*
         b. *T. rubrum* and *T. mentagrophytes* are responsible for many other types of tinea infections (e.g., tinea cruris ["jock itch"], pedis, and corporis).
      5. **Tinea versicolor** is caused by *M. furfur* and is associated with areas of hyper- and hypopigmentation after exposure to the sun; scrapings reveal the classic "**spaghetti** (hyphae) **and meatball** (yeast)" appearance.
      6. *Candida albicans* commonly produces disease involving the skin (common cause of diaper rash) and nails (onychomycosis).

Objective 2: To review maculopapular and papulosquamous disorders of the skin.

III. Maculopapular disorders
   A. These disorders are characterized by a combination of macules (flat, pigmented lesions) and papules (peaked lesions < 1 cm).
   B. Viruses are common causes of maculopapular rashes.
      1. The **human papillomavirus** (HPV) is associated with **condyloma acuminatum** (venereal wart) and the **common wart** (verruca vulgaris), which exhibit hyperkeratosis, acanthosis (thickening of the epidermis), and papillomatosis (spike-like projections from the surface).
      2. **Molluscum contagiosum** (a poxvirus) is characterized by a bowl shape with a central area of umbilication filled with keratin, within which are viral particles.
      3. **Measles (rubeola)** is associated with fever, conjunctivitis, coryza (excessive mucus production), and Koplik's spots in the mouth, followed by a maculopapular rash that begins at the hairline and extends down over the body.
      4. **German measles (rubella)**, or "3-day measles," is associated with fever, headache, arthralgias, and painful postauricular lymphadenopathy 1–2 days prior to the onset of a maculopapular rash, which begins on the head and spreads downward.
      5. **Parvovirus B19** produces **erythema infectiosum (fifth disease)**, characterized by a confluent maculopapular rash usually beginning on the cheeks (giving a "slapped face" appearance) and extending centripetally to involve the trunk.
      6. **Roseola (exanthema subitum)**, caused by herpesvirus 6, is characterized by the sudden onset of a high fever, which abates on the third to fourth day and is followed by a maculopapular rash that begins on the trunk and spreads centrifugally.
   C. Bacterial toxins may be associated with maculopapular rashes.
      1. **Toxic shock syndrome** (TSS) is due to a toxin-producing strain of *Staphylococcus aureus* and is most frequently associated with tampon-wearing menstruating women.
         a. There is a 1- to 4-day prodrome of high fever (> 39°C), mental confusion, diarrhea, hypotension, pharyngitis, and an erythematous rash that occurs during or soon after menses.
         b. The rash has a diffuse, blanching, sunburned appearance that occurs predominantly on the hands and feet and resolves with desquamation in 7–10 days.
      2. **Scarlet fever** is caused by a strain of *Streptococcus pyogenes* that generates an erythrogenic toxin.
         a. It produces an erythematous rash (having a sandpaper consistency) that begins on the trunk and limbs and then resolves with desquamation.
         b. On the face, it produces circumoral pallor and a tongue, which initially has a "white strawberry" appearance followed by a "red strawberry" appearance.
   D. **Drug reactions** (e.g., penicillin, sulfa drugs) most commonly produce maculopapular rashes and hives (urticaria; see ¶VII.A).

IV. Papulosquamous disorders
   A. An **actinic (solar) keratosis** is a premalignant skin lesion induced by UV light damage on sun-exposed areas such as the face, hands, and forearms that may progress to squamous cell carcinoma.
   B. **Lichen planus** is characterized by intensely pruritic, scaly, violaceous, flat-topped papules on the wrists, lower back, legs, and scalp; it may also occur on the oral mucosa, where it has a fine white net-like appearance (called **Wickham's striae**).
   C. **Psoriasis** is a chronic disorder characterized by erythematous plaques secondary to an unregulated proliferation of keratinocytes.
      1. Genetics, environmental factors (e.g., infection [streptococcal pharyngitis]), unregulated epidermal proliferation, and microcirculatory changes in the papillary dermis are involved in its pathogenesis.
      2. The **plaques** (scalp, pressure areas) are well-demarcated, flat, elevated salmon-colored lesions covered by silver-white scales which, when picked off, reveal pinpoint areas of bleeding (**Auspitz sign**).
      3. Pitting of the nails occurs in 50% of patients.
      4. Histologic features include hyperkeratosis, parakeratosis (persistent nuclei in the stratum corneum), focal absence of the granular layer, a regular pattern of elongation of the rete ridges (downward extensions of the basal layer), extension of the papillary dermis close to the surface epithelium, and collections of neutrophils in the stratum corneum (**Munro's microabscesses**).
   D. **Pityriasis rosea** first presents as a single, oval-shaped, scaly pink plaque on the trunk called a "**herald patch**," followed in a few days to weeks by an eruption of papules on the trunk that follow the lines of cleavage in a "**Christmas tree**" distribution.

Objective 3: To discuss vesiculobullous and pustular disorders of the skin.

V. Vesiculobullous disorders
   A. **Herpesvirus types 1 and 2 infections** are summarized in Tables 15–1 and 18–1, respectively.
   B. **Chickenpox (varicella)** presents with a rash (macules → vesicles → pustules) that begins on the trunk and extends centrifugally to involve the face and extremities.
   C. **Herpes zoster (shingles)** is the reappearance of the varicella-zoster virus (which remains dormant in sensory dorsal root ganglia after the primary infection) as an eruption of painful vesicles along the dermatome of a sensory nerve.
   D. **Impetigo**, due to *S. aureus*, begins on the face as erythematous macules and progresses to vesicles and pustules that rupture to form honey-colored, crusted lesions.
   E. The **scalded skin syndrome** is a neonatal disease that is associated with the development of bullae (blisters > 1 cm) that rupture and leave large, red areas of denuded skin; it is caused by a toxin produced by *S. aureus*.
   F. **Pemphigus vulgaris** is an immunologic disease

with IgG antibodies directed against the intercellular attachment sites (desmosomes) between keratinocytes (type II cytotoxic antibody hypersensitivity reaction).

1. It produces vesicles (blisters < 5 mm) and bullae on the skin and within the oral mucosa.
2. The vesicles are intraepidermal and have a **suprabasal location** (just above the basal cell layer), leaving the basal cells intact and looking like a row of tombstones.
3. Owing to detachment of individual keratinocytes from each other (**acantholysis**), keratinocytes are present within the vesicle fluid.
4. The bullae exhibit **Nikolsky's sign** (in which the outer epidermis separates easily from the basal layer with minimal manual pressure).

G. **Bullous pemphigoid** is an immunologic vesicular disease (IgG antibodies directed against the basement membrane) in which the vesicles are in a **subepidermal location**; Nikolsky's sign is negative, and acantholysis is not present.

H. **Dermatitis herpetiformis** is an immunologic vesicular disease characterized by the presence of IgA immunocomplexes (a type III immunocomplex reaction) located at the tips of the dermal papilla (producing **subepidermal** vesicles with neutrophils); it has a strong association with celiac disease.

I. **Erythema multiforme** is an immunologic reaction that occurs in the skin (vesicles, bullae, bull's eye lesions) and mucous membranes (**Stevens-Johnson syndrome**) in response to an infection (*Mycoplasma pneumoniae*), drugs (penicillin, sulfa drugs), various autoimmune diseases (SLE), or pregnancy.

VI. Pustular disorders

A. *S. aureus* is a gram-positive coccus that produces furuncles (boils), carbuncles (furuncles with multiple sinuses), impetigo, scalded skin syndrome, toxic shock syndrome, hidradenitis suppurativa (abscess of apocrine glands, usually in the axilla), paronychial infections, postoperative wound or stitch abscesses, and postpartum breast abscesses.

B. **Acne vulgaris** is a chronic inflammatory disorder involving the pilosebaceous unit in the skin.

1. It is subdivided into an **obstructive type**, which is characterized by **closed comedones** (whiteheads) and **open comedones** (blackheads), and an **inflammatory type** consisting of papules, pustules, nodules, cysts, and scars.
   a. The pathogenesis of the obstructive type (comedones) is related to plugging of the outlet of a hair follicle by keratin debris.
   b. The inflammatory type is associated with abnormal keratinization of the follicular epithelium, increased sebum production (androgen controlled), and bacterial lipase (derived from *Propionibacterium acnes*), with the production of irritating fatty acids that produce an inflammatory reaction.
2. Aggravating factors include hormones (e.g., testosterone, progesterone, glucocorticoids), drugs (e.g., lithium), and occupational exposures (e.g., grease).
3. Dietary factors (e.g., chocolate, nuts) do not contribute to acne.

C. **Acne rosacea** is an inflammatory disease of the pilosebaceous units on the face in middle-aged individuals.

Objective 4: To review skin disorders that present with urticaria, cellulitis, or atrophy.

VII. Urticaria, cellulitis, and atrophy

A. **Urticaria** (**hives**) is the presence of pruritic elevations of the skin secondary to the release of histamine and other chemical mediators (type I IgE-mediated reaction) due to exposure to certain foods (e.g., shellfish, peanuts), drugs (e.g., penicillin), insect bites (e.g., bee sting), and radiocontrast dyes.

B. **Angioedema**, unlike urticaria, is edema within deeper subcutaneous tissue that produces diffuse swelling of the involved tissue (e.g., **C1 esterase inhibitor deficiency**; Chapter 4).

C. **Cellulitis with lymphangitis** ("red streaks") is characteristic of *S. pyogenes* infection owing to the elaboration of hyaluronidase, which allows the inflammatory reaction to spread through the subcutaneous tissue.

D. **Erysipelas** (an *S. pyogenes* infection) is a raised, erythematous ("brawny edema"), hot cellulitis, usually on the face.

E. **Systemic lupus erythematosus** (SLE) and **chronic discoid lupus erythematosus** (DLE; primarily limited to the skin) produce skin lesions associated with epidermal atrophy.

1. The pathogenesis relates to a combination of anti-DNA antibodies directed against DNA trapped in the basement membrane (planted antigen) and DNA–anti-DNA immunocomplexes that deposit in the basement membrane of the skin.
2. The immune reaction leads to vacuolar degeneration of the basal cells along the dermal-epidermal junction and hair shafts and a lymphoid infiltrate in the same areas as well as around vessels in the papillary dermis.
3. The epidermis is atrophic, and follicular keratin plugs are noted along the surface.

Objective 5: To be familiar with nodular and cystic disorders of the skin.

VIII. Nodular disorders

A. **Subcutaneous mycoses** are usually acquired by puncture wound (traumatic implantation) of the skin and may extend into the underlying bone.

1. **Chromoblastomycosis** is a verrucous (wart-like) dermatitis associated with several pigmented fungi that elicit a granulomatous reaction; it may occur in **carpenters** (from wood splinters).
2. **Sporotrichosis** is caused by *Sporothrix schenckii* and is acquired by traumatic implantation of the fungus growing in the soil; it may occur in **rose gardeners**.
   a. It most commonly produces lymphocutaneous disease (a chain of suppurating subcutaneous nodules).
   b. Oral potassium iodide is used as treatment.

B. *Mycobacterium leprae*, an acid-fast organism, is the cause of leprosy, which is transmitted by direct contact or droplet infection.

1. The **tuberculoid type** demonstrates intact cellular immunity (positive lepromin skin test), and it causes localized skin lesions and nerve

involvement leading to skin anesthesia, muscle atrophy, and **autoamputation of digits**.

2. The **lepromatous type** demonstrates a lack of cellular immunity (negative lepromin skin test), and organisms are readily identified in tissue within macrophages (lepra cells).
   a. Patients may have the classic leonine facies.
   b. Skin biopsies reveal a narrow zone beneath the epidermis that is free of organisms (**Grenz zone**), underlying which are macrophages teeming with the organisms.
   c. Neural involvement is a late feature.

C. A **keratoacanthoma** is characterized by the rapid growth of a crateriform lesion that regresses and involutes with scarring; histologically, it may be confused with a well-differentiated squamous cell carcinoma.

D. **Erythema nodosum** is the most common cause of inflammation of subcutaneous fat (**panniculitis**).
   1. It produces raised, erythematous, painful nodules usually on the anterior portion of the shins.
   2. Common associations include streptococcal infection, sarcoidosis, tuberculosis, leprosy, drugs (e.g., sulfonamides), and coccidioidomycosis.

E. **Skin cancers** associated with UV light damage include basal cell carcinoma, squamous cell carcinoma, and malignant melanoma (see ¶X.G, below).
   1. **Basal cell carcinoma** (BCC) is the most common malignant tumor of the skin and occurs on sun-exposed, hair-bearing surfaces.
      a. BCCs are locally aggressive, infiltrating cancers arising from the basal cell layer of the epidermis and do not metastasize.
      b. They are commonly located on the face on the inner aspect of the nose, around the orbit, and on the upper lip, where they appear as raised nodules containing a central crater.
      c. The external surface of the nodular lesions is pearly colored, and prominent vascular channels are visible beneath the surface.
      d. Microscopically, cords of basophilic-staining cells originate from multiple locations along the basal cell layer that infiltrate the underlying dermis, where they form neatly arranged nests of malignant cells.
      e. Peripheral palisading of neoplastic cells occurs around the advancing margin of the tumor.
   2. **Squamous cell carcinoma** (SCC) of the skin has a low but significant potential for metastasis, which is more likely if the cancer is on a mucosal surface.
      a. SCCs are located on the face and favor areas such as the ears, nose, and lower lip (BCC targets the upper lip).
      b. Predisposing causes include UV light, arsenic poisoning, chronic skin ulcers, sinus tracts (particularly when accompanying chronic osteomyelitis), previous irradiation, burn scars, and immunosuppressive therapy.
      c. SCC is the most common overall cancer.

F. **Adnexal tumors** arise from cutaneous appendages that are capable of pilosebaceous, eccrine, or apocrine differentiation.

IX. Cystic disorders
   A. An **epidermal inclusion cyst** is derived from the epidermis of a hair follicle and contains lipid-rich debris intermixed with laminated keratin material.
   B. A **pilar cyst** (wen) is most commonly located on the scalp and is similar to an epidermal inclusion cyst except for the absence of a stratum granulosum layer in the cyst wall and absence of laminated keratin in the cyst.

======

Objective 6: To discuss melanocytic disorders of the skin.

X. Melanocytic disorders
   A. **Vitiligo** is an area of depigmentation resulting from autoimmune destruction of melanocytes.
   B. **Seborrheic keratosis** is a benign epidermal tumor that presents on the skin of middle-aged individuals.
      1. It is a raised, pigmented lesion with a verruca-like surface.
      2. Histologically, it exhibits hyperkeratosis, papillomatosis, entrapment of keratin in the epidermis (horn cysts), and proliferation of basaloid (basal cell–like) cells having increased pigmentation.
   C. **Acanthosis nigricans** is a pigmented skin lesion commonly present in the axilla that may be a phenotypic marker for an underlying adenocarcinoma of the stomach.
   D. **Freckles (ephelides)** are pigmented macular lesions that occur in sun-exposed areas of the skin; they are not premalignant and have a normal number of melanocytes along the basal cell layer but increased melanin within individual melanocytes.
   E. **Lentigo simplex** is similar to a freckle, except there are increased numbers of melanocytes along the basal layer as well as increased melanin in each melanocyte.
   F. A **nevocellular nevus** is a benign tumor of neural crest–derived cells that contain modified melanocytes of various shapes (nevus cells).
      1. Nevocellular nevi begin in early childhood as **junctional nevi** with nests of pigmented nevus cells proliferating along the basal cell layer (flat, pigmented lesions).
      2. Junctional nevi usually develop into **compound nevi** as nevus cells extend into the underlying superficial dermis, forming cords and columns of cells, so that both a junctional and an intradermal component is present (raised, pigmented, verruca-like lesions).
      3. Around puberty, the junctional component is lost, leaving only pigmented nevus cells within the dermis, hence the term **intradermal nevus**, which is the most common type in adults.
      4. A **dysplastic nevus** is more likely to develop in people who have numerous nevi spread over the entire body (dysplastic nevus syndrome); they predispose to malignant melanoma.
   G. **Malignant melanomas** derive from melanocytes.
      1. They affect both sexes equally, are more common in whites than in African Americans, and have a predilection for fair-skinned, blue-eyed persons with red or blond hair.
      2. Exposure to excessive sunlight at an early age is the single most important predisposing risk factor.
      3. Other risk factors include a history of severe sunburn, dysplastic nevus syndrome, melanoma in a first- or second-degree relative, and **xeroderma pigmentosum** (an AR disease exhibiting a lack of DNA repair enzymes).

4. They can arise *de novo*, from a preexisting lesion (e.g., congenital nevus, dysplastic nevus), or from a lentigo maligna (see ¶8).

5. Most variants have an initial **radial growth phase**, in which malignant melanocytes proliferate laterally within the epidermis, along the dermoepidermal junction, or within the papillary dermis; metastasis cannot occur in this phase.

6. There may be a **vertical growth phase**, in which malignant cells penetrate the underlying reticular dermis; metastasis can occur in this phase.

7. The **superficial spreading melanoma** is the most common type (70%) and primarily affects women over 50 years of age.
   a. The lower extremities and back are the most common locations.
   b. These are black, irregular, raised lesions that may have focal brown or red areas of discoloration, foci of depigmentation, and ulceration.

8. **Lentigo maligna melanoma** (4–10%) is an extension of a lentigo maligna (intraepidermal lesion) and primarily occurs on the sun-exposed face of an elderly person.

9. **Nodular melanomas** (15–30%) lack a radial growth phase and directly invade the dermis.

10. **Acral lentiginous melanomas** (2–8%) are located on the palms, soles, or subungual regions and may occur in African Americans.

11. The **Breslow system** of staging measures the depth of invasion from the outermost granular layer to the deepest margin of the tumor; lesions with <0.76 mm of invasion do not metastasize, whereas those > 1.7 mm of invasion have the potential for lymph node metastasis.

12. The **Clark system** subdivides invasion into levels I through V.

13. The overall 5-year survival regardless of type is ~80%.

Objective 7: To understand the pathogenesis of the most common porphyrias.

XI. Porphyria
   A. **Acute intermittent porphyria** (AIP), an AD disease, has two basic defects: increased activity of ALA synthase and decreased activity of uroporphyrinogen synthase.
      1. The net effect of the two defects is an excessive amount of δ-aminolevulinic acid (ALA) and porphobilinogen (PBG) that builds up behind the enzyme block.
      2. It is characterized by intermittent exacerbations of neurologic dysfunction including psychosis, neuropathies, and severe colicky abdominal pain that is frequently mistaken for a surgical emergency ("**bellyful of scars**.")
      3. It can be precipitated by drugs (e.g., alcohol, barbiturates) that activate the cytochrome P-450 system, hence depleting heme and the negative feedback it normally has on ALA synthase activity.
      4. When a colorless fresh-voided urine is exposed to light, over time it will turn wine-red (**windowsill test**) as porphobilinogen becomes oxidized into porphobilin.
      5. RBC uroporphyrinogen synthase activity is decreased even when the patient is asymptomatic.
      6. Periodic infusions of heme reduce the number of attacks.
   B. **Porphyria cutanea tarda** (PCT) is an acquired disease that is associated with decreased activity of uroporphyrinogen decarboxylase.
      1. The net result of this enzyme defect is increased excretion of uroporphyrin I (the urine is a wine-red color on voiding), a slight increase in the formation of coproporphyrins, and normal porphobilinogen levels.
      2. Patients have photosensitive skin lesions in sun-exposed areas, hyperpigmentation, and fragile skin with increased amounts of vellus type hair (hypertrichosis).

QUESTIONS

DIRECTIONS. (Items 1-5): Each of the numbered items or incomplete statements in this section is followed by answers or by completions of the statement. Select the ONE lettered answer or completion that is BEST in each case. Correct answers and explanations are given at the end of the chapter.

1. The lesion on this patient's face is most likely associated with

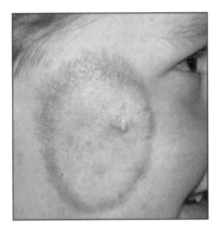

  (A) a neoplastic process
  (B) a dermatophyte infection
  (C) suprabasilar vesicles
  (D) an autoimmune disease
  (E) *Streptococcus pyogenes*

2. This skin lesion on the buttocks of a 43-year-old man most likely represents

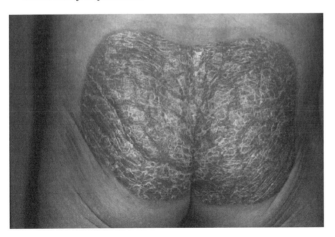

  (A) unregulated epidermal proliferation with hyperkeratosis
  (B) an autoimmune disease with spongiosis and bulla formation
  (C) a neoplastic process originating from the basal layer
  (D) a neoplastic process originating from melanocytes
  (E) an acute eczematous process with hyperkeratosis

3. The microscopic slide is of a biopsy specimen taken from the back of a hand of a 62-year-old wheat farmer. Grossly, the lesion was scaly and slightly raised. Similar lesions were present on his other hand and both forearms. This lesion is best described as a

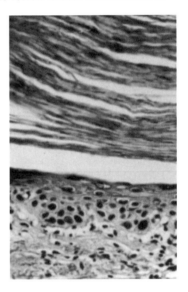

  (A) disorder of melanocytes
  (B) disorder associated with a virus
  (C) disorder associated with acantholysis
  (D) precursor lesion for basal cell carcinoma
  (E) precursor lesion for squamous cancer

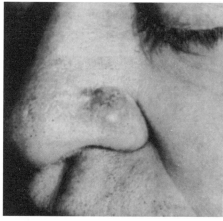
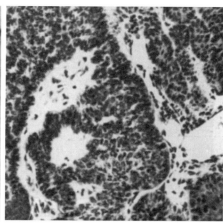

4. The section of the excisional biopsy from the lesion on this man's nose is best described as a

   (A) well-differentiated squamous cancer
   (B) viral disorder associated with poxvirus
   (C) pustular disease related to acne
   (D) neoplastic process originating from the basal cell layer
   (E) melanocytic disorder in the vertical growth phase

5. The photograph is of a skin lesion on the thigh of a 32-year-old woman. You strongly suspect that the lesion represents a

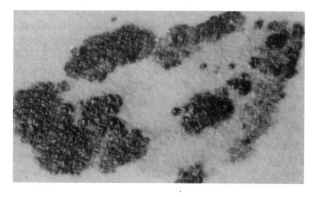

   (A) benign process associated with melanocytes
   (B) malignant process associated with squamous cells
   (C) malignant process associated with melanocytes
   (D) benign process associated with squamous cells
   (E) benign process associated with dermatophytes

ANSWERS AND EXPLANATIONS

1. The answer is B: a dermatophyte infection. The lesion is circular and shows a dark-colored leading edge and central clearing. These features are most compatible with tinea corporis, which is due to a superficial dermatophyte infection. The leading edge should be scraped and the material digested with KOH and examined under the microscope for yeast and hyphae. The circular nature of the lesion argues against a neoplastic process, an autoimmune disease (e.g., SLE), pemphigus vulgaris (suprabasilar vesicles), and impetigo (*S. pyogenes*). (Photograph reproduced, with permission, from M.A. Mir. *Atlas of Clinical Diagnosis*. Philadelphia, W.B. Saunders Co., 1995, p. 41.)

2. The answer is A: unregulated epidermal proliferation with hyperkeratosis. The photograph depicts a well-demarcated plaque-like lesion covered by silvery scales. This is most characteristic of psoriasis, which is associated with an unregulated proliferation of keratinocytes, hyperkeratosis, parakeratosis, and regular accentuation of the rete ridges. The silver scales lie close to the superficial papillary dermis, which contains vascular channels. Lifting off of a scale reveals pinpoint areas of hemorrhage, which is called the Auspitz sign. The lesion is not vesiculobullous, as in pemphigus vulgaris (choice C), oozing like acute eczema (choice E), or neoplastic. (Photograph reproduced, with permission, from J.P. Callen, K.E. Greer, A.F. Hood, et al. *Color Atlas of Dermatology*. Philadelphia, W.B. Saunders Co., 1993, p. 120.)

3. The answer is E: precursor lesion for squamous cancer. The histologic section reveals hyperkeratosis (increased thickness of the stratum corneum) and irregular, hyperchromatic nuclei in the keratinocytes. Given that the patient is a farmer with exposure to sunlight, the lesion is most representative of actinic (solar) keratosis, which is a precursor lesion for squamous cell carcinoma. UV light damage may also predispose to malignant melanoma and basal cell carcinomas; however, actinic kerato-sis most commonly is associated with squamous tumors. Acantholysis (loss of cohesion of keratinocytes) is not present in the slide, and the gross appearance and histologic features of the lesion are not compatible with verruca vulgaris (choice B). (Photomicrograph reproduced, with permission, from G.F. Murphy. *Dermatopathology*. Philadelphia, W.B. Saunders Co., 1995, p. 200.)

4. The answer is D: neoplastic process originating from the basal cell layer. The lesion on the nose is nodular, has prominent vessels along the surface, and appears to be slightly umbilicated. The histologic section reveals nests of dark-staining cells with prominent peripheral palisading characteristic of an infiltrating basal cell carcinoma. Squamous cancers do not have this histologic appearance, although these features could resemble the gross features of the tumor. A malignant melanoma is usually pigmented and would not have the orderly pattern of infiltration into the dermis noted in this case. The lesion neither grossly nor histologically represents molluscum contagiosum (choice B), nor does it resemble acne vulgaris or rosacea (choice C). (Photograph and photomicrograph reproduced, with permission, from G.F. Murphy. *Dermatopathology*. Philadelphia, W.B. Saunders Co., 1995, p. 203.)

5. The answer is C: malignant process associated with melanocytes. The lesion is pigmented, has irregular borders, and shows multifocal areas of depigmentation. This is a characteristic gross appearance of a malignant melanoma of the superficial spreading type. The areas of depigmentation are signs of regression where the patient's immune system has destroyed the cells. The process has none of the characteristic features of an actinic keratosis (choice D), squamous cancer (choice B), tinea corporis (choice E), or a benign nevus (choice A). (Photomicrograph reproduced, with permission, from G.F. Murphy. *Dermatopathology*. Philadelphia, W.B. Saunders Co., 1995, p. 247.)

DISORDERS OF THE

CENTRAL NERVOUS

SYSTEM AND SPECIAL

SENSES

SYNOPSIS

OBJECTIVES

1. To understand the pathogenesis and consequences of increased intracranial pressure.
2. To review congenital disorders of the central nervous system (CNS).
3. To summarize the most important infections of the CNS.
4. To discuss the types of injuries produced by trauma to the CNS.
5. To understand the pathophysiology of stroke.
6. To outline the common causes of demyelinating, dysmyelinating, and degenerative diseases of the CNS.
7. To review metabolic and toxic encephalopathies involving the CNS and peripheral nervous system (PNS).
8. To discuss the tumors involving the CNS and PNS.
9. To describe the types of CNS and PNS diseases associated with AIDS.
10. To be familiar with selected disorders of the peripheral nervous system.

Objective 1: To understand the pathogenesis and consequences of increased intracranial pressure.

I. Increased intracranial pressure
   A. Causes of increased intracranial pressure include a noncommunicating hydrocephalus (see below), a space-occupying mass (e.g., metastatic tumor), and cerebral edema.
   B. Cerebral edema may be intracellular (hyponatremia, ischemia) or extracellular (increased vessel permeability due to tumor, inflammation, trauma, or lead poisoning).
   C. Increased intracranial pressure may produce herniation of the cingulate gyrus, uncal herniation, or cerebellar herniation.
      1. **Uncal herniation** (herniation of the medial por-

tion of the temporal lobe) results in compression of the midbrain (which produces **Duret's lesions**), oculomotor and abducens nervus (which causes eye muscle palsies, lid lag, mydriasis), and posterior cerebral artery (which results in hemorrhagic infarction of the occipital lobe).
      2. Herniation of the **cerebellar tonsils** into the foramen magnum is followed by cardiorespiratory arrest.

Objective 2: To review congenital disorders of the central nervous system (CNS).

II. Hydrocephalus
   A. **Cerebrospinal fluid** (CSF), primarily produced by the choroid plexus in the lateral ventricles, exits the fourth ventricle through the foramina of Luschka and Magendie, enters the subarachnoid space, and is reabsorbed by the arachnoid granulations into the dural venous sinuses.
   B. **Hydrocephalus** is an increase in CSF volume with distention of the ventricles.
   C. In a **communicating hydrocephalus**, CSF has unobstructed flow between the ventricles and the subarachnoid space.
      1. This may be due to increased production of CSF (e.g., by a choroid plexus papilloma).
      2. Another possible cause is a block in the reabsorption of CSF by the arachnoid granulations (e.g., postmeningitis scarring).
   D. In a **noncommunicating hydrocephalus**, CSF flow out of the ventricles is obstructed.
      1. It may be due to stricture of the aqueduct of Sylvius (most common type in newborns).

2. Other causes include tumors in the fourth ventricle (e.g., ependymoma), Arnold-Chiari syndrome, Dandy-Walker syndrome, and blockage of CSF flow out of the foramina of Luschka and Magendie (e.g., inflammation, blood clot).

E. The ventricles dilate and enlarge the head circumference in newborns, while in adults, hydrocephalus results in progressive dementia, gait disturbances, and incontinence.

F. **Hydrocephalus *ex vacuo*** describes the appearance of the ventricles when the brain mass is decreased.

III. Open neural tube defects

A. These defects are attributed to failure of fusion of the lateral folds of the neural plate or to rupture of a previously closed tube.

B. There is an increase in maternal α-fetoprotein in the serum or amniotic fluid.

C. Folic acid taken *before* pregnancy protects the fetus from these defects.

D. **Anencephaly** is associated with complete absence of the brain, absence of the fetal adrenal cortex, a frog-like appearance, and polyhydramnios.

E. **Spina bifida** is defined as failure of the posterior vertebral arches to close on the 26th day of gestation.

   1. **Spina bifida occulta** is associated with a dimple or tuck of hair in the overlying skin of L5–S1.

   2. Spina bifida plus a cystic mass containing dura and arachnoid is called a **meningocele**; if the spinal cord is also present, it is called a **meningomyelocele**.

IV. Syringomyelia

A. Syringomyelia is due to a fluid-filled cavity (**syrinx**) within the cervical spinal cord.

B. It may be acquired later in life from ischemia, inflammation, or trauma.

C. It is associated with cervical cord enlargement, Arnold-Chiari syndrome, and neurologic deficits (loss of pain and temperature sensation [disruption of the crossed lateral spinothalamic tracts], atrophy of the intrinsic muscles of the hands [destruction of anterior horn cells]).

V. Arnold-Chiari malformation and Dandy-Walker syndrome

A. **Arnold-Chiari malformation** is associated with elongation of the medulla and cerebellar tonsils through the foramen magnum, hydrocephalus, platybasia, meningomyelocele, and syringomyelia.

B. **Dandy-Walker syndrome** consists of hypoplasia of the cerebellar vermis, cystic dilatation of the fourth ventricle, and hydrocephalus.

VI. Phakomatoses

A. Phakomatoses are **neurocutaneous syndromes** characterized by disordered growth of ectodermal tissue and malformations or tumors of the CNS (e.g., neurofibromatosis [Chapter 7], Sturge-Weber syndrome [Chapter 10], and tuberous sclerosis).

B. **Tuberous sclerosis** is an AD disease consisting of mental retardation, skin lesions, hamartomas, and benign tumors.

   1. The skin lesions consist of adenoma sebaceum and periungual fibromas.

   2. Hamartomatous proliferations of astrocytes located in subependymal portions of the brain give the appearance of "**candlestick drippings**" within the ventricles.

3. Angiomyolipomas (hamartomas) occur in the kidney and rhabdomyomas (neoplasm) in the heart.

Objective 3: To summarize the most important infections of the CNS.

VII. Infections of the CNS

A. Infections are secondary to hematogenous spread (most common), traumatic implantation, local extension from nearby infection, or ascent up the peripheral nerves or olfactory bulb (e.g., rabies or herpesvirus, respectively).

B. The most common infections include leptomeningitis, encephalitis (inflammation of the brain), and cerebral abscess.

C. **Leptomeningitis** is subdivided into acute purulent (bacterial), lymphocytic (viral), and chronic granulomatous types (primary TB, systemic fungi).

   1. Bacteria associated with acute purulent meningitis target the following age groups:

     a. **Newborns:** group B streptococci (*Streptococcus agalactiae*; most common), *Escherichia coli,* and *Listeria monocytogenes.*

     b. One month to 18 years: *Neisseria meningitidis.* (H. influenza)

     c. > 18 years: *S. pneumoniae*.

   2. CSF findings in bacterial meningitis include a neutrophil-dominant cell count, an increased protein, and a low glucose (< 40 mg/dL).

   3. Viral leptomeningitis is most often (85%) due to an enterovirus (coxsackievirus, echovirus).

   4. CSF findings in viral meningitis include a lymphocyte-dominant cell count, an elevated protein, and a normal glucose.

   5. Chronic granulomatous leptomeningitis due to primary TB favors the base of the brain, where it produces a vasculitis (danger of stroke) and extensive fibrosis (danger of hydrocephalus).

   6. *Cryptococcus neoformans* is the most common opportunistic systemic fungal infection in the CNS.

   7. Symptoms associated with leptomeningitis include fever, headache, nuchal rigidity, and an altered sensorium.

D. **Encephalitis** is characterized by impairment of mental status and drowsiness.

   1. **Inclusion bodies** are commonly found in viral encephalitis.

     a. Intracytoplasmic Negri bodies in Purkinje's cells in the cerebellum are present in 70% of patients with rabies.

     b. Intranuclear and intracytoplasmic inclusions are noted in cytomegalovirus (CMV; most common CNS viral infection in AIDS) and subacute sclerosing panencephalitis (SSPE).

     c. Intranuclear inclusions characterize herpes simplex virus type 1 (HSV-1) infection (hemorrhagic necrosis of the temporal lobes), herpes zoster, and progressive multifocal leukoencephalopathy (PML).

   2. **Arboviruses** are transmitted to humans by mosquitoes that obtain the virus from vertebrates (birds and mammals).

Reactivation of latent inf. (handwritten margin note)

a. St. Louis encephalitis is the most common encephalitis.

b. Eastern equine encephalitis has the greatest mortality.

3. **Toxoplasmosis** is the most common cause of a space-occupying lesion in the CNS in patients with AIDS. → *cysts* (handwritten)

4. **Slow virus diseases** due to a conventional agent include SSPE and PML.

   a. **SSPE** is associated with the measles (rubeola) virus either as a primary infection or as a complication of immunization against measles (live attenuated vaccine); the virus infects oligodendrocytes.

   Progressive multifocal leukoencephalopathy (handwritten margin note)

   b. **PML**, due to a papovavirus (JC virus, SV40 virus), infects and destroys oligodendrocytes, leading to primary demyelination.

5. **Creutzfeldt-Jakob (CJ) disease** is a slow virus disease transmitted by an unconventional agent (a prion, which is a protein without nucleic acid).

   a. CJ disease is a rapidly progressive dementia.

   b. It can be transmitted by corneal transplantation and is a health hazard to those working with brain tissue (e.g., neuropathologist).

   c. Microscopically, it demonstrates characteristic "bubble and holes" spongiform change in the cerebral cortex with little or no inflammatory reaction.

E. A **cerebral abscess**, usually solitary, may develop from an adjacent focus of infection (e.g., sinus, middle ear) or by hematogenous spread (e.g., cyanotic heart disease, bronchiectasis), in which case they are usually multiple.

F. **Neurosyphilis** is the tertiary stage of syphilis (*Treponema pallidum*).

   3° syphilis (handwritten margin note)

   1. The **meningovascular type** is a chronic low-grade meningitis (no visible spirochetes) with vasculitis.

   2. The **paretic type** demonstrates generalized atrophy (neuronal loss) of the frontal cortex (spirochetes present) and dementia.

   3. In **tabes dorsalis**, spirochetes attack the posterior root ganglia or the afferent sensory axons between the posterior root ganglia and the cord, leading to posterior column disease that results in

      a. Impaired joint position sense.

      b. Loss of pain and vibration sensation.

      c. Neuropathic joint (Charcot's joint).

      d. Absent deep tendon reflexes.

      e. Argyll Robertson pupil, in which the pupil constricts with a near stimulus (accommodates) but fails to react to direct light.

   4. **Laboratory findings** include a positive VDRL, positive CSF FTA-ABS, mild lymphocytosis, increased protein, and normal glucose.

Objective 4: To discuss the types of injuries produced by trauma to the CNS.

VIII. CNS trauma

A. A **cerebral concussion** is a transient loss of consciousness immediately following a nonpenetrating blunt impact to the head (e.g., in boxing) with no histologic evidence of damage to the brain.

B. Cerebral contusions and diffuse axonal injury are examples of **primary** brain injury (immediate consequence of injury).

   1. In a **cerebral contusion**, there is permanent damage to small blood vessels and the surface of the brain.

      a. It is most commonly secondary to an acceleration-deceleration injury (e.g., car accident).

      b. Contusions occurring at the site of impact are **coup injuries**, while those on the opposite side of the brain are **contrecoup injuries**.

      c. Contusions and lacerations usually occur at the tips of the frontal and temporal lobes.

   2. **Diffuse axonal injury** involves the shearing of axons located in white matter tracts or brain stem.

   3. **Meningeal tears** occur with basilar and orbital skull fractures that frequently result in loss of CSF fluid (not another body fluid) through the nose (rhinorrhea) or ears (otorrhea).

      a. CSF has a lower protein and glucose than serum.

      b. CSF has a higher chloride than serum.

C. **Traumatic intracranial hemorrhages** are most often associated with epidural or subdural hematomas.

   lucid interval (handwritten margin note)

   1. An **acute epidural hematoma** occurs when there is a fracture of the temporoparietal bone with severance of the middle meningeal artery, which lies between the dura and inner table of bone.

      a. Arterial bleeding creates a blood-filled space between the calvarium and the dura.

      b. Over the next 4–8 hours, the intracranial pressure increases, leading to herniation and death unless the clot is removed.

   2. A **subdural hematoma** is a collection of venous blood between the dura and the arachnoid membranes that is most often the result of blunt trauma. *Bridging Veins* (handwritten)

      a. It most commonly occurs in patients who have cerebral atrophy (e.g., due to dementia or chronic alcoholism).

      b. Bleeding is due to tearing of the bridging veins between the venous sinus located over the convexities of the cerebral hemispheres.

      c. Patients present with fluctuating levels of consciousness.

   3. CT is the better way to demonstrate intracranial hemorrhages in the first 48 hours, while MRI is better after 48 hours.

Objective 5: To understand the pathophysiology of stroke.

IX. Vascular injuries in the CNS

A. Neurons and neuroglial cells are very susceptible to oxygen deprivation (hypoxia) or hypoglycemia.

   1. Neurons (particularly those in the hippocampus and cerebellum [Purkinje's cells]) are most sensitive, followed next by oligodendrocytes and then by astrocytes.

   2. **Chronic ischemia**, most commonly secondary to atherosclerosis involving the internal carotid artery, may produce the following:

a. **Laminar necrosis** secondary to apoptosis of neurons in layers 3, 5, and 6 of the cerebral cortex (which eventuates in cerebral atrophy).

b. **Watershed infarcts** at junctions between major arterial territories (e.g., between the anterior and middle cerebral arteries).

c. **Cerebrovascular accidents**.

B. **Cerebrovascular accidents**, or **strokes**, can be **ischemic** (80%) or **hemorrhagic** (20%).

1. Approximately 60% of ischemic strokes are due to atherosclerosis and 10–20% to embolism (embolic stroke) from the left heart.

2. Hemorrhagic strokes are subclassified as intracerebral hemorrhage (most commonly a hypertensive stroke) and subarachnoid hemorrhage (most commonly a ruptured congenital berry aneurysm).

C. **Atherosclerotic strokes** are most commonly secondary to a thrombus overlying an atheromatous plaque in the internal carotid near the bifurcation.

1. The majority (80%) are pale infarcts in the distribution of the middle cerebral artery.

2. Reactive astrocytes (gemistocytes) proliferate at the margins of the infarct and microglial cells remove lipid debris in a process called **gliosis**.

3. Liquefactive necrosis results in the formation of a cystic area in the brain after 10 days to 3 weeks.

4. In most cases, atherosclerotic strokes are preceded by **transient ischemic attacks** (TIAs).

a. TIAs are due to embolization of platelet or cholesterol plaque material in the peripheral vessels that causes transient neurologic deficits lasting < 24 hours.

b. Deficits that do not resolve within 24 hours are called strokes.

5. The following are clinical manifestations of occlusion of the middle cerebral artery: — *Motor/Sensory*

a. Contralateral hemiparesis and sensory loss.

b. Expressive aphasia when Broca's area is involved in the dominant hemisphere.

c. Amaurosis fugax (fleeting blindness).

d. Visual field defects (contralateral inferior quadrantanopia or homonymous hemianopia).

e. Deviation of the head and eyes toward the side of the lesion.

6. Strokes involving the distribution of the vertebrobasilar arterial system are dominated by the presence of vertigo, ataxia, ipsilateral sensory loss in the face, and contralateral hemiparesis and sensory loss in the trunk and limbs.

7. The majority of patients recover (10–20% die).

D. An **embolic stroke** from thromboemboli originating in the left heart is most commonly associated with a hemorrhagic infarction in the distribution of the middle cerebral artery.

1. Owing to lysis of the thromboembolus, hemorrhage occurs into the area of infarction, usually limited to the gray matter at the periphery of the brain rather than the white matter.

2. The mortality rate is ~30%.

E. An **intracerebral hemorrhage** is most commonly secondary to vascular changes (hyaline arteriolosclerosis, fibrinoid necrosis) associated with hypertension (80%).

1. The vascular changes occur in the penetrating branches of the lenticulostriate vessels and lead to the formation of **Charcot-Bouchard microaneurysms**.

2. Rupture of the microaneurysms results in an intracerebral hemorrhage, most commonly in the basal ganglia (35–50% in the putamen), thalamus (10%), pons (10%), or cerebellar hemispheres (10%).

3. The mortality rate is 30–40%.

4. Effective treatment of hypertension has its greatest benefit in preventing strokes.

F. Most **subarachnoid hemorrhages** are secondary to a rupture of a congenital berry aneurysm (80%) in patients (usually women) between the ages of 40 and 65 years; AV malformations are a less common cause.

1. **Congenital aneurysms** are associated with an absence of the internal elastic lamina and smooth muscle in the media of cerebral vessels, particularly at branching points in the vessels.

2. Aneurysms are not present at birth but develop over time owing to normal hemodynamic stress or to enhancing factors such as essential hypertension, adult polycystic kidney disease (10–15%), and postductal coarctation of the aorta.

3. The most common aneurysm site is the junction of the anterior communicating artery with the anterior cerebral artery.

4. Patients have a sudden onset of severe occipital headache, followed by a loss of consciousness. ⟶ *worst headache ever*

5. Blood in the subarachnoid space covers the entire surface of the brain.

6. Approximately 25% die of the first bleed, and an additional 25–35% die by the end of the first year owing to rebleeds.

G. **Lacunar infarcts** are small (< 1 cm) cystic spaces that represent areas of microinfarction secondary to hypertension and, less commonly, diabetes mellitus.

1. Pure motor hemiparesis with or without dysarthria occurs when lacunar infarcts involve the internal capsule or pons.

2. Pure sensory strokes occur with infarcts in the thalamus.

Objective 6: To outline the common causes of demyelinating, dysmyelinating, and degenerative diseases of the CNS.

X. Demyelinating disorders

A. Demyelinating disorders of the white matter only directly attack myelin-synthesizing cells (oligodendrocytes in the CNS or Schwann cells in the PNS) or the myelin sheath without destroying the axon (e.g., multiple sclerosis).

B. **Multiple sclerosis** (MS), the most common demyelinating disease, is associated with autoimmune destruction of the myelin sheath.

1. It is a slightly female-predominant disease (3:2 female:male ratio) and usually targets patients between the ages of 20 and 40 years.

2. The disease may be triggered at an early age by exposure to a virus (possibly herpesvirus 6) in individuals with an HLA-DR2 haplotype.

3. Demyelinating plaques are primarily located in the white matter of the brain and spinal cord.

Meyers
100 P

a. They are sharply demarcated and have a salmon-pink, soft, gelatinous appearance.

b. Favored locations are the surface of the optic nerves and optic chiasm, cerebellar peduncles, brain stem, and angles of the ventricles.

c. They exhibit microglial cells with phagocytosed lipid, reactive gliosis, and a mild perivenular lymphoid (T cell)/plasma cell infiltrate.

4. Approximately 70% of patients present with an episodic course of neurologic dysfunction (sensory and motor dysfunction, optic neuritis, cerebellar incoordination, nystagmus) punctuated by acute relapses and remissions.

5. The CSF findings consist of a slight increase in lymphocytes (T lymphocytes), elevated γ-globulins, normal glucose, and oligoclonal bands (small bands in the γ-globulin region that are indicative of demyelinating disease).

XI. Dysmyelination disorders (leukodystrophies)

A. The leukodystrophies are genetic inborn errors of metabolism involving enzyme deficiencies that result in the synthesis of abnormal myelin (dysmyelination) in the white matter of the brain.

B. **Adrenoleukodystrophy** is an SXR disease due to a deficiency of an enzyme that results in an accumulation of long-chain fatty acids in the brain (dysmyelination) and adrenal cortex (adrenal insufficiency).

C. **Metachromatic leukodystrophy,** the most common leukodystrophy, is an AR disease characterized by a deficiency of arylsulfatase A.

D. **Krabbe's disease** is an AR leukodystrophy resulting from a deficiency of galactocerebroside β-galactosidase with accumulation of galactocerebroside in large multinucleated, histiocytic cells (globoid cells) in the CNS.

XII. Degenerative disorders

A. Degenerative diseases of the CNS are a heterogeneous group of disorders primarily involving neuronal elements.

B. **Alzheimer's disease** (AD) is responsible for ~80% of cases of dementia in both the presenile (< 65 years) and the senile (> 65 years) age bracket.

1. Its etiology is unknown, but associations have been made with the following:

a. Reduced acetylcholine levels (acetylcholine plays a role in learning).

b. Aluminum toxicity.

c. Chromosome 21 coding for an Alzheimer precursor protein (APP), part of which is β-amyloid (Aβ) protein, which is toxic to neurons.

d. Apolipoprotein gene E, allele ε4 located on chromosome 19, which makes a product that increases the neurotoxicity of Aβ protein.

e. Abnormalities on chromosome 14, which synthesizes a tau (τ) microtubule-associated protein located in neurofibrillary tangles.

f. AD is the most common cause of death in older patients with Down syndrome owing to the relationship between chromosome 21 and Aβ protein.

2. AD is characterized by cerebral atrophy owing to neuronal loss in the temporal, frontal, and parietal lobes.

a. Neuronal loss is also evident in the nucleus basalis of Meynert, amygdala, substantia nigra, brain stem, and hippocampus.

b. Histologic findings include neurofibrillary tangles (pairs of filaments coiled like a DNA helix), senile plaques (most important lesion; contain a core of Aβ amyloid surrounded by neurites), and granulovacuolar degeneration.

3. Patients have general impairment of higher intellectual function with no focal neurologic deficits.

C. **Pick's disease** exhibits pronounced cortical atrophy primarily involving the frontal and anterior portions of the temporal lobes with sparing of the posterior two-thirds of the first temporal gyrus.

D. **Idiopathic parkinsonism** is a movement disorder characterized by degeneration and depigmentation of neurons in the substantia nigra and locus ceruleus, leading to a deficiency of dopamine.

1. It generally occurs in patients over 45 years of age.

2. The substantia nigra is part of the striatal system (caudate, putamen, globus pallidus, subthalamus, thalamus), which is involved in voluntary movement of the muscles.

3. Dopamine is the principal neurotransmitter of afferent fibers in the nigrostriatal tract that connects the substantia nigra with the caudate and putamen.

4. Histologic sections of the substantia nigra reveal neuronal loss, depigmentation, and intracytoplasmic, eosinophilic bodies called **Lewy bodies**.

5. Extrapyramidal signs and symptoms include cogwheel rigidity, resting tremor ("pill rolling"), and bradykinesia (slowness of voluntary movement).

6. Patients have an expressionless face, stooped posture, and a festinating gait (progressively shortened accelerated steps).

7. Treatment targets the replacement and prevention of reuptake and metabolism of dopamine.

8. Acquired causes of Parkinson's disease include postencephalitic parkinsonism, diseases that damage the basal ganglia (e.g., ischemia, carbon monoxide, Wilson's disease), and drug use (e.g., phenothiazines, reserpine, MPTP [a meperidine analogue that damages dopaminergic neurons]).

E. **Huntington's disease** (HD) is an AD trait with a delayed appearance of symptoms until a mean age of 35–45 years.

1. It is characterized by atrophy and loss of striatal neurons in the caudate nucleus, putamen, and frontal cortex.

2. It is associated with triplet repeats of CAG on the short arm of chromosome 4.

3. There is a decrease in γ-aminobutyric acid (a false neurotransmitter), acetylcholine, and substance P.

4. HD presents with chorea, extrapyramidal signs, and dementia.

F. **Friedreich's ataxia** is an AR disease consisting of degeneration of the spinocerebellar tracts, posterior columns, pyramidal tracts, and peripheral nerves.

G. **Amyotrophic lateral sclerosis** (ALS) is associated

with loss of upper motor neurons (spasticity) and lower motor neurons (muscle atrophy, muscle fasciculations).

1. There is a defect in the zinc/copper-binding superoxide dismutase (SOD1) on chromosome 21, resulting in oxygen free radical destruction of motor neurons.
2. Atrophy of the intrinsic muscles of the hand and forearms with hand weakness and spastic changes in the lower legs are early signs.
3. The average survival is 2–3 years with respiratory failure being the most common cause of death.

Objective 7: To review metabolic and toxic encephalopathies involving the CNS and PNS.

XIII. Metabolic and toxic encephalopathies
   A. **Wilson's disease**, an AR disease with a defect in copper excretion in bile, is associated with free copper deposits in the lentiform nucleus (putamen and globus pallidus).
   B. **Hepatic encephalopathy** is associated with Alzheimer type II astrocytosis involving the globus pallidus, dentate nucleus, and caudate nucleus.
   C. **Vitamin B$_{12}$ deficiency** produces subacute combined degeneration of the spinal cord (posterior column and lateral corticospinal tract demyelination).
   D. **Alcohol abuse** is associated with cortical atrophy, Wernicke-Korsakoff syndrome complex, cerebellar atrophy (particularly of Purkinje's cells), and central pontine myelinolysis (demyelination disease associated with rapid correction of hyponatremia).
      1. **Wernicke's encephalopathy** is caused by thiamine deficiency and is characterized by the acute onset of confusion, ataxia, nystagmus, and cranial nerve palsies.
         a. There are hemorrhages with associated hemosiderin pigmentation in the mamillary bodies, third ventricle, floor of the fourth ventricle, and thalamus.
         b. In addition, there is neuronal loss and gliosis involving these same areas.
      2. **Korsakoff's psychosis** is a more advanced stage of Wernicke's encephalopathy that targets the limbic system, causing inability to form new memories (anterograde amnesia) or recall old ones (retrograde amnesia).

Objective 8: To discuss the tumors involving the CNS and PNS.

XIV. Tumors of the CNS and PNS
   A. Diseases associated with an increased incidence of brain tumors include Turcot's syndrome (AR hereditary polyposis syndrome) and neurofibromatosis (optic gliomas, meningiomas, acoustic neuromas [unilateral and bilateral]).
   B. Most primary intracranial neoplasms derive from neuroglial cells.
   C. Most **adult primary brain tumors** are supratentorial; in order of decreasing frequency, they are glioblastoma multiforme (high-grade astrocytoma), meningioma, and acoustic neuroma (schwannoma).

D. Most **childhood primary brain tumors** are infratentorial; in descending order of frequency, they are cerebellar astrocytoma, medulloblastoma, brain stem glioma, and ependymoma (in the fourth ventricle).
   E. **Astrocytomas** account for ~70% of neuroglial tumors.
      1. They are subdivided into astrocytomas (grades I and II; benign), anaplastic astrocytomas (grade III; malignant), and glioblastoma multiforme (grade IV; malignant).
      2. In children, they are more likely to be low-grade astrocytomas involving the cerebellum and brain stem, whereas in adults, they are more likely to be glioblastoma multiforme involving the cerebral cortex.
      3. **Glioblastoma multiforme** (GBM), the most common primary brain tumor in adults (40- to 70-year-old age bracket), is a highly malignant astrocytic tumor that pursues a rapidly fatal course.
         a. It has a predilection for the frontal lobes and commonly crosses the corpus callosum, producing a butterfly shape on MRI.
         b. It may arise *de novo* or represent malignant transformation of a lower grade astrocytoma.
         c. It is a hemorrhagic tumor with multifocal areas of necrosis and cystic degeneration.
         d. Prominent histologic features include hemorrhagic necrosis and pseudopalisading of neoplastic cells around areas of necrosis and vascular channels.
         e. It characteristically seeds the neuraxis but rarely metastasizes outside the CNS.
   F. **Oligodendrogliomas** are benign tumors that frequently locate in the cerebral hemispheres (frontal lobes) of adults and have calcifications that are visible on x-ray in ~40% of cases.
   G. **Ependymomas** are benign tumors that most commonly locate within the fourth ventricle (particularly in children), where they produce hydrocephalus.
      1. They are the most common intraspinal tumor (particularly in adults), having a myxopapillary pattern and involving the lumbosacral portion of the spinal cord.
      2. A characteristic finding is the orientation of ependymal cells around vascular channels (perivascular pseudorosettes).
   H. **Medulloblastomas**, the second most common brain tumor in children, are malignant primitive neuroectodermal tumors that arise in the midline of the vermis from the fetal external granular layer.
      1. They are highly infiltrative, invasive tumors that commonly spread down the neuraxis and invade the fourth ventricle.
      2. Although highly radiosensitive, they have a poor prognosis.
   I. **Meningiomas** are benign tumors arising from arachnoidal cells.
      1. They are more common in women than in men and occur between 20 and 60 years of age.
      2. Possible associations include neurofibromatosis, deletions on the long arm of chromosome 22, and a previous history of irradiation.
      3. Common locations include the convexities of the brain (parasagittal; most common location), olfactory groove, lesser wing of the sphenoid, and within the spinal cord (thoracic segment).

4. They are popcorn-shaped, firm tumors that may indent (not invade) the surface of the brain (a common cause of new-onset seizure activity in adults) or infiltrate the overlying bone (not a sign of malignancy) and cause visible hyperostosis on a skull x-ray.

5. They are composed of swirling masses of meningothelial cells, which may encompass psammoma bodies (calcified bodies).

J. **Malignant CNS lymphomas** are most commonly metastatic high-grade non–Hodgkin's lymphomas of B-lymphocyte origin.

1. Primary CNS lymphomas are more likely to be multifocal in their distribution, while metastatic lymphomas usually spread to the meninges and spare the parenchyma.

2. Primary CNS lymphomas are most often associated with AIDS and immunosuppression in renal transplant patients.

   a. The incidence has increased over the last decade owing primarily to an increase in the incidence of AIDS.

   b. They are very aggressive tumors (immunoblastic type) and are strongly associated with the presence of the Epstein-Barr virus plus HIV.

K. **Schwannomas** (neurilemomas) are benign tumors that derive from Schwann cells located on cranial nerves, spinal nerve roots, or peripheral nerves.

1. The most common intracranial site is the cerebellopontine angle with involvement of the VIIIth cranial nerve (**acoustic neuroma**).

2. Expansion of the tumor results in tinnitus (most common) and sensorineural deafness.

3. Histologically, they have very compact Antoni type A areas interspersed with loosely structured myxomatous appearing areas designated Antoni type B areas (the pattern resembles the stripes of a zebra).

L. **Metastasis** is more common than primary tumors of the CNS, with lung cancer representing the most common overall primary site of origin followed by breast cancer.

Objective 9: To describe the types of CNS and PNS diseases associated with AIDS.

XV. CNS and PNS abnormalities in AIDS

A. HIV enters the CNS via macrophages/monocytes (reservoirs of HIV) and astrocytes; microglial cells are the reservoir for HIV in the CNS.

B. HIV is associated with primary CNS lymphoma, aseptic meningitis, encephalitis, vacuolar myelopathy (resembles B_{12} deficiency), peripheral neuropathy, and opportunistic infection (CMV, toxoplasmosis, *C. neoformans*).

C. The **AIDS dementia complex** (ADC) is an encephalitis characterized by motor impairment (e.g., spasticity), cognitive or neurologic deficits (e.g., memory loss), and behavioral or neuropsychological impairment (e.g., hallucinations).

1. Affected cells include astrocytes, microglial cells (alone or in the form of multinucleated giant cells), and oligodendrocytes.

2. CNS injury is secondary to the release of cytokines from infected microglial cells and autoantibodies directed against proteins in the brain that cross-react with HIV proteins.

Objective 10: To be familiar with selected disorders of the peripheral nervous system.

XVI. Peripheral neuropathy

A. Peripheral neuropathies may result from demyelination (often segmental), axonal degeneration, or both.

B. Segmental demyelination results in sensory changes including a symmetric "glove and stocking" distribution of sensory loss ("burning foot" syndrome).

C. Axonal degeneration results in muscle atrophy and fasciculations.

D. Peripheral neuropathies may be secondary to diabetes mellitus (most common; osmotic damage of Schwann cells), toxins (e.g., alcohol, heavy metals, diphtheria), amyloidosis, drugs (e.g., isoniazid, vincristine), and nutritional deficiencies (e.g., thiamine, pyridoxine).

E. **Distal sensorimotor neuropathy** is the most prevalent type of peripheral neuropathy and is most often caused by diabetes mellitus.

F. **Guillain-Barré syndrome**, the most common cause of an acute peripheral neuropathy, presents with an ascending or descending paralysis and high CSF protein levels.

G. **Charcot-Marie-Tooth disease**, the most common genetic (AD inheritance pattern) peripheral neuropathy, primarily involves the peroneal nerve and produces atrophy of the muscles of the lower legs.

XVII. Selected disorders of the PNS

A. **Wallerian degeneration** follows transection of a nerve.

1. It is initially associated with proximal degeneration of the axon and the myelin sheath ("dying back") to the nearest node of Ranvier.

2. The distal axon and its myelin sheath also degenerate, and their breakdown products are removed by both macrophages and Schwann cells.

3. The muscle is denervated and undergoes atrophy.

4. The remaining Schwann cells begin to proliferate and form a tube that will serve to guide axon sprouts in the regeneration process.

5. Regeneration of the nerve occurs by the outgrowth of multiple axon sprouts from the proximal surviving segment of the axon.

6. These sprouts are directed distally (growth rate of 1–3 mm/d) down the tube established by the proliferating Schwann cells.

7. The sprouts are remyelinated and reestablish continuity with the motor end plate of the muscle.

8. In some cases, the regenerating axons form a tangled, often painful mass of nerve fibers called a traumatic neuroma.

B. **Idiopathic Bell's palsy** is associated with an acute onset of unilateral facial nerve (VII) paralysis.

1. Patients present with drooping of the corner of the mouth, difficulty in speaking, inability to close the eye, and drooling.

2. Known causes of Bell's palsy include Lyme disease (most common cranial nerve palsy in the disease; frequently bilateral), malignant parotid gland tumors with nerve involvement, multiple sclerosis, and HIV infection.

QUESTIONS

1. This gross autopsy specimen is from a 65-year-old man who initially presented with a right frontal headache that was present when he awoke and lasted throughout the day. The pathologic process is most closely associated with

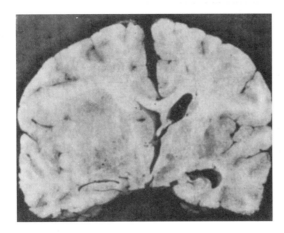

(A) a neoplastic proliferation of glial cells
(B) a demyelinating disorder
(C) an embolic stroke
(D) a degenerative disorder
(E) a hypertensive stroke

2. The photograph is a histologic section taken from an encapsulated mass removed from the cerebellopontine angle of a 29-year-old man with tinnitus. His Weber test lateralized to the right ear, and the Rinne test revealed air conduction longer than bone conduction in both ears. The mass is most likely derived from

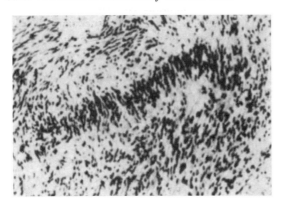

(A) ependymal cells
(B) microglial cells
(C) astrocytes
(D) arachnoidal cells
(E) Schwann cells

3. The gross photograph is an autopsy specimen removed from an afebrile 72-year-old man with a 40 pack-year (i.e., 2 packs a day for 20 years) history of smoking. He presented with headache, diastolic hypertension, sinus bradycardia, projectile vomiting, and papilledema. The pathologic process is most closely associated with

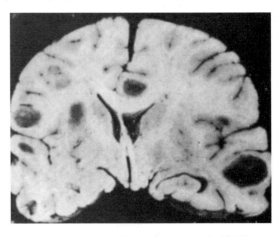

(A) hypertension
(B) infection
(C) metastasis
(D) thromboembolism
(E) atherosclerosis

4. The autopsy finding depicted in this photograph is from a 23-year-old man who died in a head-on collision with a truck. The mechanism for the pathologic process is most closely related to

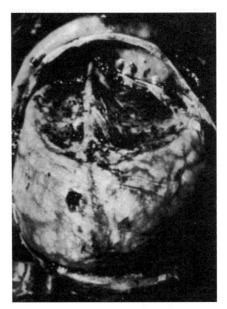

(A) tearing of the bridging veins between the dura and arachnoid
(B) tearing of the middle cerebral artery
(C) rupture of an aneurysm
(D) tearing of the middle meningeal artery
(E) a contrecoup injury to the cerebral hemispheres

5. The gross photograph is from a 55-year-old man who had a sudden onset of headache and died a few hours later. The pathogenesis of the lesion responsible for his death is most closely related to

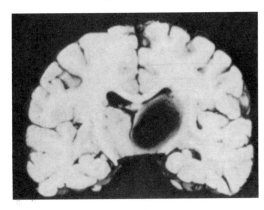

(A) atherosclerosis
(B) hypertension
(C) thromboembolism
(D) metastasis
(E) a congenital vessel defect

6. The gross photograph is from a 54-year-old woman with a long history of episodic attacks of motor weakness, sensory abnormalities, optic neuritis, nystagmus, and ataxia. The lateral ventricle is visible on the right side of the specimen. The pathologic process that produced this patient's disease is most closely associated with

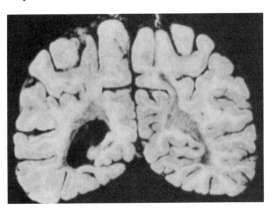

(A) dysmyelination
(B) a degenerative disorder
(C) demyelination
(D) vascular disease
(E) a slow virus disease

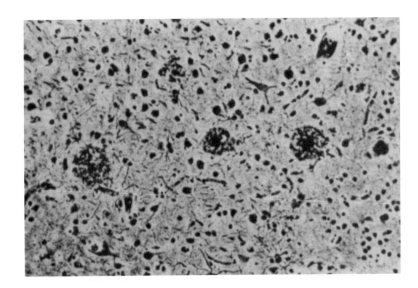

7. This is a microscopic section from the frontal lobe of a 70-year-old man with a generalized loss of higher intellectual function since age 66. His frontal, temporal, and parietal lobes were atrophic. The pathogenesis of the silver-stained structures in the photograph is most closely related to

(A) Parkinson's disease
(B) Alzheimer's disease
(C) toxoplasmosis
(D) cytomegalovirus
(E) prion disease

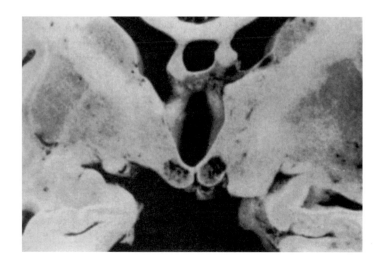

8. The photograph of brain is from a 55-year-old man with chronic liver disease and hepatic encephalopathy. The gross abnormality noted in the slide is most closely associated with

   (A) a nutritional deficiency
   (B) a hemorrhagic infarction
   (C) a defect in copper excretion
   (D) chronic exposure to carbon monoxide
   (E) a neoplastic process

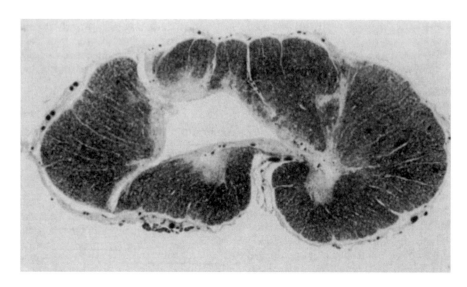

9. The photograph represents a cross-section of cervical cord removed at autopsy from a 32-year-old patient with multiple neurologic dysfunctions. The most likely diagnosis is

   (A) amyotrophic lateral sclerosis
   (B) poliomyelitis
   (C) an intraspinal ependymoma
   (D) syringomyelia
   (E) Dandy-Walker syndrome

10. Which of the following is an example of a communicating hydrocephalus?

  (A) Stricture of the aqueduct of Sylvius
  (B) Blood clot blocking the foramina of Luschka and Magendie
  (C) Blockage of the arachnoid granulations
  (D) Ependymoma infiltrating the fourth ventricle
  (E) Dandy-Walker syndrome

11. A 4-year-old child has a sudden onset of fever, nuchal rigidity, and positive Kernig's sign. Lumbar puncture reveals an elevated CSF protein, a neutrophil-dominant count, and a low CSF glucose. The Gram stain most likely revealed a gram-

  (A) negative diplococcus
  (B) positive coccus
  (C) negative rod
  (D) positive rod
  (E) positive diplococcus

12. Papilledema, lid lag and a mydriatic pupil on the right, and CT evidence of a hemorrhagic infarction of the right occipital lobe would be most consistent with

  (A) multiple sclerosis
  (B) atherosclerotic stroke
  (C) cerebellar tonsil herniation
  (D) uncal herniation
  (E) a noncommunicating hydrocephalus

DIRECTIONS. (Items 13–17): Each set of matching questions in this section consists of a list of lettered options followed by several numbered items. For each numbered item, select the ONE option that is most closely associated with it. Each lettered option may be selected once, more than once, or not at all.

  (A) Arnold-Chiari malformation
  (B) Dandy-Walker syndrome
  (C) Tuberous sclerosis
  (D) Neurofibromatosis
  (E) Sturge-Weber syndrome
  (F) Adrenoleukodystrophy
  (G) Metachromatic leukodystrophy
  (H) Krabbe's disease
  (I) Huntington's disease
  (J) Idiopathic Parkinson's disease
  (K) Amyotrophic lateral sclerosis
  (L) Meningioma
  (M) Glioblastoma multiforme
  (N) Medulloblastoma
  (O) Oligodendroglioma
  (P) Ependymoma

13. Hemorrhagic necrosis in the frontal lobe with extension across the corpus callosum to the opposite lobe in a 60-year-old man.

14. Illegible handwriting in a 65-year-old man with an expressionless face and slow movement of his arms with cerebellar function testing.

15. Cerebellar mass in a 7-year-old with extension into the fourth ventricle resulting in hydrocephalus.

16. Elongation of the medulla oblongata and cerebellum, hydrocephalus, and a myelomeningocele in a newborn.

17. Intraspinal mass involving the cauda equina in a 22-year-old man with sacral pain.

ANSWERS AND EXPLANATIONS

1. The answer is A: a neoplastic proliferation of glial cells. The specimen reveals a right-sided mass lesion in the cerebral cortex that has displaced the ipsilateral ventricles. It is most consistent with an astrocytoma, which in adults most commonly targets the cerebral hemispheres. Both embolic and hypertensive strokes are associated with intracerebral hemorrhage. Degenerative (e.g., Alzheimer's disease) and demyelinating disorders (e.g., multiple sclerosis) do not present with a unilateral mass lesion. (Photograph reproduced, with permission, from J. Poirier, F. Gray, and R. Escourolle. *Manual of Basic Neuropathology,* 3rd ed. Philadelphia, W.B. Saunders Co., 1990, p. 22.)

2. The answer is E: Schwann cells. The microscopic section shows the classic Antoni A (dark) and Antoni B (light) areas of an acoustic neuroma (schwannoma). It most likely originated from the left VIIIth nerve (sensorineural hearing loss on the left; the Weber test lateralizes to the normal ear). Acoustic neuromas derive from Schwann cells. Regarding the other choices, ependymal cells are associated with ependymomas, astrocytes with astrocytomas, and arachnoidal cells with meningiomas. Microglial cells (phagocytic cells) are not associated with neoplastic transformation. (Photomicrograph reproduced, with permission, from J. Poirier, F. Gray, and R. Escourolle. *Manual of Basic*

Neuropathology, 3rd ed. Philadelphia, W.B. Saunders Co., 1990, p. 34.)

3. The answer is C: metastasis. The photograph reveals multiple hemorrhagic lesions and displacement of both ventricles, the right more than the left. Most of the lesions are located at the junction of the gray and white matter. Given the history of smoking, metastasis from a primary lung cancer is the most likely diagnosis. The clinical findings are those of increased intracranial pressure. Hypertension and thromboembolism do not produce multifocal areas of hemorrhage. Cerebral abscesses are not hemorrhagic, and cystic spaces would be present. Atherosclerotic strokes are not multifocal and are generally pale infarcts. (Photograph reproduced, with permission, from J. Poirier, F. Gray, and R. Escourolle. *Manual of Basic Neuropathology,* 3rd ed. Philadelphia, W.B. Saunders Co., 1990, p. 49.)

4. The answer is D: tearing of the middle meningeal artery. A large blood clot is present on top of the dura, hence the patient has an epidural hematoma related to rupture of the middle cerebral artery due to a fracture of the temporoparietal bone. The location of the bleed argues against a subdural hematoma (tearing of the bridging veins) or a subarachnoid hemorrhage (rupture of an aneurysm or tearing of the middle cerebral artery). Contrecoup injuries are contusions most commonly located on the tips of the frontal and temporal

lobes. (Photograph reproduced, with permission, from J. Poirier, F. Gray, and R. Escourolle. *Manual of Basic Neuropathology,* 3rd ed. Philadelphia, W.B. Saunders Co., 1990, p. 59.)

5. The answer is B: hypertension. The photograph shows a well-circumscribed hemorrhage in the area of the basal ganglia, which is supplied by the lenticulostriate vessels. The location is classic for an intracerebral bleed from a ruptured Charcot-Bouchard microaneurysm secondary to hypertension. Atherosclerotic strokes are pale infarcts, embolic strokes are hemorrhagic and located at the periphery of the cortex, subarachnoid bleeds (aneurysm secondary to a congenital vessel defect) cover the surface of the brain, and metastases are normally multiple and favor the cerebral cortex. (Photograph reproduced, with permission, from J. Poirier, F. Gray, and R. Escourolle. *Manual of Basic Neuropathology,* 3rd ed. Philadelphia, W.B. Saunders Co., 1990, p. 68.)

6. The answer is C: demyelination. The patient's history and the gross findings of gray-colored lesions (demyelinating plaques) in a periventricular distribution within the white matter is most consistent with multiple sclerosis. Other favored locations are the optic nerves (optic neuritis), cerebellum (ataxia), and brain stem. Dysmyelination is the synthesis of abnormal myelin (e.g., metachromatic leukodystrophy). Degenerative disorders involve destruction of neurons, not myelin sheaths. Vascular disease, like atherosclerosis, targets layers 3, 5, and 6 in the cerebral cortex and the hippocampus. Slow virus diseases are very rare, although they are associated with demyelination. (Photograph reproduced, with permission, from J. Poirier, F. Gray, and R. Escourolle. *Manual of Basic Neuropathology,* 3rd ed. Philadelphia, W.B. Saunders Co., 1990, p. 128.)

7. The answer is B: Alzheimer's disease. The history and the sites of atrophy in the brain are compatible with dementia, the most common cause of which is Alzheimer's disease (AD). The well-circumscribed lesions in the photograph are senile plaques, which contain a core of β-amyloid protein surrounded by neurites. These are highly predictive of AD. Toxoplasmosis and CMV are most commonly seen in the setting of AIDS. Parkinson's disease is associated with deficiency of dopamine. Prions are the unconventional agents associated with Creutzfeldt-Jakob disease. (Photomicrograph reproduced, with permission, from J. Poirier, F. Gray, and R. Escourolle. *Manual of Basic Neuropathology,* 3rd ed. Philadelphia, W.B. Saunders Co., 1990, p. 141.)

8. The answer is A: a nutritional deficiency. The photograph exhibits the classic ring hemorrhages in the mamillary bodies associated with Wernicke's encephalopathy in a person with alcoholism and thiamine deficiency. The hemorrhages are due to rupture of capillaries (not a hemorrhagic infarction or neoplastic process). Similar findings may occur around the ventricles. Wilson's disease (a defect in copper excretion) produces degeneration in the lenticular nuclei. CO poisoning is associated with degeneration of the globus pallidus. (Photograph reproduced, with permission, from J. Poirier, F. Gray, and R. Escourolle. *Manual of Basic Neuropathology,* 3rd ed. Philadelphia, W.B. Saunders Co., 1990, p. 167.)

9. The answer is D: syringomyelia. The spinal cord exhibits a cavitating lesion encroaching upon the posterior horn and column consistent with a syrinx. The expanding lesion is commonly associated with cervical

cord enlargement and neurologic abnormalities involving the crossed lateral spinothalamic tracts, posterior columns, lateral corticospinal tracts, and anterior horn motor neurons. None of the other choices are associated with a cystic cavity in the cervical spinal cord. (Photomicrograph reproduced, with permission, from J. Poirier, F. Gray, and R. Escourolle. *Manual of Basic Neuropathology,* 3rd ed. Philadelphia, W.B. Saunders Co., 1990, p. 204.)

10. The answer is: C: blockage of the arachnoid granulations. A communicating hydrocephalus implies free flow of CSF between the ventricles and the subarachnoid space. This may occur owing to an increase in production of CSF by the choroid plexus (e.g., choroid plexus papilloma) or to blockage of reabsorption of CSF by the arachnoid granulations (e.g., postmeningeal scarring). The other choices produce a noncommunicating hydrocephalus, which prevents free access of CSF into the subarachnoid space.

11. The answer is A: negative diplococcus. The most common cause of bacterial meningitis in children between 3 months and 18 years of age is *Neisseria meningitidis,* which is a gram-negative diplococcus. *Haemophilus influenzae,* a gram-negative rod, is no longer the most common pathogen owing to immunization. The CSF findings are representative of bacterial meningitis (neutrophil-dominant count, high protein, low glucose). Kernig's sign is a test for meningeal inflammation.

12. The answer is D: uncal herniation. Papilledema indicates an increase in intracranial pressure, the eye signs (lid lag, mydriatic pupil) indicate an oculomotor nerve palsy, and a hemorrhagic infarction of the right occipital lobe is consistent with obstruction of flow in the posterior cerebral artery (PCA). All these findings are present in uncal herniations through the tentorium cerebelli with compression of the midbrain, oculomotor nerve, and PCA. The distribution of these findings would not be expected in an atherosclerotic stroke, cerebellar tonsil herniation, multiple sclerosis, or a noncommunicating hydrocephalus.

13. The answer is M: glioblastoma multiforme. GBMs, the most common primary brain tumor in adults, are grade IV astrocytomas that favor the cerebral cortex. They characteristically cross the corpus callosum, producing a butterfly shape on MRI.

14. The answer is J: idiopathic Parkinson's disease. Parkinson's disease is characterized by loss of neurons in the substantia nigra that synthesize dopamine. Extrapyramidal signs include cogwheel rigidity, bradykinesia (slow movement owing to rigidity), and a resting tremor of the hands that renders handwriting illegible.

15. The answer is N: medulloblastoma. Medulloblastomas, the second most common malignant brain tumor in children, are primitive neuroectodermal tumors that arise in the cerebellum, extend into the fourth ventricles, and seed the neuraxis.

16. The answer is A: Arnold-Chiari malformation. Elongation of the medulla oblongata and cerebellum, hydrocephalus, and a myelomeningocele in a newborn describe the Arnold-Chiari malformation. Additional findings include platybasia (flat base of the skull) and syringomyelia.

17. The answer is P: ependymoma. Ependymomas are the most common intraspinal tumor. They most often target the lumbosacral part of the spinal cord and frequently infiltrate the cauda equina, resulting in severe pain. They usually occur in adults, whereas in children ependymomas more commonly occur in the fourth ventricle.

COMPREHENSIVE

EXAMINATION

DIRECTIONS. (Items 1–132): Each of the numbered items or incomplete statements in this section is followed by answers or by completions of the statement. Select the ONE lettered answer or completion that is BEST in each case. Correct answers and explanations are given at the end of the chapter.

1. The photograph is of a 43-year-old man with long-standing alcohol abuse. Additional findings include shifting dullness on abdominal examination, bilateral gynecomastia, and scattered spider angiomas over the anterior chest. Which of the following would most likely be present in this patient?

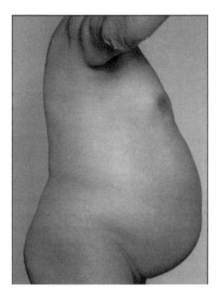

    (A) Increased effective arterial blood volume
    (B) Decreased total body sodium (TBNa)
    (C) Secondary aldosteronism
    (D) Normal plasma oncotic pressure
    (E) Normal prothrombin time

2. The finger depicted in this photograph is from a 50-year-old woman who has a strong family history of autoimmune disease. You would expect the patient to have

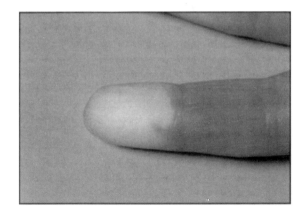

    (A) a malar rash and joint pains
    (B) dysphagia for solids and liquids
    (C) a dry mouth, dry eyes, and rheumatoid arthritis

    (D) muscle pain with an elevated serum creatine kinase
    (E) dry skin, brittle hair, and periorbital puffiness

3. The photograph is of the face of an afebrile 15-year-old boy. You expect that a Gram stain of the honey-colored crusting lesions on his face would exhibit gram-

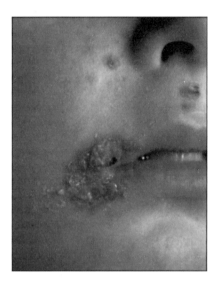

    (A) positive lancet-shaped diplococci
    (B) positive cocci in chains
    (C) negative diplococci
    (D) negative rods
    (E) positive rods

4. The photograph is of a 62-year-old woman who is being treated with chemotherapy for a malignant lymphoma. The lesion on the face is most closely associated with

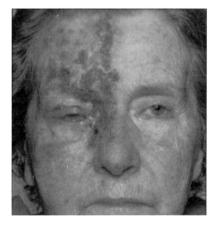

    (A) neoplastic infiltration of skin
    (B) a bacterial infection
    (C) a viral infection
    (D) a drug reaction
    (E) an autoimmune disease

5. The photograph is representative of a generalized eruption on the skin of a febrile 3-year-old boy. One week later, the child developed neurologic problems and tender hepatomegaly with an elevation in transaminases. The serum ammonia was elevated. The pathogenesis of the lesions is most closely associated with

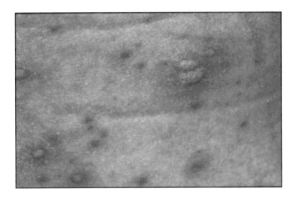

(A) a gram-positive coccus that is coagulase positive
(B) a gram-positive coccus that is catalase negative

(C) an autoimmune disorder with antibodies directed against desmosomes
(D) an autoimmune disorder with antibodies directed against the basement membrane
(E) a viral infection that often remains dormant in sensory dorsal root ganglia

6. The photograph is of a polarized sample of synovial fluid aspirated from the knee of a febrile 35-year-old man with alcoholism. The absolute neutrophil count is elevated in the fluid and in the peripheral blood. The crystals are yellow when oriented in the same direction as the slow axis of the compensator. On the basis of these findings, which of the following statements is correct?

(A) The crystals are positively birefringent
(B) The crystals represent calcium pyrophosphate
(C) There is a defect in pyrimidine metabolism
(D) There is underexcretion of uric acid by the kidney
(E) Inflammation is secondary to a direct toxic effect of alcohol

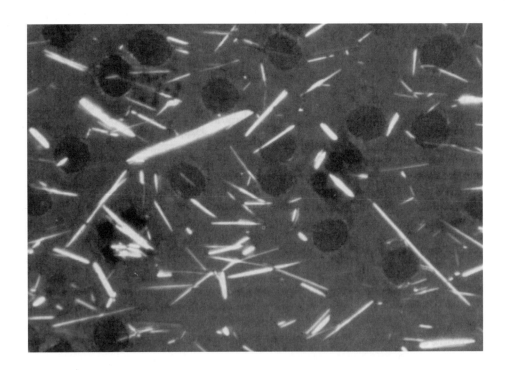

7. The gross photograph depicts a normal midbrain at top and the midbrain of a 75-year-old man at bottom.

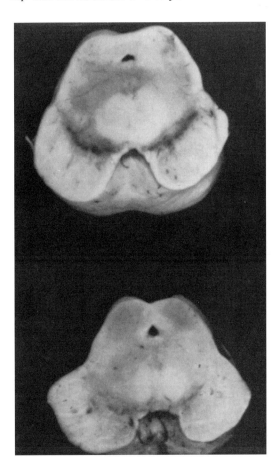

Which of the following best represents the clinical findings that were likely present in the latter?

(A) Severe headaches and papilledema
(B) Bradykinesia
(C) Confabulation
(D) Anterograde and retrograde memory deficits
(E) Transient ischemic attacks

8. The photograph is a high-power magnification of a glial cell in the brain of a patient who died of AIDS. The most likely diagnosis is

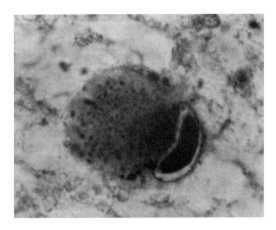

(A) cytomegalovirus encephalitis
(B) herpes type 1 encephalitis
(C) *Toxoplasma* encephalitis
(D) subacute sclerosing panencephalitis
(E) progressive multifocal leukoencephalopathy

9. The pathogenesis of the lesion in the brain of this 65-year-old African American man who died of an acute myocardial infarction is most closely related to

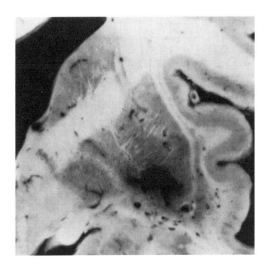

(A) diabetes mellitus
(B) essential hypertension
(C) embolic stroke
(D) atherosclerosis
(E) infection

10. The photograph of brain is from an afebrile 52-year-old woman with a long history of rheumatic heart disease. Her cardiac examination prior to death revealed an opening snap and diastolic rumble that occurred shortly after the second heart sound. P_2 was accentuated. She had an irregularly irregular pulse. The cerebral event causing her demise was unexpected and sudden. The pathogenesis of the brain lesion is most closely related to

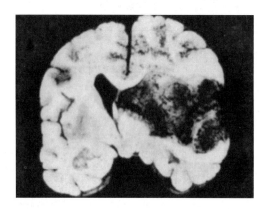

   (A) atherosclerosis
   (B) hypertension
   (C) embolism
   (D) cardiogenic shock
   (E) an infectious process

11. The photograph of brain is from an 82-year-old man who died in a nursing home of bronchopneumonia. Which of the following groupings of pathologic processes are most likely operative in the brain of this patient as either a past or a recent event?

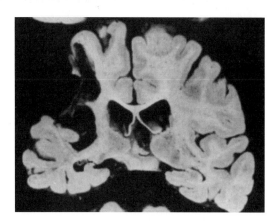

   (A) Coagulation necrosis and atrophy
   (B) Liquefactive necrosis and atrophy
   (C) Intracerebral hematoma and degenerative disease
   (D) Metastatic abscess and tissue hypoxia
   (E) Metastatic abscess and intracerebral edema

12. The autopsy finding in brain is for an 85-year-old man who was found dead in bed by his wife. The pathogenesis of the lesion in his brain is most often associated with

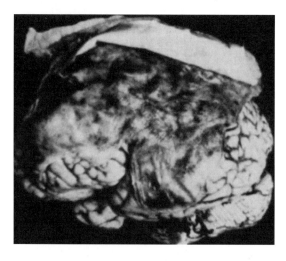

   (A) essential hypertension
   (B) a tear of the middle meningeal artery
   (C) a ruptured berry aneurysm
   (D) an embolic stroke
   (E) a tear of a bridging vein

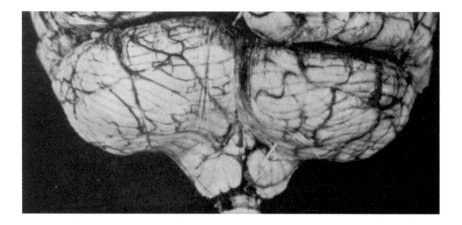

13. The gross abnormality noted in this brain removed at autopsy from a 55-year-old man is most likely the result of

    (A) intracerebral edema
    (B) a hypertonic state
    (C) bacterial meningitis
    (D) a demyelinating disease
    (E) a degenerative disease

14. This is a brain removed at autopsy from a 60-year-old man with left frontal headaches that were present upon awakening in the morning and lasted throughout the day. The pathologic process most likely responsible for his disease is

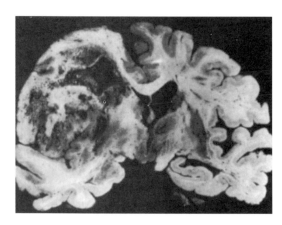

    (A) a malignant neoplasm originating from astrocytes
    (B) a malignant neoplasm originating from oligodendrocytes
    (C) an intracerebral bleed secondary to hypertension
    (D) rupture of a congenital berry aneurysm
    (E) metastatic disease from an extracranial primary site

15. The gross specimen represented in this photograph most likely came from a patient with

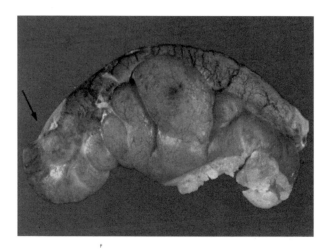

    (A) bloody diarrhea
    (B) neutrophilic leukocytosis and a left shift
    (C) crampy abdominal pain with bloody diarrhea
    (D) flushing and watery diarrhea
    (E) atypical lymphocytosis

16. Regarding the gross abnormality in this distal antrectomy specimen, you expect that a random biopsy of the gastric mucosa revealed

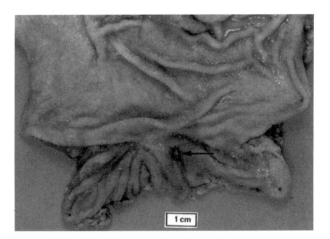

(A) an infiltrate of neoplastic signet-ring cells
(B) *Helicobacter pylori* in the mucous layer
(C) chronic atrophic gastritis
(D) hypertrophic rugae and submucosal cysts
(E) erosions secondary to NSAID use

17. The immunofluorescence (IF) pattern in this glomerulus is most consistent with

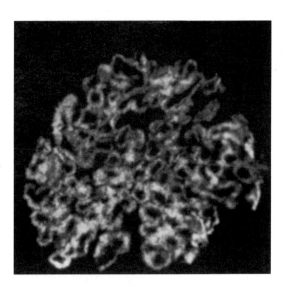

(A) focal segmental glomerulosclerosis
(B) renal amyloidosis
(C) diabetic glomerulosclerosis
(D) minimal change disease
(E) membranous glomerulonephritis

18. The most likely cause of the gross abnormality noted in this brain of a 75-year-old man is

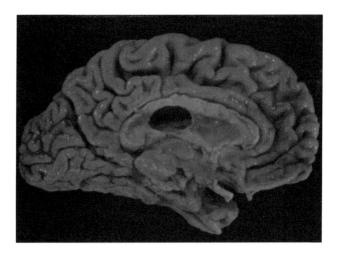

(A) a degenerative disease
(B) hypertension
(C) atherosclerosis
(D) metastasis
(E) an infectious process

19. Which of the following best describes the pathogenesis of the changes seen in the foot of this 65-year-old man with type II diabetes mellitus?

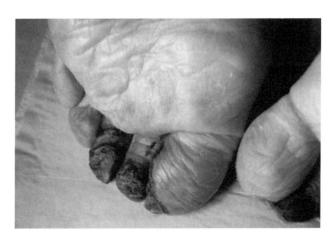

(A) Coagulation necrosis secondary to popliteal artery atherosclerosis with thrombosis
(B) Liquefactive necrosis associated with ischemic necrosis
(C) Embolization with infarction of the digits
(D) Vasculitis with infarction of the digits
(E) Infective endocarditis with embolization and infarction of the digits

20. The gross abnormality noted in this heart was most likely associated with which of the following physical findings?

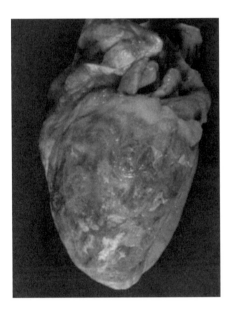

(A) S₃ heart sound
(B) Friction rub
(C) Opening snap
(D) Mid-systolic ejection click
(E) Pericardial knock

21. The electron micrograph depicts a hematopoietic cell that would most likely

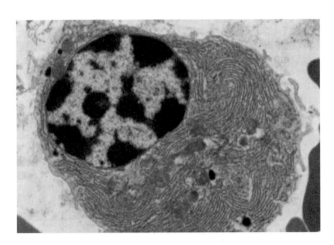

(A) release preformed histamine
(B) release major basic protein
(C) produce antibodies
(D) release muramidase
(E) release interleukin-2

22. The gross photograph and microscopic section are of a yellow, well-circumscribed, freely moveable mass removed from the forearm of a 35-year-old man. It has been present for the last 5 years. It is most likely derived from

(A) skeletal muscle
(B) smooth muscle
(C) endothelial cells
(D) adipose
(E) fibroblasts

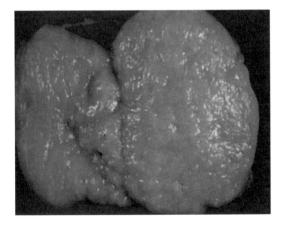

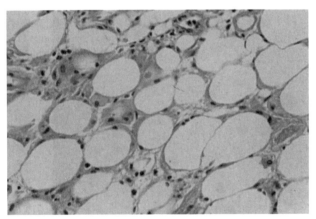

23. The electron micrograph represents cytoplasmic structures from glial cells in the brain of a child with severe mental retardation. The patient most likely had a deficiency of

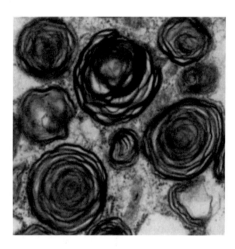

   (A) sphingomyelinase
   (B) hexosaminidase
   (C) arylsulfatase A
   (D) galactosylceramidase
   (E) α_1-iduronidase

24. The photomicrograph represents a section of lung removed at autopsy from a 4-day-old child born to a mother with gestational diabetes mellitus who had poor glycemic control during her pregnancy. The pathophysiology of the lung disorder in the baby is most closely related to

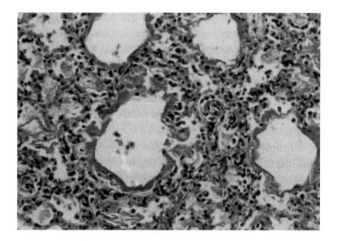

   (A) a pulmonary infection
   (B) a congenital malformation
   (C) aspiration of meconium
   (D) a perfusion disorder
   (E) a ventilation disorder

25. The gross abnormalities noted in this kidney are most likely secondary to

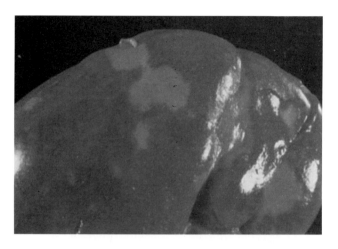

   (A) thromboembolization from the heart
   (B) ischemic acute tubular necrosis
   (C) benign nephrosclerosis
   (D) chronic pyelonephritis
   (E) malignant hypertension

26. The specimen represents a segment of small bowel removed from an elderly man with a recurrent history of severe abdominal pain 30 minutes after eating. He presented to the hospital with hypotension and bloody diarrhea. The pathologic process responsible for the gross changes in the bowel is most closely related to

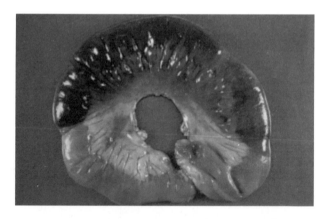

   (A) inflammatory bowel disease
   (B) bacterial enterocolitis
   (C) drug-induced enterocolitis
   (D) ischemic necrosis
   (E) angiodysplasia

27. The gross specimen represents the mitral valve viewed from the left atrium. You suspect the patient has a history of

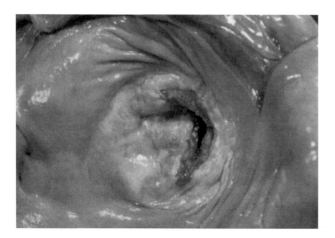

    (A) intravenous drug abuse
    (B) a carcinoid tumor of the small bowel
    (C) mitral valve prolapse
    (D) systemic lupus erythematosus
    (E) rheumatic fever

28. The photomicrograph is representative of sections taken from yellow, raised, patchy consolidations present in the left lower lobe of a 60-year-old man who died in a nursing home. The histologic findings are most consistent with

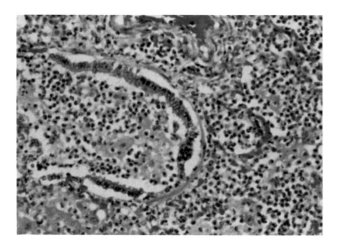

    (A) a bacterial bronchopneumonia
    (B) granulomatous inflammation
    (C) primary lung cancer
    (D) metastatic adenocarcinoma
    (E) a viral pneumonia

29. The gross specimen is of lung removed at autopsy from an afebrile retired Navy chief. He spent most of his career in naval shipyards dating back to World War II. The patient was a nonsmoker, and no other gross abnormalities were noted in sectioning of other organs. You suspect his disease is most closely associated with

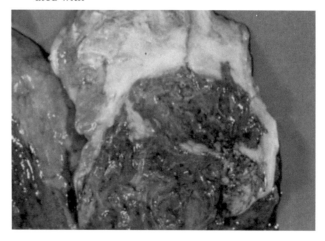

    (A) pleural spread of an underlying pneumonia
    (B) a primary small-cell carcinoma of the lung
    (C) a primary squamous cell carcinoma of the lung
    (D) reactivation tuberculosis
    (E) inhalation of asbestos fibers

30. The peripheral blood findings noted in the photomicrograph are representative of the peripheral smear in an afebrile 72-year-old man with generalized, nontender lymphadenopathy, hepatosplenomegaly, normocytic anemia, and thrombocytopenia. The total WBC count is 110,000 cells/μL. The tartrate-resistant acid phosphatase (TRAP) stain on the cells in the peripheral blood is negative. You expect the bone marrow aspirate examination reveals

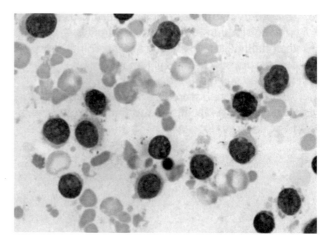

    (A) a diffuse infiltrate of neoplastic lymphocytes
    (B) > 30% myeloblasts with Auer rods present in some cells
    (C) 1–10% myeloblasts without Auer rods
    (D) a hypercellular marrow with numerous ringed sideroblasts
    (E) a fibrotic marrow with distorted megakaryocytes and islands of normal erythropoiesis

31. The photomicrograph is one of many diffusely enlarged lymph nodes in an afebrile 45-year-old man who was treated for lymphocyte-predominant Hodgkin's disease 20 years ago. The lymph node findings are most compatible with

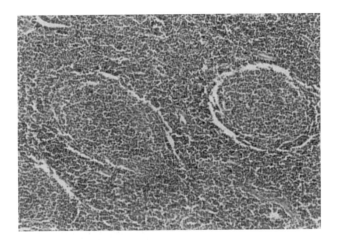

(A) metastatic carcinoma
(B) recurrent lymphocyte-predominant Hodgkin's disease
(C) nodular sclerosing Hodgkin's disease
(D) a B-cell non-Hodgkin's malignant lymphoma
(E) reactive lymph node hyperplasia

32. The gross specimen of distal esophagus and proximal stomach was removed from a 52-year-old man with alcoholism and a 40 pack-year history of cigarette smoking. He presented with weakness, weight loss, and dysphagia for solids. Biopsy of the lesion most likely revealed

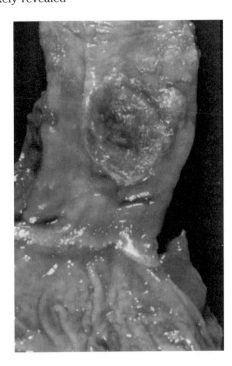

(A) ulceration secondary to a viral infection (e.g., herpes simplex type 1)
(B) glandular metaplasia with ulceration
(C) a primary squamous cell carcinoma

(D) adenocarcinoma extending into the esophagus from the stomach
(E) ulceration secondary to gastroesophageal reflux disease

33. The gross specimen represents a total colectomy performed on a 42-year-old man with a long history of bloody diarrhea. On the basis of the gross appearance of the specimen, you expect that

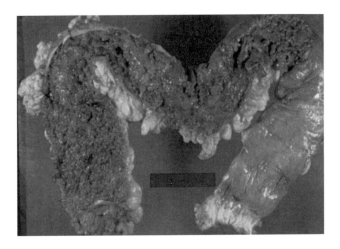

(A) there is an autosomal dominant inheritance pattern to his disease
(B) the disease began in the anal canal and spread in continuity to involve the entire colon
(C) sections revealed transmural inflammation and noncaseating granulomas
(D) sections revealed mucosal ulceration and coagulation necrosis
(E) sections exhibited inflammatory pseudopolyps and crypt abscesses

34. The photograph represents the liver removed at autopsy from a 59-year-old man who was found dead in his apartment. On the basis of the gross appearance of the liver, you suspect that the patient

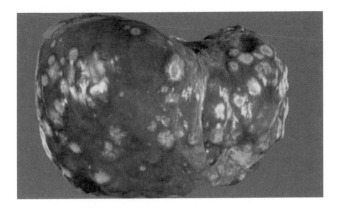

(A) had alcoholism and signs of portal hypertension
(B) had a primary cancer originating in the stomach
(C) was a smoker with a primary cancer originating in the lung
(D) had hepatocellular carcinoma
(E) had reactivation tuberculosis with miliary spread to the liver

35. The photomicrograph is representative of a section of pancreas removed at autopsy from a 40-year-old man found dead on a park bench. His liver was enlarged and had a yellow, greasy consistency. On the basis of the histologic appearance of the pancreatic tissue, you suspect that other findings in the patient included

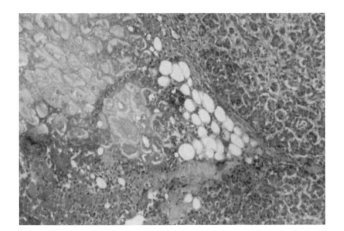

    (A) elevated serum amylase and lipase levels
    (B) metastatic liver disease secondary to pancreatic cancer
    (C) focal areas of metastatic calcification in the pancreas
    (D) normal serum transaminase and γ-glutamyltransferase levels
    (E) jaundice due to blockage of the common bile duct

36. This kidney was removed at autopsy from a 58-year-old man with hypertension and chronic renal failure requiring hemodialysis. While in the hospital, he complained of a severe occipital headache and died shortly thereafter. Examination of his brain most likely revealed

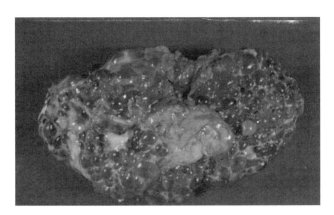

    (A) metastatic disease
    (B) a subarachnoid hemorrhage
    (C) a ruptured arteriovenous malformation
    (D) an intracerebral hematoma
    (E) a glioblastoma multiforme

37. The glomerulus depicted in this slide is representative of 70% of the glomeruli noted in a renal biopsy from a 28-year-old man with renal failure, hematuria, and RBC casts. He initially presented at the hospital one month ago with hemoptysis and then progressed to renal failure requiring hemodialysis. You suspect that the pathogenesis of his disease is most closely associated with

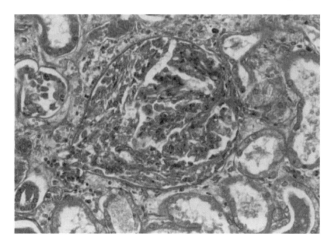

    (A) immunocomplex-related disease involving the lungs and kidneys
    (B) antibodies directed against planted antigens in the lungs and glomeruli
    (C) activation of neutrophils by c-antineutrophil cytoplasmic antibodies
    (D) activation of neutrophils by p-antineutrophil cytoplasmic antibodies
    (E) antibodies directed against the noncollagen domain of α_3 type IV collagen

38. The glomerulus depicted in this photomicrograph is representative of ~50% of the glomeruli in the kidneys removed at autopsy from a 55-year-old man with chronic renal disease. Based on the histologic appearance of the glomerulus, you suspect that the pathogenesis of his kidney disease is most closely associated with

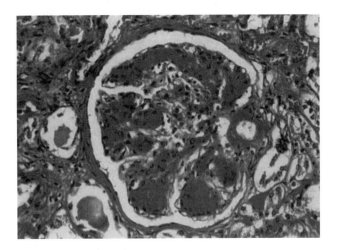

   (A) nonenzymatic glycosylation
   (B) osmotic damage
   (C) immunocomplex disease
   (D) systemic amyloidosis
   (E) antineutrophil cytoplasmic antibodies

39. The photomicrograph is representative of the histopathologic features of multiple hemorrhagic nodules in the lungs of a 75-year-old man who had cancer surgery ~20 years ago. The man has a 60 pack-year history of smoking. You suspect that the cancer removed 20 years ago was a

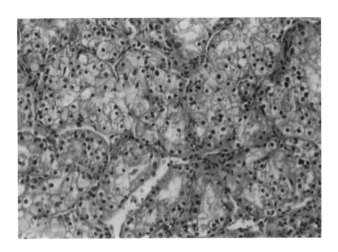

   (A) primary squamous cell carcinoma of the lung
   (B) primary small-cell carcinoma of the lung
   (C) renal adenocarcinoma
   (D) papillary adenocarcinoma of the thyroid
   (E) prostatic adenocarcinoma

40. The photomicrograph is representative of a painless testicular mass removed from a 32-year-old man. On the basis of the histopathology of the tumor, you suspect the patient has

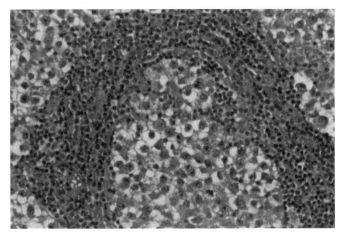

   (A) inguinal lymph node metastasis
   (B) non-Hodgkin's malignant lymphoma
   (C) an elevated serum α-fetoprotein level
   (D) a past history of tuberculosis
   (E) a past history of cryptorchidism

41. The photograph represents a total hysterectomy specimen from a 58-year-old woman with a history of postmenopausal bleeding. A cervical Pap smear taken 1 year before the surgery was reported as normal. The patient is an obese, type II diabetic with hypertension. Based on the clinical history and the gross appearance of the specimen, you would anticipate that histologic sections revealed

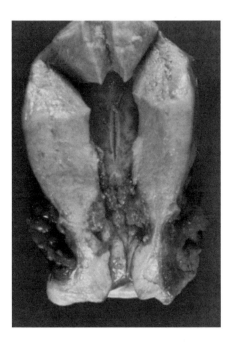

(A) a benign submucosal leiomyoma
(B) a benign endometrial polyp
(C) a benign endocervical polyp
(D) adenocarcinoma of the lower uterine segment
(E) infiltrating cervical squamous cell carcinoma with extension into the uterus

42. The photograph is a total hysterectomy specimen from a 40-year-old African American woman with a history of menorrhagia. The pathogenesis of the lesion noted in the gross specimen is most closely related to

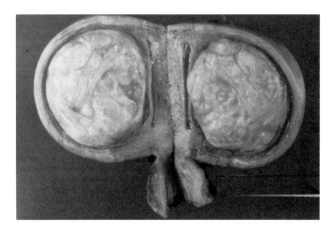

(A) neoplastic proliferation of smooth muscle
(B) adenomyosis involving the myometrial tissue
(C) neoplastic transformation of endometrial tissue
(D) cervical cancer with extension into the uterine cavity
(E) cystic hyperplasia of endometrial tissue

43. The photomicrograph is representative of a frozen section performed on tissue removed from a pelvic mass encountered during surgery on a 65-year-old woman. Preoperatively, the patient had abdominal distention, absence of shifting dullness, and the presence of induration of the pouch of Douglas on rectal examination. Which of the following best describes this patient's disease?

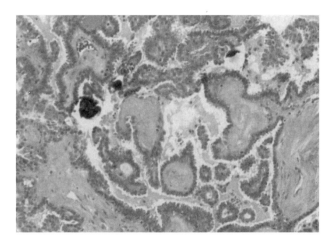

(A) Primary ovarian cancer of germ cell origin
(B) Primary ovarian cancer of sex cord–stromal origin
(C) Primary ovarian cancer derived from surface epithelium
(D) Metastatic cancer to the ovary from a primary stomach cancer
(E) Metastatic cancer to the ovary from a primary lung cancer

44. The photomicrograph is representative of sections taken through a 1.5-cm, nontender, moveable mass in the left upper outer quadrant of the breast of a 25-year-old woman whose mother died of breast cancer at age 55. There is no evidence of skin retraction overlying the mass, and the axillary examination is negative for lymphadenopathy. This mass most likely derives from

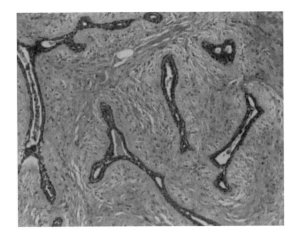

(A) the lactiferous duct
(B) the major ducts
(C) the terminal lobule
(D) breast stroma
(E) adipose tissue

45. The photograph represents a modified radical mastectomy specimen from a 62-year-old postmenopausal woman. Physical examination prior to mastectomy revealed retraction of the nipple and palpable lymph nodes in the low axillary region. On the basis of the gross appearance of the lesion, you anticipate that sections exhibited

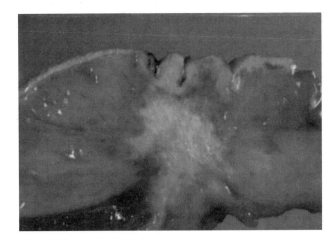

(A) in situ lobular carcinoma
(B) infiltrating ductal carcinoma
(C) intraductal carcinoma
(D) medullary carcinoma
(E) comedocarcinoma

46. The photograph is of an amputated distal right femur of a 16-year-old boy who initially complained of knee pain. X-rays of the lesion revealed a "sunburst" appearance in tissue surrounding the bone mass. You anticipate that sections of the mass revealed

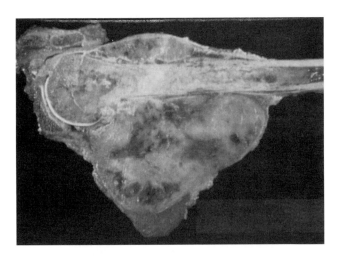

(A) malignant cells derived from cartilage
(B) small, round cells that were PAS positive
(C) numerous multinucleated giant cells
(D) small round cells that were S100 antigen positive
(E) malignant osteoblasts

47. The peripheral smear is representative of a slide prepared on a febrile 5-year-old African American boy. Scleral icterus is present. The spleen is enlarged and tender. The CBC reveals a normocytic anemia, corrected reticulocyte count of 18%, and neutrophilic leukocytosis with a left shift. Rare neutrophils demonstrate lancet-shaped diplococci in phagolysosomes. A blood culture is pending. Based on the history, CBC, and peripheral smear findings, which of the following correctly describes clinical aspects of this patient's hematologic disease?

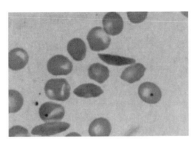

(A) Primarily intravascular hemolysis
(B) Extrinsic hemolytic anemia
(C) Conjugated hyperbilirubinemia
(D) Functional asplenia
(E) Autosomal dominant inheritance

48. The RBCs having a bull's-eye appearance in the peripheral blood are least likely to be present in a patient with

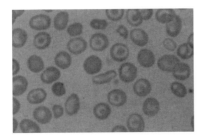

   (A) sickle cell trait
   (B) HbC disease
   (C) β-thalassemia
   (D) a splenectomy
   (E) alcoholic liver disease

49. The photomicrograph is representative of a bone marrow biopsy from a man with non-A, non-B chronic hepatitis. You anticipate that the peripheral blood findings revealed

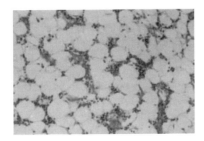

   (A) an elevated corrected reticulocyte count
   (B) pancytopenia
   (C) a microcytic anemia
   (D) polychromasia (shift cells) in the peripheral smear
   (E) circulating "blast" cells

50. The bone marrow biopsy is from a 65-year-old man who presented with abdominal distention and left upper quadrant pain. Physical examination revealed a friction rub in the left upper quadrant, a left-sided pleural effusion, and massive splenomegaly. The CBC exhibited a leukoerythroblastic smear, normocytic anemia, a total WBC count of 35,000 cells/μL, and thrombocytosis. Teardrop cells were noted. The leukocyte alkaline phosphatase (LAP) score was increased, and the Philadelphia chromosome study was negative.

Which of the following best describes this patient's condition?

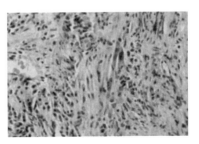

   (A) Splenomegaly secondary to extramedullary hematopoiesis
   (B) Metastatic adenocarcinoma in the bone marrow with reactive fibrosis
   (C) Primary malignant lymphoma of the spleen with bone marrow metastasis
   (D) Chronic myelogenous leukemia with reactive marrow fibrosis and splenomegaly
   (E) Portal hypertension with congestive splenomegaly

51. A 6-year-old foster child has a serum alkaline phosphatase that is 10 times higher than the normal adult range. The serum sample was hemolyzed owing to difficulties in performing the venipuncture. The elevated serum alkaline phosphatase is most likely

   (A) a false-positive test result
   (B) normal for the child's age
   (C) related to healing of bone fractures
   (D) due to trauma to his liver
   (E) due to hemolysis of the blood specimen

52. The anti-Smith (anti-Sm) antibody test for systemic lupus erythematosus (SLE) has a sensitivity of 30% and a specificity of 100%. If the prevalence of SLE is 1%, what is the chance that a patient has SLE if the test result returns positive?

   (A) 30%
   (B) 50%
   (C) 65%
   (D) 70%
   (E) 100%

53. You would expect an adult male and a nonpregnant adult female to both have the same reference intervals for

   (A) hemoglobin concentration
   (B) serum ferritin
   (C) the RBC count
   (D) percentage of HbA
   (E) the hematocrit

54. A 25-year-old man has a painless ulcer on the shaft of his penis. The serum rapid plasma reagin (RPR) test is negative, the fluorescent treponeme antibody absorption test (FTA-ABS) is positive, and the dark-field study of exudate from the ulcer is positive for spirochetes. You suspect the

    (A) negative RPR is a false negative
    (B) positive dark-field study is a false positive
    (C) positive FTA-ABS indicates old rather than current disease
    (D) ulcer is due to *Haemophilus ducreyi*
    (E) RPR has a greater specificity than the FTA-ABS

55. A test for coronary artery disease (CAD) is positive in 180 of 200 people with known CAD and negative in 140 of 200 people who do not have CAD. The sensitivity of this test for detecting CAD is

    (A) 70%
    (B) 75%
    (C) 80%
    (D) 90%
    (E) 95%

56. The sensitivity of the serum ANA in diagnosing SLE is 100%, while the specificity is 80%. You conclude from this information that

    (A) the test is best used to confirm the diagnosis of SLE
    (B) a positive test result is SLE or some other collagen vascular disease
    (C) a negative test result does not exclude SLE
    (D) the false-negative and false-positive rate are 20% and 0%, respectively
    (E) the predictive value of a positive test result is 100%

57. The mechanism of cellular swelling in tissue hypoxia most closely relates to

    (A) free radical injury of the cell
    (B) decreased apolipoprotein synthesis
    (C) calcium entering the mitochondria
    (D) irreversible injury to the cell membrane
    (E) a reduced concentration of ATP

58. A low oxygen content, normal PaO_2, and low SaO_2 (oxygen saturation) are characteristic of

    (A) anemia
    (B) respiratory acidosis
    (C) carbon monoxide poisoning
    (D) cyanide poisoning
    (E) a ventilation/perfusion mismatch

59. Which of the following cell types can undergo only hypertrophy?

    (A) Endometrial gland cell
    (B) Neuron
    (C) Smooth muscle
    (D) Hepatocyte
    (E) Skeletal muscle

60. Which of the following clinical disorders is an example of coagulation necrosis?

    (A) Acute pancreatitis
    (B) Wet gangrene of the toe in a person with diabetes
    (C) Henoch-Schönlein vasculitis
    (D) Ischemic acute tubular necrosis
    (E) Atherosclerotic infarct of the brain

61. The mechanism of fatty change in the liver in kwashiorkor is most closely associated with

    (A) decreased synthesis of apolipoprotein
    (B) free radical injury of hepatocytes
    (C) a decrease in glycolysis
    (D) an increase in β-oxidation of fatty acids
    (E) increased synthesis of VLDL

62. In which of the following groups of chemical mediators are both mediators involved in the synthesis of adhesion molecules and chemotaxis?

    (A) C3b and Hageman factor XII
    (B) LTC_4 and histamine
    (C) Bradykinin and nitric oxide
    (D) C3a and platelet-activating factor
    (E) C5a and LTB_4

63. A 6-year-old boy has recurrent infections. His nitroblue tetrazolium (NBT) dye test is normal. As a newborn, his umbilical cord did not fall off and required surgical removal. A histologic section at the base of the cord revealed no inflammatory infiltrate. His peripheral blood leukocytes are morphologically normal. Which of the following best explains the clinical findings in this patient?

    (A) Cystic fibrosis
    (B) Chronic granulomatous disease of childhood
    (C) Chédiak-Higashi syndrome
    (D) Adhesion molecule defect
    (E) Glucose-6-phosphate dehydrogenase deficiency

64. Which of the following chemical mediators contributes most to the rubor, calor, and tumor of acute inflammation?

    (A) Nitric oxide
    (B) Bradykinin
    (C) C5a
    (D) Prostaglandins
    (E) Histamine

65. Which of the following tissue/repair relationships is correctly matched?

    (A) Liver: hepatocytes stimulate fibrogenesis as a mechanism of repair
    (B) Kidney: tubules in the renal medulla have the greatest regenerative capacity
    (C) Lung: type I pneumocytes are the reserve cell responsible for repair
    (D) Brain: fibroblasts are responsible for gliosis as a mechanism of repair
    (E) Peripheral nervous system: Schwann cells are important in nerve regeneration.

66. Which of the following proteins is reduced in inflammation and useful as a marker of protein status?

    (A) C3 complement
    (B) C-reactive peptide
    (C) Haptoglobin
    (D) Transferrin
    (E) α_1-Antitrypsin

67. A pregnant woman has a positive ELISA test for human immunodeficiency virus (HIV) antibodies. With this information you would

    (A) recommend termination of the pregnancy
    (B) administer azidothymidine (AZT)
    (C) confirm the result with a Western blot assay
    (D) order a p24 antigen study
    (E) order lymphocyte cultures for HIV

68. Which of the following organs is most frequently involved in patients with AIDS?

    (A) Brain
    (B) Eyes
    (C) Lungs
    (D) Liver
    (E) Kidneys

69. You would expect an increase in plasma osmolality (Posm) and contraction of both the extracellular (ECF) and intracellular (ICF) fluid compartment in which of the following fluid derangements? Arrows indicate degree of magnitude, TBNa = total body sodium, TBW = total body water.

	Fluid	TBNa	TBW
(A)	Loss	↓	↓↓
(B)	Gain	↑	↑↑
(C)	Loss	↓	↓
(D)	Gain	↔	↑↑
(E)	Gain	↑↑	↑↑

70. In which of the following clinical situations would the effective arterial blood volume be decreased but the total extracellular fluid (ECF) volume increased?

	Fluid Tonicity	Clinical Condition
(A)	Isotonic gain of fluid	Excessive infusion of isotonic saline
(B)	Hypertonic loss of fluid	Thiazide diuretic
(C)	Hypotonic loss of fluid	Sweating
(D)	Hypotonic gain of fluid	Right heart failure
(E)	Hypotonic loss of fluid	Diabetes insipidus

71. Which of the following best represents a patient with the syndrome of inappropriate antidiuretic hormone secretion (SiADH)? Arrows indicate degree of magnitude, TBNa = total body sodium, TBW = total body water.

	Fluid	TBNa	TBW
(A)	Loss	↓	↓↓
(B)	Gain	↔	↑↑
(C)	Gain	↑	↑↑
(D)	Gain	↑↑	↑
(E)	Loss	↓↓	↓

72. In which of the following combinations do both disorders exhibit edema related to an increase in hydrostatic pressure?

    (A) Right heart failure/left heart failure
    (B) Left heart failure/celiac disease
    (C) Pleural effusion in pneumonia/ascitic fluid in cirrhosis
    (D) Cerebral edema in encephalitis/cerebral edema in hyponatremia
    (E) Swelling of tissue in a bee sting/pulmonary edema in ARDS

73. Mental retardation, cardiac disease, and dementia are most likely associated with

    (A) trisomy 16
    (B) trisomy 18
    (C) trisomy 21
    (D) an autosomal dominant disease
    (E) a sex-linked recessive disease

74. The combination of vitamin D deficiency and secondary hyperparathyroidism is most commonly the result of

    (A) malabsorption
    (B) lack of sunlight
    (C) cirrhosis
    (D) chronic renal failure
    (E) poor diet

75. Which of the following is most likely associated with a fat-soluble rather than a water-soluble vitamin deficiency?

    (A) Glossitis
    (B) Congestive cardiomyopathy
    (C) Nyctalopia
    (D) Dementia
    (E) Perifollicular hemorrhage

76. A 70-year-old widow on a tea and toast diet presents with complaints of bleeding gums after she brushes her teeth. She has a smooth red tongue, carious teeth, and inflamed gums. The pathogenesis of her disease is most closely related to

    (A) a deficiency of ATP
    (B) a cofactor deficiency in collagenase
    (C) lack of hydroxylation of lysine and proline
    (D) a cofactor deficiency in lysyl oxidase
    (E) a cofactor deficiency in the pyruvate dehydrogenase complex

77. A 25-year-old woman who has recently been admitted to an eating disorders unit is noted to have acid injury to the enamel in her teeth, bruised knuckles, and swelling of her salivary glands. You would expect her to have which of the following laboratory abnormalities?

    (A) Low arterial pH
    (B) Low $PaCO_2$
    (C) Hypokalemia
    (D) Low serum bicarbonate
    (E) Hypoglycemia

78. A person whose diet primarily consists of corn will most likely develop a deficiency associated with

    (A) ringed sideroblasts
    (B) neovascularization of the cornea
    (C) hypersegmented neutrophils
    (D) hyperpigmentation in sun-exposed areas
    (E) squamous metaplasia of the cornea

79. Which of the following may occur in both methyl alcohol poisoning and ethyl alcohol abuse?

    (A) Mallory's bodies
    (B) Hypersegmented neutrophils
    (C) Increased anion gap metabolic acidosis
    (D) Sideroblastic anemia
    (E) Optic neuritis

80. Which of the following is least likely associated with smoking?

    (A) Small for gestational age newborn
    (B) Pancreatic carcinoma
    (C) Cervical carcinoma
    (D) Dissecting aortic aneurysm
    (E) Enhancement of atherosclerosis

81. Which of the following is not associated with lead poisoning?

    (A) Microcytic anemia
    (B) Coarse basophilic stippling
    (C) Permanent damage to the CNS
    (D) Decreased RBC protoporphyrin
    (E) Nephrotoxic damage to the kidneys

82. Which of the following physical injury relationships is correct?

    (A) Motor vehicle accidents: most common cause of death between 25 and 44 years of age
    (B) Ionizing radiation: RBCs are the most vulnerable hematopoietic cell
    (C) High altitude: low atmospheric pressure reduces the PO_2
    (D) Third-degree burn: inflammation irritates nerve endings, producing pain
    (E) Electricity: wet skin decreases current

83. In which of the following sites is a primary cancer more common than metastasis?

    (A) Brain
    (B) Ovary
    (C) Bone
    (D) Liver
    (E) Lymph node

84. The second most common cause of death due to cancer in both men and women is

    (A) malignant lymphoma
    (B) malignant melanoma
    (C) lung cancer
    (D) colorectal cancer
    (E) hepatocellular carcinoma

85. Which of the following is non-neoplastic?

    (A) Solitary nodule in the lung
    (B) Moveable mass in the parotid
    (C) Ovarian mass with calcification
    (D) Tubular adenoma of the colon
    (E) Painful distal femur mass in an 18 year old

86. Which of the following is a precursor to cancer?

    (A) Leiomyoma of the uterus
    (B) Prostatic hyperplasia
    (C) Actinic keratosis
    (D) Fibroadenoma of the breast
    (E) Capillary hemangioma

87. A primary squamous cell carcinoma would most likely develop in the

    (A) kidney
    (B) true vocal cord
    (C) bladder
    (D) stomach
    (E) gallbladder

88. Seeding as a means of metastasis characteristically occurs in primary tumors of the

    (A) lung and kidney
    (B) ovary and brain
    (C) colon and uterus
    (D) liver and cervix
    (E) prostate and bladder

89. Which of the following is present in iron deficiency, lead poisoning, and β-thalassemia minor?

    (A) Abnormal serum ferritin
    (B) Abnormal total iron-binding capacity (TIBC)
    (C) Abnormal Hb electrophoresis
    (D) Microcytic RBC indices
    (E) Increased reticulocyte count

90. Which of the following differentiates pernicious anemia from other causes of B_{12} deficiency?

    (A) Abnormal proprioception
    (B) Megaloblastic bone marrow
    (C) Hypersegmented neutrophils
    (D) Pancytopenia
    (E) Anti–parietal cell antibodies

91. A 42-year-old woman presents with an episodic history of reddish-brown urine in her first morning void. Her CBC reveals a moderately severe normocytic anemia, neutropenia, thrombocytopenia, and an elevated corrected reticulocyte count. The peripheral RBC morphology is normal except for increased polychromasia (shift cells). A biochemical profile reveals a low serum iron and serum ferritin. Which of the following is the best screening test to further evaluate the cause of her anemia?

    (A) Heinz body preparation
    (B) Hb electrophoresis
    (C) Direct Coombs' test
    (D) Sugar-water test
    (E) Osmotic fragility test

92. Which of the following anemia/confirmatory test relationships is correct?

    (A) β-Thalassemia minor: free erythrocyte protoporphyrin levels
    (B) α-Thalassemia: serum ferritin
    (C) Congenital spherocytosis: Heinz body preparation
    (D) Iron deficiency: serum iron
    (E) Aplastic anemia: bone marrow examination

93. In a patient with significant blood loss within the last 2 hours, you would expect

    (A) a low Hb and Hct
    (B) a low RBC count
    (C) reticulocytosis
    (D) a normal tilt test
    (E) a normal MCV

94. An 82-year-old man with endotoxic shock has oozing of blood from every venipuncture and intravenous site. Which of the following tests has the greatest chance of being abnormal?

    (A) D-dimer assay
    (B) Platelet count
    (C) Partial thromboplastin time
    (D) Prothrombin time
    (E) Fibrinogen level

95. The most common cause of jaundice in the first 24 hours in a blood group A, Rh-negative newborn born to a blood group O, Rh-negative mother is

    (A) physiologic jaundice of the newborn
    (B) breast milk jaundice
    (C) ABO incompatibility
    (D) Rh incompatibility
    (E) neonatal hepatitis

96. A 30-year-old woman with nontender lymphadenopathy in the left cervical nodes and a mass in the anterior mediastinum most likely has

    (A) Burkitt's lymphoma
    (B) nodular sclerosing Hodgkin's disease
    (C) metastasis from another primary site
    (D) lymphocyte-predominant Hodgkin's disease
    (E) cat-scratch disease

97. A 25-year-old woman presents with a deep venous thrombosis of the right lower leg. This is her fifth admission over the last 7 years for similar problems. Her father died at 35 years of age of a pulmonary embolus and had a similar history of recurrent venous thromboses. She is not taking birth control pills. Her bleeding time, prothrombin time, activated partial thromboplastin time, and platelet count are all normal. Her activated partial thromboplastin time remained normal after she was given a loading dose of heparin. You suspect the patient has

    (A) antithrombin III deficiency
    (B) protein C deficiency
    (C) protein S deficiency
    (D) a qualitative platelet defect
    (E) von Willebrand's disease

98. A 4-year-old child presents with fever, generalized lymphadenopathy, epistaxis, and malaise. Physical examination reveals hepatosplenomegaly and bone tenderness over the sternum. A CBC exhibits a normocytic anemia, a total WBC count of 52,000 cells/μL with many "blast cells" present, and thrombocytopenia. The prognosis of this patient is most dependent on

    (A) the degree of anemia at initial presentation
    (B) the age of the patient
    (C) the number of lymphoblasts in the peripheral blood
    (D) whether the lymphoblasts are CALLA positive
    (E) the degree of thrombocytopenia at initial presentation

99. Which of the following is common to both left and right heart failure?

    (A) Normal effective arterial blood volume
    (B) Stimulation of the renin-angiotensin-aldosterone system
    (C) Increased jugular venous pressure
    (D) Dependent pitting edema
    (E) Increased pulmonary capillary wedge pressure

100. Left ventricular hypertrophy and dilatation in a heart removed at autopsy are gross findings you would expect in

    (A) restrictive cardiomyopathy
    (B) hypertrophic cardiomyopathy
    (C) aortic insufficiency
    (D) essential hypertension
    (E) mitral stenosis

101. Study the following oxygen saturation values from a patient with congenital heart disease.

	Normal Value	Patient
Right atrium	75%	75%
Right ventricle	75%	90%
Pulmonary artery	75%	90%
Pulmonary vein	95%	95%
Left atrium	95%	95%
Left ventricle	95%	95%

The patient most likely has

    (A) tetralogy of Fallot
    (B) a patent ductus arteriosus (PDA)
    (C) a ventricular septal defect (VSD)
    (D) an atrial septal defect (ASD)
    (E) complete transposition of the great vessels

102. Atherosclerosis is least likely to have a significant role in

    (A) the formation of berry aneurysms
    (B) small bowel infarction
    (C) leg claudication
    (D) transient ischemic attacks
    (E) nontraumatic amputation

103. A 65-year-old man with an acute myocardial infarction experiences dyspnea on day 5 in the coronary care unit. A pansystolic murmur is heard at the apex and bilateral wet inspiratory crackles. The serum CK-MB is elevated. The patient most likely has

    (A) heart failure secondary to aortic insufficiency
    (B) reinfarction associated with papillary muscle dysfunction
    (C) a ventricular aneurysm
    (D) reinfarction associated with pericarditis
    (E) reinfarction with rupture of the free wall of the left ventricle

104. A 42-year-old person with alcoholism and a 40 pack-year history of smoking has an abrupt onset of spiking fever, a productive cough with blood-tinged, mucoid sputum, and pleuritic chest pain. Physical examination reveals dullness to percussion, crepitant rales, and increased tactile fremitus in the right upper lobe. A chest x-ray reveals a lobar consolidation in the right upper lobe. Gram's stain of sputum is positive. You expect it showed gram-

    (A) positive rods
    (B) positive cocci in clumps
    (C) negative rods with a thick capsule
    (D) negative diplococci
    (E) positive filamentous bacteria

105. A 25-year-old woman with a history of chronic fibromyalgia, nasal polyps, and asthma is brought to the emergency department because of severe bronchospasm. With these findings, you suspect the patient has

    (A) a pulmonary embolus
    (B) cystic fibrosis
    (C) a strong family history for allergies
    (D) an immunodeficiency disorder
    (E) taken aspirin for pain

106. A 65-year-old man with a stroke and gastric aspiration develops fever, dyspnea, tachypnea, and cyanosis involving the skin and mucous membranes. Inspiratory crackles are noted in all lung fields. An arterial blood gas reveals a PaO_2 of 51 mm Hg while he breathes 40% oxygen. The PaO_2 does not significantly increase after he breathes 100% oxygen for 20 minutes. The patient most likely has

    (A) a massive pulmonary embolus
    (B) the adult respiratory distress syndrome
    (C) hypovolemic shock
    (D) lobar pneumonia
    (E) congestive heart failure

107. A 62-year-old man with a stroke develops pneumonia on the 10th hospital day. Gram's stain of sputum most likely revealed gram-

    (A) negative diplococci
    (B) positive diplococci
    (C) negative rods
    (D) positive rods
    (E) positive cocci in clusters

108. An anterior mediastinal mass in a young woman who has muscle weakness with exercise, diplopia, and lid lag is most likely

    (A) a neurogenic tumor
    (B) metastatic small cell carcinoma
    (C) a thymus-associated disorder
    (D) a malignant lymphoma
    (E) Hodgkin's disease

109. A 45-year-old real estate agent developed fever, painful nodules on his lower legs, and a pulmonary consolidation. A few weeks earlier he inspected a number of abandoned warehouses on the outskirts of Columbus, Ohio. He most likely has

    (A) cryptococcosis
    (B) coccidioidomycosis
    (C) aspergillosis
    (D) histoplasmosis
    (E) candidiasis

110. A 43-year-old man presents with increased skin pigmentation, cirrhosis, malabsorption, and diabetes mellitus. The mechanism most likely responsible for this constellation of findings is

    (A) excessive reabsorption of iron from the small bowel
    (B) a defect in the excretion of copper in bile
    (C) multisystem organ damage from alcohol
    (D) α_1-antitrypsin deficiency
    (E) multisystem organ damage from amyloid

111. A 40-year-old man presents with hepatic failure, greenish-brown deposits in Descemet's membrane of the eye, and extrapyramidal disease. The pathogenesis of this patient's disease is most likely related to

    (A) excessive iron stores in the liver
    (B) a defect in the excretion of copper into bile
    (C) a defect in the synthesis of α_1-antitrypsin
    (D) an abnormality in glycogen synthesis
    (E) an abnormality in galactose metabolism

112. A 60-year-old woman presents with numerous skin excoriations from scratching, bilateral xanthelasmas, and hepatomegaly. A biochemical profile exhibits a marked elevation of serum alkaline phosphatase and γ-glutamyltransferase, a normal total bilirubin, slightly elevated serum transaminases, and a markedly elevated serum cholesterol. An endoscopic retrograde cholangiopancreatography (ERCP) study of the common bile duct is negative. She is scheduled for a liver biopsy. Which of the following tests would be most useful in her initial workup?
    (A) Antinuclear antibody
    (B) Hepatitis B surface antigen
    (C) Serum ferritin
    (D) Anti–smooth muscle antibody
    (E) Antimitochondrial antibody

113. A febrile 10-year-old boy with chickenpox lapses into coma. Physical examination reveals hepatomegaly. The serum ammonia and transaminases are elevated, and the prothrombin time is prolonged. You expect a liver biopsy will reveal

    (A) viral hepatitis
    (B) diffuse microvesicular fatty change
    (C) α_1-antitrypsin globules
    (D) Mallory's bodies
    (E) chronic active hepatitis

114. A 26-year-old man with a long history of intravenous drug abuse and stable chronic active hepatitis B suddenly develops an increase in his prothrombin time and a drop in transaminases. Which of the following best explains these findings?

(A) Superinfection with hepatitis D
(B) Recovery from hepatitis B
(C) Vitamin K deficiency
(D) Hepatocellular carcinoma
(E) Reye's syndrome

115. Which of the following is more commonly associated with Crohn's disease than with ulcerative colitis?

(A) Toxic megacolon
(B) Crypt abscesses
(C) Obstruction
(D) Adenocarcinoma
(E) Sclerosing pericholangitis

116. Which of the following characterizes a gastric rather than a duodenal ulcer?

(A) Association with *Helicobacter pylori*
(B) Male dominance
(C) Blood group O association
(D) Association with multiple endocrine neoplasia type I
(E) Normal to low basal acid output

117. Which of the following is the most common cause of both melena and hematemesis?

(A) Gastric ulcer
(B) Duodenal ulcer
(C) Esophageal varices
(D) Gastroesophageal reflux disease
(E) Adenocarcinoma of the stomach

118. The location for the most common cancer-producing obstruction in the gastrointestinal tract is the

(A) esophagus
(B) stomach
(C) small intestine
(D) cecum
(E) rectosigmoid

119. Which of the following ovarian tumors has a different origin (derivation) from the others listed?

(A) Cystic teratoma
(B) Dysgerminoma
(C) Fibroma
(D) Endodermal sinus tumor
(E) Struma ovarii

120. The most common location for metastatic disease in the female reproductive tract is the

(A) vagina
(B) cervix
(C) endometrium
(D) ovary
(E) breast

121. Oral contraceptives protect against cancer of the

(A) liver
(B) breast
(C) ovary
(D) cervix
(E) uterus

122. Angiotensin-converting enzyme (ACE) inhibitors are useful in the treatment of diabetic nephropathy owing to their

(A) reduction of afferent arteriolar tone
(B) inhibition of aldosterone action in the kidneys
(C) direct effect on increasing the glomerular filtration rate
(D) inhibition of nonenzymatic glycosylation of glomerular capillaries
(E) inhibition of angiotensin II effect on the efferent arterioles

123. Renal papillary necrosis, the nephrotic syndrome, and a predisposition for urinary tract infection characterizes

(A) multiple myeloma
(B) systemic lupus erythematosus
(C) adult polycystic kidney disease
(D) diabetes mellitus
(E) hydronephrosis

124. Which of the following is present in both types I and II diabetes mellitus?

(A) Increased anion gap metabolic acidosis
(B) Defects in the glucose transport units
(C) Multifactorial inheritance pattern
(D) Increased production of sorbitol
(E) HLA-Dr3 and -Dr4

125. A pharmacist has an elevated serum C-peptide in a workup of a fasting hypoglycemia. The patient most likely suffers from

(A) surreptitious injection of human insulin
(B) a malignant islet cell tumor arising from α-cells
(C) a benign islet cell tumor arising from β-cells
(D) a malignant islet cell tumor arising from δ-cells
(E) a malignant islet cell tumor arising from G cells

126. In diabetic ketoacidosis, you would expect

(A) a decrease in β-oxidation of fatty acids
(B) inhibition of gluconeogenesis
(C) an increase in fatty acid synthesis
(D) activation of hormone-sensitive lipase
(E) an increase in degradation of chylomicrons and VLDL

127. Hyperplasia of the adrenal cortex is most likely associated with

(A) corticosteroid administration
(B) Addison's disease
(C) anencephaly
(D) 21-hydroxylase deficiency
(E) hypopituitarism

128. A 58-year-old man presents with a painful, hot right knee. Synovial fluid analysis reveals numerous acute inflammatory cells and needle-shaped crystals that are blue when parallel to the slow axis of the compensator. The pathogenesis of this patient's metabolic condition is most closely associated with

    (A) underexcretion of uric acid in the kidneys
    (B) overproduction of uric acid
    (C) deposition of calcium pyrophosphate in the joint
    (D) a defect in pyrimidine metabolism
    (E) HLA-B27–positive spondyloarthropathy

129. Which of the following characterizes joint disease associated with osteoarthritis rather than with rheumatoid arthritis?

    (A) Cartilage fibrillation
    (B) Pannus
    (C) IgM antibody against IgG
    (D) Fusion of the joint
    (E) Female dominance

130. Which of the following characterizes postmenopausal osteoporosis rather than osteomalacia?

    (A) Greater osteoclastic than osteoblastic activity
    (B) Osteopenia on radiologic examination
    (C) Hypocalcemia
    (D) Defect in mineralization of bone matrix
    (E) Increased thickness of osteoid seams

131. An increase in total protein concentration in a 70-year-old African American man with hypercalcemia, lytic bone lesions, anemia, and renal failure most likely denotes

    (A) a malignant plasma cell disorder
    (B) metastatic prostate carcinoma
    (C) primary hyperparathyroidism
    (D) Waldenström's macroglobulinemia
    (E) sarcoidosis

132. The mechanism of tetany in respiratory alkalosis is

    (A) increased binding of ionized calcium to globulins
    (B) lowering of the total serum calcium concentration
    (C) increased deposition of ionized calcium in bone
    (D) increased binding of ionized calcium to albumin
    (E) lowering of the serum parathormone concentration

DIRECTIONS. (Items 133–150): Each set of matching questions in this section consists of a list of lettered options followed by one or more numbered items. For each numbered item, select the ONE option that is most closely associated with it. Each lettered option may be selected once, more than once, or not at all.

Item 133

Study the following chart relating serum calcium to PTH. The square box represents normal values.

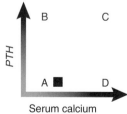

133. Patient with a renal stone, peptic ulcer disease, and constipation.

Items 134–135

	Serum T_4	T_4 BR	FT_4-I	TSH	^{131}I Uptake
(A)	Increased	Increased	Increased	Decreased	Increased
(B)	Decreased	Increased	Normal	Normal	Normal
(C)	Increased	Decreased	Normal	Normal	Normal
(D)	Decreased	Decreased	Decreased	Increased	Decreased
(E)	Increased	Increased	Increased	Decreased	Decreased
(F)	Decreased	Decreased	Decreased	Decreased	Decreased

T_4 BR = T_4 binding ratio, which is the patient's resin T_3 uptake divided by 30; FT_4-I = free T_4 index; TSH = thyroid-stimulating hormone; ^{131}I uptake = radioactive iodide-131 uptake.

134. Patient with sinus tachycardia, increased deep tendon reflexes, and a nonpalpable thyroid gland who has been taking "pills" prescribed by a weight loss clinic for the last 6 months.

135. A 23-year-old weight lifter with a normal physical examination.

Item 136

	HBsAg	HBeAg	Anti–HBc-IgM	Anti–HBc-IgG	Anti-HBs
(A)	Negative	Negative	Positive	Negative	Negative
(B)	Positive	Positive	Positive	Negative	Negative
(C)	Negative	Negative	Negative	Positive	Positive
(D)	Negative	Negative	Negative	Negative	Positive

136. Patient with hepatitis B who is in the serologic gap.

Items 137–139

	RBC Mass	Plasma Volume	SaO_2*	Erythropoietin Concentration
(A)	Increased	Normal	Normal	Increased
(B)	Normal	Decreased	Normal	Normal
(C)	Increased	Increased	Normal	Low
(D)	Increased	Normal	Low	Increased
(E)	Increased	Decreased	Variable	Variable

* SaO_2 = oxygen saturation.

137. Patient who is volume depleted after running a marathon.

138. Patient with iron overload and liver disease who develops an increase in α-fetoprotein.

139. Child with Down syndrome who has dusky cyanosis of the skin and mucous membranes.

Items 140–142

(A) Phenylketonuria
(B) Galactosemia
(C) Tay-Sachs disease
(D) Gaucher's disease
(E) Hurler's syndrome
(F) Congenital toxoplasmosis
(G) Congenital rubella
(H) Congenital syphilis
(I) Congenital herpes

140. Patient with nerve deafness, cataracts, mental retardation, and patent ductus arteriosus.

141. Adult with massive hepatosplenomegaly and macrophages having a fibrillary-appearing cytoplasm.

142. Newborn with fasting hypoglycemia, cataracts, neonatal cholestasis, and increased reducing substances in the urine.

Items 143–144

	Serum Na+ (136–145 mEq/L)	Serum Cl− (95–105 mEq/L)	Serum K+ (3.5–5.0 mEq/L)	Serum HCO₃⁻ (22–28 mEq/L)	Random UNa (<20 mEq/L)
(A)	132	86	2.6	30	>20
(B)	150	107	2.0	34	>20
(C)	128	96	5.5	20	>20
(D)	120	86	3.4	22	>20
(E)	132	94	5.8	18	>20
(F)	139	109	3.0	18	<20

143. The patient is a 25-year-old man with insulin-dependent diabetes mellitus who contracted the flu and now presents with fever and polyuria. His physical examination reveals mild hypotension, sinus tachycardia, a fruity odor to his breath, and dry mucous membranes. A urine dipstick test exhibits 4+ glucose, 3+ protein, and a strongly positive ketone reaction.

144. The patient is a 28-year-old man with diarrhea of 3 days' duration. He has had minimal fluid intake during this time. His blood pressure and pulse decrease and increase, respectively, when he moves from a supine to a sitting position. His mucous membranes are dry.

Items 145–146

Match the following sets of arterial blood gases with the appropriate clinical description.

	pH (7.35–7.45)	PaCO₂ (33–44 mm Hg)	HCO₃⁻ (22–28 mEq/L)
(A)	7.12	50	16
(B)	7.23	68	27
(C)	7.30	30	14
(D)	7.33	60	31
(E)	7.37	72	40
(F)	7.38	14	8
(G)	7.40	40	24
(H)	7.48	20	14
(I)	7.52	49	39
(J)	7.52	25	20

145. A 29-year-old woman who has a history of chronic depression is brought to the emergency room after a 911 call from her boyfriend. She is semicomatose. Undigested pills are noted in the gastric contents after her stomach has been pumped.

146. A 65-year-old man has a cardiorespiratory arrest secondary to an acute myocardial infarction.

Items 147–148

	Bleeding Time	Platelet Count	Prothrombin Time (PT)	Partial Thromboplastin Time
(A)	Prolonged	Decreased	Normal	Normal
(B)	Prolonged	Normal	Normal	Normal
(C)	Prolonged	Decreased	Prolonged	Prolonged
(D)	Prolonged	Normal	Prolonged	Prolonged
(E)	Normal	Normal	Prolonged	Normal
(F)	Normal	Normal	Normal	Prolonged
(G)	Prolonged	Normal	Normal	Prolonged
(H)	Normal	Normal	Prolonged	Prolonged

147. A 6-year-old boy with recurrent hemarthroses and a maternal grandfather with a similar problem.

148. A 48-year-old patient who takes warfarin for deep venous thrombosis.

Items 149–150

(A) Bruton's agammaglobulinemia
(B) Acquired immunodeficiency syndrome
(C) Severe combined immunodeficiency
(D) Common variable immune deficiency
(E) Wiskott-Aldrich syndrome
(F) Ataxia telangiectasia
(G) Sex-linked lymphoproliferative syndrome
(H) IgA immunodeficiency

149. Failure of B cells to mature into antibody-producing plasma cells.

150. Deficiency of adenosine deaminase with subsequent toxicity to lymphocytes.

ANSWERS AND EXPLANATIONS

1. The answer is C: secondary aldosteronism. The history of alcohol abuse and the physical examination findings of shifting dullness (which indicates ascites, as seen in the photograph), gynecomastia, and spider angiomas are all compatible with alcoholic cirrhosis (Chapter 16). Secondary aldosteronism is present owing to reduced metabolism of aldosterone by the liver. In addition, cirrhotics have a decreased synthesis of albumin, which results in pitting edema and ascites. Fluid accumulation in the interstitial space reduces venous return to the heart, thereby lowering the effective arterial blood volume (EABV; Chapter 5). A reduced EABV activates the renin-angiotensin-aldosterone system, stimulates ADH release, and increases the reabsorption of salt and water in the proximal renal tubules. The tonicity of the reabsorbed fluid is hypotonic, i.e., it contains more water than salt (↑TBNa/↑↑TBW). Owing to the reduced oncotic pressure, the reabsorbed fluid is primarily directed into the interstitial space, thus exacerbating the degree of pitting edema and ascites without increasing the EABV. Coagulation factor synthesis is decreased in cirrhosis, so the prothrombin time is usually prolonged.

2. The answer is B: dysphagia for solids and liquids. The photograph exhibits blanching of the finger secondary to Raynaud's phenomenon. This is the most common presentation for progressive systemic sclerosis (PSS) and the CREST syndrome, the latter representing a variant of PSS that has a more limited distribution of

organ pathology (Chapters 10 and 15). In both disorders, there is dysphagia for solids and liquids owing to replacement of distal esophageal smooth muscle with fibrous tissue. Choice A describes SLE; choice C, Sjögren's syndrome; choice D, dermatomyositis; and choice E, Hashimoto's thyroiditis.

3. The answer is B: positive cocci in chains. The photograph exhibits a crop of crusty lesions at the corner of the mouth consistent with impetigo due to group A β-hemolytic streptococci (gram-positive cocci that form chains; Chapter 21). *Staphylococcus aureus* (gram-positive cocci in clusters) often accompanies impetigo and adds a bullous component to the infection.

4. The answer is C: a viral infection. The photograph depicts a vesicular type of rash in the distribution of the trigeminal nerve. This is consistent with herpes zoster (shingles), due to the varicella-zoster virus (Chapter 21). After primary infection by the virus in childhood (varicella [chickenpox]), the virus remains dormant in sensory ganglia and may resurface later in life, often in association with malignant lymphoma or immunosuppressive therapy. The classic distribution of the lesion within a dermatome rules out the other answer choices.

5. The answer is E: a viral infection that often remains dormant in sensory dorsal root ganglia. The photograph depicts skin lesions at different stages of development in a patient with varicella (chickenpox; Chapter 21). Some lesions are macular and others represent vesicles and pustules. The child probably received aspirin and developed Reye's syndrome, which is manifested by neurologic problems and liver disease (microvesicular fatty change, transaminasemia, increased ammonia levels; Chapter 16).

6. The answer is D: There is an underexcretion of uric acid by the kidney. The photograph depicts monoclinic (needle-shaped) crystals, a few of which have been phagocytosed by neutrophils. Since they are yellow when parallel to the slow axis of the compensator, they represent the negative birefringent crystals of monosodium urate (Chapter 20). Gout is most frequently secondary to underexcretion of urate, a product of purine metabolism, in the kidneys. If the crystals had been blue when parallel to the axis, they would have represented the positive birefringent crystals of calcium pyrophosphate. Alcohol is not directly toxic to synovial tissue.

7. The answer is B: bradykinesia. The photographs are of midbrain with the specimen at top containing a normal substantia nigra and the one at bottom depigmentation of the substantia nigra, a characteristic feature of idiopathic Parkinson's disease (Chapter 22). Normally, the pigmented neurons in the substantia nigra synthesize dopamine, which is the principal neurotransmitter in the nigrostriatal tract that modulates impulses in the neostriatum (caudate nucleus and putamen). The defect shown at bottom leads to muscle rigidity, which is manifested by cogwheel rigidity and bradykinesia (slow movement of the extremities). Confabulation and memory deficits characterize Korsakoff's syndrome, which results from thiamine deficiency. Headache and papilledema indicate an increase in intracranial pressure. Transient ischemic attacks are not associated with depigmentation of the substantia nigra.

8. The answer is A: cytomegalovirus encephalitis. The photograph exhibits a banana-shaped intranuclear inclusion consistent with cytomegalovirus (CMV; Chapter 22). CMV is the most common cause of viral encephalitis in AIDS patients. Herpes intranuclear inclusions are smaller than those in CMV. *Toxoplasma* does not produce inclusions in glial cells; however, it is the most common cause of a space-occupying lesion in the CNS in AIDS. Subacute sclerosing panencephalitis (SSPE; link with measles virus) and progressive multifocal leukoencephalopathy (PML; papovavirus) are both slow virus diseases that have inclusions in glial cells; however, they are smaller than those seen in CMV.

9. The answer is B: essential hypertension. The photograph depicts multiple cystic lesions in the thalamus and globus pallidus in the brain. These are lacunar infarcts, which are most often secondary to hyaline arteriolosclerosis associated with essential hypertension and less commonly with diabetes mellitus. Lacunar infarcts commonly produce pure motor or pure sensory strokes (Chapter 22).

10. The answer is C: embolism. The photograph exhibits a massive hemorrhagic infarction most likely secondary to an embolism from the dilated left atrium of a person with mitral stenosis (opening snap, mid-diastolic rumble) resulting from rheumatic fever (Chapter 10). Atrial fibrillation (irregularly irregular pulse) is commonly present in mitral stenosis and may have been responsible for breaking off a piece of thrombus with subsequent embolization to the CNS. Hemorrhagic infarcts extend out to the surface of the brain owing to rupture of the weak vessels in the gray matter when blood reperfuses the area of infarction once the embolus is dissolved (Chapter 22). Atherosclerosis is associated with a pale infarct, hypertension with an intracerebral bleed, intracerebral infection (e.g., cerebral abscess) with a cystic cavity, and cardiogenic shock with the loss of neurons secondary to ischemia.

11. The answer is B: liquefactive necrosis and atrophy. The brain depicts two lesions. The left side of the brain exhibits a large cystic cavity most likely representing an old cerebral infarction, while the remaining brain reveals atrophy most likely secondary to ischemia from atherosclerosis (Chapter 22). Although degenerative diseases (e.g., Alzheimer's disease) can produce atrophy, ischemia is a more common cause of this growth alteration. The cystic lesion is very large and does not have a shaggy lining, hence excluding a metastatic abscess. Intracerebral hematomas (e.g., hypertensive bleed) are not associated with cystic cavities, which are produced by liquefactive necrosis rather than a blood clot displacing brain tissue. The brain does not undergo coagulation necrosis.

12. The answer is E: a tear of a bridging vein. The photograph exhibits a large, organized blood clot directly beneath the dura, which is reflected back from the clot. The clot represents a subdural hematoma, which is due to rupture of a bridging vein secondary to a fall or some type of trauma to the head (Chapter 22). Essential hypertension is associated with intracerebral bleeds, epidural hematomas with tears of the middle meningeal artery, hemorrhagic infarctions with embolic stroke, and subarachnoid hemorrhage with a ruptured berry aneurysm.

13. The answer is A: intracerebral edema. The brain is edematous and exhibits cerebellar coning indicative of an increase in intracranial pressure and herniation of the cerebellar tonsils into the foramen magnum (Chapter 22). Intracerebral edema is not associated with a demyelinating (e.g., multiple sclerosis) or a

degenerative disease (e.g., Alzheimer's disease). There is no exudate or congestion to suggest a meningitis. A hypertonic state produces shrinkage of the brain owing to loss of fluid from the ICF compartment by osmosis.

14. The answer is A: a malignant neoplasm originating from astrocytes. The history is suggestive of a brain tumor (headaches on waking in the morning and lasting throughout the day). There is a mass lesion in the left cerebral hemisphere with hemorrhagic necrosis consistent with a glioblastoma multiforme (high-grade astrocytoma; Chapter 22). Oligodendrogliomas are not hemorrhagic (they commonly calcify); ruptured berry aneurysms generally bleed into the subarachnoid space; intracerebral bleeds (hematomas) usually localize in the thalamus, putamen, and globus pallidus area; and metastatic disease is more likely to produce well-circumscribed masses rather than diffuse disease.

15. The answer is B: neutrophilic leukocytosis and a left shift. The specimen represents acute appendicitis evidenced by vessel engorgement, edematous fat, and exudate (grayish material). One would expect steady, right lower quadrant pain, neutrophilic leukocytosis, and a left shift, indicative of a bacterial infection (Chapter 15). Crampy pain and bloody diarrhea are more likely to occur in Crohn's disease. There is no evidence of a carcinoid tumor (choice D). Atypical lymphocytosis (choice E) most commonly accompanies viral infections.

16. The answer is B: *Helicobacter pylori* in the mucous layer. The arrow in the gross specimen points to a small, punched out, circular duodenal ulcer in the first part of the duodenum (Chapter 15). The stomach mucosa is grossly normal (no atrophy, cancer, erosions, or hypertrophic rugae are present). A random biopsy would likely reveal *H. pylori,* whereas a biopsy in the duodenum would likely be negative for the organism. One possible explanation for this discrepancy is that chemicals emitted by *H. pylori* colonizing the stomach may interfere with bicarbonate production in the mucous layer protecting the duodenal mucosa, hence exposing it to acid injury.

17. The answer is E: membranous glomerulonephritis. The IF pattern is granular ("lumpy bumpy"), indicating immunocomplex deposition in the glomerulus. Of the answer choices given, only membranous glomerulonephritis is associated with immunocomplex deposition (subepithelial deposits). This results in increased permeability of the basement membrane and proteinuria (Chapter 17). In focal segmental glomerulosclerosis and minimal change disease, there is fusion of the podocytes and loss of the negative charge in the basement membrane. In diabetic glomerulosclerosis and renal amyloidosis, nonenzymatic glycosylation and deposition of amyloid in the basement membrane, respectively, alter its permeability to proteins, hence producing proteinuria.

18. The answer is C: atherosclerosis. The brain exhibits narrow gyri and wide sulci, indicating a loss in brain mass, or atrophy (Chapter 22). The most common cause of brain atrophy is ischemia secondary to atherosclerosis, which leads to apoptosis of neurons in layers 3, 5, and 6 of the cerebral cortex and subsequent loss of brain mass. Degenerative diseases (e.g., Alzheimer's disease) and neurosyphilis (general paresis) may also cause brain atrophy; however, these are not as common as cerebrovascular atherosclerosis.

Hypertension and metastatic disease do not produce brain atrophy.

19. The answer is A: Coagulation necrosis secondary to popliteal artery atherosclerosis with thrombosis. The picture illustrates dry gangrene of the foot, which is most often secondary to atherosclerosis of the popliteal artery with thrombosis in a patient with diabetes mellitus. Dry gangrene is a type of coagulation necrosis, while wet gangrene is a superimposed anaerobic infection primarily associated with liquefactive necrosis (Chapter 2). Vasculitis in men who smoke (thromboangiitis obliterans or Buerger's disease) and embolization of material (e.g., vegetations, thrombus, atherosclerotic plaque) to the digital vessels are less likely causes of dry gangrene (Chapter 10).

20. The answer is B: friction rub. The heart shows shaggy material covering the epicardial surface consistent with fibrinous pericarditis (Chapter 10). A pericardial friction rub was most likely present owing to the noise created by separation of the visceral and parietal pericardium during the cell cycle. S_3 is heard when blood rapidly enters a ventricle with excess volume (e.g., left heart failure), an opening snap is the initial heart sound in mitral stenosis when the nonpliable valve opens, a mid-systolic ejection click is present in mitral valve prolapse, and a pericardial knock is characteristic of constrictive pericarditis.

21. The answer is C: produce antibodies. The electron micrograph reveals a "cartwheel" chromatin pattern, an eccentric nucleus, and an extensive amount of rough endoplasmic reticulum (site of protein synthesis) representing a plasma cell, the antibody-producing cells in the body (Chapters 3 and 4). Mast cells and basophils release histamine, eosinophils release major basic protein, monocytes release muramidase, and CD4 T helper cells release interleukin-2.

22. The answer is D: adipose. The tumor represents a lipoma, which is the most common benign soft tissue tumor in adults (Chapter 20). It is derived from adipose cells (empty spaces in the histologic section). Benign counterparts for the other answer choices include rhabdomyoma (skeletal muscle), leiomyoma (smooth muscle), hemangioma (endothelial cells), and fibroma (fibroblasts).

23. The answer is B: hexosaminidase. The electron micrograph exhibits myelin figures composed of whorled configurations of concentric membranes that characterize the accumulation of G_{M2} ganglioside in lysosomes in Tay-Sachs disease secondary to a deficiency of hexosaminidase α_2-subunit (Chapter 7). Sphingomyelinase is deficient in Niemann-Pick disease, arylsulfatase A in metachromatic leukodystrophy, galactosylceramidase in Krabbe's disease, and α_1-iduronidase in Hurler's syndrome. None of these four demonstrate these configurations.

24. The answer is E: a ventilation disorder. The lung section reveals spaces lined by hyaline membranes and atelectatic (collapsed) alveoli consistent with a diagnosis of respiratory distress syndrome (RDS; Chapter 11). Owing to the loss of surfactant (lecithin), the surface tension is reduced and the alveoli collapse (ventilation disorder), hence producing massive intrapulmonary shunting of blood rather than a perfusion defect. The relationship of RDS with maternal diabetes is that hyperglycemia in the mother also occurs in the fetus. The fetus responds with insulin release, which inhibits surfactant synthesis. The histologic findings in the lung and the relationship of the newborn's lung

disease with maternal diabetes essentially exclude infection, meconium aspiration, and a congenital malformation.

25. The answer is A: thromboembolization from the heart. The kidney exhibits sharply circumscribed, pale areas on the cortical surface consistent with cortical infarcts (pale infarcts with coagulation necrosis; Chapter 17). The majority of emboli (e.g., thrombus, vegetation) in the systemic circulation derive from the left heart. Ischemic ATN is associated with enlarged diffusely pale kidneys. Benign nephrosclerosis (kidney of hypertension) has a coarsely granular surface, while malignant hypertension has a "flea-bitten" cortical surface from necrotizing arteriolitis of the afferent arterioles. Chronic pyelonephritis (chronic interstitial nephritis) demonstrates U-shaped cortical scars that overlie blunt calyces.

26. The answer is D: ischemic necrosis. The small bowel exhibits a hemorrhagic infarction most likely secondary to thrombosis overlying an atherosclerotic plaque in the superior mesenteric artery (Chapter 15). The history of abdominal pain 30 minutes after eating represents mesenteric angina and the bloody diarrhea with hypotension the ischemic event that resulted in the transmural infarction represented on the slide. The previous history of abdominal pain associated with eating, the gross appearance of the bowel, and the sudden onset of bloody diarrhea with hypotension exclude inflammatory bowel disease, bacterial enterocolitis, drug-induced pseudomembranous colitis (large bowel disease), and angiodysplasia (vascular lesions in the cecum with blood loss).

27. The answer is E: rheumatic fever. The mitral valve demonstrates the classic fish-mouth appearance of mitral stenosis, which is most commonly secondary to repeated attacks of rheumatic fever (Chapter 10). Intravenous drug abuse leads to infective endocarditis, valvular vegetations, and insufficiency type murmurs rather than stenosis. Carcinoid heart disease is most often associated with liver metastasis from a small bowel carcinoid tumor and the release of serotonin into the venous system. Serotonin is fibrogenic and results in right-sided valvular disease, namely tricuspid insufficiency and pulmonic stenosis. Mitral valve prolapse exhibits redundant valvular material with the potential for mitral insufficiency rather than stenosis. SLE is associated with Libman-Sacks endocarditis which does not progress to mitral stenosis.

28. The answer is A: a bacterial bronchopneumonia. The slide exhibits bronchopneumonia with a bronchus destroyed by neutrophils that spill into the subjacent lung parenchyma (Chapter 11). This is an example of liquefactive necrosis. There is no evidence of granulomatous inflammation (granulomas with multinucleated giant cells) or cancer. Viral pneumonias have an interstitial pattern of inflammation rather than an alveolar exudate, and lymphocytes are the inflammatory cells rather than neutrophils.

29. The answer is E: inhalation of asbestos fibers. The lung is partially encased by a thick, white tissue that focally infiltrates the lung parenchyma. Given the history of working in a shipyard, the patient most likely inhaled asbestos fibers used as insulation around pipes. Asbestos exposure in the absence of smoking predisposes to a mesothelioma arising from the pleura rather than primary lung cancer, which is most often associated with asbestos exposure plus smoking (Chapter 11). Primary squamous and small-cell carcinomas are centrally located tumors with a strong relationship to smoking. There is no evidence of cavitation to suggest reactivation TB or a pneumonic process in the parenchyma with spread to the pleura.

30. The answer is A: a diffuse infiltrate of neoplastic lymphocytes. The age, physical examination findings, and presence of large numbers of "mature-appearing" lymphocytes in the peripheral blood associated with a normocytic anemia and thrombocytopenia are consistent with chronic lymphocytic leukemia (CLL; Chapter 12). CLL is the most common leukemia and cause of generalized lymphadenopathy in patients ≥ 60 years of age. The age of the patient and the morphology of the cells argue against acute and chronic myelogenous leukemia (choices B and C). Myelodysplasia with ringed sideroblasts (choice D) is common in this age bracket; however, pancytopenia is the rule in addition to a megaloblastoid marrow. Agnogenic myeloid metaplasia (choice E) demonstrates peripheralization of the marrow elements (leukoerythroblastic smear) rather than a lymphocyte-predominant WBC count.

31. The answer is D: a B-cell non-Hodgkin's malignant lymphoma. The biopsy reveals a monomorphic proliferation of cells with a nodular pattern consistent with a poorly differentiated nodular lymphocytic lymphoma (follicular lymphoma) of B-cell origin (Chapter 13). This is a common second malignancy in patients with previous Hodgkin's disease (HD) who are treated with alkylating agents. Nodular sclerosing HD exhibits broad bands of collagen and lacunar spaces within which are Reed-Sternberg (RS) equivalents (lacunar cells). Recall that the malignant cell in HD is the RS cell, hence one would not expect a monomorphic infiltrate of cells (in this case, lymphocytes) in HD. Reactive hyperplasia has sharply demarcated germinal centers and a proliferation of many different cell types. There is no evidence of metastasis.

32. The answer is C: a primary squamous cell carcinoma. The specimen reveals an isolated, large, ulcerated mass in the distal esophagus. Although this is not the most common location for squamous cell carcinoma of the esophagus (which is more common in the mid-esophagus), it is not an extension from cancer in the proximal stomach, primary adenocarcinoma arising from Barrett's esophagus (choice B), or ulceration consistent with gastroesophageal reflux disease, since the gastroesophageal junction and proximal stomach have no visible lesions (Chapter 15). In addition, the patient has two risk factors for esophageal cancer—alcohol and smoking—which act as cocarcinogens. Herpes esophagitis produces odynophagia and not dysphagia for solids.

33. The answer is E: sections exhibited inflammatory pseudopolyps and crypt abscesses. The specimen reveals numerous pseudopolyps and areas of ulceration between the pseudopolyps consistent with ulcerative colitis (Chapter 15). Crypt abscesses were likely present on microscopic examination (not granulomas as in Crohn's disease) and also inflammatory changes limited to the mucosa and submucosa (not transmural as in Crohn's disease). Ulcerative colitis begins in the rectum and generally spares the anus. Crohn's disease commonly involves the anus (ulcers and fistulas). Infarction of the entire colon is uncommon owing to multiple blood supplies. Familial polyposis (autosomal dominant) is not associated with ulceration and bloody diarrhea.

34. The answer is C: was a smoker with a primary cancer

originating in the lung. The liver exhibits multiple umbilicated nodular lesions consistent with metastasis (Chapter 16). The primary sites, in order of decreasing incidence, of metastasis to the liver are lung, colon, pancreas, breast, and stomach. Granulomatous hepatitis secondary to miliary TB is associated with millet seed–sized infiltrates rather than large umbilicated lesions. Primary hepatocellular carcinoma develops in the setting of cirrhosis, which is not evident in the liver.

35. The answer is A: elevated serum amylase and lipase levels. The photomicrograph reveals ghost-like areas of enzymatic fat necrosis secondary to acute pancreatitis (Chapter 16). The gross description of the liver is consistent with a fatty liver, hence the patient was most likely an alcoholic with acute pancreatitis. Acute pancreatitis is associated with an elevation of amylase and lipase. Areas of enzymatic fat necrosis frequently undergo dystrophic calcification (not metastatic), which may be visualized on x-ray. The serum AST and GGT are both elevated in people with alcoholism, the former released from alcohol damage to mitochondria, which is the primary location of AST, and the latter from alcohol induction of the cytochrome P-450 system. Blockage of the common bile duct (e.g., stone or carcinoma of the head of pancreas) produces a green discoloration of the liver. There is no evidence of pancreatic cancer.

36. The answer is B: a subarachnoid hemorrhage. The kidney exhibits complete replacement by cysts, hence the patient has adult polycystic kidney disease (APKD). The occipital headache and death of the patient are most likely secondary to a subarachnoid bleed from a ruptured berry aneurysm, which occurs in 10–30% of patients with APKD (Chapter 17). Hypertension is not the cause of the patient's death, since hypertension produces intracerebral bleeds (hematomas) usually within the distribution of the lenticulostriate vessels. There is no association of primary cancer (choice E) or arteriovenous malformation (choice C) with APKD.

37. The answer is E: antibodies directed against the noncollagen domain of α_3 type IV collagen. The biopsy reveals crescent formation within Bowman's capsule consistent with crescentic glomerulonephritis. The renal biopsy findings along with the history of lung disease in a young man is consistent with Goodpasture's syndrome (Chapters 11 and 17). It is a type II cytotoxic antibody reaction against the noncollagen domain of α_3 type IV collagen in both the pulmonary and glomerular capillary basement membranes. The immune reaction is not against planted antigens (e.g., bacterial products, DNA), since type IV collagen is the primary collagen in basement membranes. Anti-cANCA and -pANCA antibodies are associated with Wegener's granulomatosis and polyarteritis nodosa, respectively. Nonenzymatic glycosylation occurs in diabetes mellitus (choice A).

38. The answer is A: nonenzymatic glycosylation. The glomerulus exhibits globular ("Christmas ball") mesangial deposits and a prominent arteriole with hyaline arteriolosclerosis. These findings are consistent with a diagnosis of nodular glomerulosclerosis, which is the nephropathy of diabetes mellitus (Kimmelstiel-Wilson syndrome; Chapters 10, 17, and 19). Nonenzymatic glycosylation is the primary cause of the arteriolar disease and also contributes to the glomerular capillary alterations that increase permeability to protein

and proteinuria. Osmotic damage may contribute to the glomerular disease as well. Although the mesangial deposits resemble those of renal amyloidosis, the arteriolar changes are more characteristic of diabetes mellitus. Furthermore, diabetic nephropathy is the most common cause of chronic renal disease in the United States. Neither immunocomplex disease nor antineutrophil cytoplasmic antibodies are operative in diabetic nephropathy.

39. The answer is C: renal adenocarcinoma. The sections reveal nests of clear cells with tubule formation. Among the choices given, a renal adenocarcinoma is the only malignancy that has this appearance and the tendency for hemorrhagic metastasis (Chapter 17). Smoking is a major risk factor for renal adenocarcinoma.

40. The answer is E: a past history of cryptorchidism. The section reveals large clear cells with prominent nucleoli surrounded by benign lymphocytes. The age of the patient and the histologic features of the lesion are characteristic of a seminoma, which may arise from a cryptorchid testis or a normal testis (Chapter 17). A small percentage of these tumors secrete β-hCG. Since the testes migrate from the abdominal cavity into the scrotum, metastasis is to intra-abdominal lymph nodes rather than inguinal lymph nodes. α-Fetoprotein is produced by yolk sac tumors (endodermal sinus tumors). Though well circumscribed, the process is neoplastic and not a granuloma (no multinucleated giant cells) representing TB. Malignant lymphomas involving the testes are generally metastatic tumors and are more common in elderly men.

41. The answer is D: adenocarcinoma of the lower uterine segment. The specimen reveals a polypoid, necrotic mass in the lower uterine segment, which along with the patient's age and history of obesity, hypertension, and diabetes is consistent with endometrial adenocarcinoma (Chapter 18). The cervix is grossly normal (which rules out choice E), and no endometrial polyps, endocervical polyps, or leiomyomas are present in the gross specimen.

42. The answer is A: neoplastic transformation of smooth muscle. The specimen exhibits a large, well-circumscribed leiomyoma filling the endometrial cavity and distorting the shape of the uterus (Chapter 18). On cut section, the leiomyoma has a whorled appearance and no areas of hemorrhage and necrosis. The gross findings are virtually diagnostic of a leiomyoma and would not be confused with endometrial or cervical cancer, cystic hyperplasia of endometrial tissue, or adenomyosis, which involves the presence of benign glands and stroma within myometrial tissue.

43. The answer is C: primary ovarian cancer derived from surface epithelium. The sections reveal a papillary tumor with dark concretions representing psammoma bodies. With the presence of induration in the rectal pouch, the tumor has already metastasized (seeding). The tumor is a serous cystadenocarcinoma of the ovary, which is the most common primary cancer of the ovary (Chapter 18). Psammoma bodies and bilaterality are prominent features of this tumor, which is derived from surface epithelial cells. Primary germ cell and sex cord–stromal tumors are not papillary and do not contain psammoma bodies. Metastatic stomach cancer (Krukenberg's tumor) usually features signet-ring cells. Primary lung cancer does not have psammoma bodies.

44. The answer is D: breast stroma. The histologic section

reveals the characteristic features of a fibroadenoma with proliferation of stromal cells and compression of the ducts into slit-like spaces (Chapter 18). The neoplastic cell in fibroadenomas derives from the stroma. There is no relationship between the fibroadenoma and the history of breast cancer in the mother.

45. The answer is B: infiltrating ductal carcinoma. The gross specimen exhibits retraction of the nipple by an indurated mass with irregular borders and a chalky appearance consistent with an infiltrating ductal carcinoma, which is the most common cancer of the breast (Chapter 18). Lobular cancers are not usually indurated and are more likely to be discovered by mammography. Comedocarcinomas have necrotic debris emanating from the cut surface of the tumor. Medullary carcinomas are large, bulky tumors with pushing rather than infiltrating borders. Intraductal carcinomas do not have an infiltrative pattern.

46. The answer is E: malignant osteoblasts. The location of the tumor, the "sunburst" appearance on x-ray (bone formation in soft tissue), and the age of the patient all indicate that the tumor is an osteogenic sarcoma, the second most common primary bone cancer (multiple myeloma is the most common primary cancer). These sarcomas derive from osteoblasts (Chapter 20). Chondrosarcomas usually occur in an older age bracket and have a cartilaginous appearance on cut section. Ewing's sarcomas have small, round cells that are PAS positive and are more often present in younger children. Giant cell tumors of bone originate in the epiphysis, whereas osteogenic sarcomas arise in the metaphysis of bone. Neuroblastomas have small round cells that are S100 antigen positive, indicating their neural crest origin. They are more common in young children as a metastasis from a primary site in the adrenal medulla.

47. The answer is D: functional asplenia. The peripheral smear reveals sickle cells and Howell-Jolly bodies (nuclear remnants). Even though the patient's spleen is enlarged owing to trapping of sickle cells, the presence of Howell-Jolly bodies and *Streptococcus pneumoniae* septicemia (gram-positive diplococci) indicate that it is nonfunctional. Eventually, it will be autosplenectomized after repeated infarctions. Sickle cell disease is AR and an intrinsic type of hemolytic anemia with extravascular hemolysis, the latter associated with an unconjugated hyperbilirubinemia (Chapter 12).

48. The answer is A: sickle cell trait. Target cells have an excess of RBC membrane that bulges in the center, giving a bull's-eye appearance to the cells (Chapter 12). They are excellent markers of alcohol-related liver disease (owing to alteration of the cholesterol in the RBC membrane) and hemoglobinopathies (e.g., HbC disease, β-thalassemia, sickle cell disease [not trait]). Absence of the spleen is also associated with target cells, since macrophages normally remove excess membrane from RBCs.

49. The answer is B: pancytopenia. The bone marrow is hypoplastic and because of the history of NANB viral hepatitis, the patient most likely has aplastic anemia. Pancytopenia, reticulocytopenia, absence of shift cells, and a normocytic to slightly macrocytic anemia are expected CBC findings.

50. The answer is A: splenomegaly secondary to extramedullary hematopoiesis. The patient has agnogenic myeloid metaplasia, a myeloproliferative disease that begins in the bone marrow and moves to the spleen, which then takes over the function of hematopoiesis

(extramedullary hematopoiesis; Chapter 12). Reactive fibrosis occurs in the marrow owing to secretion of growth factors by megakaryocytes that promote fibroblast synthesis of collagen. Unlike in chronic myelogenous leukemia, the LAP score is high and the Philadelphia chromosome is absent. RBCs that are synthesized in the bone marrow are deformed by the fibrotic tissue, hence they appear as teardrops in the peripheral blood. Splenic infarctions are common with subsequent production of a pleural effusion. There is no evidence of metastatic disease in the bone marrow. Primary malignant lymphomas of the spleen are extremely rare. Portal hypertension with congestive splenomegaly is not associated with marrow fibrosis.

51. The answer is C: related to healing of bone fractures. Hemolysis of a blood sample falsely increases the serum lactate dehydrogenase (LDH), serum potassium, and serum aspartate aminotransferase (AST). It has no effect on the serum alkaline phosphatase (AP). Serum AP is normally higher in growing children than in adults owing to bone growth; however, a higher value than normal in a child who may be a victim of abuse most likely represents healing bone fractures. The serum γ-glutamyltransferase (GGT) would be normal if the AP is of bone origin and increased if the AP is derived from the liver (Chapter 16).

52. The answer is E: 100%. When the specificity of a test is 100% (no false positives; specificity = TN/TN + FP), the predictive value of a positive test (PV+ = TP/TP + FP) is always 100%. Hence, the anti-Sm antibody test is more useful in confirming the diagnosis of SLE than as a screening test, since the sensitivity (positivity in disease; TP/TP + FN) is so low (Chapter 1).

53. The answer is D: percentage of HbA. Since women have fewer iron stores than men (owing to menses, childbearing) the serum iron, ferritin, RBC count, Hb, and Hct are lower than in the male (Chapter 1). However, the percentage of HbA in each RBC is the same in both sexes.

54. The answer is A: the negative RPR is a false negative. Although the RPR is the initial screening test for syphilis, it has a sensitivity of only 75% in primary disease, and an FN is possible (Chapters 1 and 18). The FTA-ABS has close to 100% specificity for all stages of syphilis, hence a positive test is likely to be a TP, especially when a painless chancre is present. It has a much higher specificity than the RPR, which is often positive in SLE and other diseases. However, the FTA-ABS does not distinguish active from inactive disease. Dark-field microscopy is the gold standard for diagnosing primary and secondary syphilis and has a high specificity. *Haemophilus ducreyi* produces painful ulcers.

55. The answer is D: 90%. The sensitivity of disease, or the percent chance that the test is positive in a patient with the disease, is calculated as follows: TP/TP + FN (Chapter 1). Since the test is positive in 180 of 200 people with known CAD, the sensitivity is 90% (180/180 + 20). The specificity is 70% (TN/TN + FP; 140/140 + 60). The PV+ is 75% (TP/TP + FP; 180/180 + 60). The PV− is ~88% (TN/TN + FN; 140/140 + 20). The prevalence of disease is 50% (people with disease [TP + FN] divided by the total population studied [TP + FP + TN + FN]; 200/400).

56. The answer is B: a positive test result is SLE or some other collagen vascular disease. When the sensitivity of a test is 100% (no FNs), the PV− test result repre-

senting a TN must be 100%. However, if the test is positive, the test result may be a TP or an FP (Chapter 1). Therefore, highly sensitive tests are most useful in screening for disease, since a negative test excludes disease, while a positive test does not differentiate a TP from an FP. When the specificity of a test is 100% (no FPs), the PV+ test result representing a TP must be 100%; however, if it is negative, the test result may be a TN or an FN. Hence, tests with high specificity are useful in confirming rather than screening for disease. Therefore, if the test for SLE has a sensitivity of 100% (PV− must be 100%) and a specificity of 80%, it is a better screen (FN rate = 0%) than a confirmatory test (FP rate = 20%), since a positive test may be SLE or some other collagen vascular disease.

57. The answer is E: a reduced concentration of ATP. In tissue hypoxia, the lack of oxygen in tissue affects oxidative phosphorylation in the mitochondria (oxygen is the last reaction in electron transfer), hence ATP depletion is the primary problem (Chapter 2). ATP is important in maintaining the sodium/potassium-ATPase pump; therefore, the lack of ATP allows sodium entry into the cell with subsequent cellular swelling (cloudy swelling). ATP depletion also decreases synthesis of proteins, such as apolipoproteins; however, this produces fatty change in the liver, since VLDL cannot be secreted without its protein coat. The other answer choices result in irreversible injury to the cell.

58. The answer is C: carbon monoxide poisoning. All the choices listed produce tissue hypoxia (inadequate oxygenation of tissue); however, not all do so by lowering the oxygen content (1.34 [Hb] × SaO_2 + PaO_2; Chapters 2 and 8). In CO poisoning, CO rather than oxygen attaches to heme, hence the oxygen saturation (SaO_2) is decreased without affecting the amount of oxygen dissolved in plasma (PaO_2). The oxygen content is decreased in anemia owing to the reduction in Hb concentration (not the PaO_2 or SaO_2), whereas in respiratory acidosis, both the SaO_2 and the PaO_2 are reduced, since less alveolar oxygen is present for gas exchange when the alveolar CO_2 is increased. Cyanide blocks cytochrome oxidase without affecting the oxygen content. A ventilation/perfusion mismatch reduces both the PaO_2 and the SaO_2.

59. The answer is E: skeletal muscle. Skeletal muscle (also cardiac muscle) is a permanent cell (it cannot enter the cell cycle) and is the only cell type listed that can undergo only hypertrophy. Skeletal muscle hypertrophy occurs in response to an increase in workload (Chapter 2). Hepatocytes, endometrial cells, and smooth muscle cells are stable cells that may undergo both hyperplasia and hypertrophy. Neurons are permanent cells that cannot undergo either hypertrophy or hyperplasia.

60. The answer is D: ischemic acute tubular necrosis. In ischemic acute tubular necrosis, the renal tubular cells undergo coagulation necrosis and then slough off into the lumen, hence contributing to oliguria (Chapters 2, 5, and 17). Acute pancreatitis is an example of enzymatic necrosis, wet gangrene of liquefactive necrosis, Henoch-Schönlein vasculitis of fibrinoid necrosis, and an atherosclerotic infarct of the brain of liquefactive necrosis.

61. The answer is A: decreased synthesis of apolipoprotein. Kwashiorkor is characterized by a low protein intake in the presence of a normal total caloric intake consisting primarily of carbohydrates. Hypoproteine-

mia leads to apolipoprotein depletion, hence VLDL cannot be secreted from the hepatocyte without its protein coat (Chapter 2). Although choices B, D, and E may produce fatty change in the liver, they are not responsible for the fatty liver of kwashiorkor. Decreased glycolysis does not produce a fatty liver.

62. The answer is E: C5a and LTB_4. An additional function of C5a is as an anaphylatoxin along with C3a. LTB_4 is the only leukotriene that does not affect vessel permeability or caliber (Chapter 3). Regarding the other choices, C3b is an opsonin; Hageman factor XII activates the intrinsic clotting pathway, the kinin system (produces bradykinin), and the fibrinolytic system (produces plasmin); LTC_4 increases vessel permeability and is a bronchoconstrictor and vasoconstrictor; histamine is a vasodilator and increases vessel permeability; bradykinin increases vessel permeability, is a vasodilator, and produces pain; nitric oxide is a vasodilator; C3a is an anaphylatoxin; and platelet-activating factor is a vasodilator (low concentration) and a vasoconstrictor (high concentration), increases vessel permeability, is a chemotactic agent, and increases adhesion molecule synthesis.

63. The answer is D: adhesion molecule defect. The patient has an adhesion molecule defect, most likely a deficiency of β_2-integrin in the CD11/CD18 complex. Since neutrophils cannot adhere to the endothelium, they cannot emigrate into tissue. In newborns, this results in failure of the umbilical cord to separate and in recurrent bacterial infections (Chapter 3). Cystic fibrosis may present with meconium ileus at birth and has no leukocyte defects. Chronic granulomatous disease of childhood (SXR disease with a deficiency of NADPH oxidase) is ruled out by the normal NBT dye test, indicating a normal respiratory burst mechanism. Normal peripheral blood leukocytes rule out the Chédiak-Higashi syndrome (AR disease with a defect in the polymerization of microtubules and giant lysosomes in leukocytes). G6PD deficiency presents with neonatal jaundice due to hemolysis of RBCs.

64. The answer is E: histamine. Histamine, the most important chemical mediator of acute inflammation, is a vasodilator (it produces rubor [redness] and calor [warmth of the skin]) and increases vessel permeability (tumor [swelling]) of inflammation (Chapter 3). Refer to the discussion of question 62 regarding choices A, B, and C. Prostaglandins produce vasodilatation, increased vessel permeability, and pain.

65. The answer is E: Schwann cells are important in nerve regeneration. When a peripheral nerve is transected, the proliferation of Schwann cells serves as a guide for the axonal sprouts that arise from the proximal stump and extend distally to reunite with the muscle (Chapters 3 and 22). In the liver, Ito cells are responsible for stimulating fibrogenesis as a mechanism of repair. The renal cortical tubules have the greatest oxygen supply and regenerative capacity in response to injury. Type II pneumocytes are the reserve cell responsible for repair in the lungs as well as for surfactant synthesis. Astrocytes are the "fibroblast" of the CNS and provide some structural support in the brain with their cell processes when there is injury and repair (called gliosis).

66. The answer is D: transferrin. Transferrin, the binding agent for iron, is reduced in inflammation owing to the synthesis of other acute-phase reactants in the liver (Chapter 3). Since transferrin is measured as the total iron-binding capacity (TIBC), it is decreased in the

anemia of inflammation. Transferrin has a half-life of 10 days, hence its usefulness as a marker of protein reserve. All the other proteins listed are increased in inflammation as acute-phase reactants, and none serve as a marker of protein status.

67. The answer is C: confirm the result with a Western blot assay. The ELISA test for HIV antibody, which detects the anti-gp120 antibody, is only a screen and must be confirmed by Western blot assay, which measures more than one antibody. If the Western blot test is positive, the positive ELISA test is a true positive and the patient is a candidate for AZT. The p24 antigen is a marker of disease activity and is increased in the initial infection and prior to development of AIDS. Lymphocyte cultures for HIV are reserved for equivocal cases and for workups of newborns born to HIV-positive mothers (Chapter 4).

68. The answer is C: lungs. Although all the organs listed can be involved in AIDS, the lungs are most frequently targeted. Acute bronchitis; *P. carinii, S. pneumoniae,* and *M. avium-intracellulare* pneumonia; and CMV pneumonitis are commonly observed (Chapter 4).

69. The answer is A: loss of fluid, ↓ TBNa, ↓↓ TBW. To increase the plasma osmolality (hypernatremia) and decrease both the ECF and ICF volume, there must be a loss of hypotonic fluid in the following proportions (↑ serum sodium ≅ ↓ TBNa/ ↓↓ TBW; Chapter 5). Only a loss of salt produces a recognizable loss of volume in the ECF, hence a loss of pure water will not reduce ECF volume unless it is an extreme loss. Choices B and D produce hyponatremia and an increase in volume in both compartments; choice C produces an isotonic loss of fluid with no change in the serum sodium and contraction limited to the ECF compartment; choice E increases the serum sodium and ECF volume while decreasing the ICF volume.

70. The answer is D: hypotonic gain of fluid/right heart failure. When the EABV does not match the ECF volume, there must be an alteration in Starling's forces (increased hydrostatic pressure or decreased plasma oncotic pressure; Chapter 5). This results in interstitial edema, which traps fluid in that space and reduces the venous return to the heart with a subsequent drop in the cardiac output and EABV. Hence, the ECF volume is increased owing to excess fluid in the interstitial space, while the arterial volume is decreased. In all the other answer choices, the EABV matches the ECF compartment volume.

71. The answer is B: gain of fluid, ↔TBNa, ↑↑ TBW. SiADH results in the reabsorption of free water without any salt, hence the serum sodium is decreased, there is no change in TBNa, and the TBW is increased (Chapter 5). Most of the water is in the ICF compartment. Regarding the other fluid alterations, choice A is a hypotonic loss of both water and salt (via osmotic diuresis, sweat), choice C is a hypotonic gain of both water and salt (fluid absorption in the edema states), choice D is a hypertonic gain of more salt than water (infusion of hypertonic saline), and choice E is a hypertonic loss of more salt than water (diuretic use).

72. The answer is A: right heart failure/left heart failure. An increase in hydrostatic pressure is an alteration in Starling's forces resulting in the production of a transudate (Chapter 5). In right heart failure, the venous system is volume overloaded and the hydrostatic pressure is increased, leading to pitting edema, whereas in left heart failure, the pulmonary venous system is overloaded, leading to pulmonary edema.

Celiac disease is a malabsorption syndrome resulting in a drop in oncotic pressure due to the loss of albumin. A pleural effusion in pneumonia, cerebral edema in encephalitis, swelling of tissue in a bee sting, and pulmonary edema in ARDS are examples of edema secondary to inflammation, hence an exudate rather than a transudate is produced. Ascitic fluid in cirrhosis is a combination of increased hydrostatic pressure (portal hypertension) and decreased oncotic pressure (hypoalbuminemia from reduced liver synthesis of albumin). Cerebral edema in hyponatremia is due to an osmotic shift of water into the ICF compartment. This is not a Starling's force alteration.

73. The answer is C: trisomy 21. Down syndrome (trisomy 21), the most common genetic cause of mental retardation, is also associated with endocardial cushion defects (ASD and VSD) and dementia, if the patient lives into adulthood (Chapter 7). Dementia is due to the production of β-protein by chromosome 21, which is converted into amyloid that is toxic to neurons in the CNS. Trisomies 16 and 18 are associated with cardiac defects and mental retardation; however, there is no increased incidence of dementia. No AD or SXR disease is associated with this combination of abnormalities.

74. The answer is D: chronic renal failure. The second hydroxylation step in vitamin D metabolism utilizing 1α-hydroxylase occurs in the proximal tubules of the kidneys (Chapter 6). Overall, chronic renal failure is the most common cause of hypovitaminosis D. Since vitamin D is important in the reabsorption of calcium and phosphorus in the small bowel, hypocalcemia occurs and is a potent stimulus for the secretion of parathormone, leading to secondary hyperparathyroidism. The other choices (decreased sunlight, poor intake, malabsorption, cirrhosis) do result in hypovitaminosis D but are not the most common cause of hypovitaminosis D.

75. The answer is C: nyctalopia. Nyctalopia, or night blindness, is the first clinical sign of vitamin A deficiency (Chapter 6). Vitamin A is important in maintaining visual purple in both the rods (night vision) and cones (daytime vision). Glossitis is most commonly associated with water-soluble vitamin deficiencies (vitamin C, riboflavin), congestive cardiomyopathy with thiamine deficiency, dementia with niacin deficiency, and perifollicular hemorrhage with vitamin C deficiency.

76. The answer is C: lack of hydroxylation of lysine and proline. The clinical history is classic for scurvy secondary to vitamin C deficiency (Chapter 6). Vitamin C is critical in the hydroxylation of lysine and proline in collagen synthesis, since these are the sites for cross-linkage by lysyl oxidase to increase the strength of collagen. A deficiency of ATP is noted in niacin, riboflavin, and thiamine deficiencies; zinc is a cofactor in collagenase; copper is a cofactor in lysyl oxidase; and thiamine is a cofactor in the pyruvate dehydrogenase complex.

77. The answer is C: hypokalemia. The clinical history is classic for bulimia, in which patients binge on food and then self-induce vomiting (Chapter 6). Electrolyte abnormalities are most commonly observed owing to the vomiting (e.g., hypokalemia, metabolic alkalosis [increased pH, increased bicarbonate, increased PaCO$_2$ as compensation]). Glucose abnormalities are not present in bulimia.

78. The answer is D: hyperpigmentation in sun-exposed areas. Corn is deficient in tryptophan, an essential

amino acid used in the synthesis of niacin. A diet deficient in niacin leads to pellagra, which is characterized by diarrhea, dementia, and dermatitis (pigmentation in sun-exposed areas). Ringed sideroblasts are associated with pyridoxine deficiency (sideroblastic anemia), neovascularization of the cornea with riboflavin deficiency, hypersegmented neutrophils with B_{12} and folate deficiency, and squamous metaplasia of the cornea with vitamin A deficiency.

79. The answer is C: increased anion gap metabolic acidosis. Methyl alcohol is converted to formic acid, which causes an increased anion gap (AG) metabolic acidosis and optic neuritis leading to blindness (Chapters 5 and 8). Ethyl alcohol is associated with lactic and ketoacidosis owing to the increase in NADH in alcohol metabolism (pyruvate to lactate, acetyl-CoA to β-hydroxybutyrate). Choices A, B, and D are primarily noted in ethyl alcohol abuse.

80. The answer is D: dissecting aortic aneurysm. Although chemicals in smoke produce endothelial injury that predisposes to atherosclerosis, atherosclerosis is not a predisposing cause of a dissecting aortic aneurysm, which is associated with elastic tissue fragmentation and cystic medial necrosis (Chapters 8 and 10). All the other answer choices are associated with smoking.

81. The answer is D: decreased RBC protoporphyrin. Lead blocks ferrochelatase and ALA dehydrase in heme synthesis, resulting in a microcytic anemia with ringed sideroblasts (Chapters 8 and 12). The block in ferrochelatase increases the RBC protoporphyrin levels, which formerly was a screening test of choice for lead poisoning. Ferrochelatase enhances the reaction that combines iron with protoporphyrin to form heme. All the other findings listed are associated with lead poisoning.

82. The answer is C: high altitude: low atmospheric pressure reduces the PO_2. The percent oxygen at high altitudes is still 21%; however, the atmospheric pressure is less than 760 mm Hg, which lowers the alveolar PO_2, resulting in hypoxemia (Chapter 8). AIDS is the most common cause of death between 25 and 44 years of age in black men and women. Lymphocytes are the most vulnerable hematopoietic cells to ionizing radiation. Third-degree burns are nonpainful owing to destruction of the nerves. Wet skin increases current by lowering the resistance of skin.

83. The answer is B: ovary. Serous cystadenocarcinomas are the most common cancers in the ovary, while breast cancer is the most common metastatic tumor to the ovary (Chapters 9 and 18). In all the other sites, metastasis (primary site in parenthesis) is more common than a primary cancer: brain (lung), bone (breast and prostate), liver (lung followed by colon), and lymph node (most common organ metastasized to, usually by carcinomas).

84. The answer is D: colorectal cancer. Lung cancer is the most common cause of death due to cancer in both men and women, while colorectal cancer is second (Chapter 9). Breast cancer is the second most common cause of death due to cancer in women and prostate cancer in men; however, colorectal cancer has the greatest overall combined mortality.

85. The answer is A: solitary nodule in the lung. Greater than 75% of solitary coin lesions in the lung are benign, with granulomas representing the greatest percentage of the disorders (Chapter 11) A moveable mass in the parotid is most likely a pleomorphic adenoma (mixed tumor). An ovarian mass with calcifica-

tion may be a teratoma, fibroma, or gonadoblastoma (Chapter 18). A tubular adenoma of the colon is neoplastic but rarely progresses to cancer (Chapter 15). A painful distal femur mass in an 18-year-old is most likely osteogenic sarcoma (Chapter 20).

86. The answer is C: actinic keratosis. An actinic keratosis is sun-damaged skin that has a propensity for progression to squamous cell carcinoma of the skin (Chapter 9). A leiomyoma rarely if ever progresses to leiomyosarcoma of the uterus. Prostatic hyperplasia does not progress to prostate carcinoma but is commonly in the same vicinity as prostate cancer. Fibroadenoma of the breast may be associated with breast cancer, but it does not progress to a breast cancer. Capillary hemangiomas do not progress to a vessel cancer.

87. The answer is B: true vocal cord. The true vocal cord is normally lined by pseudostratified columnar epithelium. Smoking causes squamous metaplasia of the cords, which can progress to squamous cancer (Chapter 11). Adenocarcinomas are the most common cancers of the kidney, gallbladder, and stomach, while transitional cell carcinomas are the most common cancer in the bladder (Chapter 9).

88. The answer is B: ovary and brain. Tumors that seed are usually located near cavities (Chapter 9). Hence, ovarian and colon cancers may seed in the abdominal cavity. CNS tumors that may seed include glioblastoma multiforme, ependymoma, and medulloblastoma. The other tumors listed spread by direct extension or by the lymphatic route.

89. The answer is D: microcytic RBC indices. Iron deficiency, lead poisoning, and β-thalassemia minor are all microcytic anemias, since they all demonstrate a reduction in the synthesis of Hb, which causes extra mitoses in developing RBCs in the bone marrow (Chapter 12). Iron deficiency and lead poisoning are associated with abnormal iron studies: iron deficiency—low ferritin, high TIBC;, lead poisoning—increased ferritin, low TIBC. β-Thalassemia minor demonstrates abnormal Hb electrophoresis (low HbA, increased HbA_2 and HbF). None of the three anemias is associated with an increased reticulocyte count except for anemia produced by lead poisoning, which may, in some cases, have a hemolytic component.

90. The answer is E: anti–parietal cell antibodies. Pernicious anemia (PA), an autoimmune disease with immune destruction of parietal cells by autoantibodies against parietal cells and intrinsic factor, is the most common cause of B_{12} deficiency (Chapter 12). However, other causes of B_{12} deficiency (e.g., chronic pancreatitis, fish tapeworm, terminal ileal disease, bacterial overgrowth) are not autoimmunities and do not have autoantibodies. Choices A, B, C, and D occur in B_{12} deficiency due to any cause.

91. The answer is D: sugar-water test. The history of episodic hemoglobinuria in a morning urine void and a hemolytic anemia is strongly suggestive of paroxysmal nocturnal hemoglobinuria (PNH). PNH is an acquired stem cell disorder with a deficiency of decay-accelerating factor (which normally increases complement degradation on cell membranes) on all hematopoietic cells, rendering them susceptible to complement destruction at night (the reason for pancytopenia) when a mild respiratory acidosis enhances complement activity. The sugar-water test is the best screening test, while the acidified serum test (Ham test) is confirmatory. Enough hemoglobin may be lost in the urine to result in iron deficiency, as in this patient. There is

an increased incidence of leukemia and hepatic vein thrombosis, the latter owing to destruction of platelets and release of thromboxane A_2, a platelet aggregator. Heinz body preparations are used in the diagnosis of quiescent G6PD deficiency, Hb electrophoresis in the diagnosis of thalassemia and other types of hemoglobinopathy, the direct Coombs' test in the diagnosis of autoimmune hemolytic anemia, and the osmotic fragility test in the diagnosis of congenital spherocytosis.

92. The answer is E: aplastic anemia: bone marrow examination. The diagnosis of aplastic anemia, which is associated with pancytopenia, must always be confirmed by a bone marrow study, since other anemias may also exhibit pancytopenia (e.g., B_{12}/folate deficiency, PNH; Chapter 12). Hb electrophoresis is the confirmatory test for β-thalassemia minor (free erythrocyte protoporphyrin levels are normal). α-Thalassemia is most often a diagnosis of exclusion once β-thalassemia minor is ruled out by a normal Hb electrophoresis (serum ferritin is normal). Congenital spherocytosis is confirmed by an increased osmotic fragility test, while a Heinz body preparation is confirmatory for G6PD deficiency. Iron deficiency is confirmed by a low serum ferritin or in equivocal cases by absent iron stores in the bone marrow. Serum iron is decreased in anemia of inflammation and therefore cannot be used as a confirmatory test for iron deficiency.

93. The answer is E: normal MCV. Acute blood loss within 2 hours will produce signs of hypovolemia (positive tilt test, sinus tachycardia) only if the blood loss is significant (Chapter 12). Since both plasma and RBC are lost in equal proportions, the Hb, Hct, RBC count, and MCV remain normal. Reticulocytosis does not occur until the marrow is able to produce and release reticulocytes (5–7 days). The anemia is unmasked when the plasma begins to be replaced over the ensuing days.

94. The answer is A: D-dimer assay. The history of endotoxic shock and oozing of blood from all puncture sites is classic for DIC (Chapter 5). The tests with the highest sensitivity as initial screens are those that detect secondary fibrinolysis, one of which is the D-dimer test and the other fibrin(ogen) degradation products (FDPs). The former detects cross-linked fragments indicating the presence of fibrin clots, while the latter detects X, Y, D, and E fragments derived from fibrinogen alone or fibrin clots. The other tests listed are also useful in DIC; however, they do not have as good a sensitivity as D dimers and FDPs and are frequently normal.

95. The answer is C: ABO incompatibility. With an O mother who is Rh negative and an A baby who is Rh negative, the baby will have a hemolytic anemia secondary to ABO incompatibility, since mothers who are blood group O normally have IgG anti-A,B antibodies in their serum (Chapter 14). Therefore, IgG antibodies will cross the placenta and attach to fetal A and/or B cells, causing their extravascular removal by macrophages in the fetal spleen. Jaundice will develop soon after birth in the newborn, since the liver conjugating enzymes cannot handle the excessive unconjugated bilirubin load. Since the baby is Rh negative, there is no danger of Rh sensitization in the mother. Physiologic jaundice and breast milk jaundice do not develop in the first 24 hours. Neonatal hepatitis is unlikely with this history.

96. The answer is B: nodular sclerosing Hodgkin's disease.

In this woman's age bracket, the presence of abnormal lymph nodes in the neck and an anterior mediastinal mass has a high predictive value for Hodgkin's disease, particularly nodular sclerosing HD, the most common type of HD in women (not lymphocyte-predominant HD; Chapter 13). Burkitt's lymphoma is more common in children, metastasis from another primary site to the anterior mediastinum is unlikely in this woman's age bracket, and cat-scratch disease produces painful adenopathy and would not be expected to involve the mediastinum.

97. The answer is A: antithrombin III deficiency. A history of deep venous thrombosis and pulmonary emboli in a young woman who has a family history of similar events is highly suggestive of a hereditary disorder associated with hypercoagulability (Chapter 5). Since the PTT was not prolonged when heparin was administered, the patient most likely has antithrombin III deficiency, since ATIII is necessary for the action of heparin in neutralizing coagulation factors. Proteins C and S deficiencies also produce thrombosis; however, the PTT would have become prolonged with heparin therapy. Von Willebrand's disease and a qualitative platelet defect produce a bleeding diathesis and not a hypercoagulable state.

98. The answer is D: whether the lymphoblasts are CALLA positive. The patient has acute lymphoblastic leukemia. Although all the factors listed as choices have importance in the prognosis of the patient, the most important is whether the lymphoblasts are positive for the common ALL antigen (CALLA), which portends a more favorable prognosis than a negative antigen study.

99. The answer is B: stimulation of the renin-angiotensin-aldosterone system. Both left and right heart failure demonstrate a reduction in cardiac output, which reduces the EABV with subsequent stimulation of the renin-angiotensin-aldosterone system (direct stimulation by the sympathetic nervous system plus reduced renal blood flow). This is called secondary aldosteronism (Chapters 5 and 10). Increased jugular venous pressure and dependent pitting edema from increased hydrostatic pressure in the venous system are characteristic of right heart failure. Similarly, with left heart failure, the left ventricular end diastolic volume and hydrostatic pressure in the pulmonary veins are increased, which is reflected by an increase in the pulmonary capillary wedge pressure.

100. The answer is C: aortic insufficiency. Left ventricular hypertrophy (LVH) may result from an increase in afterload (concentric hypertrophy; essential hypertension) or from volume overload with increased work in ejecting the blood from the ventricle (Chapter 10). The latter may occur from valvular insufficiency (mitral or aortic valve) or increased return of blood to the left heart (left-to-right shunts). Restrictive cardiomyopathy is associated with difficulty in filling of the heart (e.g., amyloidosis, iron overload), while hypertrophic cardiomyopathy is similar to aortic stenosis in that there is obstruction to blood flow out of the left ventricle. Mitral stenosis has underfilling of the left ventricle.

101. The answer is C: a ventricular septal defect. There is a step-up of oxygen in the right ventricle and pulmonary artery, indicating a left-to-right shunt at the level of the ventricles (ventricular septal defect; Chapter 10). An ASD would have a step-up of oxygen in the right atrium as well, while a PDA would only have a step-up

of oxygen in the pulmonary artery. In tetralogy of Fallot, a cyanotic congenital heart disease (CHD), unoxygenated blood is directed into the left ventricle through a VSD, leading to a drop in oxygen saturation in the left ventricle. In transposition of the great vessels, another cyanotic CHD, there is a step-up of oxygen in the right atrium, right ventricle, and pulmonary artery from an ASD with a left-to-right shunt. The aorta empties part of this mixture of unoxygenated and oxygenated blood from the right ventricle into the systemic circulation, resulting in cyanosis. In addition, some of the blood from the right ventricle is shunted across a VSD into the left ventricle, which drops the oxygen saturation in this chamber from normal. The left ventricle is emptied by the pulmonary artery, which directs the blood to the lungs for oxygenation.

102. The answer is A: the formation of berry aneurysms. Berry aneurysms are most commonly congenital, in that the vessels lack an internal elastic membrane and muscle wall at the base of the aneurysm (Chapter 10). All the other choices are commonly associated with atherosclerosis: small bowel infarction (superior mesenteric artery), leg claudication (aorta and iliac artery), transient ischemic attacks (carotid artery), and nontraumatic amputation (popliteal artery).

103. The answer is B: reinfarction associated with papillary muscle dysfunction. The patient has reinfarction owing to the reappearance of an elevated CK-MB (Chapter 10). A pansystolic murmur with wet rales indicates mitral valve insufficiency leading to left heart failure. This is most likely due to papillary muscle rupture or dysfunction secondary to a right coronary artery thrombosis, which supplies the posteromedial papillary muscle. Aortic insufficiency is a diastolic murmur after S_2. A ventricular aneurysm is not associated with a murmur and does not develop in the first week. Pericarditis is associated with a friction rub, not a murmur. Ruptures of the free wall with tamponade do not produce murmurs owing to muffling of all heart sounds.

104. The answer is C: negative rods with a thick capsule. The physical findings and chest x-ray are consistent with bacterial pneumonia. The mucoid sputum with blood streaks in an alcoholic is highly suggestive of *Klebsiella pneumoniae*, which is a thick, gram-negative rod with a thick gelatinous capsule. *S. pneumoniae* also has mucoid strains; however, it is a gram-positive diplococcus, which is not given as an answer choice.

105. The answer is E: taken aspirin for pain. The history of a patient with a chronic pain syndrome, asthma, and a nasal polyp is most likely triad asthma induced by aspirin taken to relieve pain (Chapter 11). Aspirin blocks the prostaglandin pathway, leaving the leukotriene pathway open for production of LTC_4-D_4-E_4, which are potent bronchoconstrictors. A pulmonary embolus is not associated with nasal polyps. Cystic fibrosis is associated with nasal polyps; however, asthma is not present in these patients. Allergic polyps and asthma may occur together, but the question implies that the asthma and polyps are associated with a pain syndrome. IgA deficiency is not associated with polyps.

106. The answer is B: the adult respiratory distress syndrome. Aspiration of gastric juice has a high association with ARDS (Chapter 11). The lower the pH of the gastric juice, the greater the likelihood of ARDS. The low PaO_2 even after the patient is given 100% oxygen indicates massive intrapulmonary shunting of blood

owing to atelectasis from neutrophil injury to the type II pneumocytes. The relationship of the patient's respiratory problems with aspiration essentially excludes the other answer choices. In addition, administration of oxygen in the other conditions listed would increase the PaO_2.

107. The answer is C: negative rods. Nosocomial (hospital-acquired) pneumonias are most frequently secondary to gram-negative organisms that colonize the upper respiratory tract. *E. coli* and *P. aeruginosa*, which are gram-negative rods, are most commonly implicated. followed by *S. aureus*, a gram-positive coccus.

108. The answer is C: a thymus-associated disorder. The history of muscle weakness and lid lag suggest myasthenia gravis, an autoimmune disorder with antibodies directed against acetylcholine receptors (Chapters 11 and 20). The thymus is thought to be the source of the antibody production. In the majority of cases, the thymus exhibits hyperplasia with germinal follicle formation, while in 10–15% of cases, a thymoma is present. The relationship of the thymic mass to myasthenia gravis excludes the other choices.

109. The answer is D: histoplasmosis. Abandoned warehouses are frequently occupied by bats, which are associated with histoplasmosis (Chapter 11). Pigeons are more likely to produce cryptococcosis. The painful nodules on the lower legs represent erythema nodosum, which may occur with systemic fungal infections. The other systemic fungal infections listed are not associated with bats or birds. Coccidioidomycosis occurs in the southwestern United States.

110. The answer is A: excessive reabsorption of iron from the small bowel. The patient most likely has hemochromatosis ("bronze diabetes"), an AR disease associated with excessive reabsorption of iron from the small bowel with subsequent deposition in the liver (pigment cirrhosis), pancreas (causing malabsorption, diabetes mellitus), heart (causing restrictive cardiomyopathy), skin (increasing melanin synthesis, leading to hyperpigmentation), and other organs (Chapter 16). Iron initiates the formation of free radicals, which damage the tissue. Alcohol-related disease comes close to all these findings; however, increased skin pigmentation does not occur as a sign of the disease.

111. The answer is B: a defect in the excretion of copper into bile. The patient has Wilson's disease, an AR disease with a defect in the excretion of copper in bile and subsequent accumulation of copper in the liver (Chapter 16). In the liver, it produces chronic active hepatitis, which may progress to a micronodular cirrhosis. The synthesis of ceruloplasmin, the binding protein for copper, is reduced owing to chronic liver disease, hence the total copper level (bound plus free) is decreased, while the free copper level is increased. The excess free copper deposits in the cornea of the eye, producing the Kayser-Fleischer ring, and in the lenticular nuclei, leading to extrapyramidal disease. None of the other diseases listed are associated with the triad of chronic liver disease, deposits in the cornea, and extrapyramidal disease. However, all of them target the liver as a primary manifestation of the disease (e.g., iron overload, glycogenoses, AAT deficiency, galactosemia).

112. The answer is E: antimitochondrial antibody. The patient has primary biliary cirrhosis, an autoimmune disease with granulomatous destruction of the bile duct radicles in the portal triads (Chapter 16). Initially, bile salts are deposited in the skin and produce severe

pruritus. The cholestasis enzymes alkaline phosphatase and GGT are markedly elevated in the absence of jaundice, which is a late manifestation of the disease. The antimitochondrial antibody is increased in the majority of cases. ERCP is useful in excluding extrahepatic obstruction (e.g., a stone in the common bile duct, primary sclerosing cholangitis). Antinuclear antibody and anti–smooth muscle antibody tests are useful in diagnosing autoimmune hepatitis, HBsAg is useful in ruling out chronic hepatitis B, and serum ferritin is useful in ruling out iron overload disease. However, these diseases are not associated with cholestatic liver disease.

113. The answer is B: diffuse microvesicular fatty change. The patient has Reye's syndrome, which is associated with aspirin ingestion in the setting of influenza or chickenpox infections (Chapter 16). The CNS and liver are primarily involved in the disease, leading to cerebral edema (drowsiness, convulsions, coma) and microvesicular steatosis in the liver with subsequent jaundice and prolongation of the prothrombin time (decreased synthesis of coagulation factors). Salicylates damage the mitochondria and disrupt urea metabolism in the liver, hence ammonia is not properly metabolized. Ammonia contributes to encephalopathy. Although viral hepatitis is one of the most common causes of fulminant liver failure with hepatic encephalopathy, the relationship of this child's disease with chickenpox favors Reye's syndrome as the most likely diagnosis. Mallory's bodies are associated with alcoholic liver disease, and AAT deficiency is an AR disease that would have presented at an early age with liver abnormalities. The acuteness of the disease argues against chronic active hepatitis.

114. The answer is A: superinfection with hepatitis D. The hepatitis B virus is not cytolytic to infected hepatocytes; however, it does alter the class I antigens, resulting in destruction of the cells by CD8 cytotoxic T cells. Hepatitis D requires HBsAg to replicate and is cytolytic once it is able to replicate within a hepatocyte. Hence, superinfection with HDV leads to massive destruction of hepatocytes infected with HBV and fulminant liver failure, evidenced in this patient by an increase in the PT and a decrease in serum transaminases. The acute nature of the events in this patient argue against vitamin K deficiency, recovery from HBV infection, and hepatocellular carcinoma. Reye's syndrome is not likely in an adult and has no relationship to chronic HBV liver disease.

115. The answer is C: obstruction. Crohn's disease (CD) is characterized by transmural inflammation, which commonly results in repair by fibrosis, narrowing of the lumen (particularly in the terminal ileum), and obstruction (Chapter 15). Ulcerative colitis (UC) involves the mucosa and submucosa and is not associated with obstruction; however, it is associated with crypt abscesses and has a higher incidence of adenocarcinoma, toxic megacolon, and sclerosing pericholangitis than does CD.

116. The answer is E: normal to low basal acid output. Owing to an association with type B chronic atrophic gastritis and a reduction in acid secretion from damage to gastrin-producing G-cells, the basal acid output is either normal or low in gastric ulcers, whereas it is usually elevated in duodenal ulcers (Chapter 15). In addition, duodenal ulcers are more likely to be associated with blood group O (gastric ulcers with blood group A), MEN type I, male sex, and *H. pylori* infection than are gastric ulcers.

117. The answer is B: duodenal ulcer. Duodenal ulcers are the most common cause of hematemesis, followed by gastric ulcers and esophageal varices (Chapter 15). In addition, they are the most common cause of melena, which is the presence of black, tarry stools that in most cases originate from bleeds above the ligament of Treitz. The black color is due to conversion of Hb to hematin by acid. Gastroesophageal reflux disease and adenocarcinoma of the stomach are not common causes of either hematemesis or melena.

118. The answer is E: rectosigmoid. Cancers in the GI tract commonly obstruct in the esophagus, small bowel, and rectosigmoid; however, of the three locations, the rectosigmoid is the most common primary site for not only obstruction but also cancer of the GI tract in general (Chapter 15). Stomach cancers most commonly develop on the lesser curvature and are more likely to present with weight loss, epigastric pain, anorexia, and vomiting. Cecal lesions are more likely to bleed.

119. The answer is C: fibroma. Ovarian fibromas are of stromal origin, while cystic teratomas, dysgerminomas, endodermal sinus tumors (yolk sac tumors), and struma ovarii (thyroid tissue in a cystic teratoma) are of germ cell origin (Chapter 18). Fibromas are the most common of the stromal tumors and may be associated with Meigs' syndrome (ascites, right-sided pleural effusion).

120. The answer is D: ovary. Although the ovary is more likely to have primary cancer as the most frequent malignancy (serous cystadenocarcinoma), it is a more common site of metastasis than the vagina, cervix, endometrium, or breast (Chapter 18). Breast cancer is the most common primary malignancy to metastasize to the ovaries. Stomach cancers also frequently spread to the ovaries (Krukenberg's tumor).

121. The answer is C: ovary. Oral contraceptives reduce the incidence of ovarian cancer by inhibiting ovulation, which is associated with a reparative process that may activate oncogenes (Chapter 18). Oral contraceptives have been implicated as a cause of hepatocellular carcinoma and cervical cancer. There is neither an increased nor a decreased risk for developing uterine cancer in those using oral contraceptives.

122. The answer is E: inhibition of angiotensin II effect on the efferent arterioles. ACE inhibitors (e.g., captopril) block the formation of angiotensin II, which is a vasoconstrictor of the efferent arterioles, the first site of involvement by hyaline arteriolosclerosis in diabetic nephropathy (Chapter 17). Therefore, blocking ATII vasodilates the lumen of the efferent arteriole and reduces the increase in pressure on the glomerular capillaries, whose basement membranes are more permeable to protein (microalbuminuria) owing to nonenzymatic glycosylation.

123. The answer is D: diabetes mellitus. Hyaline arteriolosclerosis, the small-vessel disease of diabetes mellitus (DM), reduces intrarenal blood flow, hence rendering the renal medulla, normally the least well perfused part of the kidneys, subject to ischemia and the potential for renal papillary necrosis (Chapter 17). Nonenzymatic glycosylation of glomerular capillary basement membranes increases their permeability to proteins, which is first manifested by microalbuminuria and later by significant proteinuria (nodular glomerulosclerosis), often in the nephrotic range (> 3.5 g/dL). Glu-

cosuria is conducive to urinary tract infection. None of the other answer choices predispose to renal papillary necrosis or urinary tract infection; however, SLE may present with the nephrotic syndrome.

124. The answer is D: increased production of sorbitol. Both types I and II DM are associated with osmotic damage to tissue induced by the conversion of glucose into sorbitol by aldolase reductase in tissues such as the lens, Schwann cells, and pericytes around retinal vessels. Sorbitol establishes an osmotic gradient favoring the movement of water into the cells, resulting in damage (e.g., cataracts, peripheral neuropathy, microaneurysms, respectively). Increased anion gap metabolic acidosis and HLA-Dr3/-Dr4 are present in type I DM, while defects in the glucose transport units (GLUTs) and multifactorial inheritance are features of type II DM.

125. The answer is C: a benign islet cell tumor arising from β-cells. Proinsulin is cleaved into C peptide and insulin in the Golgi apparatus of the β-cells in the islets, hence providing a marker of endogenous production of insulin. Since the patient has an elevation of C peptide along with hypoglycemia, the C peptide must be coming from β-islet cells, in this case, an insulinoma, which is not only the most common islet cell tumor but also the one that is most likely to be benign. Surreptitious injection of insulin lowers the C peptide, since hypoglycemia suppresses the patient's own endogenous production of insulin. The other types of islet cell tumors listed, except tumors derived from G-cells (Zollinger-Ellison syndrome), are more likely to produce hyperglycemia, not hypoglycemia. ZE syndrome produces excess gastrin and is not associated with problems with glucose.

126. The answer is D: activation of hormone-sensitive lipase. In DKA, the absence of insulin results in activation of hormone-sensitive lipase by glucagon with the release of fatty acids and glycerol. Fatty acids undergo β-oxidation owing to the loss of the inhibitory effect of malonyl-CoA on carnitine acyltransferase. Glucagon also enhances gluconeogenesis, which is primarily responsible for hyperglycemia in DKA. Fatty acid synthesis is inhibited owing to the absence of insulin. Chylomicrons and VLDL accumulate in the plasma, since insulin normally increases the synthesis of capillary lipoprotein lipase, which removes fatty acids and glycerol from these circulating lipoprotein fractions.

127. The answer is D: 21-hydroxylase deficiency. In 21-hydroxylase deficiency, the most common cause of the AR adrenogenital syndrome, the block in cortisol production leads to an increase in ACTH, with subsequent stimulation of the adrenal cortex to produce more cortisol (Chapter 7). Unfortunately, the gland responds with hyperplasia of the cells, but the enzyme block still prevents cortisol synthesis. Corticosteroid administration and hypopituitarism lead to atrophy of the adrenal cortex (particularly the zona fasciculata and reticularis; Chapter 19). In anencephaly, there is absence of the fetal adrenal cortex (Chapter 22). Addison's disease is associated with autoimmune destruction of the adrenal cortex, leading to hypocortisolism and deficiency of mineralocorticoids.

128. The answer is C: deposition of calcium pyrophosphate in the joint. The patient has pseudogout as evidenced by the presence of needle-shaped crystals (calcium pyrophosphate crystals) that are blue when parallel to the slow axis of the compensator (positive birefringence). Monosodium urate crystals are yellow when parallel to the axis of the compensator (negative birefringence). Most cases of gout, a defect in purine metabolism, are secondary to underexcretion rather than overproduction of uric acid (Chapter 20). Pseudogout is not associated with HLA-B27–related disorders.

129. The answer is A: cartilage fibrillation. Osteoarthritis (OA), the most common joint disease, is due to degeneration of articular cartilage, one manifestation of which is perpendicular clefts in the cartilage called cartilage fibrillation (Chapter 20). Pannus (hyperplastic synovial tissue growing over the articular cartilage), rheumatoid factor (IgM antibody against IgG), and ankylosis (fusion of the joint) are features of rheumatoid arthritis. Both diseases are female dominant.

130. The answer is A: greater osteoclastic than osteoblastic activity. In postmenopausal osteoporosis, the lack of estrogen leaves interleukin-1 (osteoclast activating factor) release by the osteoblasts unchecked, hence osteoclastic activity is greater than osteoblastic activity, leading to an overall reduction in bone mass. Osteopenia (loss of bone density) on radiologic examination is common to both osteoporosis and osteomalacia, the latter a defect in the mineralization of bone (increased thickness of osteoid seams) owing to hypovitaminosis D and subsequent development of hypocalcemia.

131. The answer is A: a malignant plasma cell disorder. The constellation of hyperproteinemia, hypercalcemia, lytic bone lesions, anemia, and renal failure characterizes multiple myeloma, the most common primary malignancy of bone. Malignant plasma cells produce osteoclast activating factor, which lyses the bone and releases calcium into the blood and excessive amounts of γ-globulin (usually IgG), leading to an increase in total protein. Renal failure is most commonly secondary to obstruction of the tubules by Bence Jones protein and an inflammatory reaction directed against the protein. Anemia is the result of diffuse marrow infiltration by malignant plasma cells. Metastatic prostate carcinoma produces osteoblastic metastases and is not usually associated with renal failure. Primary hyperparathyroidism is associated with hypercalcemia, lytic lesions, and the potential for renal failure (nephrocalcinosis); however, it is not associated with hyperproteinemia. Waldenström's macroglobulinemia is characterized by the production of excessive amounts of IgM by malignant lymphoplasmacytoid cells. It is not associated with lytic bone lesions. Sarcoidosis may be associated with hypercalcemia and renal failure.

132. The answer is D: increased binding of ionized calcium to albumin. Alkalosis increases the number of negative charges on proteins, particularly albumin (Chapter 19). The total calcium represents calcium bound to albumin (40%), other anions (17%), and ionized calcium (47%). Hence, in alkalosis, the increased number of negative charges allows albumin to bind more calcium than normally at the expense of the ionized calcium fraction, leading to tetany. However, the total calcium concentration remains normal, since calcium has been shifted from one compartment to another, causing the ionized calcium concentration to decrease.

133. The answer is C: PTH increased, serum calcium increased. Primary hyperparathyroidism, most often due to a parathyroid adenoma, is associated with hypercalcemia, which increases the secretion of gastrin, hence increasing acid production, causing peptic ulcer disease. Hypercalcemia also results in constipation.

134. The answer is E: serum T_4 increased, T_4BR increased, FT_4-I increased, TSH decreased, ^{131}I uptake decreased. The patient has developed hyperthyroidism owing to overmedication with thyroid hormone (Chapter 19). As a result of suppression of the patient's TSH by thyroid hormone excess, the gland is understimulated, hence it undergoes atrophy and is unable to take up ^{131}I. In Graves' disease, the gland is enlarged and the ^{131}I uptake is increased.

135. The answer is B: serum T_4 decreased, T_4 BR increased, FT_4-I normal, TSH normal, ^{131}I uptake normal. Anabolic steroids reduce the concentration of TBG, hence reducing the T_4 concentration (Chapter 19). The resin T_3 uptake (RTU) is increased, since excess radioactive T_3 is left over to bind with the resin owing to the reduction in TBG concentration and available binding sites. The T_4 BR is also increased ($\uparrow$RTU/control RTU). When the high T_4 BR is multiplied by the low T_4 to calculate the FT_4-I, the result is normal, indicating that a normal free hormone level is present and that the low total T_4 was secondary to an alteration in TBG concentration. The TSH and ^{131}I are normal, since the free hormone level is normal.

136. The answer is A: HBsAg negative, HBeAg negative, anti–HBc-IgM positive, anti–HBc-IgG negative, anti-HBs negative. When a patient recovers from hepatitis B, the HBeAg disappears first, followed by HBsAg; however, the anti–HBc-IgM remains positive for a few more weeks before converting to anti–HBc-IgG (Chapter 16). Since the anti-HBs antibody does not develop immediately after HBsAg disappears, the anti–HBc-IgM is the only marker remaining during this brief time interval, or serologic gap (window).

137. The answer is B: RBC mass normal, plasma volume decreased, SaO_2 normal, erythropoietin concentration normal. Volume depletion reduces the plasma volume and hemoconcentrates the RBCs, hence the RBC count is increased, since it is expressed in terms of the number of cells per microliter (Chapter 12). However, the RBC mass is normal, since it reflects the total number of RBCs regardless of the status of the plasma volume. As expected, the SaO_2 and erythropoietin levels are normal.

138. The answer is A: RBC mass increased, plasma volume normal, SaO_2 normal, erythropoietin concentration increased. The patient has developed hepatocellular carcinoma arising from pigment cirrhosis secondary to iron overload.

139. The answer is D: RBC mass increased, plasma volume normal, SaO_2 low, erythropoietin concentration increased. Children with Down syndrome often have congenital heart defects, most commonly an endocardial cushion defect (ASD + VSD; Chapters 10 and 12). This condition is associated with the mixing of arterial and venous blood, hence the SaO_2 is reduced, erythropoietin is increased, the RBC mass is increased, and the plasma volume is normal (hence the findings in choice D).

140. The answer is G: congenital rubella. Congenital rubella is transmitted transplacentally, and it is more teratogenic the earlier in the pregnancy it is contracted. Nerve deafness is the most common abnormality (Chapter 7).

141. The answer is D: Gaucher's disease. Gaucher's disease is a lysosomal storage disease exhibiting a deficiency of glucocerebrosidase, hence glucocerebroside accumulates in the cells (Chapter 7). In macrophages, the material has a fibrillary appearance (it looks like crumpled newspaper).

142. The answer is B: galactosemia. Galactose results from the metabolism of lactose (glucose + galactose). In galactosemia, there is a total lack of galactose-1-phosphate uridyl transferase (GALT), which catalyzes the following reaction:

$$\text{Galactose} \xrightarrow{\textit{Galactokinase}} \text{Galactose 1-phosphate}$$

$$\xrightarrow{\textit{GALT + UDP-glucose}} \text{Glucose 1-phosphate + UDP-galactose}$$

Glucose 1-phosphate is converted by phosphoglucomutase to the six-carbon intermediate glucose 6-phosphate, which may be utilized as a substrate for glycolysis or as a substrate in gluconeogenesis to produce glucose via glucose-6-phosphatase. Excess galactose may be converted to the polyol (alcohol sugar) galactitol, which produces osmotic damage in the lens, nerve tissue, liver, and CNS. Galactose 1-phosphate is toxic to tissues and causes neonatal cholestasis (jaundice due to a fatty liver, which may progress to cirrhosis), CNS damage (mental retardation), and renal damage (aminoaciduria). Neonatal hypoglycemia occurs owing to a lack of glucose 6-phosphate (Chapter 7).

143. The answer is E: serum sodium 132, serum chloride 94, serum potassium 5.8, serum bicarbonate 18, random urine sodium > 20. Patients with DKA have an increased anion gap metabolic acidosis (AG = 20 mEq/L; AG = 133 − [94 + 18]). The serum sodium is reduced owing to the osmotic gradient created by hyperglycemia, which favors the movement of water out of the ICF compartment into the ECF compartment with subsequent dilution of the serum sodium (Chapter 5). Hyperkalemia is due to the movement of potassium out of the cells in response to hydrogen ions moving into the cells for intracellular buffering. The UNa is > 20 mEq/L, since glucosuria results in a loss of both water and salt by osmotic diuresis.

144. The answer is F: serum sodium 139, serum chloride 109, serum potassium 3.0, serum bicarbonate 18, random urine sodium < 20. Diarrhea produces a normal anion gap metabolic acidosis owing to the loss of bicarbonate in the stool (Chapter 5). The AG for this patient is 12 mEq/L (AG = 139 − [109 + 18]). Note how chloride ions replace the loss in bicarbonate, hence maintaining a normal AG. Hypokalemia results from the loss of potassium in diarrhea fluid. The UNa is decreased, since the EABV is decreased from volume loss (patient has a positive tilt test) and the kidney is reabsorbing sodium to offset the loss in the stool.

145. The answer is B: pH 7.23, $PaCO_2$ 68, HCO_3 27. The patient has taken an overdose of a drug that has depressed her respiratory center, hence she has retained CO_2 and has acute respiratory acidosis without compensation, since the bicarbonate has not extended outside the normal range (Chapter 5).

146. The answer is A: pH 7.12, $PaCO_2$ 50, HCO_3 16. In cardiorespiratory arrest, the absence of breathing results in respiratory acidosis, and cardiac arrest leads to anaerobic metabolism with accumulation of lactic acid and subsequent increased anion gap metabolic acidosis (Chapter 5). Two acidoses will have a cumulative effect, resulting in a very low pH.

147. The answer is F: normal bleeding time, normal platelet count, normal prothrombin time, prolonged partial

thromboplastin time. The patient most likely has hemophilia A, an SXR disease demonstrating a deficiency of factor VIII:C (Chapter 5). Since factor VIII is in the intrinsic system, the PTT is prolonged (PTT evaluates XII → XI → IX → **VIII** → X → V → II → I → clot), while the PT is normal (VII → X → V → II → I → clot). The bleeding time and platelets are not affected in hemophilia.

148. The answer is H: normal bleeding time, normal platelet count, prolonged prothrombin time, prolonged partial thromboplastin time. Warfarin blocks epoxide reductase, which maintains vitamin K in its active K_1 form (Chapter 5). Hence, the vitamin K–dependent factors II, VII, IX, and X cannot be activated and the patient's blood is anticoagulated. Both the PT and PTT are prolonged because both utilize the final common pathway factors (X, V, II, and I).

149. The answer is D: common variable immune deficiency. CVID is a heterogeneous group of diseases with no recognizable pattern of inheritance. It first presents between 15 and 35 years of age with recurrent sinopulmonary infections secondary to decreased immunoglobulin (Ig) production. There is an intrinsic defect in the maturation of B cells into antibody-producing plasma cells. Patients are prone to chronic diarrhea (commonly due to giardiasis), malabsorption disorders (e.g., celiac sprue, lactose intolerance), and autoimmune disease (e.g., pernicious anemia).

150. The answer is C: severe combined immunodeficiency. SCID is a heterogeneous group of conditions characterized by deficiencies of both B and T cells. Children have either an SXR or AR pattern of inheritance. Approximately 50% of children with the AR pattern have a deficiency of adenosine deaminase. Absence of this enzyme results in an accumulation of adenine, which is toxic to both B and T lymphocytes. Children with SCID present with life-threatening infections associated with protracted diarrhea, vomiting, and pneumonia secondary to *P. carinii*.

ANSWER KEY

Chapter Examinations

Question No. \ Chapter No.	1	2	3	4	5	6	7	8	9	10	11	12	13	14	15	16	17	18	19	20	21	22
1	D	B	A	D	E	C	C	E	B	D	B	C	A	A	C	C	E	D	D	D	B	A
2	B	A	E	B	A	B	A	B	E	B	D	A	E	D	D	E	A	A	C	C	A	E
3	B	D	C	A	E	D	E	D	B	D	E	E	B	C	A	A	D	B	A	A	E	C
4	B	E	B	D	B	A	B	C	A	C	A	E	D	D	D	B	D	B	B	B	D	D
5	B	C	C	E	D	E	A	A	C	B	C	B	C	E	E	D	E	E	B	E	C	B
6	A	D	A	E	B	D	B	B	E	A	D	E	D	C	C	A	C	E	E	A		C
7	B	A	B	A	A	D	D	A	D	B	E	B	D	C	B	B	A	B	D	C		B
8	A	C	D	C	D	C	C	D	C	C	B	C	A		A	C	B	A	B	D		A
9		A	B	B	A		C		A	B	C	D	A		C	E	A	C	A	D		D
10		E	D	A	C		H		E	B	A	B	B		D	A	D	D	B	C		C
11		B	A	A	D		G		B	C	E	D			B	A	C	E	A	I		E
12		C	I	H	B		L		D	A	E	A			D	B	C	C	D	A		D
13		B	F	E	D		K		E	E	D	A			B	G	E	D	A	N		M
14		B			C				B	B	E	D			E	A	B	D	E			J
15		E			A				C	C	B	B			E	H	K	A	C			N
16		A			D				E	E	B	C			A	E	O	E	B			A
17		D			I				B	B	B	A			C	L	R	C	D			P
18					J					D		D										
19					C					D		C										
20					C					A		E										
21					G					D		H										
22					E					E		C										
23					A					B		F										
24					G					B												
25					B					C												
26					A					A												
27					A					D												
28										A												
29										F												
30										H												

Comprehensive Examination

1.	C	51.	C	101.	C
2.	B	52.	E	102.	A
3.	B	53.	D	103.	B
4.	C	54.	A	104.	C
5.	E	55.	D	105.	E
6.	D	56.	B	106.	B
7.	B	57.	E	107.	C
8.	A	58.	C	108.	C
9.	B	59.	E	109.	D
10.	C	60.	D	110.	A
11.	B	61.	A	111.	B
12.	E	62.	E	112.	E
13.	A	63.	D	113.	B
14.	A	64.	E	114.	A
15.	B	65.	E	115.	C
16.	B	66.	D	116.	E
17.	E	67.	C	117.	B
18.	C	68.	C	118.	E
19.	A	69.	A	119.	C
20.	B	70.	D	120.	D
21.	C	71.	B	121.	C
22.	D	72.	A	122.	E
23.	B	73.	C	123.	D
24.	E	74.	D	124.	D
25.	A	75.	C	125.	C
26.	D	76.	C	126.	D
27.	E	77.	C	127.	D
28.	A	78.	D	128.	C
29.	E	79.	C	129.	A
30.	A	80.	D	130.	A
31.	D	81.	D	131.	A
32.	C	82.	C	132.	D
33.	E	83.	B	133.	C
34.	C	84.	D	134.	E
35.	A	85.	A	135.	B
36.	B	86.	C	136.	A
37.	E	87.	B	137.	B
38.	A	88.	B	138.	A
39.	C	89.	D	139.	D
40.	E	90.	E	140.	G
41.	D	91.	D	141.	D
42.	A	92.	E	142.	B
43.	C	93.	E	143.	E
44.	D	94.	A	144.	F
45.	B	95.	C	145.	B
46.	E	96.	B	146.	A
47.	D	97.	A	147.	F
48.	A	98.	D	148.	H
49.	B	99.	B	149.	D
50.	A	100.	C	150.	C